Management Dilemmas at the Junction of Neurocritical Care and Neurosurgery: What Is the Evidence?

Notice

Management Dilemmas at the Junction of Neurocritical Care and Neurosurgery: What Is the Evidence?

Kevin T. Huang, MD
Assistant Professor
Department of Neurosurgery
Mass General Brigham
Harvard Medical School
Boston, Massachusetts

Wenya Linda Bi, MD, PhD
Associate Professor
Department of Neurosurgery
Mass General Brigham
Harvard Medical School
Boston, Massachusetts

Saef Izzy, MD, MBChB
Assistant Professor of Neurology
Divisions of Neurocritical Care and Cerebrovascular Diseases
Department of Neurology
Mass General Brigham
Harvard Medical School
Boston, Massachusetts

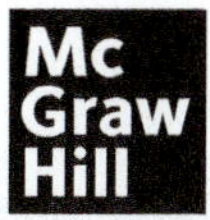

Management Dilemmas at the Junction of Neurocritical Care and Neurosurgery: What Is the Evidence?

1 2 3 4 5 LBC 28 27 26 25 24

ISBN 978-1-260-14341-6
MHID 1-260-14341-4

This book was set in Adobe Garamond by KnowledgeWorks Global Ltd.
The editors were Timothy Y. Hiscock and Christina M. Thomas.
The production supervisor was Catherine Saggese.
Project management was provided by Tasneem Kauser, KnowledgeWorks Global Ltd.

Library of Congress Cataloging-in-Publication Data

Names: Huang, Kevin T., editor. | Bi, Wenya Linda, editor. | Izzy, Saef, editor.
Title: Management dilemmas at the junction of neurocritical care and neurosurgery : what is the evidence? / [edited by] Kevin T. Huang, Wenya Linda Bi, Saef Izzy.
Description: New York : McGraw Hill, [2024] | Includes bibliographical references and index. | Summary: "An evidence-based review of landmark studies in the management and treatment of common acute neurological illnesses"—Provided by publisher.
Identifiers: LCCN 2023054698 | ISBN 9781260143416 (paperback) | ISBN 9781260143423 (ebook)
Subjects: MESH: Nervous System Diseases—surgery | Nervous System Diseases—therapy | Neurosurgical Procedures—methods | Trauma, Nervous System | Critical Care—methods | Evidence-Based Emergency Medicine—methods | Case Reports
Classification: LCC RD593 | NLM WL 140 | DDC 617.4/8—dc23/eng/20240126
LC record available at https://lccn.loc.gov/2023054698

Contents

SECTION VI

TUMOR 263

SECTION VII

SPINE 283

Contributors

Muhammad M. Abd-El-Barr, MD, PhD
Department of Neurosurgery, Duke University Hospital
Durham, North Carolina

Yasmin Aghajan, MD
Department of Neurology, Brigham and Women's Hospital, Harvard Medical School
Boston, Massachusetts

Feras Akbik, MD, PhD
Department of Neurology and Neurosurgery, Division of Neurocritical Care, Emory University School of Medicine
Atlanta, Georgia

Ozan Akca, MD
Neuroscience Critical Care Division, Departments of Neurology, Neurosurgery, and Anesthesiology and Critical Care Medicine, Johns Hopkins University School of Medicine
Baltimore, Maryland

Ayham Alkhachroum, MD
Department of Neurology, Neurocritical Care Division, University of Miami, Miller School of Medicine, Jackson Memorial Hospital and Clinics
Miami, Florida

Sulaiman Almohaish, PharmD, BCPS
Department of Pharmacotherapy & Outcomes Science, School of Pharmacy, Virginia Commonwealth University
Richmond, Virginia
Department of Pharmacy Practice, Clinical Pharmacy College, King Faisal University
Al-Ahsa, Saudi Arabia

Safwan Alomari, MD
Department of Neurosurgery, Johns Hopkins University School of Medicine
Baltimore, Maryland

Hussein Alshammari, MD
Department of Neurology, Duke University Hospital
Durham, North Carolina

Ronald Alvarado-Dyer, MD
Neurocritical Care Unit, Departments of Neurology and Neurosurgery, The University of Chicago Medical Center
Chicago, Illinois

Fatten El Ammar, MD
Neurocritical Care Unit, Departments of Neurology and Neurosurgery, The University of Chicago Medical Center
Chicago, Illinois

Omar Arnaout, MD
Department of Neurosurgery, Brigham and Women's Hospital, Harvard Medical School
Boston, Massachusetts

Neeraj Badjatia, MD, MSc
Department of Neurology, Program in Trauma, Division of Neurocritical Care and Emergency Neurology, University of Maryland School of Medicine
Baltimore, Maryland

Shawn Banash, MD
Department of Neurologic Surgery, UC Davis
Sacramento, California

Brooke Barlow, PharmD
Department of Pharmacy, Memorial Hermann Woodlands Medical Center
Woodlands, Texas

Megan E. Barra, PharmD
Department of Pharmacy, Massachusetts General Hospital
Boston, Massachusetts

Carolina G. Benjamin, MD, FAANS
Department of Neurological Surgery, University of Miami Miller School of Medicine
Miami, Florida

Wenya Linda Bi, MD, PhD
Department of Neurosurgery, Brigham and Women's Hospital, Harvard Medical School
Boston, Massachusetts

Manuel Melo Bicchi, MD
Department of Neurology, Comprehensive Epilepsy Center and Neurohospitalist Division, University of Miami, Miller School of Medicine
Jackson Memorial Hospital and Clinics
Miami, Florida

Sherri A. Braksick, MD
Department of Neurology,
Mayo Clinic School of Medicine
Rochester, Minnesota

Gretchen M. Brophy, PharmD, BCPS, FCCP, FCCM, FNCS, MCCM
Department of Pharmacotherapy & Outcomes Science,
School of Pharmacy, Virginia Commonwealth University
Richmond, Virginia

Matthew Brown, MD
Farber Hospitalist Service,
Department of Neurological Surgery,
Thomas Jefferson University
Philadelphia, Pennsylvania

Karol P. Budohoski, MD, PhD
Department of Neurosurgery,
Clinical Neurosciences Center
University of Utah
Salt Lake City, Utah

Joseph D. Burns, MD
Section of Neurocritical Care, Division of Neurology,
Lahey Hospital and Medical Center
Burlington, Massachusetts
Department of Neurology, and Department of
Neurosurgery, Tufts University School of Medicine
Boston, Massachusetts

Ali Bydon, MD
Department of Neurosurgery,
Johns Hopkins University School of Medicine
Baltimore, Maryland

Stefanie P. Cappucci, MD
Department of Neurology, Yale School of Medicine
New Haven, Connecticut

J. Ricardo Carhuapoma, MD
Departments of Neurology, Anesthesiology &
Critical Care Medicine,
The Johns Hopkins University School of Medicine
Baltimore, Maryland

Anna Cervantes-Arslanian, MD
Department of Neurology, Boston Medical Center
Boston, Massachusetts

Henry Chang, MD, PhD
Neuroscience Critical Care Division, Departments of
Neurology, Neurosurgery, and Anesthesiology and
Critical Care Medicine, Johns Hopkins University
School of Medicine
Baltimore, Maryland

Antoinette Charles, BS
Duke University School of Medicine
Durham, North Carolina

Sung-Min Cho, DO, MHS
Neuroscience Critical Care Division,
Departments of Neurology, Neurosurgery, and
Anesthesiology and Critical Care Medicine,
Johns Hopkins University School of Medicine
Division of Cardiac Surgery, Department of Surgery,
Johns Hopkins University School of Medicine,
Baltimore, Maryland

Jameson Cooper, MS, CCC-SLP
Department of Speech, Language & Swallowing
Disorders, Massachusetts General Hospital
Boston, Massachusetts

Joacir G. Cordeiro, MD, PhD
Department of Neurosurgery, University of Miami,
Miller School of Medicine
Miami, Florida

Justine Cormier, MD
Department of Neurology, Yale School of Medicine
New Haven, Connecticut

Rene Daniel, MD, PhD
Farber Hospitalist Service, Department of Neurological
Surgery, Thomas Jefferson University
Philadelphia, Pennsylvania

Alvin S. Das, MD
Department of Neurology, Beth Israel Deaconess
Medical Center, Harvard Medical School
Boston, Massachusetts

Carlos David, MD
Department of Neurosurgery, University of North
Carolina School of Medicine
Chapel Hill, North Carolina

Hormuzdiyar Dasenbrock, MD, MPH
Department of Neurosurgery, Boston Medical Center
Boston, Massachusetts

Elliana K. Devore, MD
Department of Otolaryngology-Head and Neck Surgery,
Massachusetts Eye and Ear, Harvard Medical School
Boston, Massachusetts

Ian F. Dunn, MD, FACS, FAANS
Department of Neurosurgery, University of Oklahoma
Health Sciences Center
Oklahoma City, Oklahoma

Turki Elarjani, MD
Department of Neurological Surgery,
University of Miami Miller School of Medicine
Miami, Florida

Eddy Fan, MD, PhD
Interdepartmental Division of Critical Care Medicine,
University of Toronto
Department of Medicine,
University Health Network
Toronto, Ontario, Canada

Salia Farrokh, PharmD
Neuroscience Critical Care Division, Departments of Neurology, Neurosurgery, and Anesthesiology and Critical Care Medicine,
Johns Hopkins University School of Medicine
Baltimore, Maryland

Pouneh K. Fazeli, MD, MPH
Neuroendocrinology Unit, Division of Endocrinology and Metabolism, Department of Medicine,
University of Pittsburgh School of Medicine
Pittsburgh, Pennsylvania

Arthur Formanek, MD
Department of Anesthesiology, Perioperative and Pain Management, Brigham and Women's Hospital,
Harvard Medical School
Boston, Massachusetts

William D. Freeman, MD
Department of Neurology
Department of Critical Care Medicine,
Mayo Clinic
Jacksonville, Florida
Department of Neurosurgery, Mayo Clinic
Jacksonville, Florida

Kevin Furlong, DO
Division of Endocrinology, Department of Medicine,
Thomas Jefferson University
Philadelphia, Pennsylvania

Paul A. Gardner, MD
Department of Neurological Surgery, University of Pittsburgh School of Medicine
Pittsburgh, Pennsylvania

Emily J. Gilmore, MD, FNCS, FACNS
Department of Neurology, Division of Neurocritical Care and Emergency Neurology,
Yale School of Medicine, New Haven,
Connecticut Department of Neurology,
Yale Comprehensive Epilepsy Center,
Yale School of Medicine
New Haven, Connecticut

Tessa Goldsmith, MA, CCC-SLP
Department of Speech, Language & Swallowing Disorders, Massachusetts General Hospital
Boston, Massachusetts

C. Rory Goodwin, MD, PhD
Duke University School of Medicine
Durham, North Carolina

Ramesh Grandhi, MD
Department of Neurosurgery, Clinical Neurosciences Center, University of Utah
Salt Lake City, Utah

Diana Greene-Chandos, MD, FNCS
Department of Neurology, University of New Mexico School of Medicine
Albuquerque, New Mexico

Saksham Gupta, MD
Department of Neurosurgery,
Brigham and Women's Hospital,
Harvard Medical School
Boston, Massachusetts

Elan L. Guterman, MD, MAS
Department of Neurology,
University of California San Francisco
San Francisco, California

Daniel S. Harrison, MD
Department of Neurology, Harvard Medical School,
Brigham and Women's Hospital,
Massachusetts General Hospital
Boston, Massachusetts

Jafar Hashem, MD
Department of Neurology,
The Edward B. Bromfield Epilepsy Program,
Brigham and Women's Hospital, Harvard Medical School
Boston, Massachusetts

Sara Hocker, MD
Professor of Neurology, Mayo Clinic College of Medicine, Chair, Division of Neurocritical Care and Hospital Neurology, Associate Chair, Department of Neurology, Hospital Practice
Rochester, Minnesota

Samantha E. Hoffman, BS
Department of Neurosurgery, Brigham and Women's Hospital, Harvard Medical School
Boston, Massachusetts

Sukwoo Hong, MB
International Fellow, Department of Neurological Surgery, Mayo Clinic Rochester
Rochester, Minnesota

Mariyam Humayun, MBBS
Departments of Neurology, Neurosurgery and Anesthesiology & Critical Care Medicine, Division of Neurosciences Critical Care, The Johns Hopkins University School of Medicine
Baltimore, Maryland

David Y. Hwang, MD
Department of Neurology, Neuroscience Intensive Care Unit, University of North Carolina Medical Center
Chapel Hill, North Carolina

Saef Izzy, MD, MBChB
Department of Neurology, Brigham and Women's Hospital, Harvard Medical School
Boston Massachusetts

Casey Jarvis, MD
Department of Neurosurgery, Brigham and Women's Hospital, Harvard Medical School
Boston, Massachusetts

T. Jayde Nail, MD
Department of Neurosurgery,
Tufts University School of Medicine
Boston, Massachusetts

Hera A. Kamdar, MD
Department of Neurology
The Ohio State University
Columbus, Ohio

Ulrick S. Kanmounye, MD, MSc
Department of Neurosurgery, Geisinger Health System
Danville, Pennsylvania

Jennifer A. Kim, MD, PhD
Department of Neurology, Yale School of Medicine
New Haven, Connecticut

Nora C. Kim, MD
Department of Neurosurgery,
NYU Langone Medical Center
New York, New York

May Kim-Tenser, MD, MHA, FAHA
Associate Professor of Neurology, Medical Director/Chief of the Neurosciences ICU at Keck Hospital of USC, Associate Chair of Neurology, Keck Hospital of USC
Los Angeles, California

Evan M. Krueger, DO, MSc
Department of Neurosurgery,
University of Miami—Miller School of Medicine
Miami, Florida

Christopher M. Kyper, MD
Department of Neurology, Mayo Clinic
Department of Critical Care Medicine, Mayo Clinic
Jacksonville, Florida

Pui Man Rosalind Lai, MD
Department of Neurosurgery, Brigham and Women's Hospital, Harvard Medical School
Boston, Massachusetts

Christos Lazaridis, MD, EDIC
Neurocritical Care Unit, Departments of Neurology and Neurosurgery, The University of Chicago Medical Center
Chicago, Illinois

Jong Woo Lee, MD, PhD
Department of Neurology, The Edward B. Bromfield Epilepsy Program, Brigham and Women's Hospital, Harvard Medical School
Boston, Massachusetts

David P. Lerner, MD
Lahey Clinic, Department of Neurology
Burlington, Massachusetts
Department of Neurology, Division of Neurocritical Care, Brookdale Hospital and Medical Center
Department of Neurology,
SUNY Downstate Medical Center
Brooklyn, New York

Ariane Lewis, MD
Department of Neurosurgery,
Department of Neurology,
NYU Langone Medical Center
New York, New York

Mary Jane Lim-Fat, MD, MSc, FRCPC
Department of Neurology, Harvard Medical School
Center for Neuro-Oncology, Dana Farber Cancer Institute
Boston, Massachusetts

David J. Lin, MD
Center for Neurotechnology and Neurorecovery, Division of Neurocritical Care, and Stroke Service; Department of Neurology, Massachusetts General Hospital; Harvard Medical School
Boston, Massachusetts
Center for Neurorestoration and Neurotechnology, Rehabilitation Research and Development Service, Department of Veterans Affairs
Providence, Rhode Island

David D. Liu, MD
Department of Neurosurgery, Brigham and Women's Hospital, Harvard Medical School
Boston, Massachusetts

Victor Lopez-Rivera, MD
Department of Neurosurgery, Boston Medical Center
Boston, Massachusetts

Emily Luo, BS
Duke University School of Medicine
Durham, North Carolina

Sean Lyne, MD
Department of Neurosurgery, Brigham and Women's Hospital, Harvard Medical School
Boston, Massachusetts

Hussain Mahmud, MD
Neuroendocrinology Unit,
Division of Endocrinology and Metabolism,
Department of Medicine University of Pittsburgh School of Medicine
Pittsburgh, Pennsylvania

Hinna Malik, MD
Department of Anesthesiology, Perioperative and Pain Management, Brigham and Women's Hospital, Harvard Medical School
Boston, Massachusetts

Jody Manners, MD
Department of Neurology, Program in Trauma, University of Maryland School of Medicine
Baltimore, Maryland
LCDR, MC, Naval Medical Leader and Professional Development Command
Bethesda, Maryland

Ryan M. Martin, MD
Department of Neurologic Surgery
Department of Neurology, UC Davis
Sacramento, California

Rohan Mathur, MD, MPA
Departments of Neurology, Neurosurgery and Anesthesiology & Critical Care Medicine,
Division of Neurosciences Critical Care,
The Johns Hopkins University School of Medicine
Baltimore, Maryland

Victoria McCredie, MBChB, PhD
Interdepartmental Division of Critical Care Medicine, University of Toronto
Department of Medicine,
University Health Network
Toronto, Ontario, Canada

James Tanner McMahon, MD
Department of Neurosurgery, Brigham and Women's Hospital, Harvard Medical School
Boston, Massachusetts

Anthony N. Mefford, MD
Department of Neurology, University of California, San Francisco
San Francisco, California

Newton Mei, MD
Farber Hospitalist Service, Department of Neurological Surgery, Thomas Jefferson University
Philadelphia, Pennsylvania

Timothy Miller, MD
Department of Diagnostic Radiology and Nuclear Medicine, University of Maryland School of Medicine
Baltimore, Maryland

Bradley J. Molyneaux, MD, PhD
Department of Neurology, Brigham and Women's Hospital, Harvard Medical School
Boston, Massachusetts

Kelly D. Nahum, DO
Department of Surgery / Surgical Critical Care, Ohio State University Wexner Medical Center
Columbus, Ohio

Michael A Mooney, MD
Department of Neurosurgery,
Brigham and Women's Hospital
Boston, Massachusetts

Nicholas A. Morris, MD
Department of Neurology, Program in Trauma, University of Maryland School of Medicine
Baltimore, Maryland

Kelly R. Wackerle, MD
Department of Neurosurgery, Duke University Hospital
Durham, North Carolina

Matthew R. Naunheim, MD, MBA
Head and Neck Surgery, Department of Otolaryngology, Massachusetts Eye and Ear, Harvard Medical School
Boston, Massachusetts

Lauren K. Ng, MD
Department of Neurology
Department of Critical Care Medicine
Department of Neurosurgery, Mayo Clinic
Jacksonville, Florida

Vanessa Ogundipe, MD
Internal Medicine and Geriatrics, MercyOne Siouxland
Sioux City, Iowa

Ebubechi Okwumabua, MD
Department of Orthopaedic Surgery, McGovern School of Medicine, The University of Texas Health Science Center
Houston, Texas

K. O'Phelan, MD
Department of Neurology, Division of Neurocritical Care, University of Miami—Miller School of Medicine
Miami, Florida

Marcey L. Osgood, DO
Department of Neurology, UMass Memorial Medical Center
Burlington, Massachusetts

Donato Pacione, MD
Department of Neurosurgery,
NYU Langone Medical Center
New York, New York

Nirav J. Patel, MD
Department of Neurosurgery, Brigham and
Women's Hospital, Harvard Medical School
Boston, Massachusetts

Jamie E. Podell, MD
Department of Neurology, Program in Trauma, Division
of Neurocritical Care and Emergency Neurology,
University of Maryland School of Medicine
Baltimore, Maryland

Meghan Price, MD
Duke University School of Medicine
Durham, North Carolina

Alejandro A. Rabinstein, MD
Department of Neurology, Mayo Clinic School of Medicine
Rochester, Minnesota

Daniel M. S. Raper, MBBS
Department of Neurological Surgery,
University of California
San Francisco, California

Michael Reznik, MD
Department of Neurosurgery
Division of Neurocritical Care, Department of
Neurology, The Warren Alpert School of Medicine,
Brown University
Providence, Rhode Island

Emerson Rhudy, RN
Neuroscience Intensive Care Unit,
University of North Carolina Medical Center
Chapel Hill, North Carolina

Kent R. Richter, MD
Department of Neurosurgery, Geisinger Health System
Danville, Pennsylvania

Ofer Sadan, MD, PhD
Department of Neurology and Neurosurgery,
Division of Neurocritical Care,
Emory University School of Medicine
Atlanta, Georgia

Walid K. Salah, BA
Spencer Fox Eccles School of Medicine
University of Utah
Salt Lake City, Utah

Rahul A. Sastry, MD
Department of Neurosurgery, The Warren Alpert School
of Medicine, Brown University
Providence, Rhode Island

Clemens M. Schirmer, MD, PhD
Department of Neurosurgery, Geisinger Health System
Danville, Pennsylvania

Andreas Seas, BS
Duke University School of Medicine
Durham, North Carolina

Shreyansh Shah, MD
Depatment of Neurology, Duke University Hospital,
Durham, North Carolina

Kiarash Shahlaie, MD, PhD
Department of Neurologic Surgery
Department of Neurology, UC Davis
Sacramento, California

Aya Shnawa, MD
Department of Neurology,
Tufts University School of Medicine
Boston, Massachusetts

James Edward Showery, MD
Department of Orthopaedic Surgery,
McGovern School of Medicine,
The University of Texas Health Science Center
Houston, Texas

Max Shutran, MD
Department of Neurosurgery, Beth Israel Deaconess
Medical Center, Harvard Medical School
Boston, Massachusetts

Neel S. Singhal, MD, PhD
Department of Neurology,
University of California San Francisco
San Francisco, California

Michael Silva, MD
Department of Neurological Surgery,
University of Miami Miller School of Medicine
Miami, Florida

Samuel B. Snider, MD
Department of Neurology, Brigham and Women's
Hospital, Harvard Medical School
Boston, Massachusetts

Priya Srikanth, MD, PhD
Center for Neurorestoration and Neurotechnology;
Rehabilitation Research and Development Service;
Department of Veterans Affairs
Providence, Rhode Island
Center for Neurotechnology and Neurorecovery,
Division of Neurocritical Care, and Stroke Service,
Department of Neurology, Massachusetts General
Hospital, Harvard Medical School
Department of Neurology, Brigham and Women's Hospital
Boston, Massachusetts

Tamara A. Strohm, MD
Department of Neurology, Neuroscience Intensive Care Unit, University of North Carolina Medical Center
Chapel Hill, North Carolina

Jose I. Suarez, MD
Division of Neurosciences Critical Care;
Departments of Neurology, Neurosurgery and Anesthesiology & Critical Care Medicine;
The Johns Hopkins University School of Medicine
Baltimore, Maryland

David A.W. Sykes, BA
Duke University School of Medicine
Durham, North Carolina

Troy Q. Tabarestani, BA
Duke University School of Medicine
Durham, North Carolina

Shaurya Taran, MD
Interdepartmental Division of Critical Care Medicine, University of Toronto
Department of Medicine, University Health Network
Toronto, Ontario, Canada

Fawaz Tarzi, MD
Neurocritical Care Fellow, Neurosciences Critical Care/Stroke Division, University of Southern California/Keck School of Medicine
Los Angeles, California

Sherwin A. Tavakol, MD, MPH
Department of Neurosurgery, University of Oklahoma Health Sciences Center
Oklahoma City, Oklahoma

Shelly D. Timmons, MD, MPh
Department of Neurosurgery
University of Oklahoma Health Sciences Center
Oklahoma City, Oklahoma

Jose A. Torres, BS
Department of Orthopaedic Surgery, McGovern School of Medicine, The University of Texas Health Science Center
Houston, Texas

Brett M. Tracy, MD
Department of Surgery/Surgical Critical Care, Ohio State University Wexner Medical Center
Columbus, Ohio

Steven Tobochnik, MD
Department of Neurology, Brigham and Women's Hospital
Boston, Massachusetts

Henrikas Vaitkevicius, MD
Marinus Pharma
Boston, Massachusetts

Juan C. Vicenty-Padilla, MD
Department of Neurosurgery, Brigham and Women's Hospital, Harvard Medical School
Boston, Massachusetts

Jeffrey R. Vitt, MD
Department of Neurologic Surgery
Department of Neurology, UC Davis
Sacramento, California

Patrick Y. Wen, MD
Department of Neurology, Harvard Medical School
Boston, Massachusetts
Center for Neuro-Oncology, Dana Farber Cancer Institute
Boston, Massachusetts

Alexander G. Yearley, BA
Department of Neurosurgery, Brigham and Women's Hospital, Harvard Medical School
Boston, Massachusetts

Mohamed A. Zaazoue, MD, MSc
Department of Neurological Surgery
Indiana University School of Medicine
Indianapolis, Indiana

Georgios A. Zenonos, MD
Neuroendocrinology Unit, Division of Endocrinology and Metabolism, Department of Medicine, University of Pittsburgh School of Medicine
Pittsburgh, Pennsylvania

Kahli Zietlow, MD
Division of Geriatrics and Palliative Medicine, Department of Internal Medicine, University of Michigan
Geriatrics Research, Education and Clinical Center, Veterans Affairs
Ann Arbor, Michigan

Lara L. Zimmermann, MD
Department of Neurologic Surgery
Department of Neurology, UC Davis
Sacramento, California

Preface

This book is one born of practicality. Neurosurgeons and neurointensivists work closely together to tackle some of the most challenging cases in the hospital. But with the passion and dedication that characterize both specialties inevitably come debate. In our ICU at Brigham and Women's Hospital, it is a common sight for us to be haggling over many clinical management issues, ranging from sodium goals to blood pressure management to DVT prophylaxis. Though much of our debates often focus on the specifics of the patient at hand, inevitably, we reach a common refrain, "Is there any evidence for that?"

This book is our attempt at an answer. Over time, we have come to realize that similar debates are likely erupting in NeuroICUs across the United States and the rest of the world. They tend to feature topics that are some of the hardest to deal with—those with either incomplete or inconsistent bodies of evidence where obvious answers elude us. It is exactly for those problems that we felt a book was the most appropriate answer. Currently, it is possible to have near-instant access to any number of systematic reviews and metanalyses on the Internet with the click of a button. However, it was only in a book where we could get world-leading experts to review, opine on, and synthesize the available data on many controversial management topics, stacked one right after the other.

In the following chapters, we have gathered the opinions of some of the most respected and well-published researchers and thought leaders from a wide range of fields, including not just neurosurgeons and neurointensivists, but also otolaryngologists, anesthesiologists, pharmacists, and orthopedic surgeons. In each chapter, we have asked them a nearly impossible question—typically one without any clear answers or consensus—and implored them to answer it (and succinctly no less!). We have been stunned by the quality of their responses. What shines through in their writing is both their command of a difficult body of evidence and the higher-level synthesis of that evidence, which is the marker of true expertise.

It has been our absolute pleasure to read and engage with our authors on these challenging subjects—and we hope you will too. By highlighting and structuring the key controversies in our field, we hope that our readers will be better prepared to resolve them. It is often said that in cutting-edge fields, research is obsolete from the time it is published. This could be said doubly so for a book seeking to review current evidence. But on that day, we would be proud to look back and see that this book helped make itself obsolete just a little bit faster.

Kevin T. Huang, MD
Wenya Linda Bi, MD, PhD
Saef Izzy, MD, MBChB
Mass General Brigham
Harvard Medical School
Boston, MA
April 17, 2023

SECTION I MONITORING AND GENERAL CARE

CHAPTER

1

Do Post-Operative Elective Craniotomy Patients Routinely Need the ICU?

Saksham Gupta, MD, Samantha E. Hoffman, BS, & Omar Arnaout, MD

Case

A 43-year-old woman without other comorbidities undergoes an elective craniotomy for a growing left temporal meningioma. The surgery was uncomplicated intraoperatively. Should this patient be admitted to an intensive care unit (ICU) for immediate postoperative care?

Key Points

- Not all patients need to be admitted to an ICU after elective cranial surgery.
- Neurosurgery departments and hospitals can benefit from shorter lengths of stay and decreased resource utilization without increasing adverse events through the development and implementation of clinical protocols that bypass the ICU after elective cranial surgery.
- Protocol details will vary by each hospital's staffing and room availability, so a multidisciplinary approach is needed to tailor the protocol to each hospital's resources.

BACKGROUND

Patients undergoing elective craniotomies traditionally stay overnight in intensive care units (ICUs) including specialized neurologic ICUs to monitor for acute postoperative complications including hemorrhage and ischemic stroke. The workforce and equipment in ICUs allow for closer postoperative monitoring, so postoperative complications that require urgent medical or surgical attention can be identified and intervened upon more quickly. The risk profiles of certain neurosurgery operations mandate postoperative ICU admission. For instance, patients should go to the ICU after surgery for all vascular malformations and urgent cranial operations given tenuous neurologic and hemodynamic status after these operations. Even elective treatment of aneurysms and arteriovenous malformations is associated with a 5% to 20% risk of adverse perioperative neurologic and medical events.[1–3] However, the value of routine ICU admission after elective craniotomies for nonvascular pathologies has recently come under question. ICU admissions are expensive and unequipped to provide physical and occupational therapy. ICU beds can be scarce and need to be allocated thoughtfully.

A cadre of postoperative clinical protocols designed to bypass the ICU after elective craniotomies has been reported. In this chapter, we review the evidence on which patients undergoing elective craniotomies for nonvascular pathologies need postoperative ICU admission. We focus on elective brain tumor surgery specifically given the robust evidence that exists on postoperative pathways in neuro-oncology.

EVIDENCE AND REVIEW

Hospitals and wards vary in the scope of their ICUs, postanesthesia care units (PACUs)/stepdown wards, and floor wards. For the purposes of this chapter, we define three levels of care as described in Table 1–1. Briefly, ICUs have lower nurse-patient ratios, dedicated critical care teams, and can monitor patients frequently. PACU and stepdown wards have similar capability as ICUs but cannot provide care overnight. Floor wards have higher nurse-patient ratios and provide less frequent neurologic exams. Some hospitals will have specialized neurologic ICUs, PACUs/stepdown wards, and floor wards. When available, patients undergoing cranial neurosurgery should be admitted to specialized neurologic units to optimize postoperative monitoring.[4] Hospitals may also have nuanced criteria about the perioperative care admissible in differing units, such as whether specific intracranial drains are permissible on a floor.

Nearly a dozen studies have been published describing clinical protocols about bypassing ICU care after craniotomies for brain tumors and other pathologies (Table 1–2). These studies have differing methodologies, ranging from observational cohorts to quasi-experimental designs. All protocols include supratentorial craniotomies for brain tumors, five protocols

TABLE 1–1 Definition and scope of ICU, PACU/stepdown, and floor levels of care.

	ICU	PACU/Stepdown	Floor
Maximum time allowed	None	4-8 h	None
Maximum nurse-patient ratio	1:2	1:2	1:4
Invasive blood pressure monitoring	Yes	Yes	No
IV drip medications	Yes	Temporarily	No
Frequency of neurologic exams	Every hour	Every hour	Every 4 h
Dedicated critical care team	Yes	Yes	No

(45%) include infratentorial craniotomies for brain tumors, three protocols (27%) include infratentorial craniotomies for microvascular decompression, and two protocols (18%) include supratentorial craniotomies for nonurgent subdural hematoma and infratentorial craniectomy for Chiari malformation. Two protocols (18%) include pediatric patients. Protocols differed in the postoperative monitoring periods and destinations. Eight protocols (73%) involved transfer to a PACU for 2 to 4 hours after surgery, while three protocols (27%) involved direct admission to a floor. Two of the eight protocols involving transfer to PACU also included a pathway for same-day discharge after brain tumor surgery with no complications, specifically. Five (45%) and three (27%) protocols included cutoffs for operative time and intraoperative blood loss to qualify for bypassing the ICU, respectively. The rate of ICU transfer ranged from 0% to 24% in the studies.

We have conducted our own subanalysis of brain tumor cases within the postoperative PACU to floor protocol at our institution. Inclusion into the protocol required an operative time under 5 hours, an estimated blood loss under 500 mL, and no operative complications (including intraoperative seizures and postoperative neurologic deficits). We included craniotomies for subdural hematoma evacuation, Chiari malformations, and microvascular decompression in our protocol but analyzed craniotomies for brain tumors specifically against a matched historic cohort. We found that our protocol led to decreased overall length-of-stay, faster time-to-imaging, and lower hospital charges compared to matched controls (Figure 1–1). These benefits were observed regardless of operative time or day, and regardless of the distance of a patient's home from the hospital. By bypassing the ICU, critical care resource utilization was improved by freeing 0.95 ICU days per patient. Only 2.5% of patients needed to be transferred to the ICU for medical necessity, and our pathway demonstrated noninferiority in terms of perioperative complications, discharge disposition, and 30-day emergency room evaluations or readmissions.

Ours and others' experiences suggest that not all patients undergoing elective craniotomies need to go to the ICU postoperatively. Clinical pathways that bypass the ICU can improve patient outcomes, reduce hospital costs, and free more ICU beds for critical patients. Maintaining sufficient ICU bed availability directly impacts outcomes across the health system; reduced ICU bed census has been correlated with increases in morbidity, mortality, and ICU readmission rates for patients with coronavirus disease-19 (COVID-19), cardiac arrest, and beyond.[5-7] ICU bed scarcity also restricts triage decision-making and can result in denial of intensive care to some patients with significant need or redirection to palliative measures.[8-11] The United States continues to grapple with persistently high demand for healthcare resources and an ever-growing shortage of ICU staffing capacity, protocols to bypass the ICU will become increasingly vital to maintaining patient access to acute medical and surgical care.[12,13]

The implementation of postoperative PACU or floor admissions protocols will vary by hospital. We propose that the minimum requirements for a protocol to bypass the ICU include the capability to perform frequent nursing neurologic exams and

TABLE 1–2 Results of selective protocols and care pathways designed to bypass overnight admission to the ICU.

Author	Methodology	Study Size* (n)	Pathway Criteria	Protocol	ICU Time Reduction per Patient (days)	Length of Stay Reduction (days)	ICU Admissions/ Transfers	Cost Savings per Patient	Pathway Readmission	Comparison Group	Comparison Findings
Hoffman (2022) (*unpublished*)	Retrospective cohort	202 (adult brain tumor resection)	Supratentorial craniotomy for brain tumor/SDH, infratentorial craniotomy for Chiari/MVD, operative time under 5 h, EBL under 500 cc	4-h observation in PACU with q1 neurologic checks then transfer to floor	0.95	0.7	3.4%	$13,448	19% (30-day, includes ER visits)	Historical controls	Decreased time to MRI, time to PT, LOS, and hospital charge for pathway
Vallejo (2022)[14]	Single-surgeon prospective cohort	37 (adult brain tumor resection)	Supratentorial brain tumor under 4 cm, operative time under 3 h, EBL under 300 cc, start time before 8:30 a.m.	3-h observation in PACU, followed by MRI, then 3-h ICU monitoring, then PT evaluation followed by discharge	–	–	0.0% (14.0% admitted to floor)	–	11%	–	–
Young (2021)[15]	Case-control	94 (adult brain tumor resection, MVD, and Chiari malformation)	Age under 65 years, supratentorial craniotomy for brain tumor under 3 cm, infratentorial craniotomy for Chiari/MVD, case length < 6 h, EBL <500 cc	4-h observation in PACU with q2 neurologic checks then transfer to floor	1	0.25	0.0%	$4,000	1% (30-day)	Concurrent patients	Decreased LOS and hospital charge for pathway
ter Laan (2019)[16]	Retrospective cohort	109 (adult brain tumor resection)	Supratentorial craniotomy for brain tumor, operative time under 6 h	Routine admission to ward unless surgery >6 h or significant cardiopulmonary co-morbidities	0.2	1	24.0%	E1,953	–	Historical controls	Decreased length of ICU stay, perioperative complications, and hospital charge
Mirza (2018)[17]	Retrospective cohort	355 (adult and pediatric brain tumor resection)	Supratentorial craniotomy for intra-axial brain tumor	2-4-h observation in PACU, then transfer to floor	–	–	0.1%	–	–	–	–

(*Continued*)

TABLE 1–2 Results of selective protocols and care pathways designed to bypass overnight admission to the ICU. (Continued)

Author	Methodology	Study Size* (n)	Pathway Criteria	Protocol	ICU Time Reduction per Patient (days)	Length of Stay Reduction (days)	ICU Admissions/ Transfers	Cost Savings per Patient	Pathway Readmission	Comparison Group	Comparison Findings
Florman (2017)[18]	Retrospective cohort	200 (adult brain tumor resection and biopsy)	Supratentorial craniotomy for brain tumor	4-h observation in PACU with transfer to floor	–	4	2.5%	–	–	Concurrent patients	Decreased LOS and increased likelihood of discharge home
Gabel (2016)	Retrospective cohort	61 (pediatric brain tumor resection)	Supra- and infratentorial craniotomy for brain tumor	Routine floor admission	–	–	9.8%	–	–	–	–
Venkataghavan (2016)[19]	Single-surgeon retrospective cohort	198 (adult brain tumor resection)	Supratentorial craniotomy for brain tumor, operative time under 4 h, caregiver ability overnight within 1 h of hospital	2-h observation in PACU, CT scan 4-h postoperatively, 2-h observation in day surgery unit	–	–	0.0% (11.6% admitted to floor)	–	3%	–	–
Bui (2011)[20]	Retrospective cohort	394 (adult brain tumor resection and biopsy, ventricolustomy, and vascular lesion management)	Supra- and infratentorial brain tumor, pituitary tumors, hydrocephalus undergoing ETV	2-3-h observation in PACU, then 6-h observation on floor with q1 neurologic and vital sign checks, then routine floor care	–	2.9	13% (2% planned, 11% unplanned)	–	–	–	–
Boulton (2008)[21]	Single-surgeon retrospective cohort	145 (adult brain tumor resection)	Supratentorial craniotomy for intra-axial brain tumor	Routine admission to PACU with plan for discharge home POD0	–	–	–	–	–	–	–
Beauregard (2003)[22]	Single-surgeon retrospective cohort	132 (adult brain tumor resection and trigeminal neuralgia)	Supra- and infratentorial brain tumor, pituitary tumors, trigeminal neuralgia	Routine admission to floor	–	3.3	–	$4,026	–	Concurrent patients of other attending surgeons	Decreased LOS and hospital charge

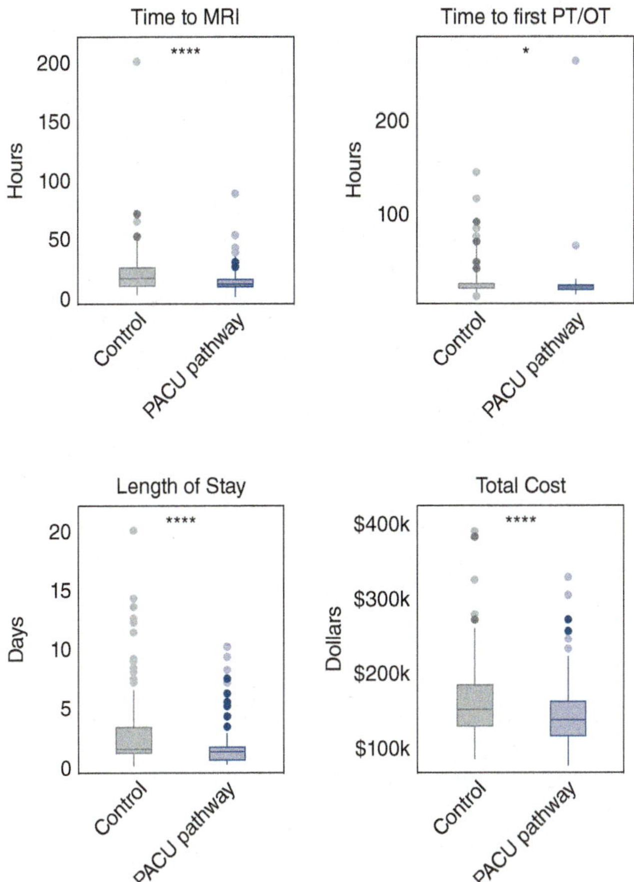

FIGURE 1–1 Comparison of patient hospital course between PACU pathway patients and historic controls. ns = not significant; * = $P < .05$, **** = $P < .0001$.

vital signs checks for 2 to 4 hours in a PACU/stepdown unit postoperatively and a resident or advanced practice provider to perform an early exam and escalate care to an ICU if needed. We suggest the following criteria for pathways to bypass the ICU when appropriate resources are available:

1. **Restriction by pathology.** We suggest restricting protocols to elective craniotomies for brain tumors, subdural hematomas, Chiari malformations, and trigeminal neuralgia.
2. **Restriction by operative time.** We suggest restricting protocols to operations under 5 hours.
3. **Restriction by blood loss.** We suggest restricting protocols to operations with an estimated blood loss under 500 cc and no intraoperative blood transfusions.
4. **Restriction by operative complications.** We suggest excluding patients with intraoperative seizures, neurovascular injuries, sustained changes in electrophysiologic neuromonitoring signals, electrocardiogram changes, significant laboratory derangements, and complicated extubation.
5. **Restriction by postoperative status.** We suggest excluding patients with new neurologic deficits that are not rapidly improving, new postoperative seizures, persistent intravenous (IV) drip medication requirement to keep blood pressure under systolic blood pressure of 150 mm Hg, and a high oxygen requirement (ie, above 3 L through a nasal cannula).

REFERENCES

1. Alshekhlee A, Mehta S, Edgell RC, et al. Hospital mortality and complications of electively clipped or coiled unruptured intracranial aneurysm. *Stroke.* 2010;41(7):1471–1476.
2. Davidson AS, Morgan MK. How safe is arteriovenous malformation surgery? A prospective, observational study of surgery as first-line treatment for brain arteriovenous malformations. *Neurosurgery.* 2010;66(3):498–504.
3. Kameda-Smith MM, Klurfan P, van Adel BA, et al. Timing of complications during and after elective endovascular intracranial aneurysm coiling. *J Neurointerv Surg.* 2018;10(4):374–379.
4. Jeong JH, Bang J, Jeong W, et al. A dedicated neurological intensive care unit offers improved outcomes for patients with brain and spine injuries. *J Intensive Care Med.* 2019;34(2):104–108.
5. Santos AC, de Oliveira SLF, Macedo VLM, et al. Intensive care unit prioritization: the impact of ICU bed availability on mortality in critically ill patients who requested ICU admission in court in a Brazilian cohort. *J Crit Care.* 2021;66:126–31.
6. Town JA, Churpek MM, Yuen TC, Huber MT, Kress JP, Edelson DP. Relationship between ICU bed availability, ICU readmission, and cardiac arrest on the general wards. *Crit Care Med.* 2014;42(9):2037.
7. Hosey MM, Needham DM. Survivorship after COVID-19 ICU stay. *Nat Rev Dis Primers.* 2020;6(1):1–2.
8. Robert R, Coudroy R, Ragot S, et al. Influence of ICU-bed availability on ICU admission decisions. *Ann Intensive Care.* 2015;5(1):1–7.
9. Stelfox HT, Hemmelgarn BR, Bagshaw SM, et al. Intensive care unit bed availability and outcomes for hospitalized patients with sudden clinical deterioration. *Arch Intern Med.* 2012;172(6):467–474.
10. Gooch RA, Kahn JM. ICU bed supply, utilization, and health care spending: an example of demand elasticity. *JAMA.* 2014;311(6):567–568.
11. Sinuff T, Kahnamoui K, Cook DJ, Luce JM, Levy MM. Rationing critical care beds: a systematic review. *Crit Care Med.* 2004;32(7):1588–1597.
12. Goel NJ, Bird CE, Hicks WH, Abdullah KG. Economic implications of the modern treatment paradigm of glioblastoma: an analysis of global cost estimates and their utility for cost assessment. *J Med Econ.* 2021;24(1):1018–1024.
13. Bradley S, Sherwood PR, Donovan HS, et al. I could lose everything: understanding the cost of a brain tumor. *J Neurooncol.* 2007;85(3):329–338.
14. Vallejo FA, Eichberg DG, Morell AA, et al. Same-day discharge after brain tumor resection: a prospective pilot study. *J Neurooncol.* 2022;157(2):345–353.
15. Young JS, Chan AK, Viner JA, et al. A safe transitions pathway for post-craniotomy neurological surgery patients: high-value care that bypasses the intensive care unit. *J Neurosurg.* 2020;134(5):1386–1391.
16. ter Laan M, Roelofs S, van Huet C, Adang EMM, Bartels R. In reply: selective intensive care unit admission after adult supratentorial tumor craniotomy: complications, length of stay, and costs. *Neurosurgery.* 2020;86(6):E574.
17. Mirza FA, Wang C, Pittman T. Can patients safely be admitted to a ward after craniotomy for resection of intra-axial brain tumors? *Br J Neurosurg.* 2018;32(2):201–205.
18. Florman JE, Cushing D, Keller LA, Rughani AI. A protocol for postoperative admission of elective craniotomy patients to a non-ICU or step-down setting. *J Neurosurg.* 2017;127(6):1392–1397.
19. Venkatraghavan L, Bharadwaj S, Au K, Bernstein M, Manninen P. Same-day discharge after craniotomy for supratentorial tumour surgery: a retrospective observational single-centre study. *Can J Anaesth.* 2016;63(11):1245–1257.
20. Bui JQ, Mendis RL, van Gelder JM, Sheridan MM, Wright KM, Jaeger M. Is postoperative intensive care unit admission a prerequisite for elective craniotomy? *J Neurosurg.* 2011;115(6):1236–1241.
21. Boulton M, Bernstein M. Outpatient brain tumor surgery: innovation in surgical neurooncology. *J Neurosurg.* 2008;108(4):649–654.
22. Beauregard CL, Friedman WA. Routine use of postoperative ICU care for elective craniotomy: a cost-benefit analysis. *Surg Neurol.* 2003;60(6):483–489.

CHAPTER

2

Do Specialized Neurocritical Care Units Improve Outcomes?

Hera A. Kamdar, MD &
Bradley J. Molyneaux, MD, PhD

Case

A 32-year-old man presents to the emergency room following a high-speed motor vehicle crash. He has two rib fractures, a comminuted tibial fracture, and a Glasgow Coma Score of 6 upon arrival. Head CT demonstrates bifrontal contusions, and a left subdural hemorrhage without significant midline shift. An emergent intracranial pressure monitor is placed. What is the best unit for this patient to be admitted to?

Key Points

- Specialized neurocritical care units (NCCUs) have been shown to improve outcomes for a diverse range of neurologic pathologies, with as much as a 17% relative risk reduction in all-cause mortality or adverse outcomes.
- Neurointensivists serve as important resources for comprehensive general critical care.
- Adoption of dedicated NCCUs is still variable in different parts of the world, but increased adoption can help provide high quality, specialized care for all acute neurologically ill patients.

BACKGROUND

Over the past two decades, intensive care units (ICUs) that specialize in the complex management of neurological illness have become more established, widespread, and valued. A once commonly employed, general ICU model across the nation has evolved into a specialty focused model that is divided based on the type of disease and its management with allocation of management to be led by those with expertise within each field. Amongst these has emerged the neurocritical care unit (NCCU), which specializes in perioperative neurosurgical patients, as well as primary neurological diseases that are at high risk for neurological deterioration including neuromuscular weakness, intracranial hypertension, cerebral edema, brain herniation, cerebral ischemia, cerebral hemorrhage, cerebral vasospasm, and status epilepticus. Furthermore, as recent years have shown significant progress in both the acute management of neurological disease and multimodal neurological monitoring, there has been an even greater need for established NCCUs to deliver the highest quality of care to neurologically ill patients to allow for the best opportunity for recovery.

Patient Population

The NCCU has historically been home to primarily complex perioperative neurosurgical patients, for example those with large brain tumors. However, with the advancement of treatment and multimodal neurological monitoring techniques, this population has grown to include acute neurological illnesses, such as ischemic stroke, intracerebral hemorrhage, subarachnoid hemorrhage (SAH), acute nontraumatic weakness, traumatic brain injury (TBI), traumatic spinal cord injury or spinal cord compression, anoxic brain injury, coma, meningitis or encephalitis, and status epilepticus.[1]

Infrastructure

Over the years, many types of organizational models have been used to deliver neurocritical care, of which the open or closed models predominate.[2] An open model delineates the responsibility of the primary care of the patient to be delivered by the neurosurgeon or neurologist, while intensivist and other subspecialists are utilized on a consultative basis.[2] In a closed model the team is overseen, and the patient is primarily provided for by the intensivist.[2]

In 2018, a guideline describing the standard of a NCCU was published by the Neurocritical Care Society (NCS).[1] General infrastructure of the unit should include a distinct location within the medical center where there is ability to allocate specialized staff familiar with management and monitoring of acute neurological illness, as well as a proximity to the emergency department, operating rooms, imaging, and the laboratory to allow for streamlining efficient care.[1] Alongside the organization of the unit, a highly specialized and qualified multidisciplinary team is required for the success of a NCCU. Neurointensivists and neurocritical care nurses are key experts who have received specialty training to recognize, treat, and prevent neurological disease as well as practice critical care that are paramount to the care of critically ill neurological patients.[2] Additional members of the team vital to providing comprehensive quality care include neurosurgeons, neurointerventionalists, subspecialty trained epileptologists and neurovascular neurologists, specialty-trained advance care providers, pharmacists, respiratory therapists, physical/occupational/speech and language therapists, and dieticians.[1,2]

EVIDENCE AND REVIEW

Specialized NCCU on Improving Outcomes

Observational studies have reported improvement in the clinical outcome of acute brain injury patients treated within these specialized NCCUs as early as 1991.[3] Further studies have shown this positive impact on patient outcomes through lower mortality rates, decreased length of stay, and increased rate of discharge disposition to home.[4] Patient and family experience reported through satisfaction scores have also improved.[5] Moreover, despite certain studies reporting higher Acute Physiologic Assessment and Chronic Health Evaluation scores in patients with critical neurological illness, 30-day mortality rates are concurrently reported as significantly lower with neurointensivist comanagement.[6] A meta-analysis conducted in 2022 including 26 studies with 55,792 patients reported an improvement in all-cause mortality at longest follow-up until 6 months with relative risk reduction of 17% (RR 0.83; 95% CI 0.75-0.92; $P = .001$) in those receiving specialized neurocritical care.[7] A subsequent sub-group analysis divided based on disease presentation including acute ischemic stroke (AIS), intracranial hemorrhage (ICH), SAH, and TBI was completed with no significant difference seen between differing diseases.[7] Secondary outcomes focused on eight studies including 4,667 patients, also demonstrated a 17% relative risk reduction (RR, 0.83; 95% CI, 0.70-0.97; $P = .03$) in unfavorable outcomes with those patients treated within subspecialized neurocritical care settings.[7]

NCCUs on Providing General Critical Care

While fellowship trained neurointensivists have a range of backgrounds, NCCUs in the United States are predominantly staffed by clinicians with residency training in neurology with additional comprehensive critical care training. However, some continue to argue on these providers' ability to provide standardized general critical care for patients without specific neurologic disease. With the surge in critical care needs during the COVID-19 pandemic and transformation of many NCCUs to COVID-19 medical ICUs, Philips et al. were able to comment on the ability of a neurointensivist to provide general critical care.[8] The study compared units staffed by general intensivists versus neurointensivists and found there was no significant difference in the use of mechanical ventilation, renal replacement therapy, vasopressors, or in-hospital mortality.[8] This continues to show how neurointensivists are salient resources for comprehensive general critical care, in addition to their specific neurologic expertise.[8]

Practice Patterns Across the Globe

Despite the evidence-based approach to support the implementation of NCCUs, there remains a lack of universal specialized neurocritical care both domestically and globally, leading to a wide variety of practice patterns in treating acute neurological disease. The PRINCE Study Part 1 was performed in 257 hospitals across 47 countries and sought to understand and describe the commonalities, differences, and gaps with neurocritical care globally.[9,10] Nearly half of the responding sites were in North America (46.3%), followed by Europe (17.2%), Asia (13.3%), Latin America (13.3%), Oceania (5.5%), and then the Middle East (3.5%).[10] They found most NCCUs were in academic institutions within large urban centers with most participants reporting dedicated NCCUs (67% overall), which may be skewed given the highest percentage in North America (82%) making up nearly half (46.3%) of responding sites.[10] The PRINCE Study Part 2 analyzed data from 1,545 patients admitted in 147 hospitals across 31 countries to better understand practice patterns.[11] They found significant variability within the treatment team with differences in nursing staff ratios, and resource allocation in terms of general versus specialized NCCUs across the globe.[11] As we now know the benefit of these specialized NCCUs, collaborative next steps must be taken to implement such paradigms within the infrastructure of intensive care to provide the most comprehensive and high-quality care for all acute neurologically ill patients.

REFERENCES

1. Moheet AM, Livesay SL, Abdelhak T, et al. Standards for neurologic critical care units: a statement for healthcare professionals from The Neurocritical Care Society. *Neurocrit Care*. 2018;29(2):145–160.
2. Kramer AH, Zygun DA. Do neurocritical care units save lives? Measuring the impact of specialized ICUs. *Neurocrit Care*. 2011;14(3):329–333.
3. Wärme PE, Bergström R, Persson L. Neurosurgical intensive care improves outcome after severe head injury. *Acta Neurochir (Wien)*. 1991;110(1-2):57–64.
4. Varelas PN, Conti MM, Spanaki MV, et al. The impact of a neurointensivist-led team on a semiclosed neurosciences intensive care unit. *Crit Care Med*. 2004;32(11):2191–2198.
5. Ko MA, Lee JH, Kim JG, et al. Effects of appointing a full-time neurointensivist to run a closed-type neurological intensive care unit. *J Clin Neurol*. 2019;15(3):360–368.
6. Kim SH, Yum KS, Jeong JH, et al. Impact of neurointensivist co-management in a semiclosed neurocritical-care unit. *J Clin Neurol*. 2020;16(4):681–687.

7. Pham X, Ray J, Neto AS, et al. Association of Neurocritical Care Services With Mortality and Functional Outcomes for Adults With Brain Injury: a systematic review and meta-analysis. *JAMA Neurol.* 2022;79(10):1049–1058.
8. Philips S, Shi Y, Coopersmith CM, et al. Surge capacity in the COVID-19 era: a natural experiment of neurocritical care in general critical care. *Neurocrit Care.* 2022;1–6.
9. Kramer AH, Couillard P. Neurocritical care: a growing international collaborative. *Neurocrit Care.* 2020;32(1):80–83.
10. Suarez JI, Martin RH, Bauza C, et al. Worldwide Organization of Neurocritical Care: Results from the PRINCE Study Part 1. *Neurocrit Care.* 2020;32(1):172–179.
11. Venkatasubba Rao CP, Suarez JI, Martin RH, et al. Global Survey of Outcomes of Neurocritical Care Patients: Analysis of the PRINCE Study Part 2. *Neurocrit Care.* 2020;32(1):88–103.

CHAPTER

3

What Is the Role of Invasive Multimodal Monitoring in Neurosurgical Patients?

Evan M. Krueger, DO, MSc, Joacir G. Cordeiro, MD, PhD, Ayham Alkhachroum, MD, & K. O'Phelan, MD

Case

A 37-year-old man with no known past medical history, presented after a motor vehicle crash, with an initial Glasgow Coma Scale (GCS) score of 6, without eye opening and withdrawing from noxious stimulation bilaterally. Computed tomography (CT) head demonstrated skull fractures of the right frontal bone, frontal sinus, and orbital roof, with traumatic subarachnoid hemorrhage (SAH) and interpeduncular hemorrhage. Computed tomography angiography (CTA) of the neck demonstrated a grade 4 right carotid dissection (Figures 3–1 to 3–3). CT perfusion was with perfusion deficit or infarct, and transcranial Doppler study demonstrated decreased flow velocity over the right middle cerebral artery (MCA) territory, which was improved partially with increasing BP. Is $PbtO_2$ monitoring safe and feasible?

Key Points

- Brain monitoring is a cornerstone of the management of patients with acute brain injury.
- Multimodal Monitoring (MMM) is a natural evolution of earlier intracranial monitoring algorithms. The extensive data and patient centered outcomes needed to ultimately decide the best therapeutic targets are not yet completely collected.
- MMM has not yet been widely adopted as a standard of care. There are two important randomized control trials (Best TRIP and BOOST-II) that evaluated the role of MMM in traumatic brain injury patients with initial GCS 3 to 8.
- The BOOST-II trial showed that $PbtO_2$ monitoring is safe and feasible. $PbtO_2$ + ICP goal-directed therapies reduced both the time spent with $PbtO_2 < 20$ mm Hg and the depth of $PbtO_2$ measured, as compared to ICP directed therapies alone.
- As technology advances and we can learn about the specific physiology of each individual patient, clinicians will be able to tailor therapy to their needs and improve functional recovery.

BACKGROUND

Multimodal monitoring (MMM) is an integral component of modern neurocritical care (NCC) that combines sophisticated physiologic measurements with emerging technologies. Implementation of MMM has been recommended by various societies and guidelines including the Neurocritical Care Society and Brain Trauma Foundation,[1,2] although MMM has not yet been widely adopted as a standard of care. The challenges to broader implementation of MMM include uncertainty about which type of physiologic monitoring is preferred and whether MMM utilization directly translates to improved neurologic outcomes. This chapter will explore the role and controversies surrounding invasive MMM in neurosurgical patients and provide critical analysis of how the currently available literature should be properly applied in patient care. Noninvasive MMM devices such as ultrasonography to measure optic nerve sheath diameter, noninvasive transcutaneous intracranial pressure (ICP) monitors, transcranial Doppler ultrasonography, pupillometry, tympanometry, visual-evoked potentials, electroencephalography, and near-infrared spectroscopy are beyond the scope of this chapter; but likely do play an important role in the future clinical management.

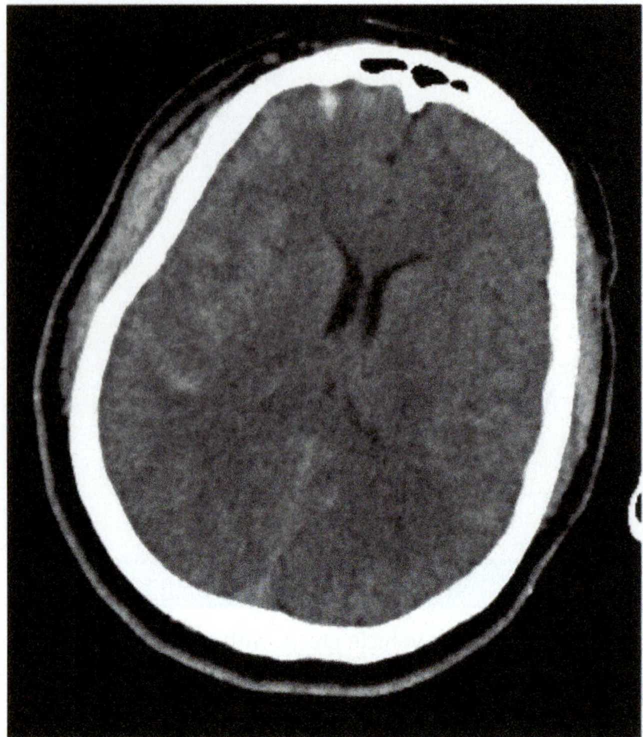

FIGURE 3–1 Noncontrast CT of the head demonstrating traumatic subarachnoid hemorrhage and small right frontal contusion.

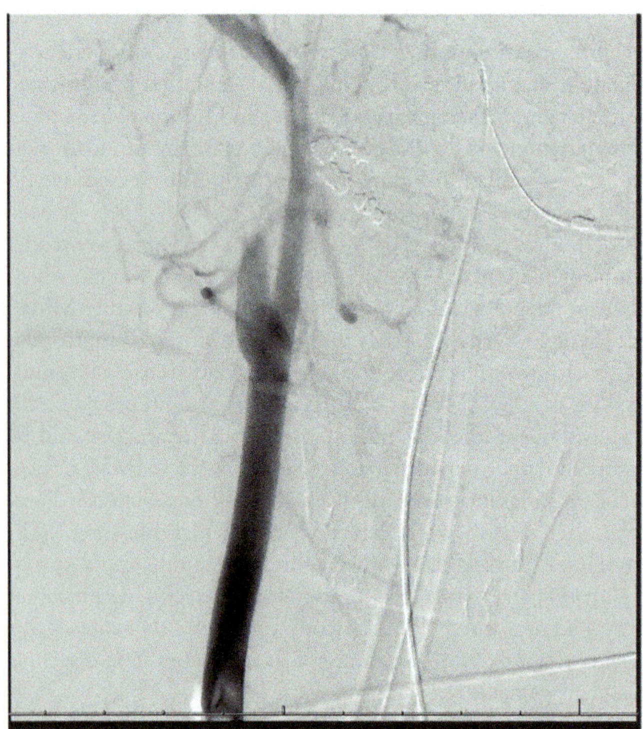

FIGURE 3–2 Digital subtraction angiography demonstrating grade 4 internal carotid dissection.

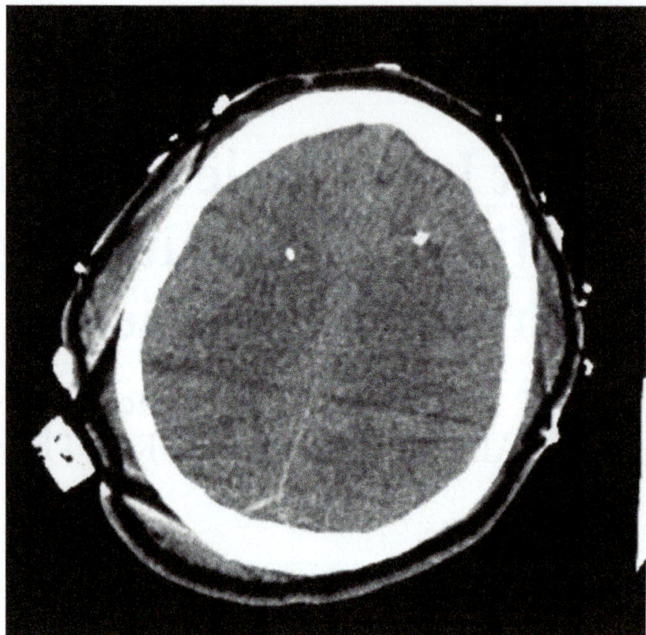

FIGURE 3–3 Noncontrast CT of the brain demonstrates placement of left frontal ICP monitor and right frontal $PbtO_2$ probe.

EVIDENCE AND REVIEW

Principles of Invasive Multimodal Monitoring

A core tenet of NCC is identifying vulnerable tissue and optimizing various parameters to prevent permanent damage. An invasive MMM device provides a tool to guide clinicians to hypothetically achieve these goals. An ideal MMM device is described below; unfortunately, no singular MMM device has all these characteristics (Table 3–1).

Invasive MMM devices allow clinicians to measure various physiologic parameters including ICP, cerebral blood flow (CBF), oxygenation, electrical activity, and metabolism. Clinicians should

TABLE 3–1 Ideal MMM device characteristics.

• Point-of-care, does not interfere with other patient care.	• High spatial and temporal resolution.	• Correlates with other clinical and radiographic findings.
• Low risk to patients and staff.	• High sensitivity and specificity for regional and global information.	• Can be used independently without reliance on other devices or measurements.
• Durable, reliable. Repeatable, not user-dependent.	• Can detect real-time adjustable parameters. These parameters have identifiable causes and effects.	• Affordable. Readily available.

consider individual measurements as well as dynamic trends in the context of clinical and radiographic variables. This allows for the development of precise, individualized, goal-directed therapies.

In general, hesitation to use invasive MMM devices is based on a determination of unacceptable risk benefit profile. The hypothetical benefits are relatively less well supported by evidence and will largely be the focus of the subsequent sections. Alternatively, the risks associated with placement of invasive MMM devices are well described. The incidence of hemorrhage and infection associated with external ventricular drain (EVD) usage have been reported as high as 8.4% and 7.9%, respectively.[3] Fiberoptic parenchymal monitors have significantly lower risks of hemorrhage (0.8%) and infection (0.8%) as compared to EVDs.[4] It should be noted however that these risks may be higher if an invasive MMM device is to be placed in injured or vulnerable tissue. There are additional concerns with the applicability of regional monitoring for more diffuse disease processes. Lastly, consideration should be given to the fiscal cost as well as increased labor and staffing associated with usage of invasive MMM devices.

Landmark Trials

Presently, MMM literature is composed primarily of observational studies. Thus, most clinical decision making is informed by lower power evidence. However, two important randomized control trials—the "A Trial of Intracranial-Pressure Monitoring in Traumatic Brain Injury (Best TRIP)" and "Brain Tissue Oxygen Monitoring and Management in Severe Traumatic Brain Injury (BOOST-II): a Phase II Randomized Trial" studies are summarized below (Table 3–2).[5,6]

Intracranial Pressure and Cerebral Perfusion Pressure

Persistently elevated ICP has consistently been shown to be associated with impaired cerebral perfusion (CPP), infarction, and mortality. Importantly, the findings of the Best TRIP trial do not suggest that ICP monitoring should not be used; instead, it questions whether a protocol based on imaging and clinical exam, or a protocol based on data obtained from ICP monitoring is the more efficacious way to improve neurologic outcomes. The third edition of the Brain Trauma Foundation (BTF) guidelines previously recommended placement of an ICP monitoring device for severe Traumatic Brain Injury (TBI) (ie, GCS ≤ 8) in patients with a normal CT scan when ≥2 of the following features were noted: age > 40 years, unilateral or bilateral motor posturing, or systolic blood pressure < 90 mm Hg.[7] These were removed from the most recent BTF fourth edition guidelines published in 2016 due to more stringent criteria for included recommendations, rather than due to the presence of new contrarian evidence.[2] A consensus statement was put forth in 2019 by the Seattle International Brain Injury Consensus Conference (SIBICC) supporting a tier-based algorithm toward the treatment of ICP in severe TBI patients. This resource for practical bedside management of patients with ICP monitoring devices, describes the assessment of cerebral autoregulation (CA) via interpretation of ICP changes when mean arterial pressure (MAP) is modified in order to determine individualized CPP goals.[8] Knowing the appropriate CPP goal for a dynamic disease process such traumatic injury is challenging since a low CPP risks cerebral ischemia, whereas an excessively high CPP risks cardiopulmonary injury and cerebral hyperemia. In a multicenter randomized control trial, Tas et al. showed that treatment using individualized CA was able to maintain dynamic target CPP goals significantly more often than fixed target CPP goals of 60 to 70 mm Hg (per current BTF guidelines).[9] There were no differences in adverse safety events, but also no differences in long-term neurologic outcomes.[9] Other options for evaluating CA to inform CPP targets include the use of transcranial Doppler, Doppler flowmetry, and invasive cerebral perfusion monitoring.

TABLE 3–2 Recent TBI clinical trials.

Trial	Design	Population	Intervention	Results	Critiques
Best TRIP[6]	Multi-center, randomized control trial	$n = 324$. Included: age > 13, initial GCS 3-8. Excluded: initial GCS 3 and fixed dilated pupils, nonsurvivable injury	Guideline based management treatment based on ICP (as obtained with ICP monitor or EVD), or treatment based on imaging and clinical exam.	No significant differences in 6-month composite outcomes, mortality, and total ICU length of stay. The imagining and clinical exam-based treatment group had more days in ICU receiving brain-specific treatments.	Trial should not be interpreted as whether to monitor or not. Data may not be applicable to all countries with varying care delivery systems.
BOOST-II[5]	Multi-center, randomized control trial	$n = 119$. Included: age > 13, initial GCS 3-8. Excluded: penetrating injury, secondary oxygen concerns, non-survivable injury.	All patients had both ICP and $PbtO_2$ monitors placed within 12 hours of injury. Randomized to receive therapy for ICP only, or therapy for ICP and $PbtO_2$ measurements.	Better proportion of time (0.16 ICP+$PbtO_2$ *versus* ICP 0.45, $p < 0.001$) and depth (1.0 ICP+$PbtO_2$ *versus* 3.6 ICP, $p < 0.0001$) below $PbtO_2$ <20 mm Hg. No differences in 6-month GOS-E scores, protocol deviations, or serious adverse events.	Trial stopped early; as a phase II was powered for safety and not efficacy.

Cerebral Oxygenation

Ultimately ICP and CPP are imperfect surrogates of CBF and energy homeostasis. Sources of cerebral hypoxia are not just limited to ischemia. Cerebral oxygenation is another potential target and has brought forth interest in brain interstitial O_2 tension ($PbtO_2$) monitoring. Adequate cerebral oxygenation is dependent on sufficient oxygen delivery (a product of CBF and oxygen content) to meet metabolic demands as well as effective mitochondrial function to use the delivered substrate. Therefore, there are multiple strategies to improve cerebral oxygenation. The BOOST-II trial showed that $PbtO_2$ monitoring is safe and feasible. Additionally, $PbtO_2$ + ICP goal-directed therapies reduced both the time spent with $PbtO_2 < 20$ mm Hg and the depth of $PbtO_2$ measured, as compared to ICP-directed therapies alone. As a phase II study, the BOOST II trial was not powered to evaluate efficacy and there were ultimately no differences in long-term neurologic outcomes.[5] The BOOST III study is currently enrolling subjects to address this question. Jugular bulb oximetry also provides clinicians information about global cerebral oxygen extraction. However, this device carries risk of thromboembolic complications, and it can be challenging to distinguish between changes in oxygen demand or delivery if jugular bulb oximetry is used as a stand-alone measure.

Other Measurements—Cerebral Metabolism

Cerebral microdialysis is an invasive neuromonitoring technique that provides a continuous measure of various molecules important for cellular energy metabolism. In 2014, an international committee put forth a consensus statement suggesting a tiered importance of various metabolites measured by microdialysis catheters. Tier 1 consisted of high- or low-glucose concentrations, and a high or low lactate/pyruvate ratios associated with poor outcomes or impaired oxygen delivery, respectively; tier 2 consisted of excessive glutamate observed in ischemia; and tier 3 consisted of high glycerol associated with oxidative stress.[10] Unfortunately, adoption is slow and microdialysis catheters are still not widely used. This is likely because they are labor and cost intensive and provide regional information which is specific to the area of tissue in which the monitor is placed. These monitors provide hourly measurements which illuminate cellular level responses to physiologic changes and clinical treatments.

Other Measurements—Spreading Depolarizations

Spreading depolarizations (SD) are a result of noxious stimuli that produce pathologic waves throughout the gray matter, are thought to be a major source of excitotoxic injury, and a possible therapeutic target. A multicenter prospective trial of 138 patients requiring neurosurgical intervention for traumatic brain injury showed repetitive SD occurred in 37% of patients, and these SD were associated with worse long-term neurologic outcomes.[11] Presently, the invasive methods to detect SD are subdural strip typically placed via craniotomy for aneurysm clipping or hematoma evacuation, and percutaneous intracortical electrodes. There are data showing that SD related to TBI and SAH can be effectively controlled with medications[12] (eg, ketamine). Nevertheless, evidence for efficacious and targeted treatment of SD is still being collected in other clinical trials.

Other Measurements—Cerebral Blood Flow

Theoretically, CBF provides the most direct physiologic measurement of the degree of oxygen delivery. Probes should be placed in the subcortical white matter in the vessel territory of interest and can provide real-time measurements. However, this remains a relatively new technology with minimal supporting clinical evidence. CBF measurements are regional and will not detect abnormal perfusion in distant areas of the brain. They must also be used in conjunction with other measurements due to confounding effects of level of consciousness and sedating medications that may alter ischemic thresholds.

AVAILABLE GUIDELINES

Implementation of MMM has been recommended by various societies and guidelines including the Neurocritical Care Society and Brain Trauma Foundation,[1,2] although MMM has not yet been widely adopted as a standard of care.

REFERENCES

1. Le Roux P, Menon DK, Citerio G, et al. Consensus summary statement of the International Multidisciplinary Consensus Conference on Multimodality Monitoring in Neurocritical Care: a statement for healthcare professionals from the Neurocritical Care Society and the European Society of Intensive Care Medicine. *Intensive Care Med.* Sep 2014;40(9):1189–1209. doi:10.1007/s00134-014-3369-6
2. Carney N, Totten AM, O'Reilly C, et al. Guidelines for the Management of Severe Traumatic Brain Injury, Fourth Edition. *Neurosurgery.* 2016;80(1): 6–15. doi:10.1227/neu.0000000000001432
3. Dey M, Stadnik A, Riad F, et al. Bleeding and infection with external ventricular drainage: a systematic review in comparison with adjudicated adverse events in the ongoing Clot Lysis Evaluating Accelerated Resolution of Intraventricular Hemorrhage Phase III (CLEAR-III IHV) trial. *Neurosurgery.* Mar 2015;76(3):291–300; discussion 301. doi:10.1227/neu.0000000000000624
4. Dimitriou J, Levivier M, Gugliotta M. Comparison of complications in patients receiving different types of intracranial pressure monitoring: a retrospective study in a single center in Switzerland. *World Neurosurg.* May 2016; 89:641–646. doi:10.1016/j.wneu.2015.11.037
5. Okonkwo DO, Shutter LA, Moore C, et al. Brain Oxygen Optimization in Severe Traumatic Brain Injury Phase-II: A Phase II Randomized Trial. *Crit Care Med.* Nov 2017;45(11):1907–1914. doi:10.1097/ccm.0000000000002619
6. Chesnut RM, Temkin N, Carney N, et al. A trial of intracranial-pressure monitoring in traumatic brain injury. *N Engl J Med.* Dec 27 2012; 367(26):2471–2481. doi:10.1056/NEJMoa1207363
7. Guidelines for the management of severe traumatic brain injury. *J Neurotrauma.* 2007;24 Suppl 1:S1–S106. doi:10.1089/neu.2007.9999
8. Hawryluk GWJ, Aguilera S, Buki A, et al. A management algorithm for patients with intracranial pressure monitoring: the Seattle International Severe Traumatic Brain Injury Consensus Conference (SIBICC). *Intensive Care Med.* Dec 2019;45(12):1783–1794. doi:10.1007/s00134-019-05805-9

9. Tas J, Beqiri E, van Kaam RC, et al. Targeting autoregulation-guided cerebral perfusion pressure after traumatic brain injury (COGiTATE): a feasibility randomized controlled clinical trial. *J Neurotrauma*. Oct 15 2021; 38(20):2790–2800. doi:10.1089/neu.2021.0197
10. Hutchinson PJ, Jalloh I, Helmy A, et al. Consensus statement from the 2014 International Microdialysis Forum. *Intensive Care Med*. Sep 2015; 41(9):1517–1528. doi:10.1007/s00134-015-3930-y
11. Hartings JA, Andaluz N, Bullock MR, et al. Prognostic value of spreading depolarizations in patients with severe traumatic brain injury. *JAMA Neurol.* Apr 1 2020;77(4):489–499. doi:10.1001/jamaneurol.2019.4476
12. Carlson AP, Abbas M, Alunday RL, et al. Spreading depolarization in acute brain injury inhibited by ketamine: a prospective, randomized, multiple crosssover trial. *J Neurosurg*. 2018 May 25;1–7. doi:10.3171/2017

CHAPTER

4

How Should Delirium Be Managed in the NeuroICU?

Vanessa Ogundipe, MD & Kahli Zietlow, MD

Case

An 83-year-old man is admitted to the neurointensive care unit (neuroICU) following a fall down the stairs, leading to traumatic brain injury featuring several hemorrhagic contusions. Based on his clinical and radiographic progress, he is managed nonoperatively. During the first 48 hours of admission, he becomes increasingly agitated and disoriented, yelling at hospital staff and tugging and pulling at his lines and tubes. How should such a patient be managed?

Key Points

- Delirium is a frequent complication in the neuroICU, and can lead to devastating consequences, including long-term functional and cognitive impairment, and increased risk of mortality.
- Prevention is key, and includes management of pain, nutrition, sleep, environmental triggers, and avoidance of potentially problematic medications.
- Once recognized, delirium is best managed by treating the underlying causes. Antipsychotics have not been shown to reduce duration of delirium, ICU/hospital stay, or mortality, and are reserved for patients with distressing symptoms and those at risk for harm.

BACKGROUND

Delirium is an acute change in mental status that typically develops over hours to days. It is common in the inpatient setting and particularly in intensive care units. One systematic review estimated that 31.8% of all patients admitted to an intensive care unit are diagnosed with delirium.[1] Similar rates exist for patients in the neuroICU, with an estimated 12% to 43% of patients impacted.[2] Delirium is associated with several adverse outcomes, including increased length of hospital stay and duration of mechanical ventilation, increased rate of discharge to facility (versus home), and increased mortality. Although delirium is typically thought to resolve as underlying risk factors are addressed, patients who experience delirium may suffer long lasting functional and cognitive impairment.[1]

EVIDENCE AND REVIEW

Risk Factors and Prevention

Advancing age, sensory impairment, underlying cognitive impairment, and structural brain disease are common preexisting risk factors for delirium. There are many modifiable risk factors that can precipitate delirium in patients admitted to the hospital (summarized in Table 4–1).[3] Medications are a common causative factor. Physiologic changes of aging including diminished hepatic and renal clearance, sarcopenia, and increased adiposity alter drug metabolism and increase susceptibility to adverse drug effects. In patients with delirium, all medications should be critically assessed, especially medications with anticholinergic or psychotropic effects. Pharmacists can facilitate age-appropriate dosing, rapid identification of problematic medications, and consideration of safer alternatives.

Screening and Differential Diagnosis

In any ICU setting, standardized screening tools such as the confusion assessment method (CAM) and intensive care delirium screening checklist (ICDSC) can be rapidly utilized by clinicians to screen for and identify delirium.[4] The CAM-ICU is a modified assessment tool that is used in patients receiving mechanical ventilation or who are otherwise nonverbal.[5] Screening can be performed by providers or nursing staff and should be performed frequently given its high prevalence and fluctuating course.

There is a broad differential diagnosis for delirium. For instance, hypoactive delirium may masquerade as depression. Some forms of dementia, including Lewy body dementia and frontotemporal dementia, are characterized by hallucinations, falls, and personality changes, and could be mistaken for

TABLE 4–1 Risk factors that can precipitate delirium in patients admitted to the ICU.

Medications*	Metabolic
Anticholinergic medications	Uremia
Antidepressants	Hypoglycemia, hyperglycemia
Antiepileptics	Hyponatremia
Anxiolytics	Hypercalcemia, hypocalcemia
Cefepime	Hyperosmolar, hypo-osmolar
Ciprofloxacin	**Endocrine disturbance**
Digoxin	**Nutritional**
Dopamine agonists	B_{12} deficiency
First-generation antihistamines	Wernickes/Thiamine deficiency
Gabapentin, pregabalin	**Cardiovascular**
Histamine-2 receptor blockers	Hypotension, orthostasis
Lithium	Arrhythmias
Muscle relaxants	Heart failure
Sedatives	Acute coronary syndrome
Medication/Substance Withdrawal	**Respiratory**
Alcohol	Hypoxemia
Benzodiazepine	Hypercapnia
Nicotine	**Brain disease**
Opioid	Hypertensive emergency
Intoxication	Traumatic brain injury
Infection	Intracranial hemorrhage
Kidney injury	Edema
Liver injury	Encephalitis/meningitis
Hypothermia, hyperthermia	Brain abscess
Pain	Nonconvulsive status epilepticus
Dysregulated circadian rhythm	**Urinary retention**
	Constipation

*Almost any new medication may cause altered mental status; any new medication in a patient with delirium should be critically evaluated.

delirium; however, onset is not as rapid. Behavioral disturbance secondary to dementia may also mimic delirium, but these symptoms usually develop more insidiously and may occur reliably with certain triggers (eg, sundowning in the early evening). Collateral history from family, including a thorough assessment of the patient's baseline cognitive status, can help differentiate delirium from other neuropsychiatric disorders. Metabolic disturbances, particularly hypoglycemia, may cause an abrupt change in mental status.

In the neuroICU, the differential diagnosis is even broader, and many factors can contribute to a patient's delirium. In particular, nonconvulsive seizures, intracranial hemorrhage, infection, and ischemia can all occur subacutely, mimicking both the insidious onset and waxing/waning characteristics of delirium. Moreover, these factors can predispose a patient to delirium due to reduced cognitive reserve. A thorough neurologic exam to exclude focal deficits, as well as laboratory and imaging studies, are important to screen for other causes before settling on a diagnosis of delirium. Moreover, many medications used in the neuroICU setting are deliriogenic (see again Table 4–1), particularly those used to control seizures, pain, and agitation. It is important to consider further workup with electroencephalogram (EEG) and/or advanced neurologic imaging such as MRI or PET-CT based on clinical findings to further evaluate for structural cause of delirium.

Relatively little evidence exists to guide delirium screening protocols in the neuroICU setting. In a 2019 systematic review analyzing seven prospective cohort studies with a total of 1,173 patients compared delirium assessment tools in the neuroICU.[2] Five of these studies used CAM-ICU, while the others used the ICDSC, 4-A Test, and CAM. When compared to a Diagnostic and Statistical Manual of Mental Disorders (DSM-IV) reference standard, these common ICU screening methods demonstrated moderate sensitivity (62%-76%), higher specificity (74%-98%), and relatively high positive and negative predictive values (PPV: 63%-91%, NPV: 70%-94%). A 2018 study of 74 neuroICU patients compared delirium assessment performed by bedside nurses using ICDSC and CAM-ICU to psychiatrist assessment.[6] They found that the CAM-ICU had a lower sensitivity (59% vs. 85%), positive predictive value (71% vs. 88%), negative predictive value (43% vs. 71%), and overall accuracy (58% vs. 82%) than the ICDSC. Overall, these studies, although limited, demonstrate that in neuroICU patients, standardized assessment tools can be used effectively to assess delirium.

Management

Once acute delirium has been diagnosed, a multimodal approach to treatment with an emphasis on nonpharmacologic interventions should be employed. Multicomponent interventions focusing on cognitive stimulation, pain management, sleep, and mobility have shown to reduce delirium, ICU length of stay, and hospital mortality. The American Society of Critical Care Medicine created the ABCDEF bundle to address the need to optimize delirium prevention in ICU patients. The bundle includes **A**ssess, Prevent and Manage Pain, **B**oth Spontaneous Awakening Trials (SAT) and Spontaneous Breathing Trials (SBT), **C**hoice of analgesia and sedation, **D**elirium: Assess, Prevent and Manage, **E**arly mobility and Exercise, and **F**amily engagement and empowerment.[7] Another commonly used strategy is the Hospital Elder Life Program, a multicompartmental approach that has taken root in many hospitals throughout the United States. It consists of clinical nurse specialists and trained volunteers who engage with older adults at risk for delirium, through the implementation of daily visits, stimulating activities, early mobilization, feeding support, assistance with vision and hearing aids, and sleep enhancement.[8] This program is effective in reducing delirium and falls in the hospital, as well as reducing length of stay and institutionalization.

Patients with underlying cognitive impairment are at particular risk for delirium. As such, interventions to enhance contextual awareness, including use of cognitive stimulation, music, clocks, calendars, and frequent reorientation by family and caregivers are very useful. Moreover, family presence offers comfort to the patient and allows family members to advocate for the needs and preferences of their loved ones. Presence of family may also lessen the burden of ICU staff, as family can assist with activities of daily living such as feeding and promote supervised mobility. It is also important to address sensory deficits that are common in older adults. Patients should continue to use their corrective eyewear and hearing aids if possible. If hearing aids are not readily available, personalized sound amplifiers are an economical alternative. Communication boards and white boards can also help facilitate communication in those with impaired speech.

Critically ill patients are at high risk for deconditioning and functional impairment due to prolonged immobility and underlying disease processes. Early mobilization may help to prevent functional decline and mitigate acute delirium. Patients must achieve cardiovascular, respiratory, and neurologic stability prior to engaging in therapy. Early mobilization is particularly important after cerebral infarct and has been shown to improve functional capacity and reduce morbidity.[9] Monitors, continuous IV fluids, urinary catheters, sequential compression devices, and other items that tether patients to the bed limit mobility and should be discontinued as soon as medically appropriate.

Adequate assessment and management of pain improves patient comfort and reduces incidence of delirium by as much as 10% to 20%.[10,11] Assessment of pain may be difficult in critically ill patients; the behavioral pain scale and critical care pain observation tool allows measurement of pain in individuals unable to self-report.[12] Acetaminophen should be considered a first-line option and can reduce or obviate the need for opioids. For those without contraindications, Non-steroidal anti-inflammatory drugs (NSAIDs) can also be an effective alternative to opioids. Membrane stabilizers and muscle relaxants can be effective, but should be used cautiously given their sedative effects. Opioids should be used at the lowest effective dose and should be used with caution in renal impairment. All patients on opioids should be frequently assessed for constipation and urinary retention, which can also precipitate delirium.

Choice of sedation is important in preserving cognitive function in the ICU. Several studies have shown an increased risk of delirium with benzodiazepine use, and a comparative reduction in delirium with dexmedetomidine, though this effect is of borderline significance in a pooled meta-analysis of large trials (RR 0.81, 95% CI: 0.60-1.08).[12] Daily spontaneous awakening trials can minimize sedation requirements and have been shown to decrease duration of mechanical ventilation and ICU length of stay.[7]

Sleep disruption is common in the ICU and is associated with increased risk of delirium. Critically ill patients spend a greater proportion of time in light sleep and a smaller proportion in deep sleep; they are also prone to fragmented sleep. Factors reported by patients to be disruptive to sleep include environmental (noise, lights), physiologic (pain, nausea), care-related (nursing procedures, restriction from lines and catheters, monitors), and psychologic (fear, anxiety, disorientation). Evidence to support routine use of medications to enhance sleep such as dexmedetomidine, tricyclic antidepressants, sedative-hypnotics and atypical antipsychotics is inconclusive, with no agent having shown a consistent ability to improve subjective sleep quality or circadian rhythm alteration.[12] Melatonin has been associated with reduced incidence of delirium on medical wards and has minimal risk of adverse events, thus scheduled melatonin 1 hour prior to bedtime may be appropriate in older adults at risk of delirium.[13] Tricyclic antidepressants, sedative-hypnotics, and atypical antipsychotics are often used for their sedating effects; however, there is insufficient research to support their efficacy in delirium prevention and these medications may paradoxically precipitate delirium.[12] Use of a formalized, nonpharmacologic sleep protocol has demonstrated reduced incidence of delirium in hospitalized patients in limited studies.[12] Components of such a sleep protocol may include reducing sedation, minimizing light and noise, offering earplugs and eye shades to appropriate patients, using relaxing music, and clustering care to avoid nighttime interruptions.

Two large, randomized trials have recently examined the use of antipsychotic medication for the prophylaxis of delirium in critical care patients (REDUCE and MIND-USA). These trials did not show any decrease in the incidence of delirium, the duration of mechanical ventilation, or the length of ICU stay.[9] The MIND-USA trial demonstrated no significant reduction in duration of delirium in ICU patients who received haloperidol or ziprasidone compared to those who did not.[14] The REDUCE trial showed no improvement in survival in critically ill patients at high risk for delirium who received haloperidol.[15] A meta-analysis showed no association between antipsychotic use for treatment of delirium with duration or severity of delirium, ICU or hospital length of stay, or mortality.[16] As such, we advocate that antipsychotic usage in delirium be reserved for patients who experience significant distress related to symptoms of delirium, such as anxiety, hallucinations, or delusions, or patients who pose a threat to themselves or others due to violent behavior. Common adverse effects of antipsychotics include QTc prolongation, sedation, and extrapyramidal symptoms (see Table 4–2). Benzodiazepines have a limited role as they can prolong delirium and are poorly tolerated in older adults. However, they are first-line agents for alcohol and benzodiazepine withdrawal, and may have a role in severe, refractory agitation, particularly in patients who cannot tolerate antipsychotics due to cardiac or extrapyramidal effects. Valproic acid is emerging as a potential adjunct agent in the treatment of refractory, agitated delirium, but there is a paucity of evidence to support its use.[17] Patients on valproic acid should be monitored for hyperammonemia, liver dysfunction, and thrombocytopenia.

TABLE 4–2 Medications to treat severe agitation in delirious patients.[a]

Agent	Dose	Benefits	Adverse Events
Risperidone	0.25-0.5 mg po q4h PRN; Max dose:[b] 2 mg/24 h	Relatively nonsedating	Slightly fewer EPS than haloperidol; less cardiac toxicity
Olanzapine	2.5-5 mg po/ IM q12h (should not be given IV) Maximum dosage:[b] 20 mg/24 h	Fewer EPS than risperidone	More sedating than risperidone
Quetiapine	12.5-25 po q12h; maximum dosage:[b] 50 mg/24 h	Fewer EPS than risperidone; can be used in patients with Parkinsonism	More sedating than risperidone; hypotension
Ziprasidone	5-10 mg IM, 20 mg capsule po; maximum dosage:[b] 20 mg/24 h	Fewer EPS than haloperidol; moderate sedation	Risk of cardiac arrhythmia, heart failure, agranulocytosis
Haloperidol	0.25-0.5 mg po/ IM/IV q4h PRN; maximum dosage:[b] 3 mg/24 h	Relatively nonsedating	EPS, especially if >3 mg/d
Lorazepam	0.25-0.5 mg po/ IV q8h PRN	Use in sedative and alcohol withdrawal; history of neuroleptic malignant syndrome	More paradoxical excitation and respiratory depression than haloperidol
Pimavanserin	34 mg po daily	Approved for use of psychosis in Parkinson disease, may be appropriate for acute agitation in patients with Parkinsonism	GI upset, peripheral edema. Very limited data regarding use in delirium.

[a]*Geriatrics Review Syllabus.* Nielsen Bookdata; 2022.

[b]Maximum dose per 24 h is the recommended total cumulative dose threshold to minimize risk of adverse events in frail older adults. Younger patients may be able to tolerate somewhat higher doses.

Adapted with permission from Harper GM, Lyons WL, Potter JF. The Geriatrics Review Syllabus: A Core Curriculum in Geriatric Medicine, 11th Ed. American Geriatrics Society; 2022.

REFERENCES

1. Salluh JI, Wang H, Schneider EB, et al. Outcome of delirium in critically ill patients: systematic review and meta-analysis. *BMJ*. 2015;350.
2. Patel MB, Bednarik J, Lee P, et al. Delirium monitoring in neurocritically ill patients: a systematic review. *Crit Care Med.* 2018 Nov;46(11):1832–1841. PMID: 30142098
3. Marcantonio ER. Delirium in hospitalized older adults. *N Engl J Med.* 2017;377(15):1456–66.
4. Inouye SK, van Dyck CH, Alessi CA, et al. Clarifying confusion: the confusion assessment method: a new method for detection of delirium. *Ann Intern Med.* 1990 Dec 15;113(12):941–8.
5. Ely EW, Margolin R, Francis J, et al. Evaluation of delirium in critically ill patients: validation of the Confusion Assessment Method for the Intensive Care Unit (CAM-ICU). *Crit Care Med.* 2001 Jul 1;29(7):1370–9.
6. Larsen LK, Frokjaer VG, Nielsen JS, Sket al. Delirium assessment in neurocritically ill patients: a validation study. *Acta Anaesthesiologica Scandinavica* 2019 Mar;63(3):352–9.
7. Marra A, Ely EW, Pandharipande PP, et al. The ABCDEF bundle in critical care. *Crit Care Clin.* 2017 Apr;33(2):225–43. doi: 10.1016/j.ccc.2016.12.005. PMID: 28284292; PMCID: PMC5351776.
8. Hshieh TT, Yang T, Gartaganis SL, et al. Hospital elder life program: systematic review and meta-analysis of effectiveness. *Am J Geriatr Psychiatry.* 2018;26(10):1015–33. doi: 10.1016/j.jagp.2018.06.007. Epub 2018 Jun 26. PMID: 30076080; PMCID: PMC6362826.
9. Reznik ME, Slooter AJC. Delirium management in the ICU. *Curr Treat Options Neurol.* 2019 Nov 14;21(11):59. doi: 10.1007/s11940-019-0599-5. PMID: 31724092.
10. Lynch EP, Lazor MA, Gellis JE, et al. The impact of postoperative pain on the development of postoperative delirium. *Anesth Analg.* 1998 Apr; 86(4):781–5.
11. Vaurio LE, Sands LP, Wang Y, et al. Postoperative delirium: the importance of pain and pain management. *Anesth Analg.* 2006 Apr;102(4):1267–73.
12. Devlin JW, Skrobik Y, Gélinas C, et al. Clinical Practice Guidelines for the Prevention and Management of Pain, Agitation/Sedation, Delirium, Immobility, and Sleep Disruption in Adult Patients in the ICU. *Crit Care Med.* 2018 Sep;46(9):e825–e873. doi: 10.1097/CCM.0000000000003299. PMID: 30113379.
13. Chen S, Shi L, Liang F, et al. Exogenous melatonin for delirium prevention: a meta-analysis of randomized controlled trials. *Mol Neurobiol.* 2016 Aug; 53(6):4046–53.
14. Girard TD, Exline MC, Carson SS, et al.; MIND-USA Investigators. Haloperidol and ziprasidone for treatment of delirium in critical illness. *N Engl J Med.* 2018 Dec 27;379(26):2506–16.
15. van den Boogaard M, Slooter AJC, Brüggemann RJM, et al. Effect of haloperidol on survival among critically ill adults with a high risk of delirium: The REDUCE Randomized Clinical Trial. *JAMA.* 2018 Feb 20;319(7):680–90.
16. Neufeld KJ, Yue J, Robinson TN, et al. Antipsychotic medication for prevention and treatment of delirium in hospitalized adults: a systematic review and meta-analysis. *J Am Geriatr Soc.* 2016 Apr;64(4):705–14.
17. Cuartas CF, Davis M. Valproic acid in the management of delirium. *Am J Hospice Palliat Med.* 2022 May;39(5):562–9.

CHAPTER

5

How Do We Achieve Adequate Pain Control in Neurosurgical Patients?

Arthur Formanek, MD & Hinna Malik, MD

Case

A 59 year-old woman with a history of substance abuse disorder is scheduled to undergo a two-stage posterior fossa meningioma resection. How can we better understand her intraoperative pain management and its implications for immediate postoperative pain management?

Key Points

- Neurosurgical patients require unique anesthetic considerations due to the frequent need for neuromonitoring signals, as well as the need for accurate neurologic examination in the postoperative period.
- Intraoperative narcotic medication is the mainstay of intraoperative anesthesia, but adjuncts can ease the transitions in the perioperative period.
- Regional anesthesia is a powerful tool for targeted pain control, but care should be taken to differentiate potential postoperative complications related to regional blockade from intracranial pathology.

BACKGROUND

Postoperative care of the neurosurgical patient is unique in that maintaining adequate mental status is paramount to enabling a high-quality neurologic examination. The intraoperative course may affect downstream neurologic exam and analgesia. Providing minimum, but adequate, levels of opioid administration to control pain while optimizing mental status is key. Additional modalities such as regional anesthesia and adjuncts are also greatly beneficial.

EVIDENCE AND REVIEW

Intraoperative Management and Immediate Postoperative Pain Implications

Intraoperative goals for providing adequate analgesia in craniotomy procedures should also consider duration of action, potential for delay of the postoperative neurologic exam, and negative functional effects of medications in addition to just providing analgesia. The ideal anesthetic regimen should allow for expedient postoperative neurologic exams while also avoiding potential side effects of certain medications including decreased respiratory drive and delirium.

As many craniotomy procedures are done utilizing intraoperative monitoring of evoked potentials (sensory, motor, visual, auditory, etc.), anesthetic plans are tailored to allow for as little interference with neuromonitoring as possible. This includes utilizing no greater than 0.5 to 0.75 MAC of volatile anesthetic, with higher levels having been shown to increase SSEP latency and decrease SSEP amplitude, while supplementing with intravenous opioids such as the short-acting remifentanil and commonly propofol, which can have similar effects to volatile anesthetics on waveforms in large doses.[1]

During the surgical resection, short-acting opioids and sedatives are frequently used to preserve the respiratory drive at the conclusion of the craniotomy.[2] Remifentanil is easily and quickly titratable to deepen the level of anesthesia, blunt coughing, and reduce respiratory drive without accumulation.[3] Consequently, while the rapid metabolism of remifentanil speeds emergence and aids in extubation, the rapid metabolism will ensure no longer-lasting effect and may result in hyperalgesia. Hydromorphone or morphine may be administered at the end of the case for longer-duration algesia depending upon the alertness of the patient. Especially if the patient has a history of chronic pain and a procedure with a higher forecasted postoperative pain level is performed, a longer-acting opioid infusion such as fentanyl or sufentanil may be used in lieu of remifentanil to avoid hyperalgesia.

Opioids

Opioids remain the mainstay of intraoperative and some acute postoperative pain but the effect of mental status depression is problematic. Intravenous (IV) hydromorphone and morphine are generally functionally equivalent with hydromorphone having fewer pruritic side effects. Of note, if pruritis is encountered after synthetic opioid administration, it is likely μ-receptor related and antihistamines will be ineffective.[4] Patient-controlled analgesia (PCA) has been shown to provide superior analgesia but increases opioid use.[5] Once the patient may take oral opioids, oxycodone has a longer duration of action. If longer duration IV opioids are desired, IV methadone is highly effective, especially for patients with chronic opioid use because of its N-methyl-D-aspartate (NMDA) receptor antagonism, but care should be taken because of its long duration and nonlinear dose conversion.

If infusions are required during mechanical ventilation, a fentanyl infusion offers analgesia, suppression of respiratory drive and coughing, synergy with a hypnotic infusion, and predictable pharmacodynamics. Alternatively, sufentanil may be used for a shorter duration of action or hydromorphone may be used for longer half-life. Rotation of opioids may be required if prolonged infusion is necessary.

Adjuncts

The use of preoperative gabapentin as both an analgesic and as antiseizure prophylaxis for craniotomy patients has been studied, with a reported decreased consumption of postoperative opioids, but the caveat of potential delayed tracheal extubation and increased sedation.[6,7] Preoperative use of acetaminophen also provides intra and postoperative analgesia but is not sufficient on its own to provide adequate pain relief. Preoperative celecoxib has been shown to decrease postoperative opioid consumption and has minimal sedating effects compared to gabapentin, but its use in neurosurgery patients is controversial in its potential to increase bleeding.[8]

Intraoperative utilization of lidocaine and dexmedetomidine infusions can also augment analgesia, with the added benefit of limited effect on evoked potential monitoring. Our group has had good results in early tracheal extubation using both infusions as adjuncts to minimize the use of both propofol and volatile anesthetic during the dura and skin closure portions of craniotomies. Both lidocaine and dexmedetomidine have analgesic properties, minimal sedating effects, and avoid respiratory drive depression.[8] These infusions can also be continued in the postoperative setting for intubated and extubated patients.

NMDA antagonists may also be useful adjuncts (Table 5–1). While ketamine preserves ventilatory drive, it is generally a poor choice because of its potential to alter the patient's consciousness and produce delirium. Magnesium, which may act partially through NMDA antagonism, has been demonstrated to reduce pain scores and opioid consumption in the first 24 hours postoperatively.[9]

Regional Anesthesia and Scalp Block

A scalp block provides inhibition of nociception to both superficial and deep soft tissues.[6] Compared to surgical site infiltration, the scalp block reduces pain scores and opioid consumption in the early postoperative period (up to 24-48 hours after surgery).[14,15]

A total of six nerves bilaterally generally are blocked: the greater occipital nerve, the lesser occipital nerve, the auriculotemporal nerve, the zygomaticotemporal nerve, the supraorbital nerve, and the supratrochlear nerve. A unilateral scalp block is not frequently performed so that contralateral Mayfield pin sites may be covered, although some anesthesiologists use lower concentration local anesthetic on the nonoperative side if toxicity is of concern.

Use of lidocaine, ropivacaine, bupivacaine, and levobupivacaine in scalp blocks have been published, with no study published that investigates superiority of a specific local anesthetic, concentration.[6] In our practice, we prefer 0.25% bupivacaine with epinephrine, dexmedetomidine, and dexamethasone (either IV or in the block mixture) for immediate postoperative pain to provide a long-acting (approximately 24 hours) block.

The scalp block generally consists of 12 injections, and caution must be exercised in calculating maximum dose of local anesthetic because of the large volume delivered (in addition to any local anesthetic delivered in the field). In addition, care must be taken to diligently aspirate for blood before injecting because of the highly vascular nature of the scalp and the risk of direct injection of arrhythmia-inducing agents into the venous system.

The greater occipital nerve innervates the posterior aspect of the head extending to the vertex and is located approximately midway between the occipital protuberance and mastoid process, where it courses medial to the occipital artery.[16–18] The greater occipital nerve is located by palpating the occipital artery in the medial one-third to midpoint between the occipital protuberance and mastoid process or using ultrasound. The needle is then inserted perpendicularly to the skin and advanced until cranium is contacted: 4 to 5 mL of local anesthetic medial to the artery is injected as the needle is slowly withdrawn.[19,20]

The lesser occipital nerve innervates the skin behind the ear and courses approximately 2.5 cm lateral to the greater occipital nerve and 7 cm lateral to the greater occipital protuberance.[21] The block is performed by injecting 4 to 5 mL of local anesthetic approximately 2.5 cm lateral to the greater occipital block along the superior nuchal line.

The auriculotemporal nerve innervates the anterior ear and posterior forehead.[22] The needle is inserted 1 cm superior to the tragus behind the superior temporal artery to block it.[23] Injection of 2 to 3 mL of local anesthetic above and below the temporalis fascia is typically sufficient.[28]

The zygomaticotemporal nerve innervates the posterior portion of the forehead.[21] It is performed by finding the notch along the zygomatic arch behind the lateral canthus of the eye, and advance the needle until a pop or resistance change is noted as the temporalis fascia is pierced. The nerve ramifies through the temporalis fascia, so 2 to 3 mL of local anesthetic should be placed in total to cover both above and below the fascia.[19,20]

The supraorbital nerve innervates the scalp from the upper eyelid to the lambdoid suture and the supraorbital notch is easily palpated in the medial third of the supraorbital ridge.[24] Inserting the needle close to but not into the supraorbital notch is important to avoid the supraorbital artery:[20] 2 to 3 mL of local anesthetic is typically sufficient.

TABLE 5–1 Analgesics and adjuncts.[10–13]

Drug	Dosing	Duration of Action/ Half Life	Benefits	Drawbacks
Remifentanil	0.05-0.2 mcg/kg/min infusion	Terminal ½ life 10-20 min	Intraoperative analgesia; minimal effect on neuromonitoring	Respiratory depression; hyperalgesia; intraoperative use only
Sufentanil	0.2-0.5 mcg/kg/h infusion	Elimination half-life 164 min	Reliable intraop analgesia	Respiratory depression, long duration of action, intraoperative use only
Fentanyl	25-100 mcg bolus; 50-150 mcg/h infusion	20-30 min	Rapid onset of action, reliable analgesia	Short duration of action as a bolus; respiratory depression; tachyphylaxis
Hydromorphone	0.25-2 mg bolus (IV)	Elimination half-life 2.5 h	Reliable analgesia; can be utilized as a PCA or bolus	Respiratory depression, prolonged duration of action, nausea, vomiting
Morphine	2.5-10 mg bolus (IV)	Terminal half-life 2-4 h	Intra and postoperative analgesia	Respiratory depression; pruritis, nausea, vomiting
Oxycodone	5-20 mg (PO)	3-6 h (immediate release)	Intra and postoperative analgesia; can decrease IV opiate consumption when given preoperatively	Respiratory depression, nausea, vomiting
Lidocaine	1-1.5 mg/kg bolus followed by 1-4 mg/kg/h infusion	2 h	Intra and postoperative analgesia; preservation of respiratory drive	Risk for toxicity with prolonged infusion, requires daily lidocaine level monitoring
Dexmedetomidine	0.2-0.7 mcg/kg/h infusion	Terminal half-life approx. 2 h	Intra and postoperative analgesia; preservation of respiratory drive	Potential hypotension and bradycardia
Ketamine	3-5 mcg/kg/min infusion	half-life 45 min	Preservation of respiratory drive, safe for extubated patients	Can increase ICP, impaired neuro exams from delirium
Gabapentin	300 mg preoperatively	Elimination half-life 6.5 h	Analgesia with antiseizure activity, opioid-sparing	Sedation, increased time to tracheal extubation
Magnesium	500 mg-2 g bolus (IV), 0.5 g/h infusion	4 h	Opioid-sparing	Hypotension, risk for magnesium toxicity with repeated or prolonged use
Acetaminophen	1000 mg q4-6 h	4-6 h	Opioid-sparing, nonsedating	Large quantities may impair liver function
Ketorolac	7.5-30 mg q6h (IV)	4-6 h	Opioid-sparing, nonsedating	Theoretical risk of increased bleeding (not supported by meta-analyses), nephrotoxicity with prolonged use
Ibuprofen	200-600 mg q6h (po)	Half-life 1-2 h	Opioid-sparing, nonsedating	Risk for nephrotoxicity and gastric ulceration with prolonged use

The supratrochlear nerve innervates the skin of the lower forehead and is located in the superomedial angle of the orbit. It may be blocked by injecting 2 to 3 mL of anesthetic above the eyebrow, 1 cm medial to the supraorbital notch.[20]

Sphenopalatine Ganglion Block

Because dura is not covered by the traditional scalp block, the afferent branches of the trigeminal nerve traversing through sphenopalatine ganglion are an attractive target to block.[25] Activation of the trigeminal-autonomic reflex may also release vasoactive peptides and present clinically as a headache.[26–28] However, large studies evaluating the perioperative utility of sphenopalatine ganglion block for postsurgical pain remain to be published.

A sphenopalatine ganglion block is generally performed by placing a wick (a Q-tip or commercial applicator) into each nare and advance past the middle turbinate to the posterior nasopharynx. Cases with ropivacaine, bupivacaine, mepivacaine, and cocaine have been published, but 2 to 4 mL in each nare of 1% to 4% lidocaine is frequently utilized.[25,29]

Complications of Regional Anesthesia

Care must be taken to differentiate adverse effects of regional anesthesia from intracranial pathology, such as focal deficits or seizures caused by local anesthetic toxicity. Bradycardia from trigeminal cardiac reflex activation has also been observed during blockade of the supratrochlear nerve.[30] Mechanical ptosis caused by edema from local anesthetic volume or hematoma has also been described, and the presence of Horner syndrome or other physical exam finding should be noted.[31] If the auriculotemporal nerve block injection is made too close to the facial nerve or a large volume of anesthetic is used, inadvertent facial nerve paralysis may occur.[32,33] By injecting 1 cm cephalad to the tragus, this risk is minimized.[23] Because of the vascular nature of the scalp, one must also be cautious of local anesthetic toxicity.

REFERENCES

1. Goettel N, Bharadwaj S, Venkatraghavan L, Mehta J, Bernstein M, Manninen PH. Dexmedetomidine vs propofol-remifentanil conscious sedation for awake craniotomy: a prospective randomized controlled trial. *Br J Anaesth*. 2016;116(6):811–821. doi:10.1093/bja/aew024
2. Weinzierl MR, Reinacher P, Gilsbach JM, Rohde V. Combined motor and somatosensory evoked potentials for intraoperative monitoring: intra- and postoperative data in a series of 69 operations. *Neurosurg Rev*. 2007;30(2):109–116; discussion 116. doi:10.1007/s10143-006-0061-5
3. Tung A, Fergusson NA, Ng N, Hu V, Dormuth C, Griesdale DEG. Medications to reduce emergence coughing after general anaesthesia with tracheal intubation: a systematic review and network meta-analysis. *Br J Anaesth*. Published online February 22, 2020. doi:S0007-0912(20)30012-X [pii]
4. Ganesh A, Maxwell LG. Pathophysiology and management of opioid-induced pruritus. *Drugs*. 2007;67(16):2323–2333. doi:10.2165/00003495-200767160-00003
5. Hudcova J, McNicol E, Quah C, Lau J, Carr DB. Patient controlled opioid analgesia versus conventional opioid analgesia for postoperative pain. *Cochrane Database Syst Rev*. 2006;(4):CD003348. doi:10.1002/14651858.CD003348.pub2
6. Guilfoyle MR, Helmy A, Duane D, Hutchinson PJ. Regional scalp block for postcraniotomy analgesia: a systematic review and meta-analysis. *Anesth Analg*. 2013;116(5):1093–1102. doi:10.1213/ANE.0b013e3182863c22
7. Türe H, Sayin M, Karlikaya G, Bingol CA, Aykac B, Türe U, The analgesic effect of gabapentin as a prophylactic anticonvulsant drug on postcraniotomy pain: a prospective randomized study. *Anesth Analg*. 2009;109(5):1625–1631. doi:10.1213/ane.0b013e3181b0f18b
8. Shlobin NA, Rosenow JM. Nonopioid postoperative pain management in neurosurgery. *Neurosurg Clin N Am*. 2022;33(3):261–273. doi:10.1016/j.nec.2022.02.004
9. Albrecht E, Kirkham KR, Liu SS, Brull R. Peri-operative intravenous administration of magnesium sulphate and postoperative pain: a meta-analysis. *Anaesthesia*. 2013;68(1):79–90. doi:10.1111/j.1365-2044.2012.07335.x
10. Arianpour K, Allen M, Ashman P, Folbe AJ. Perioperative analgesia in cranial and skull base surgery. In: Svider PF, Pashkova AA, Johnson AP, eds. *Perioperative Pain Control: Tools for Surgeons*. Springer International Publishing; 2021:207–222. doi:10.1007/978-3-030-56081-2_13
11. Tobias JD, Goble TJ, Bates G, Anderson JT, Hoernschemeyer DG. Effects of dexmedetomidine on intraoperative motor and somatosensory evoked potential monitoring during spinal surgery in adolescents. *Paediatr Anaesth*. 2008;18(11):1082–1088. doi:10.1111/j.1460-9592.2008.02733.x
12. Grathwohl KW, Black IH, Spinella PC, et al. Total intravenous anesthesia including ketamine versus volatile gas anesthesia for combat-related operative traumatic brain injury. *Anesthesiology*. 2008;109(1):44–53. doi:10.1097/ALN.0b013e31817c02e3
13. Crosby V, Wilcock A, Corcoran R. The safety and efficacy of a single dose (500 mg or 1 g) of intravenous magnesium sulfate in neuropathic pain poorly responsive to strong opioid analgesics in patients with cancer. *J Pain Symptom Manage*. 2000;19(1):35–39. doi:10.1016/s0885-3924(99)00135-9
14. Akcil EF, Dilmen OK, Vehid H, Ibisoglu LS, Tunali Y. Which one is more effective for analgesia in infratentorial craniotomy? The scalp block or local anesthetic infiltration. *Clin Neurol Neurosurg*. 2017;154:98–103. doi:S0303-8467(17)30026-4 [pii]
15. Yang X, Ma J, Li K, et al. A comparison of effects of scalp nerve block and local anesthetic infiltration on inflammatory response, hemodynamic response, and postoperative pain in patients undergoing craniotomy for cerebral aneurysms: a randomized controlled trial. *BMC anesthesiology*. 2019;19(1):91–94. doi:10.1186/s12871-019-0760-4
16. Prigge L, Schoor AN van, Bosenberg AT. Anatomy of the greater occipital nerve block in infants. *Paediatr Anaesthes*. 2019;29(9):945–949. doi:10.1111/pan.13693
17. Won HJ, Ji HJ, Song JK, Kim YD, Won HS. Topographical study of the trapezius muscle, greater occipital nerve, and occipital artery for facilitating blockade of the greater occipital nerve. *PloS one*. 2018;13(8):e0202448. doi:10.1371/journal.pone.0202448
18. Allen SM, Mookadam F, Cha SS, Freeman JA, Starling AJ, Mookadam M. Greater occipital nerve block for acute treatment of migraine headache: a large retrospective cohort study. *J Am Board Fam Med*. 2018;31(2):211–218. doi:10.3122/jabfm.2018.02.170188
19. Osborn I, Sebeo J. "Scalp block" during craniotomy: a classic technique revisited. *J Neurosurg Anesth*. 2010;22(3):187–194. doi:10.1097/ANA.0b013e3181d48846
20. Rosenblatt MA, Lai Y. *Scalp Block and Cervical Plexus Block Techniques*. Vol. 2019; 2019. https://www.uptodate.com
21. Kemp 3rd WJ, Tubbs RS, Cohen-Gadol AA. The innervation of the scalp: a comprehensive review including anatomy, pathology, and neurosurgical correlates. *Surgical Neurology International*. 2011;2:178. Epub 2011 Dec 13. doi:10.4103/2152-7806.90699
22. Janis JE, Hatef DA, Ducic I, et al. Anatomy of the auriculotemporal nerve: variations in its relationship to the superficial temporal artery and implications for the treatment of migraine headaches. *Plast Reconstr Surg*. 2010;125(5):1422–1428. doi:10.1097/PRS.0b013e3181d4fb05
23. Bebawy JF, Bilotta F, Koht A. A modified technique for auriculotemporal nerve blockade when performing selective scalp nerve block for craniotomy. *J Neurosurg Anesth*. 2014;26(3):271–272. doi:10.1097/ANA.0000000000000032
24. Nanayakkara D, Manawaratne R, Sampath H, Vadysinghe A, Peiris R, Supraorbital nerve exits: positional variations and localization relative to surgical landmarks. *Anat Cell Biol*. 2018;51(1):19–24. doi:10.5115/acb.2018.51.1.19
25. Nair AS, Rayani BK. Sphenopalatine ganglion block for relieving postdural puncture headache: technique and mechanism of action of block with a narrative review of efficacy. *Korean J Pain*. 2017;30(2):93–97. doi:10.3344/kjp.2017.30.2.93
26. Cohen S, Levin D, Mellender S, et al. Topical sphenopalatine ganglion block compared with epidural blood patch for postdural puncture headache management in postpartum patients: a retrospective review. *Reg Anesth Pain Med*. 2018;43(8):880–884. doi:10.1097/AAP.0000000000000840
27. Lv X, Wu Z, Li Y. Innervation of the cerebral dura mater. *Neuroradioly J*. 2014;27(3):293–298. doi:10.15274/NRJ-2014-10052
28. Mojica J, Mo B, Ng A. Sphenopalatine ganglion block in the management of chronic headaches. *Curr Pain Headache Rep*. 2017;21(6):27. doi:10.1007/s11916-017-0626-8
29. Candido KD, Massey ST, Sauer R, Darabad RR, Knezevic NN. A novel revision to the classical transnasal topical sphenopalatine ganglion block for the treatment of headache and facial pain. *Pain Phys*. 2013;16(6):769.
30. Chowdhury T, Baron K, Cappellani RB. Severe bradycardia during scalp nerve block in patient undergoing awake craniotomy. *Saudi J Anaesth*. 2013;7(3):356–357. doi:10.4103/1658-354X.115344
31. Hassan MH, Wan WMHN, Kandasamy R, Chong SE. Unilateral complete ptosis after scalp block for awake craniotomy: a rare complication. *J Neuroanaesth Crit Care*. 2018;05(02):111–113. doi:10.1055/s-0038-1665545
32. McNicholas E, Bilotta F, Titi L. Chandler J, Rosa G, Koht A. Transient facial nerve palsy after auriculotemporal nerve block in awake craniotomy patients. *A & A Case Rep*. 2014;2(4):40–43. doi:10.1097/ACC.0b013e3182a8ee71
33. Sargin M, Samancioglu H, Uluer MS. Transient facial nerve palsy after the scalp block for Burr hole evacuation of subdural hematoma. *Turk J Anaesthesiol Reanim*. 2018;46(3):238–240. doi:10.5152/TJAR.2018.58219

CHAPTER

6

What Are Special Considerations for Goals of Care Discussions in the NeuroICU?

Stefanie P. Cappucci, MD, Emerson Rhudy, RN, Tamara A. Strohm, MD, & David Y. Hwang, MD

Case

A 75-year-old man has been admitted to the neuroICU for over 2 weeks for complications after a large left MCA infarct. His medical complications include a ventilator-associated pneumonia and renal failure requiring continuous renal replacement therapy. Are there any special considerations for discussing goals of care with the family in such a scenario?

Key Points

- Discussions around goals of care, patients' and families' values, and prognostication are a daily part of work in a neurocritical care unit.
- Communication amongst care team members and with surrogate decision makers should be frequent, acknowledge and normalize the uncertainty in prognostication, and attempt to elicit patient's values and preferences, while simultaneously avoiding common bias pitfalls.

BACKGROUND

The neuroICU takes care of a heterogeneous population of systemically and neurologically ill patients, many of whom are unable to participate in discussions about their care. There exists an expanding body of work regarding communication and end-of-life care in the general ICU population. However, for the purposes of this chapter, we will highlight the mounting evidence for patients specifically afflicted by severe neurologic illnesses, aiming to highlight evidence that is specific to this population and their disease states.

There are five overlapping tenets that must be considered when caring for and discussing the trajectory of patients with severe neurologic injury: (1) the acuity of injury and immediacy of cognitive and functional decline; (2) the role of surrogate decision makers; (3) the possibility of survival with a level of disability inconsistent with the patient's values; (4) the degree of uncertainty in prognostication; and (5) the application of ethical tenets.

EVIDENCE AND REVIEW

Acuity of Injury

The nature of most severe brain injury is that of immediate and precipitous decline, followed by an undulating course (usually in hospital or acute care facility), with little assurance as to the ultimate outcome (Figure 6–1).[1] This stands in contrast to other disease courses, such as acute on chronic decline, slow progression, or recurrent chronic episodes of improvement and decline.

The initial severe brain injury typically results in a significant and near instantaneous departure from the patient's baseline functionality, often leaving the patient unable to participate in their own decision-making, and the family in a state of shock. Neurologic injury tends to impact the perception of personhood in ways that nonneurologic injury may not, and in most instances impedes attempts at including the patient in communication. Previously completed advanced directives rarely account for the nuances that surrogate decision makers are asked to navigate. Often family members, even those with significant medical literacy, may struggle to make complex decisions with neurointensive and neurosurgical teams while trying to process new realities. This must be accounted for with sensitivity, especially early in the hospitalization, when attempting to counsel surrogates about possible treatment options.

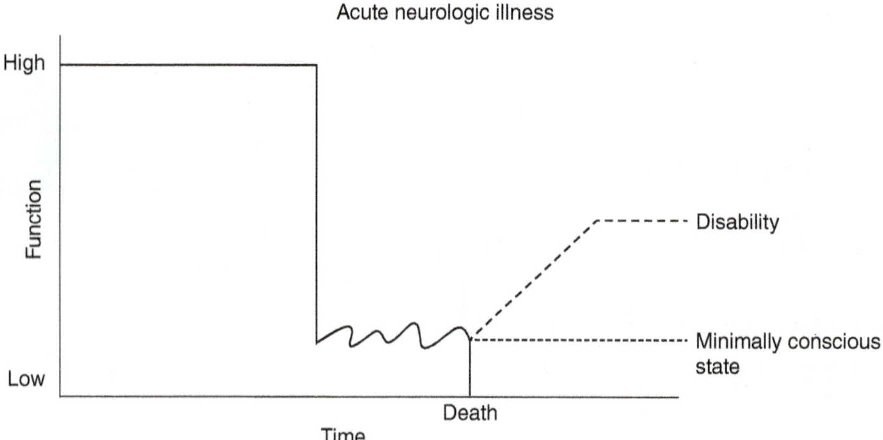

FIGURE 6–1 Illness trajectory in acute neurologic injury. Figure adapted from: Frontera JA, Curtis JR, Nelson JE, Campbell M, Gabriel M, Hays RM, et al. Integrating Palliative Care into the Care of Neurocritically Ill Patients: A Report from The IPAL-ICU (Improving Palliative Care in the Intensive Care Unit) Project Advisory Board and the Center to Advance Palliative Care. Crit Care Med. 2015;43:1964–77.

Role of the Surrogate Decision Maker

Despite the challenges of families adjusting to a new, foreign environment in the neuroICU, shared decision-making is an essential component of critical care and neurosurgical practice.[2,3] Organizing an early family meeting within 72 hours of patient's admission (and ideally held within the first 24 hours) has been correlated with family satisfaction.[4] Similarly, deliberative collaboration, as contrasted with paternalistic or rigid recommendations, between the care team and the surrogates has also been correlated with family satisfaction.[5]

Emphasis should be placed on substituted judgement; that is, making decisions aligned with the patient's values as opposed to what is desired by surrogates. All members of the care team must consider their own biases and understand how their perception of disability impacts their communication with surrogate decision-makers. Implementation of substituted judgement may mitigate the impact of these biases in the goals of care process. Additionally, recovery is a dynamic process, and attempts should be continuously made to engage the patient as clinical status changes, acknowledging that this may require adaptive communication tools and an investment in time to establish the patient's role in their own decision-making.

While early family meetings are essential, surrogates are not always prepared to receive prognostic information. Surrogate readiness should be assessed prior to discussing prognosis, and families should be prepared to transition from the information sharing phase to prognostic conversations. This should be an iterative process, especially if there is initial reluctance on the part of the surrogate to discuss prognostic information.

Evidence suggests that openness and frequency of communication[4] have a strong impact on surrogate experience. In the case of discussing tracheostomy for patients with acute brain injury, open communication was the most important factor when surrogate decision-makers were reflecting on this decision, regardless of the patient's outcome.[6] Practically speaking, family meetings should be important and frequent occurrences and can be considered a procedural skill with key steps to follow for best practices. Planning the meeting, a brief pre-meeting huddle, the meeting itself, and a postmeeting debrief are all essential to success (Figure 6–2).[2,7–9]

There are no validated measures to aid in decision-making in the neurocritically ill population. However, several have gone through feasibility studies and are actively being developed. Validated measures and decision aids may alleviate the burden and decisional stress experienced by surrogate decision-makers.[11]

Finding Concordance Between Patient Values and Potential Disability

Advances in critical care and life-sustaining therapies have grown exponentially in the last several decades, which have made the issue of acceptable functional outcomes all the more salient for patients and their surrogates. While most neurocritically ill patients can be medically or surgically supported to survive their acute injury, their functional outcome or prognosis may not justify continuation of life-sustaining care according to the patient's wishes and values. There are many treatment decisions that act as larger benchmarks in care, such as surgical decompression, mechanical ventilation and/or tracheostomy placement, and placement of a nasogastric or gastrostomy tube for nutrition.[10] Choosing these treatments may increase the likelihood of survival, but may also be misaligned with the patient's values.

Thus, it becomes integral to elicit value preference in an early and iterative fashion. Onus should not be placed on the surrogates to make decisions in a vacuum, but rather surrogates should be guided toward focus on the values of the patient, the things that were important to them, and those aspects of functionality that they would be unwilling to sacrifice.[11] Collectively, this act of predicting how a patient might feel in the future based off of a current decision is known as affective forecasting.[10]

- Planning the meeting
  - 24–72 h after admission
  - Who should attend? (SW, bedside RNs, subspecialists)
  - Time and Location, need for interpreter or chaplain
- Pre-Meeting huddle
  - Review clinical data
  - Ensure agreement amongst team-members
  - Assign roles
  - Anticipate challenges
- Meeting
  - Introductions
  - State explicit goals or headline of the meeting
  - Explain surrogate's role as an advocate as opposed to sole decision-maker
  - Probe surrogate's preferred role
  - Brief medical summary using simple language
  - Acknowledge uncertainty and discuss prognosis
  - Best case and worst case scenario
  - Elicit patient preferences, what did the patient enjoy and value
  - Describe treatment options
  - Re-elicit surrogate's preferred role
  - Summarize and make a recommendations with support
  - Inquire about concerns and fears
  - Respond to emotions
  - Summarize, clarify misconceptions, reassurance against patient suffering
  - Make joint treatment decision
  - Arrange a follow-up meeting
- Post-Meeting huddle
  - Discuss what was successful and areas for improvement
  - Future goals/strategies
  - Consider scheduled nursing, chaplain or SW check-in with surrogates

FIGURE 6–2 Outline for conducting a family meeting.

There are several biases (Figure 6–3) that come into play with this form of prediction.[7] It is particularly important to be aware of the "disability paradox" when participating in affective forecasting with surrogate decision-makers; that is, patients with disability often report a higher quality of life when compared to healthy participants asked to imagine a scenario in which they are living with significant, persistent disability.[10] This phenomenon emphasizes the need for the care team to examine their own biases about disability and interrogate how these biases effect their communication with families and surrogate decision-makers.

Uncertainty

Uncertainty is a large part of any challenging conversation in the neurocritical care unit regarding prognostication after acute brain injury. Much of this uncertainty is fueled by a lack of long-term outcome data (ie, studies of most major neurocritical care intervention outcomes have primary endpoints only at 90 days). Thus, there is a discordance between the individualized nature of these decisions (ie, eliciting value-preferences) and the broad scope of population-based data often used to guide a potential range of outcome for surrogates.[12] Perhaps most strikingly, and in contrast with other critical care populations, a withdrawal bias in the available evidence-based-medicine affects the applicability of this data. Even in well-designed observational and interventional studies, there are variable rates of withdrawal of life-sustaining therapy, thus dramatically affecting the population that is studied.[12] As such, in the cases of acute stroke, for example, the American Heart Association (AHA) recommends refraining from altering a patient's preexisting code status before the second full day of admission.[13]

Despite critical limitations in currently available population-based clinical grading scale data, surrogates do report that that numerical estimates of prognosis are helpful aids in decision-making.[14] Given the challenges of providing such concrete figures for many neuroICU patients, current recommendations focus on utilizing a best-case, worst-case framework[15] when presenting surrogates with a range of possible outcomes, to create structure for these discussions.

Time-limited trials refer to a strict time period (such as several months in the future) after which certain decisions will be revisited and made (ie, withdrawal or continuation of mechanical ventilation). This can be helpful to "wait and see" given the degree of uncertainty in prognostication. This tool can be employed in many critical care settings to allow families time to digest the range of possible outcomes.[16,17] Normalizing and embracing the uncertainty when discussing prognosis with surrogate decision-makers, and resolutely avoiding early nihilism can be difficult but effective.[12]

Recall bias Surrogates are apt to remember a patient as being healthier and more independent than he/she was before the hospitalization; this can impact their decision-making
Disability parabox People with disabilities report greater quality of life than surrogates without disabilities imagine they would report, so surrogates can be biased about how much a given disability would affect a patient
Response shift Surrogates may not be aware that patients can adapt to disability over time by adjusting their standards, values, and perception of quality of life
Focusing illusion Surrogates without disability fail to imagine the degree of patients' adaptability to disability, by focusing on aspects which will change rather than aspects that will remain the same, they can introduce bias into decision-making

FIGURE 6–3 Cognitive bias during affective forecasting. Adapted from Knies AK, Hwang DY. Palliative Care Practice in Neurocritical Care. Semin Neurol. 2016;36:631–41.

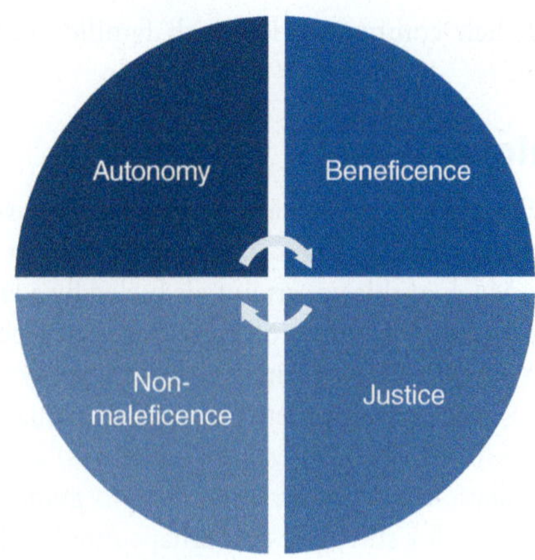

FIGURE 6–4 Ethical considerations.

Applying Ethical Considerations

Balancing traditional ethical principles for the neuroICU population can be particularly difficult, as this patient population often lacks capacity or has difficulty participating in discussion without specific accommodations (Figure 6–4). Ensuring the patient's and surrogate's rights to participate in shared decision-making, autonomy, is paramount.[8] Beneficence is the provider's effort to act in the patient's best interest. This is often paired with the principle of nonmaleficence or "do no harm." Providers must balance the tension between providing futile care versus premature withdrawal of care in applying these ethical tenets; open communication between the neurosurgery and critical care team is critical to minimize individual provider biases and provide united messages to patients' families.[18] The final tenet, justice, involves treating all patients fairly and with equitable use of health resources. Awareness of inequity in palliative care delivery and of the barriers to delivery of care for patients that live with disability, is an important component of value-based discussion needed for this patient and family population.[19]

REFERENCES

1. Frontera JA, Curtis JR, Nelson JE, et al. Integrating palliative care into the care of neurocritically ill patients: a report from the IPAL-ICU (Improving Palliative Care in the Intensive Care Unit) Project Advisory Board and the Center to Advance Palliative Care. *Crit Care Med.* 2015;43:1964–1977.
2. Curtis JR, White DB. Practical guidance for evidence-based ICU family conferences. *Chest.* 2008;134:835–843.
3. Khan MW, Muehlschlegel S. Shared decision-making in neurocritical care. *Neurosurg Clin N Am.* 2018;29:315–321.
4. Weber U, Zhang Q, Ou D, et al. Predictors of family dissatisfaction with support during neurocritical care shared decision-making. *Neurocrit Care.* 2021;35:714–722.
5. Sahgal S, Yande A, Thompson BB, et al. Surrogate satisfaction with decision making after intracerebral hemorrhage. *Neurocrit Care.* 2021;34:193–200.
6. Lou W, Granstein JH, Wabl R, Singh A, Wahlster S, Creutzfeldt CJ. Taking a chance to recover: families look back on the decision to pursue tracheostomy after severe acute brain injury. *Neurocrit Care.* 2021;1–7.
7. Knies AK, Hwang DY. Palliative care practice in neurocritical care. *Semin Neurol.* 2016;36:631–641.
8. Cai X, Robinson J, Muehlschlegel S, et al. Patient preferences and surrogate decision making in neuroscience intensive care units. *Neurocrit Care.* 2015;23:131–141.
9. Billings JA, Block SD. The end-of-life family meeting in intensive care part III: a guide for structured discussions. *J Palliat Med.* 2011;14:1058–10 64.
10. Creutzfeldt CJ, Holloway RG. Treatment decisions after severe stroke. *Stroke.* American Heart Association; 2012;43:3405–3408.
11. Ge C, Goss AL, Crawford S, et al. Variability of prognostic communication in critically ill neurologic patients: a pilot multicenter mixed-methods study. *Crit Care Explor.* 2022;4:e0640.
12. Hemphill JC, White DB. Clinical nihilism in neuro-emergencies. *Emerg Med Clin North Am.* 2009;27:27-37.
13. Powers WJ, Rabinstein AA, Ackerson T, et al. Guidelines for the early management of patients with acute ischemic stroke: 2019 update to the 2018 guidelines for the early management of acute ischemic stroke: a guideline for healthcare professionals from the American Heart Association/American Stroke Association. *Stroke* [Internet]. 2019 [cited 2022 Nov 14];50. Available from: https://www.ahajournals.org/doi/10.1161/STR.0000000000000211
14. Quinn T, Moskowitz J, Khan MW, et al. What families need and physicians deliver - contrasting communication preferences between surrogate decision-makers and physicians during outcome prognostication in critically-ill TBI patients. *Neurocrit Care.* 2017;27:154–162.
15. Hwang DY, Knies AK, Mampre D, et al. Concerns of surrogate decision makers for patients with acute brain injury. *Neurology.* 2020;94:e2054– e2068.
16. Quill TE, Holloway R. Time-limited trials near the end of life. *JAMA.* 2011;306:1483–1484.
17. Chang DW, Neville TH, Parrish J, et al. Evaluation of time-limited trials among critically ill patients with advanced medical illnesses and reduction of nonbeneficial ICU treatments. *JAMA Intern Med.* 2021;181:786–794.
18. Taylor LP, Besbris JM, Graf WD, et al. Clinical guidance in neuropalliative care: an AAN position statement. *Neurology.* 2022;98:409–416.
19. Johnsen A, Siegler M, Winslade W. *Clinical Ethics: A Practical Approach to Ethical Decisions in Clinical Medicine*, 9e | AccessMedicine | McGraw Hill Medical [Internet]. McGraw Hill Medical; [cited 2022 Oct 24]. Available from: https://accessmedicine.mhmedical.com/book.aspx?bookID=3130

CHAPTER 7

How Should We Manage Hyponatremia in Neurosurgical Patients?

Sulaiman Almohaish, PharmD, BCPS &
Gretchen M. Brophy, PharmD, BCPS, FCCP, FCCM, FNCS, MCCM

Case

A 49-year-old woman presented to the emergency department (ED) with the worst headache of her life. Computed tomography (CT) head showed diffuse subarachnoid hemorrhage (SAH). CT angiogram revealed a posterior communicating aneurysm which was later successfully coiled. During her stay in the neuroscience ICU, she developed worsening hydrocephalus managed by an external ventricular drain, and severe vasospasm treated with intra-arterial verapamil. Despite an attempt to maintain euvolemia, on hospital day 6, the bedside nurse reported that patient urine output increased to 500 mL/h for the last 3 hours. A stat set of labs revealed Na of 130 mmol/L, which previously was 141 mmol/L. Serum osmolality is 272 mOsm/kg. A set of stat urine studies was sent: UNa: 42 mmol/L, urine osmolality 201 mOsm/kg. How should we manage hyponatremia in neurosurgical patients?

Key Points

- Hyponatremia is very common among neurosurgical patients with up to 60% risk of mortality in traumatic brain injury (TBI) patients.
- Hyponatremia is classified based on the patient's volume status and serum osmolality. It's defined by a serum sodium of <135 mEq/L but is often treated at <140 mEq/L in neurosurgical patients.
- The most common reasons of hyponatremia in neurosurgical patients are syndrome of inappropriate antidiuretic hormone (SIADH), cerebral salt wasting syndrome (CSWS), and medications.
- The treatment strategy for hyponatremia is based on symptom severity. Asymptomatic patients can be further assessed until the cause of hyponatremia is known before starting therapy. Patients with severe symptoms from hyponatremia should be start on HS therapy immediately.
- Limit sodium correction to 8 to 10 mEq/L in 24 hours to avoid rapid sodium overcorrection and prevent osmotic demyelination syndrome (ODS).
- Patients with SIADH are often managed with volume restriction; however, euvolemia should be the goal for all neurosurgical patients. Consider the use of fludrocortisone in patients with CSWS.

BACKGROUND

The central nervous system (CNS) plays a major role in regulating sodium and water homeostasis. Sodium disturbances are very common in patients with neurological disease or trauma.[1,2] Hyponatremia, serum sodium concentration of <135 mEq/L, presents in 38% to 54% in neurologically injured patients.[1,2] In TBI, hyponatremia can increase risk of death up to 60%.[3] Hyponatremia occurs when there is imbalance between intracellular fluid (ICF) and extracellular fluid (ECF) concentration of water and sodium.[4,5] Therefore, measuring osmolality and sodium concentration is helpful to determine the cause of sodium disturbances. Hyponatremia is considered acute when it occurs for <48 hours and chronic when it persists for >48 hours. The symptoms of hyponatremia may vary based on severity of the hyponatremia: (1) mild hyponatremia, Na concentration between 130 and 135 mEq/L; moderate hyponatremia, Na concentration between 120 and 129 mEq/L; severe hyponatremia, Na concentration <120 mEq/L (Table 7–1).[4,5] Symptoms of mild to moderate hyponatremia may include nausea and vomiting, fatigue, gait instability and falls, and/or attention deficits, while symptoms of severe hyponatremia progress to headache, seizures, respiratory arrest, coma, or death. Finally, it is important to recognize if patients have chronic hyponatremia or acute hyponatremia as the aggressiveness of treatment strategies and therapeutic goals vary between them. In neurocritical care and neurosurgical patients, hyponatremia may increase brain edema which will elevate intracranial pressure (ICP), and cause or worsen other neurological symptoms such as delirium, tremor, seizure, agitation, and/or coma (Table 7–1). This chapter will discuss the common causes and management of hyponatremia in neurosurgical patients.

EVIDENCE AND REVIEW

Classification, Causes, and Diagnosis

Hyponatremia patients can be classified based on volume status and or serum osmolality (Table 7–2). Common causes of hyponatremia in neurosurgical patients are CSWS, SIADH, and drug-induced hyponatremia.[6-8]

TABLE 7–1 Hyponatremia severity and symptoms.[4,5]

Category	Serum Concentration	Symptoms
Mild hyponatremia	130-135 mEq/L (<140 mEq/L in neurosurgical patients)	Nausea and vomiting, fatigue, gait instability and falls, and/or attention deficits
Moderate hyponatremia	120-129 mEq/L	Nausea and vomiting, fatigue, gait instability and falls, and/or attention deficits
Severe hyponatremia	<120 mEq/L	Nausea and vomiting, headache, seizures, respiratory arrest, coma, death

TABLE 7–2 Common causes of hyponatremia in neurosurgical patients.

• Cerebral salt wasting syndrome (CSWS) • Syndrome of inappropriate antidiuretic hormone (SIADH) • Drug-induced hyponatremia	
Classifications of hyponatremia	
Based on volume status	• **Hypovolemic hyponatremia**—a decrease in total body water along with sodium concentration • **Euvolemic hyponatremia**—a decrease in sodium while total body water remains unchanged • **Hypervolemic hyponatremia**—an abnormal retention of total body water which results in a decrease in sodium concentration due to dilution
Based on serum osmolality	• **Hypotonic hyponatremia**, serum osmolality <275 mOsm/kg • **Isotonic hyponatremia**, serum osmolality 275-295 mOsm/kg • **Hypertonic hyponatremia**, serum osmolality >295 mOsm/kg

SIADH versus CSWS

The pathophysiology of CSWS is still unclear; however, one suggested theory is an increase in natriuretic peptides which causes a loss of sodium from the renal distal tubules.[9] The other possible mechanism is sympathetic nervous system impairment which may cause disruption of the renin and aldosterone release and a reduction in proximal sodium reabsorption.[10] Neurosurgical patients with trauma, infection, or tumors may develop hyponatremia due to CSWS.[11–16] In patients with SIADH, the body is unable to regulate antidiuretic hormone (ADH) production resulting in hyponatremia and impaired water excretion.[4,5,17] Several diseases and events could lead to SIADH in neurosurgical patients which include ischemic or hemorrhagic stroke, trauma, infection, cancer, postsurgical patients.[17]

Typically, CSWS is categorized as a hypovolemic hyponatremia whereas SIADH patients are often euvolemic or hypervolemic, with all other laboratory findings being similar (Table 7–3).[2,4,5,17] Thus, it is essential to assess patient volume status to differentiate between the two hyponatremic states.

Drug-Induced Hyponatremia

Multiple medications can induce hyponatremia via different pathways. Some may increase sodium excretion such as diuretics and others may cause SIADH which will lead to hyponatremia. Drugs that may induce hyponatremia and are commonly used in neurosurgical patients include thiazide and loop diuretics, mannitol, tricyclic antidepressants, selective serotonin reuptake inhibitors (SSRIs), antiseizures (carbamazepine, oxcarbazepine, lamotrigine, and valproate sodium), nonsteroidal anti-inflammatory drugs (NSAIDs), antibiotics

TABLE 7–3 Diagnostic laboratory criteria for SIADH versus CSWS[2,4,5,17]

	SIADH	CSWS
Volume status	Euvolemic	Hypovolemic
Serum sodium	<135 mEq/L	<135 mEq/L
Serum osmolality	<275 mOsm/kg	<275 mOsm/kg
Urine osmolality	>100 mOsm/kg	>100 mOsm/kg
Urinary sodium	>30 mEq/L	>30 mEq/L

(trimethoprim-sulfamethoxazole and ciprofloxacin), and antiarrhythmics (amiodarone) (Table 7–4).[18]

Assessment and Management of Hyponatremia

When assessing a patient with hyponatremia (Na < 135 mEq/L, or <140 mEq/L in neurosurgical patients), the first step is to determine if it is a true hyponatremia. Sodium concentrations can be falsely decreased in patients with hyperglycemia; therefore, a corrected sodium concentration must be calculated as sodium decreases by 1.6 mEq/L for every 100 mg/dL that glucose is above 100 mg/dL. Next, check the patients' medication list for any possible drugs that could cause hyponatremia and assess their severity by the presenting symptoms. If severe symptoms are present, obtain a serum sodium concentration and start therapy immediately, correcting sodium up to 1 to 2 mEq/L/h within the first few hours. It is recommended to start these patients on 150 mL of 3% NaCl, also referred to as hypertonic saline (HS), infused over 20 minutes or 100 mL of 3% HS infused over 10 minutes (Figure 7–1).[4,5,7] Serum sodium concentrations should be checked approximately 1 after the first infusion to allow for redistribution of sodium and determine if additional doses are necessary and then every 4 hours to prevent overcorrection and to confirm the sodium concentration has been stabilized. The correction of sodium within the first 24 hours should not exceed 8 to 10 mEq/L (Figure 7–1).[4,5]

In asymptomatic patients, monitoring volume status, serum osmolality, urine osmolality, and urine sodium is also important in the acute setting.[4,5,19]

TABLE 7–4 Medications associated with hyponatremia.[17-19]

Drug Name*		
Thiazide or loop diuretics	Carbamazepine	Methotrexate
Indapamide	Oxcarbazepine	Opiates
Hypotonic fluids	Valproate sodium	Chlorpropamide
Amitriptyline	Lamotrigine	Desmopressin or vasopressin
Protriptyline	Vincristine	NSAIDs
Desipramine	Vinblastine	Venlafaxine
SSRIs	Cisplatin	Amiodarone
Monoamine Oxidase Inhibitors	Carboplatin	Ciprofloxacin
Phenothiazines	Cyclophosphamide	Trimethoprim-sulfamethoxazole
Butyrophenones	Ifosfamide	IVIG
Amlodipine	Duloxetine	Bupropion
Angiotensin-converting enzyme inhibitors	Proton pump inhibitors	Fluorescein angiography

*Some of these medications may cause SIADH which will cause hyponatremia

Effects of Mannitol on Serum Sodium

Patients who receive mannitol for the treatment of cerebral edema may develop hyponatremia but maintain a serum osmolality >300 mOsm/kg due to the large mannitol molecule being included in the osmolality measurement.[4,5,20] Thus, consider switching therapy for cerebral edema to HS when managing patients with elevated ICP, or a sodium chloride/acetate combination therapy in patients with elevated ICP and hyperchloremia.[21]

Treatment for SIADH and CSWS

The treatment for SIADH and CSWS is based on severity of the symptoms (Figure 7–1). Severe symptoms of hyponatremia caused by SIADH or CSWS are typically treated with HS as first-line therapy; however, salt tablet administered orally/enterally can also be considered if tolerable. In mild CSWS cases, 0.9% saline (normal saline) is sufficient to restore volume and sodium level, and it is helpful as a maintenance therapy in patients with CSWS and severe symptoms once the sodium goal is reached.[4] Additionally, fludrocortisone can be beneficial to decrease sodium loss due to its mineralocorticoid effects, but requires monitoring for adverse effects such as hypokalemia, fluid overload and hypertension.[23]

Fluid restriction therapy for SIADH should be used cautiously if used for neurosurgical patients with TBI or SAH as it may lead to hypovolemia and a reduction in cerebral perfusion pressure (CPP).[4] Medications that inhibit ADH (arginine vasopressin) receptors can also be considered for the treatment of chronic mild SIADH. Conivaptan has been studied in neurointensive care patients and showed significant increase in the sodium concentration; however, whether it will help to improve patients' symptoms is unclear.[22] In refractory cases, clinicians may consider a trial of demeclocycline, but its effects can be delayed up to 1 week.[4,7,8]

Patients with serum sodium concentration of <120 mEq/L for more than 48 hours are at high risk of ODS due to rapid sodium overcorrection.[4] Therefore, identifying the duration of hyponatremia is essential for determining the aggressiveness of the sodium correction treatment strategy.[4] To avoid sodium overcorrection in these patients, reduced sodium correction goal to 4 to 8 mEq/L per day, check sodium concentration more frequently, and consider administering desmopressin after sodium correction.[4]

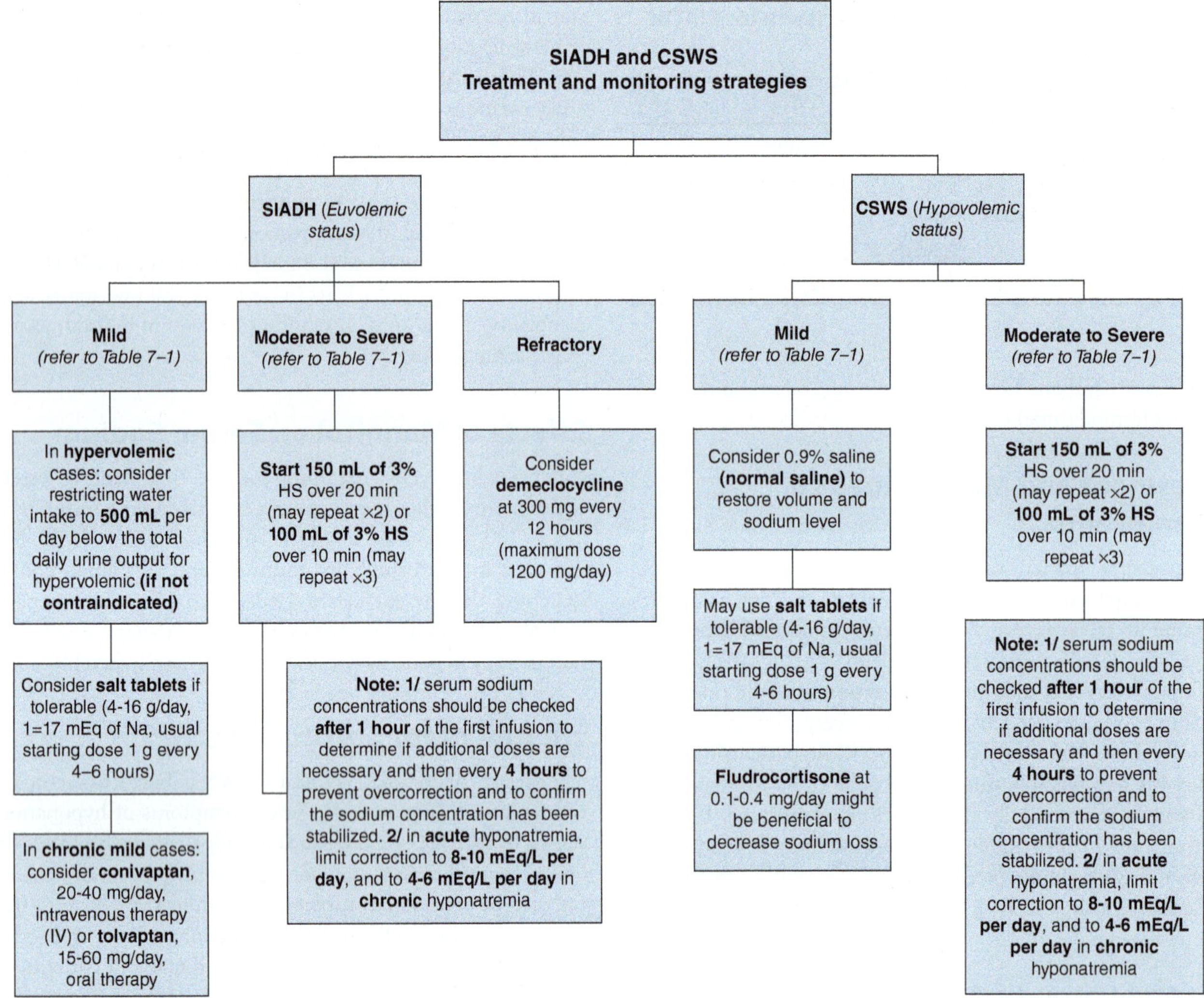

FIGURE 7–1 SIADH and CSWS treatment and monitoring strategies.[4,5,8,23]

REFERENCES

1. Human T, Cook AM, Anger B, et al. Treatment of hyponatremia in patients with acute neurological injury. *Neurocrit Care.* 2017;27(2):242–248. doi:10.1007/s12028-016-0343-x
2. Yee AH, Burns JD, Wijdicks EFM. Cerebral salt wasting: pathophysiology, diagnosis, and treatment. *Neurosurg Clin N Am.* 2010;21(2):339–352. doi:10.1016/j.nec.2009.10.011
3. Diringer MN, Zazulia AR. Hyponatremia in neurologic patients: consequences and approaches to treatment. *The Neurologist.* 2006;12(3):117–126. doi:10.1097/01.nrl.0000215741.01699.77
4. Verbalis JG, Goldsmith SR, Greenberg A, et al. Diagnosis, evaluation, and treatment of hyponatremia: expert panel recommendations. *Am J Med.* 2013;126(10):S1–S42. doi:10.1016/j.amjmed.2013.07.006
5. Spasovski G, Vanholder R, Allolio B, et al. Clinical practice guideline on diagnosis and treatment of hyponatraemia. *Eur J Endocrinol.* 2014;170(3):G1–G47. doi:10.1530/EJE-13-1020
6. Cole CD, Gottfried ON, Liu JK, Couldwell WT. Hyponatremia in the neurosurgical patient: diagnosis and management. *Neurosurg Focus.* 2004;16(4):1–10. doi:10.3171/foc.2004.16.4.10
7. Lerner DP, Shepherd SA, Batra A. Hyponatremia in the neurologically ill patient: a review. *The Neurohospitalist.* 2020;10(3):208–216. doi:10.1177/1941874419895124
8. Manzanares W, Aramendi I, Langlois PL, Biestro A. Hyponatremia in the neurocritical care patient: an approach based on current evidence. *Med Intensiva.* 2015;39(4):234–243. doi:10.1016/j.medin.2014.11.004
9. Wijdicks EF, Ropper AH, Hunnicutt EJ, Richardson GS, Nathanson JA. Atrial natriuretic factor and salt wasting after aneurysmal subarachnoid hemorrhage. *Stroke.* 1991;22(12):1519–1524. doi:10.1161/01.str.22.12.1519
10. Bitew S, Imbriano L, Miyawaki N, Fishbane S, Maesaka JK. More on renal salt wasting without cerebral disease: response to saline infusion. *Clin J Am Soc Nephrol.* 2009;4(2):309–315. doi:10.2215/CJN.02740608
11. Gutierrez OM, Lin HY. Refractory hyponatremia. *Kidney Int.* 2007;71(1):79–82. doi:10.1038/sj.ki.5001845
12. Filippella M, Cappabianca P, Cavallo LM, et al. Very delayed hyponatremia after surgery and radiotherapy for a pituitary macroadenoma. *J Endocrinol Invest.* 2002;25(2):163–168. doi:10.1007/BF03343981
13. Sengupta K, Ali U, Andankar P. Cerebral salt wasting. *Indian Pediatr.* 2002;39(5):488–491.
14. Ti LK, Kang SC, Cheong KF. Acute hyponatraemia secondary to cerebral salt wasting syndrome in a patient with tuberculous meningitis. *Anaesth Intensive Care.* 1998;26(4):420–423. doi:10.1177/0310057X9802600413
15. Erduran E, Mocan H, Aslan Y. Another cause of hyponatraemia in patients with bacterial meningitis: cerebral salt wasting. *Acta Paediatr Oslo Nor 1992.* 1997;86(10):1150–1151. doi:10.1111/j.1651-2227.1997.tb14830.x

16. Oster JR, Perez GO, Larios O, Emery WE, Bourgoignie JJ. Cerebral salt wasting in a man with carcinomatous meningitis. *Arch Intern Med.* 1983;143(11):2187–2188.
17. Ellison DH, Berl T. Clinical practice. The syndrome of inappropriate antidiuresis. *N Engl J Med.* 2007;356(20):2064–2072. doi:10.1056/NEJMcp066837
18. Liamis G, Milionis H, Elisaf M. A review of drug-induced hyponatremia. *Am J Kidney Dis Off J Natl Kidney Found.* 2008;52(1):144–153. doi:10.1053/j.ajkd.2008.03.004
19. Kirkman MA, Albert AF, Ibrahim A, Doberenz D. Hyponatremia and brain injury: historical and contemporary perspectives. *Neurocrit Care.* 2013;18(3):406–416. doi:10.1007/s12028-012-9805-y
20. Manninen PH, Lam AM, Gelb AW, Brown SC. The effect of high-dose mannitol on serum and urine electrolytes and osmolality in neurosurgical patients. *Can J Anaesth J Can Anesth.* 1987;34(5):442–446. doi:10.1007/BF03014345
21. Cook AM, Morgan Jones G, Hawryluk GWJ, et al. Guidelines for the acute treatment of cerebral edema in neurocritical care patients. *Neurocrit Care.* 2020;32(3):647–666. doi:10.1007/s12028-020-00959-7
22. Naidech AM, Paparello J, Liebling SM, et al. Use of conivaptan (vaprisol) for hyponatremic neuro-ICU patients. *Neurocrit Care.* 2010;13(1):57–61. doi:10.1007/s12028-010-9379-5
23. Misra UK, Kalita J, Kumar M. Safety and efficacy of fludrocortisone in the treatment of cerebral salt wasting in patients with tuberculous meningitis: a randomized clinical trial. *JAMA Neurol.* 2018;75(11):1383–1391. doi:10.1001/jamaneurol.2018.2178

CHAPTER

8

What Blood Glucose Levels Should We Target in Neurologically Injured Patients?

Matthew Brown, MD, Kevin Furlong, DO, Newton Mei, MD, & Rene Daniel, MD, PhD

Case

A 58-year-old man with a long-standing history of type 2 diabetes mellitus is admitted to the neurolCU (NICU) following a high-speed motor vehicle collision resulting in a severe traumatic brain injury (TBI). The medical record indicates that his last hemoglobin A1c was 10.4 at a clinic visit several months ago and that he requires basal and mealtime insulin as part of his home therapy. How should we think about managing his blood glucose during his intensive care stay?

Key Points

- In the noncritical care setting, most guidelines agree that a premeal blood glucose < 140 mg/dL and a random blood glucose of <180 mg/dL is recommended.[37]
- Recommendations for glycemic targets in the critical care setting differ only slightly[37] with overarching consensus to target a blood glucose to 140 to 180 mg/dL while avoiding hypoglycemia.[35]

BACKGROUND

In the general inpatient population, both high blood glucose levels and low glucose levels are associated with unfavorable outcomes.[1,2] Hyperglycemia and diabetes are also common in the neurosurgical population and have been associated with increased postoperative complications, length of stay, higher mortality rates, and hospital costs.[3,4] The stress of neurological illness and surgery can activate a neuroendocrine response that antagonizes insulin activity.[5] This is mediated by an increase in hormones such as epinephrine and cortisol, as well as an increase in proinflammatory cytokines.[6] However, it is still debated whether hyperglycemia is a surrogate marker for worse outcomes or an underlying cause.[7] While many studies have associated hyperglycemia with worse outcomes, there is a paucity of data showing that intensive glucose control provides benefit and may result in increased incidence of hypoglycemia. Below, we will review the relevant evidence and provide evidence-based goals where available.

Hyperglycemia is common in the critical care setting and has long been associated with adverse outcomes. There have been multiple trials comparing conventional glucose management (CGM) to intensive insulin therapy (IIT) in this setting. Differences in patient population, center experience, nutritional supplementation methods, severity of illness, and outcome measures make this a heterogeneous group of studies.

EVIDENCE AND REVIEW

Historical Studies

Data from a clinical trial by Van Den Berghe et al. in 2001 showed benefit to intensive glucose control in surgical ICU patients who were receiving mechanical ventilation.[8] A total of 1,548 patients were enrolled and randomly assigned to either IIT with a goal blood glucose goal of 80 to 110 mg/dL or to CGM with a goal blood glucose level of 180 to 200 mg/dL. Only 4% of these patients were admitted to the ICU for neurologic disease, cerebral trauma, or brain surgery. IIT reduced mortality during intensive care from 8% to 4.6% ($P < .04$). The benefit of IIT was attributable to its effect on mortality among patients who remained in the ICU for more than 5 days. IIT also reduced overall in-hospital mortality, blood stream infections, acute renal failure requiring dialysis or hemofiltration, the medium number of red-cell transfusions, and critical illness polyneuropathy.

After this trial was published, many centers developed insulin protocols with more intensive glucose goals. However, subsequent, multicenter studies were performed in an attempt to investigate and verify these results, but many have failed to find a benefit for IIT. The Volume Substitution and Insulin Therapy in Severe Sepsis (VISEP) study and Glucontrol study were two such multicenter prospective randomized trials, but notably neither showed significant difference in mortality in IIT versus CGM.[9,10] However, they did show increased episodes of severe hypoglycemia in the IIT arms.

The NICE-SUGAR study was a large multicenter randomized control trial which enrolled 6,104 patients.[11] It compared an intensive glucose target of 80 to 108 mg/dL to a conventional target of 180 mg/dL or less. Mortality in the IIT group was 27.5% compared to 24.9% in the CGM group ($p = .02$). The incidence of severe hypoglycemia was 6.8% in the IIT group versus 0.5% in the CGM group ($P < .001$). This lack of detectable benefit and possibility of increased harm has led to a more relaxed glucose goal in the critical care setting in more recent times.

Ischemic Stroke

There have been several studies evaluating the effects of IIT in acute ischemic stroke patients with hyperglycemia, and while multiple of which have shown a correlation between hyperglycemia and increased infarct size, stroke severity and poor outcome, prospective clinical trials evaluating IIT have failed to find a benefit for tighter control.[12,13]

The THIS trial by Bruno et al. compared IIT (goal BS of <130) versus conventional therapy (goal BS of <200 mg/dL).[14] There was no difference at outcomes in 3 months; however, there was a 35% rate of hypoglycemia in the IIT group.

The Intensive versus Subcutaneous Insulin in Patients with Hyperacute Stroke (INSULINFARCT) trial, a prospective, randomized, unblinded trial including patients with hyperacute stroke, was designed to determine if IIT with continuous insulin infusion would improve glucose control and reduce subsequent infarct growth on magnetic resonance imaging.[15] The authors found that patients in the IIT group had improved overall glucose control within the first 24 hours of stroke, but this was in fact associated with *larger* infarct growths.

The SHINE trial randomized patients with acute ischemic stroke and hyperglycemia to intensive treatment (581 patients, target BG 80-130) versus standard therapy (570 patients, target BG 80-179) for up to 72 hours. There was no significant difference in favorable functional outcome at 90 days and severe hypoglycemia occurred only among patients in the intensive treatment group.[16]

Subarachnoid Hemorrhage

Hyperglycemia has been recognized as a poor prognostic factor in subarachnoid hemorrhage (SAH) and is associated with increased risk for vasospasm following aneurysmal SAH, longer length of stay in the NICU, and worse outcome at discharge.[17,18] However, there is no evidence that strict glucose control improves outcomes. A trial of 834 patients by Theile et al. showed no difference in mortality with IIT (BG < 120) but an increased risk of hypoglycemia ($P < .001$). Hypoglycemia was associated with a substantially increased risk of death on multivariate analysis ($P = .009$; OR = 3.818).[19]

Traumatic Brain Injury

Similarly, hyperglycemia has been shown to be an independent predictor of worse outcome in TBI.[20,21] There are several studies evaluating the use of IIT in the treatment of these patients. In one study, persistent hyperglycemia was identified as an independent risk factor for mortality (OR = 4.91; $P < .0001$) after adjusting for significant risk factors.[21] One study found no effect of IIT on sepsis rates, neurological outcome, or duration of ICU stay.[22] Another study showed IIT shortened ICU stays but had no effect on infection rates or mortality.[23] A further study found that IIT decreased infection rates, days spent in the ICU, and neurologic outcome at the 6-month follow-up.[24] In a small study by Wang et al., IIT decreased infection rate and reduced duration of ICU stay but mortality rates were similar between the two groups.[25]

Neurosurgery

Hyperglycemia and diabetes are common in neurosurgical patients. Surgical procedures themselves are known to induce intraoperative hyperglycemia[26] and volatile anesthetics have been shown to worsen stress-induced hyperglycemia by inhibition of insulin secretion and glucose utilization.[27,28] A retrospective study of 918 patients undergoing craniotomy and spine-related neurosurgical procedures demonstrated that preoperative hyperglycemia (blood glucose > 120 mg/dL) was associated with increased risk of postoperative complications at all levels of care.[29] Similarly, diabetes and hyperglycemia in surgical patients (blood glucose > 200 mg/dL) on the day of procedure were independent predictors of morbidity after brain biopsy in a retrospective study.[30]

Diabetes has been shown to be an independent risk factor for postoperative infection. Meng et al. showed an OR of 2.04 in patients with diabetes versus those without.[31] In another study, individuals with diabetes with an A1c < 7% had a 0% chance of infection, whereas patients with an A1c > 7% had a 35.5% infection rate.[32] Despite the association of hyperglycemia with increased infection, a recent systematic review reached the conclusion that there remains insufficient evidence that strict glucose control is advantageous over conventional management for the prevention of surgical site infection.[33]

NICU Patient Meta-Analyses

In a meta-analysis, Kramer et al. examined 1,248 neurocritical care patients in 16 randomized clinical trials with TBI, ischemic or hemorrhagic stroke, anoxic encephalopathy, central nervous system infections, or spinal cord injury. A comparison of protocols

	AACE/ADA (2009)	ADA (2014)	ENDO (2012)	ACP (2011)	SCCM (2012)	SAMBA (2010)	STS (2009)
Glycemic targets							
Non-ICU							
• Premeal	<140	<140	<140	N/A	N/A	N/A	N/A
• Random	<180	<180	<180	N/A	N/A	N/A	N/A
ICU							
• Majority of patients	140-180	140-180	N/A	140-200	<150	N/A	<180
• Select patients	Lower targets may be appropriate, but <110 mg/dL not recommended	110-140	N/A		100-150 in stroke; <180	N/A	<150

FIGURE 8–1 Glycemic targets in inpatient settings per different studies.[1-12]

that used tight glycemic targets (70-140 mg/dL) versus protocols that kept the glucose levels below 144 to 300 mg/dL[34] revealed several conclusions. First, tight glucose control resulted in better neurological outcomes, but had no effect on mortality. Second, hypoglycemic episodes were far more common in the tightly controlled group. Third, although the "loose control" protocols were associated with worse neurological outcomes, these were observed only when glucose levels were above 200 mg/dL. Outcomes for the range between 140 and 180 mg/dL were not as bad as those in the tight glucose control group (Figure 8–1).

Similar results were obtained by Ooi et al. in another meta-analysis comparing tight glucose control versus conventional glucose control in critically ill neurological and neurosurgical patients.[35] Nine studies were included in the analysis, five of which were restricted to neurosurgical patients and four including neurological patients. The results showed that tight glucose control improved the neurological outcomes and reduced rates of infection. Again however, mortality was not affected by the tight glucose control and it did result in more hypoglycemic events. These results did not enable the authors to determine the optimal glucose targets, which means the question of appropriate glycemic targets remains to a certain degree open.[35] Nevertheless, the available evidence suggests that the glycemic goal between 140 and 180 mg/dL appears to be appropriate for critically ill neurosurgical patients.[34-36]

AVAILABLE GUIDELINES

Several major guidelines and consensus statements *now recommend a glucose goal of 140 to 180 mg/dL in the ICU setting.*[37] Studies of IIT in subtypes of neurologic injury are scarcer but so far have resulted in similar recommendations. In cases of acute ischemic stroke, the American Heart Association Stroke guidelines recommend that it is reasonable to target glucose levels between 140 and 180 mg/dL.[38] Meanwhile, for patients with acute TBI, currently there are no formal guidelines for glucose management.

REFERENCES

1. ADA, Standards of medical care in diabetes—2016. Diabetes Care, 2016. 39 (Supplement 1):S99–S104.
2. Clement S, Braithwaite SS, Magee MF, et al., Management of diabetes and hyperglycemia in hospitals. *Diabetes Care*, 2004;27(2):553–591.
3. Capes SE, Hunt D, Malmberg K, Pathak P, Gerstein HC. Stress hyperglycemia and prognosis of stroke in nondiabetic and diabetic patients: a systematic overview. *Stroke*. 2001;32(10):2426–2432.
4. Jeremitsky E, Omert LA, Dunham CM, Wilberger J, Rodriguez A. The impact of hyperglycemia on patients with severe brain injury. *J Trauma*. 2005;58(1):47–50.
5. McCowen KC, Malhotra A, Bistrian BR. Stress-induced hyperglycemia. *Crit Care Clin*. 2001;17(1):107–124.
6. Nylen E, Muller B. Endocrine changes in critical illness. *J Intensive Care Med*. 2004;19(2):67–82.
7. Atkins J, Smith D. A review of perioperative glucose control in the neurosurgical population. *J Diabetes Sci Technol*. 2009;3(6):1352–1364.
8. Van Den Berghe G, Wouters P, Weekers F, et al. Intensive insulin therapy in critically ill patients. *N Engl J Med*. 2001;345:1359–1367.
9. Brunkhorst FM, Engel C, Bloos F, et al. Intensive insulin therapy and pentastarch resuscitation in severe sepsis. *N Engl J Med*. 2008;358(2):125–139.
10. Preiser J.-C., Devos P, Ruiz-Santana S, et al. A prospective randomised multi-centre controlled trial on tight glucose control by intensive insulin therapy in adult intensive care units: the Glucontrol study. *Intensive Care Med*. 2009;35(10):1738–1748.
11. NICE-SUGAR Study Investigators; Finfer S, Chittock DR, Yu-Shuo Su S, et al. Intensive versus conventional glucose control in critically ill patients. *N Engl J Med*. 2009;360(13):1283–1297.
12. Pulsinelli WA, Levy DE, Sigsbee B, Scherer P, Plum F. Increased damage after ischemic stroke in patients with hyperglycemia with or without established diabetes mellitus. *Am J Med*.1983;74(4):540–554.
13. Parsons MW, Barber PA, Desmond PM, et al. Acute hyperglycemia adversely affects stroke outcome: a magnetic resonance imaging and spectroscopy study. *Ann Neurol*. 2002;52(1):20–28.
14. Bruno A, Kent TA, Coull BM, et al. Treatment of hyperglycemia in ischemic stroke (THIS): a randomized pilot trial. *Stroke*. 2008;39(2):384–389.
15. Rosso C, Corvol J.-C., Pires C, et al. Intensive versus subcutaneous insulin in patients with hyperacute stroke: results from the randomized INSULINFARCT trial. *Stroke*. 2012;43(9):2343–2349.
16. Intensive vs standard treatment of hyperglycemia and functional outcome in patients with acute ischemic stroke: the SHINE randomized clinical trial. Johnston KC, Bruno A, Pauls Q, et al.; Neurological Emergencies Treatment Trials Network and the SHINE Trial Investigators. *JAMA*. 2019;322(4):326.
17. Inagawa T, Yahara K, Ohbayashi N. Risk factors associated with cerebral vasospasm following aneurysmal subarachnoid hemorrhage. *Neurol Med Chir (Tokyo)*. 2014;54(6):465–473.

18. Badjatia N, Topcuoglu MA, Buonanno FS, et al. Relationship between hyperglycemia and symptomatic vasospasm after subarachnoid hemorrhage. *Crit Care Med.* 2005;33(7):1603.
19. Thiele RH, Pouratian N, Zuo Z, et al. Strict glucose control does not affect mortality after aneurysmal subarachnoid hemorrhage. *Anesthesiology.* 2009;110(3):603–610.
20. Shi J, Dong B, Mao Y, et al. Review: Traumatic brain injury and hyperglycemia, a potentially modifiable risk factor. *Oncotarget,* 2016;7(43):71052–71061.
21. Salim A, Hadjizacharia P, Dubose J, et al. Persistent hyperglycemia in severe traumatic brain injury: an independent predictor of outcome. *Am Surg.* 2009;75(1):25–29.
22. Coester A, Neumann C, Schmidt M. Intensive insulin therapy in severe traumatic brain injury: a randomized trial. *J Trauma.* 2010;68:904–911.
23. Bilotta F, Caramia R, Cernak I, et al. Intensive insulin therapy after severe traumatic brain injury: a randomized clinical trial. *Neruocrit Care.* 2008;9:159–166.
24. Yang M, Guo Q, Zhang X, et al. Intensive insulin therapy on infection rate, days in NICU, in-hospital mortality and neurological outcome in severe traumatic brain injury patients: a randomized controlled trial. *Int J Nurs Stud.* 2009;46:753–758.
25. Wang Y, Li J.-P., Song YL, Zhao QH. Intensive insulin therapy for preventing postoperative infection in patients with traumatic brain injury. *Medicine.* 2017;96:13(e6458).
26. Sudhakaran S, Surani SR. Guidelines for perioperative management of the diabetic patient. *Surg Res Pract.* 2015;2015:284063.
27. Tanaka T, Nabatame H, Tanifuji Y. Insulin secretion and glucose utilization are impaired under general anesthesia with sevoflurane as well as isoflurane in a concentration-independent manner. *J Anesth.* 2005;19(4):277–281.
28. Tanaka K, Tsutsumi YM. [Glucose metabolism: stress hyperglycemia and glucose control]. *Masui.* 2016;65(5):495–502.
29. Davis MC, Ziewacz JE, Sullivan SE, El-Sayed AM. Preoperative hyperglycemia and complication risk following neurosurgical intervention: a study of 918 consecutive cases. *Surg Neurol Int.* 2012;3:49.
30. McGirt MJ, Woodworth GF, Coon AL, et al. Independent predictors of morbidity after image-guided stereotactic brain biopsy: a risk assessment of 270 cases. *J Neurosurg.* 2005;102(5):897–901.
31. Meng F, Cao J, Meng X. Risk factors for surgical site infections following spinal surgery. *J Clin Neurosci.* 2015;22(12):1862–1866.
32. Hikata T, Iwanami A, Hosogane N, et al. High preoperative hemoglobin A1c is a risk factor for surgical site infection after posterior thoracic and lumbar spinal instrumentation surgery. *J Orthop Sci.* 2014;19(2):223–228.
33. Kao LS, Meeks D, Moyer VA, Lally KP. Peri-operative glycaemic control regimens for preventing surgical site infections in adults. *Cochrane Database Syst Rev.* 2009;(3):1–24.
34. Kramer AH, Roberts DJ, Zygun DA. Optimal glycemic control in neurocritical care patients: a systematic review and meta-analysis. *Crit Care.* 2012;16(5):R203.
35. Ooi YC, Dagi TF, Maltenfort M, et al. Tight glycemic control reduces infection and improves neurological outcome in critically ill neurosurgical and neurological patients. *Neurosurgery.* 2012;71(3):692–702; discussion 702.
36. Bilotta F, Rosa G. Optimal glycemic control in neurocritical care patients. *Crit Care.* 2012;16(5):163.
37. Mathioudakis N, Golden S. A comparison of inpatient glucose management guidelines: implications for patient safety and quality. *Curr Diab Rep.* 2015;15:13.
38. Powers WJ, Rabinstein AA, Ackerson T, et al. 2018 guidelines for the early management of patients with acute ischemic stroke. *Stroke.* 2018;49 (3):e46–e110.

CHAPTER

9

When Is Fever a "Central Fever"?

Sukwoo Hong, MB & Sara Hocker, MD

Case

A 54-year-old man with a history of smoking and hypertension is admitted to the intensive care unit (ICU) after an acute onset headache, followed rapidly by confusion and lethargy. Computed tomography (CT) head on presentation to the emergency department (ED) showed diffuse subarachnoid hemorrhage (SAH) and was found to have an anterior communicating artery aneurysm s/p coil. Post-bleed day 4, the patient started to develop a persistent fever. Infectious workup, including CT chest, abdomen, and pelvis and repeated cultures, has been unrevealing. Is this central fever (CF)?

Key Points

- Fever occurs in between a quarter and half of patients admitted to neurosciences intensive care unit (NICU). CF typically occurs earlier and is associated with a higher fever burden when compared with infectious fever in NICU.
- CF is a diagnosis of exclusion. Maximum temperature, leukocytosis, and the presence of systemic inflammatory response criteria do not differentiate between central and infectious fever. However, a left shift of white blood cells can be used to help differentiate discern central from infectious fever and eosinophilia, elevated transaminases, or rash may suggest underlying drug-related fever.
- In a patient with acute neurologic illness, however, fever can lead to secondary injury by increasing metabolic demand, worsening cerebral edema, and provoking seizures.
- Data on the use of biomarkers to differentiate CF is limited.
- Controlling fever is important given its detrimental effects on the brain. There is no evidence base on which to recommend one treatment strategy over another.

BACKGROUND

Fever, Hyperthermia, & Hyperpyrexia: What's the Difference?

Fever, hyperpyrexia, and hyperthermia all refer to an elevation in core body temperature (CBT). Fever is typically defined as a CBT of ≥38.3°C or 101°F. No strict cutoff criteria exist because normal body temperatures demonstrate variance between people and a diurnal pattern of temperature occurs such that a person's normal body temperature will differ depending on the time of day it is measured. Hyperpyrexia is a very high fever, again variably defined as a CBT ≥ 41°C (106°F).[1] Fever and hyperpyrexia are caused by elevation of the hypothalamic thermoregulatory set point and are adaptive responses to a pyrogen which may be endogenous (ie, cytokines), or exogenous (ie, bacterium). Hyperthermia is an elevation in CBT caused by either (a) heat production or (b) absorption that exceeds body's ability to dissipate heat. Hyperthermia is often caused by noninfectious etiology such as excessive heat exposure or muscle activity, as can be seen in neuroleptic malignant syndrome, malignant hyperthermia, and serotonin syndrome. This mechanism of elevated CBT is poorly responsive to antipyretics or antibiotics.[2] Figure 9–1 and Table 9–1 summarize the differences between fever, hyperthermia, and hyperpyrexia.

Pathogenesis of Central Fever

CF is simply any elevated CBT resulting from central nervous system pathology. CBT is usually controlled within ± 0.5 to 1°C around 37°C through homeostasis maintained by the central thermoregulatory network.[3] While the functional organization of this network has been fairly comprehensibly elucidated, the mechanism of neurogenic fever remains poorly understood.[1,4–9] When functioning normally, the preoptic area (POA) of the hypothalamus, spinothalamocortical pathways, and the lateral parabrachial nucleus in the pons interact with each other to control CBT.[10] The POA is important and sensitive to pyrogenic mediators such as prostaglandin E_2.[11] Humoral change (progesterone, prostaglandins) may also modify the firing rate of heat-sensitive neurons in the medial preoptic nucleus in the POA.[2] POA controls CBT setpoint. When pyrogens or other fever mediators inhibit preoptic heat-sensitive neurons, the setpoint gets elevated and vasoconstriction occurs. This causes shivering,

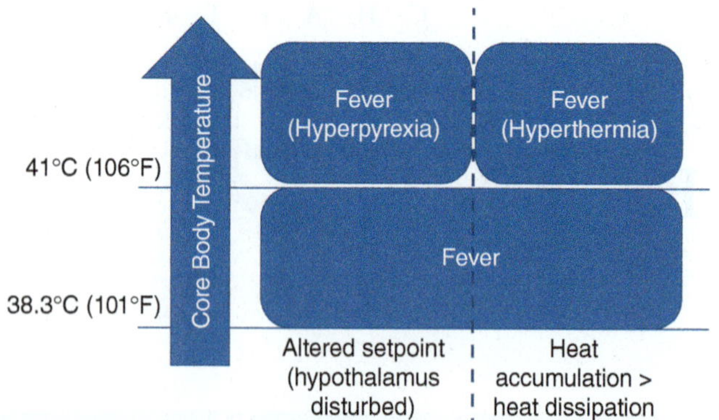

FIGURE 9–1 Core body temperature at or above 38.3 degrees Celsius is defined as fever. If core body temperature is at or above 41 degrees Celsius due to problems in the hypothalamus, it can be called hyperpyrexia; whereas if it is due to heat imbalance, where the heat accumulation is more than the heat dissipation, it can be called hyperthermia.

resulting in higher CBT through heat production. When pyrogens get decreased, the setpoint returns to normal and vasodilatation and sweating occur, dissipating heat and lowering CBT.[12,13]

Increase in the sympathetic tone and inflammation in the first 24 hours after brain injury,[14] and damage to thermoregulatory centers in the hypothalamus and pons cause elevated temperature. The mechanism through the hypothalamus is well known, whereas that of the pons is less well understood; however, if the pons is damaged, for example by strokes, this pathway may be affected resulting in hyperthermia without shivering.[15] Damage to thermoregulatory centers may also be caused by extravasated blood in the subarachnoid space or ventricle.[16] Some propose that CF is induced by the cold hypothalamus.[17] This pathway is associated with gamma-aminobutyric acid (GABA) neurons. When cold is sensed by the POA, signals are relayed to the dorsomedial hypothalamus, then the GABAergic neurons of the rostroventral medulla in the brainstem, followed by sympathetic outflow to the tissue.[10] Several hypothalamic signaling pathways have been identified that can increase sympathetic output to adipose tissue, including leptin receptors in the ventromedial hypothalamus and POA. Another hypothesized mechanism is that necrotic products of a brain tumor and/or blood may lead to irritation of leptomeninges triggering increased temperature.[18] These mechanisms may explain high CBT in SAH, intraventricular hemorrhage (IVH), and brain tumors.

EVIDENCE AND REVIEW

Temperature Elevations in the Neuroscience ICU

Fever occurs in between a quarter and half of patients admitted to NICU,[16,19–23] and between 52% and 67% are due to infection.[16,19,21] Variance can largely be attributed to differences in methodology (especially exclusion of patients admitted <48 hours), and patient populations between studies (diagnosis mix). A NICU admission <24 hours has been associated with a fever frequency of 15%.[22] All of the typical hospital-acquired infections in general critical care can occur

TABLE 9–1 Fever, Hyperpyrexia, and Hyperthermia.

	Fever, Hyperpyrexia	Hyperthermia
Possible mechanism	• Change in hypothalamic setpoint • Anterior hypothalamus stimulation results in vasodilation and increased BT[61] • Posterior hypothalamus stimulation results in vasoconstriction and decreased BT[12] • Due to pyrogens/immune system/coordination of autonomic/endocrine/ behavioral responses[62,63] • Well-known pathology	• No change in hypothalamic setpoint (thermoregulatory center remains intact) • Exogeneous heat exposure • Endogenous heat production[62] • BT elevates above the setpoint[64]
Clinical manifestation	• Shivering (due to vasoconstriction) → heat production • Sweating (due to vasodilatation) → heat dissipation	• No shivering
Examples	• Stroke, SAH, brain tumor, TBI • Infection • Venous thrombosis	• Heat stroke, malignant hyperthermia, thyrotoxicosis, adrenal crisis, PCC, SS, NMS, drug
Medications	• Antipyretics • Antibiotics • Difficult to manage if neurogenic causes[65]	• Poor response to antipyretics or antibiotics • **Treat underlying cause** • Baclofen • Bromocriptine • Dantrolene • Cyproheptadine (SS)

Abbreviations: BT, body temperature; NMS, neuroleptic malignant syndrome; PCC, pheochromocytoma; SAH, subarachnoid hemorrhage; SS, serotonin syndrome; TBI, traumatic brain injury.

in the neurocritical care population and must be sought out and treated before determining that a fever is central in origin. Some of the noninfectious, noncentral fevers can be attributed to venous thrombosis, drugs, or malignancy, although in up to a third of patients, a cause is never identified.[20] CF most commonly occurs in acute brain injury, especially intracerebral hemorrhage, IVH, and SAH, traumatic brain injury (TBI), brain tumors, and cardiac arrest.[21,24] Risk factors for CF include disease severity, subarachnoid or intraventricular blood, and depressed level of consciousness.[16,25] About 70% of patients with SAH or TBI develop fever in the first 72 hours.[20] In SAH, disease severity, volume of subarachnoid blood, and the presence of IVH, are strong risk factors for the development of fever.[16] In addition, the febrile response has been associated with and implicated in the development of delayed cerebral ischemia after SAH.[26–29] In TBI, patients with lower Glasgow coma scale (GCS) scores tend to have higher CBT than those with higher scores, with the majority peaking in the first day and normalizing over 3 weeks, although CF may persist for weeks to months in up to 37% of patients.[8,14] CF is more common in hemorrhagic than ischemic stroke.[30] Fever occurs in 23% to 38% of stroke patients, and between 33% and 39% are central in origin.[31] It is uncommon for CF to reach its peak after 96 hours of a stroke.[14] Therefore, when a fever spike occurs after 96 hours of stroke or during 1 to 3 weeks' convalescent period, evaluation for other causes should be pursued. In the brain tumor population, CF is more frequently associated with tumors located in the sella, diencephalon, and intraventricular regions.[21,32] The occurrence of fever in the first 72 hours after cardiac arrest is very common and is independently associated with poor outcome.[33,34] CF may also accompany paroxysmal sympathetic hyperactivity, a complication of severe acute brain injuries, which manifests as stereotyped episodes of tachycardia, tachypnea, hypertension, sweating, fever, and dystonic posturing.[35]

While fever can be seen during convulsive status epilepticus, its occurrence after the convulsive phase is more likely to be infectious in origin with pneumonia accounting for the majority of infections in this population.[36] Fever is more likely to be infectious in spinal cord injury (SCI) as well; common causes include pneumonia, urinary tract infection (UTI), and soft tissue infections (eg, decubitus ulcer).[22,25,37] CF has been reported to occur in 8% of patients with SCI in one study, and is more frequent in cervical or thoracic injuries,[38] and in complete SCI (89%) compared with incomplete (11%).[39]

CF typically occurs earlier and is associated with a higher fever burden when compared with infectious fever in a purely NICU.[19,21,30] Maximum temperature, leukocytosis, and the presence of systemic inflammatory response criteria do not differentiate between central and infectious fever.[21] However, a left shift of white blood cells has been shown to be rare in a population of mixed hemorrhagic and ischemic stroke patients and can be used to help differentiate discern central from infectious fever, at least in this population.[13] Data on the use of biomarkers to differentiate CF is limited. Procalcitonin appears to be a poor predictor of noninfectious fever in the neurocritical care unit. In one study of 73 patients with intracranial hemorrhage, procalcitonin did not differentiate infectious from noninfectious fever.[40] Procalcitonin has also been shown to be elevated in moderate to severe TBI without extracranial injuries and may be a marker of disease severity in that population.[41] Serum lactate has not been adequately studied with respect to this question. Caution should thus be exercised in extrapolating from the general critical care literature to other acute neurologic disease states. Table 9–2 classifies common diseases based on central versus noncentral cause and infectious versus noninfectious cause.

TABLE 9–2 Classification of fever based on central or non-central and infectious or noninfectious origins.[49] Causes discussed in this chapter are bolded.

	Central	Noncentral
Infectious	Encephalitis, meningitis, empyema, brain abscess, ventriculitis[66]	Pneumonia, UTI, bloodstream infection, Clostridium difficile diarrhea, sinusitis, SSI, CRBSI, CLABSI
Noninfectious	**Stroke (hemorrhagic, ischemic), SAH, DCI, brain tumor, TBI, DAI, SCI, paroxysmal sympathetic hyperactivity,** delirium	**VTE, drug fever,** drug withdrawal, allergy (transfusion, contrast), CTD, MI, pancreatitis, acalculous cholecystitis, ischemic bowel, GI bleed, (pseudo)gout, transplant rejection, hematoma, cirrhosis, decubitus ulcer, thrombophlebitis, **neoplastic fever,** pheochromocytoma, thyrotoxicosis, adrenal insufficiency

Abbreviations: CLABSI, central line-associated blood stream infection; CRBSI, catheter-related blood stream infection; CTD, connective tissue disease; DAI, diffuse axonal injury; DCI, delayed cerebral ischemia; GI, gastrointestinal; MI, myocardial infarction; SAH, subarachnoid hemorrhage; SCI, spinal cord injury; SSI, surgical site infection; TBI, traumatic brain injury; UTI, urinary tract infection; VTE, venous thromboembolism.

Secondary Neurologic Injury: Impact of Fever and Hyperthermia on Brain and Spinal Cord

Fever has been shown to be bactericidal in the setting of infection and thus is not universally treated in critical care settings. In a patient with acute neurologic illness, however, fever can lead to secondary injury by increasing metabolic demand, worsening cerebral edema, and provoking seizures,[42–47] and a meta-analysis of all brain injury types found that fever is related to morbidity and mortality.[48] As such, fever is detrimental to the acutely injured brain,[49–51] and should be treated in patients with these pathologies. In one study of acute stroke patients, maximum CBT ≥ 37.9°C during the first 7 days was an independent risk factor for a worse outcome.[52] And in a separate study of patients with acute stroke, an average temperature increase of 1°C resulted in increase of odds ratio of 2.2 (95% CI 1.4-3.5) of having a poor outcome.[53] In hemorrhagic stroke, CF has been shown to be a poor prognostic factor for outcome,[53] and duration of time with a CBT ≥ 37.5°C in the first 72 hours was linearly related to poor outcome.[51] Similar findings have been demonstrated in SAH[54,55] and TBI.[56] Although human data on the impact of fever on outcomes in SCI is lacking, some animal studies showed detrimental effects of fever.[57] CF is more associated with morbidity and mortality than non-CF which may imply that it can be viewed as a marker of severity of injury.[30,31]

Diagnostic Evaluation

Differentiating between infectious and noninfectious temperature elevation, and in the case of the latter, central and noncentral, will determine the clinical response. CF is a diagnosis of exclusion. Fever occurrence early after an acute brain injury, in addition to a negative evaluation for infection raises the possibility of CF. For patients admitted to neurologic ICU, meeting the following three criteria predicted CF with 90% probability: (1) fever onset within 72 hours of admission, (2) negative cultures and CXR, and (3) presence of SAH, IVH, or brain tumor.[21] For patients with strokes, CF was likely if all three of the following criteria are met: (1) BT > 39°C within 24 hours after stroke onset, (2) no infectious fever in the past week, and (3) negative evaluation (chest x-ray, blood, sputum, and urine cultures) for infectious origin.[13] Noncentral, noninfectious causes of fever must also be considered including deep venous thrombosis, pulmonary embolism, and drug fever. Drug fever may be differentiated by its late onset (1-2 weeks from initiation of the medication), relative bradycardia, and in some cases by the presence of eosinophilia, elevated transaminases, or rash. It is frequently a matter of trial and error to identify the culprit drug. The fever usually disappears within 3 days of stopping the offending drug.[49,58]

Management of Central Fever

There is no evidence base on which to recommend one treatment strategy over another. Controlling fever is important given its detrimental effects on the brain. Available methods include fans, sponging, surface cooling devices, and pharmacologic methods (acetaminophen, acetylsalicylic acid, and other nonsteroidal anti-inflammatory medications and corticosteroids).[59,60] Other drugs with reported efficacy include morphine, baclofen, bromocriptine, chlorpromazine, and growth hormone.[49] However, the evidence supporting the use of these drugs are limited to case reports and should be used cautiously.

AVAILABLE GUIDELINES

A good practice statement developed using GRADE methodology by the European Resuscitation Council and European Society of Intensive Care Medicine recommending the active prevention of fever (defined as a temperature > 37.7°C) for at least 72 hours in post-cardiac arrest patients who remain comatose.[23]

REFERENCES

1. Little RA. Heat production after injury. *Br Med Bull.* 1985;41(3):226–231.
2. Ge X, Luan X. Uncontrolled central hyperthermia by standard dose of bromocriptine: a case report. *World J Clin Cases.* 2020;8(23):6158–6163.
3. Huang YS, Hsiao MC, Lee M, Huang YC, Lee JD. Baclofen successfully abolished prolonged central hyperthermia in a patient with basilar artery occlusion. *Acta Neurol Taiwan.* 2009;18(2):118–122.
4. Przelomski MM, Roth RM, Gleckman RA, Marcus EM. Fever in the wake of a stroke. *Neurology.* 1986;36(3):427–429.
5. Powers JH, Scheld WM. Fever in neurologic diseases. *Infect Dis Clin North Am.* 1996;10(1):45–66.
6. Thompson HJ. Elevated body temperature in the neuroscience intensive care unit. *Crit Care Med.* 2005;33(7):1672.
7. Thompson HJ, Pinto-Martin J, Bullock MR. Neurogenic fever after traumatic brain injury: an epidemiological study. *J Neurol Neurosurg Psychiatry.* 2003;74(5):614–619.
8. Thompson HJ, Tkacs NC, Saatman KE, Raghupathi R, McIntosh TK. Hyperthermia following traumatic brain injury: a critical evaluation. *Neurobiol Dis.* 2003;12(3):163–173.
9. Lee HC, Kim JM, Lim JK, Jo YS, Kim SK. Central hyperthermia treated with baclofen for patient with pontine hemorrhage. *Ann Rehabil Med.* 2014;38(2): 269–272.
10. Morrison SF, Nakamura K. Central mechanisms for thermoregulation. *Annu Rev Physiol.* 2019;81:285–308.
11. Nakamura K, Kaneko T, Yamashita Y, et al. Immunocytochemical localization of prostaglandin EP3 receptor in the rat hypothalamus. *Neurosci Lett.* 1999;260(2):117–120.
12. Lenhardt R, Kurz A, Sessler DI. Thermoregulation and hyperthermia. *Acta Anaesthesiol Scand Suppl.* 1996;109:34–38.
13. Sung CY, Lee TH, Chu NS. Central hyperthermia in acute stroke. *Eur Neurol.* 2009;62(2):86–92.
14. Young AB, Ott LG, Beard D, Dempsey RJ, Tibbs PA, McClain CJ. The acute-phase response of the brain-injured patient. *J Neurosurg.* 1988;69(3):375–380.
15. Clapham JC. Central control of thermogenesis. *Neuropharmacology.* 2012;63(1):111–123.
16. Commichau C, Scarmeas N, Mayer SA. Risk factors for fever in the neurologic intensive care unit. *Neurology.* 2003;60(5):837–841.
17. Rango M, Arighi A, Arighi L, Bresolin N. Central hyperthermia, brain hyperthermia and low hypothalamus temperature. *Clin Auton Res.* 2012;22(6):299–301.
18. Soffer D. Brain tumors simulating purulent meningitis. *Eur Neurol.* 1976;14(3):192–197.
19. Rabinstein AA, Sandhu K. Non-infectious fever in the neurological intensive care unit: incidence, causes and predictors. *J Neurol Neurosurg Psychiatry.* 2007;78(11):1278–1280.
20. Albrecht RF, Wass CT, Lanier WL. Occurrence of potentially detrimental temperature alterations in hospitalized patients at risk for brain injury. *Mayo Clin Proc.* 1998;73(7):629–635.
21. Hocker SE, Tian L, Li G, Steckelberg JM, Mandrekar JN, Rabinstein AA. Indicators of central fever in the neurologic intensive care unit. *JAMA Neurol.* 2013;70(12):1499–1504.
22. Kilpatrick MM, Lowry DW, Firlik AD, Yonas H, Marion DW. Hyperthermia in the neurosurgical intensive care unit. *Neurosurgery.* 2000;47(4):850–5; discussion 855–856.
23. Stocchetti N, Rossi S, Zanier ER, Colombo A, Beretta L, Citerio G. Pyrexia in head-injured patients admitted to intensive care. *Intensive Care Med.* 2002;28:1555–1562.
24. Badjatia N. Hyperthermia and fever control in brain injury. *Crit Care Med.* 2009;37(7)(Suppl.).
25. Fishburn MJ, Marino RJ, Ditunno JF Jr. Atelectasis and pneumonia in acute spinal cord injury. *Arch Phys Med Rehabil.* 1990;71(3):197–200.
26. Weir B, Disney L, Grace M, Roberts P. Daily trends in white blood cell count and temperature after subarachnoid hemorrhage from aneurysm. *Neurosurgery.* 1989;25:161–165.
27. Simpson RK Jr, Fischer DK, Ehni BL. Neurogenic hyperthermia in subarachnoid hemorrhage. *South Med J.* 1989;82:1577–1578.
28. Oliveira-Filho J, Ezzeddine MA, Segal AZ, et al. Fever in subarachnoid hemorrhage: relationship to vasospasm and outcome. *Neurology.* 2001;56:1299–1304.
29. Dorhout Mees SM, Luitse MJA, van den Bergh WM, Rinkel GJE. Fever after aneurysmal subarachnoid hemorrhage: relation with extent of hydrocephalus and amount of extravasated blood. *Stroke.* 2008;39:2141–2143.

30. Georgilis K, Plomaritoglou A, Dafni U, Bassiakos Y, Vemmos K. Aetiology of fever in patients with acute stroke. *J Intern Med.* 1999;246(2):203–209.
31. Morales-Ortiz A, Jiménez-Pascual M, Pérez-Vicente JA, Monge-Arguiles A, Bautista-Prados J. [Fever of central origin during stroke]. *Rev Neurol.* 2001;32(12):1111–1114.
32. Clar HE. Clinical and morphological studies of pituitary and diencephalic space-occupying lesions before and after operation, with special reference to temperature regulation. *Acta Neurochir (Wien).* 1979;50:153–199.
33. Takasu A, Saitoh D, Kaneko N, Sakamoto T, Okada Y. Hyperthermia: is it an ominous sign after cardiac arrest? *Resuscitation.* 2001; 49:273–277.
34. Zeiner A, Holzer M, Sterz F, et al. Hyperthermia after cardiac arrest is associated with an unfavorable neurologic outcome. *Arch Intern Med.* 2001;161:2007–2012.
35. Scott RA, Rabinstein AA. Paroxysmal sympathetic hyperactivity. *Semin Neurol.* 2020;40(5):485–491.
36. Hawkes MA, Hocker SE. Systemic complications following status epilepticus. *Curr Neurol Neurosci Rep.* 2018;18(2):7.
37. Sugarman B, Brown D, Musher D. Fever and infection in spinal cord injury patients. *JAMA.* 1982;248(1):66–70.
38. Savage KE, Oleson CV, Schroeder GD, Sidhu GS, Vaccaro AR. Neurogenic fever after acute traumatic spinal cord injury: a qualitative systematic review. *Global Spine J.* 2016;6(6):607–614.
39. Colachis SC 3rd, Otis SM. Occurrence of fever associated with thermoregulatory dysfunction after acute traumatic spinal cord injury. *Am J Phys Med Rehabil.* 1995;74(2):114–119.
40. Halvorson K, Shah S, Fehnel C, et al. Procalcitonin is a poor predictor of non-infectious fever in the neurocritical care unit. *Neurocrit Care.* 2017;27(2):237–241.
41. Wang R, Hua Y, He M, Xu J. Prognostic value of serum procalcitonin based model in moderate to severe traumatic brain injury patients. *J Inflamm Res.* 2022;15:4981–4993.
42. Takagi K, Ginsberg MD, Globus MY, Martinez E, Busto R. Effect of hyperthermia on glutamate release in ischemic penumbra after middle cerebral artery occlusion in rats. *Am J Physiol.* 1994;267:H1770–H1776.
43. Chopp M, Welch KM, Tidwell CD, Knight R, Helpern JA. Effect of mild hyperthermia on recovery of metabolic function after global cerebral ischemia in cats. *Stroke.* 1988;19:1521–1525.
44. Chen Q, Chopp M, Bodzin G, Chen H. Temperature modulation of cerebral depolarization during focal cerebral ischemia in rats: correlation with ischemic injury. *J Cereb Blood Flow Metab.* 1993;13:389–394.
45. Morimoto T, Ginsberg MD, Dietrich WD, Zhao W. Hyperthermia enhances spectrin breakdown in transient focal cerebral ischemia. *Brain Res.* 1997;746:43–51.
46. Kim Y, Truettner J, Zhao W, Busto R, Ginsberg MD. The influence of delayed postischemic hyperthermia following transient focal ischemia: alterations of gene expression. *J Neurol Sci.* 1998;159:1–10.
47. Sharma HS, Hoopes PJ. Hyperthermia induced pathophysiology of the central nervous system. *Int J Hyperthermia.* 2003;19:325–354.
48. Greer DM, Funk SE, Reaven NL, Ouzounelli M, Uman GC. Impact of fever on outcome in patients with stroke and neurologic injury: a comprehensive meta-analysis. *Stroke.* 2008;39:3029–3035.
49. Goyal K, Garg N, Bithal P. Central fever: a challenging clinical entity in neurocritical care. *J Neurocrit Care.* 2020;13(1):19–31.
50. Ginsberg MD, Busto R. Combating hyperthermia in acute stroke: a significant clinical concern. *Stroke.* 1998;29(2):529–534.
51. Schwarz S, Häfner K, Aschoff A, Schwab S. Incidence and prognostic significance of fever following intracerebral hemorrhage. *Neurology.* 2000; 54(2):354–361.
52. Azzimondi G, Bassein L, Nonino F, et al. Fever in acute stroke worsens prognosis. A prospective study. *Stroke.* 1995;26(11):2040–2043.
53. Honig A, Michael S, Eliahou R, Leker RR. Central fever in patients with spontaneous intracerebral hemorrhage: predicting factors and impact on outcome. *BMC Neurol.* 2015;15:6.
54. Fernandez A, Schmidt JM, Claassen J, et al. Fever after subarachnoid hemorrhage: risk factors and impact on outcome. *Neurology.* 2007;68(13): 1013–1019.
55. Zhang G, Zhang JH, Qin X. Fever increased in-hospital mortality after subarachnoid hemorrhage. *Acta Neurochir Suppl.* 2011;110(pt 1):239–243.
56. Jiang JY, Gao G-Y, Li W-P, Yu MK, Zhu C. Early indicators of prognosis in 846 cases of severe traumatic brain injury. *J Neurotrauma.* 2002;19(7):869–874.
57. Yu CG, Jagid J, Ruenes G, Dietrich WD, Marcillo AE, Yezierski RP. Detrimental effects of systemic hyperthermia on locomotor function and histopathological outcome after traumatic spinal cord injury in the rat. *Neurosurgery.* 2001;49(1):152–158; discussion 158–159.
58. Johnson DH, Cunha BA. Drug fever. *Infect Dis Clin North Am.* 1996;10(1):85–91.
59. Henker R, Rogers S, Kramer DJ, Kelso L, Kerr M, Sereika S. Comparison of fever treatments in the critically ill: a pilot study. *Am J Crit Care.* 2001;10: 276–280.
60. Steele RW, Tanaka PT, Lara RP, Bass JW. Evaluation of sponging and of oral antipyretic therapy to reduce fever. *J Pediatr.* 1970;77:824–829.
61. Molitch ME. 230—neuroendocrinology and the neuroendocrine system. In *Goldman's Cecil Medicine*, 24th ed, Goldman L, Schafer AI, editors, W.B. Saunders: Philadelphia, 2012; 1425–1431.
62. Fauci A, Braunwald E, Kaspe D, et al. *Harrison's Principles of Internal Medicine*, 17th ed, McGraw-Hill Professional. New York, 2008, p. 2958.
63. Saper CB, Breder CD. The neurologic basis of fever. *N Engl J Med.* 1994;330(26):1880–1886.
64. Achaiah NC, Ak AK. Fever in the intensive care patient. In *StatPearls*. 2022, StatPearls Publishing Copyright © 2022, StatPearls Publishing LLC.: Treasure Island (FL).
65. Samudra N, Figueroa S. Intractable central hyperthermia in the setting of brainstem hemorrhage. *Ther Hypothermia Temp Manag.* 2016;6(2):98–101.
66. Alshahrani AM, Al-Said YA, Mamoun IA, Streletz LJ. Central fever due to hypothalamic lesion in a patient with tuberculous meningitis. *Neurosciences (Riyadh).* 2002;7(4):301–303.

CHAPTER

10

How Do We Distinguish Between and Treat Postoperative TACO and TRALI?

Hera A. Kamdar, MD &
Diana Greene-Chandos, MD, FNCS

Case

A 49-year-old woman with a past medical history of scoliosis presents for corrective surgery with multilevel posterior fusion. During the prolonged case a massive transfusion protocol is ordered given large volume blood loss. On arrival to the neurocritical care unit, the patient remains intubated on pressure support settings. On evaluation her heart rate is 111, respiratory rate is 29, and blood pressure is 145/89. Chest radiograph reveals diffuse bilateral pulmonary edema (Figure 10–1). What is the diagnosis and how will you treat the patient?

Key Points

- Transfusion-associated circulatory overload (TACO) and transfusion-related acute lung injury (TRALI) are amongst the leading causes of transfusion-related morbidity and mortality.
- Cardiovascular disease (eg, congestive heart failure or coronary artery disease) and chronic kidney disease are risk factors TACO, while substance abuse (eg, chronic alcohol use, tobacco use) and shock are risk factors for TRALI.
- TACO occurs in the setting of increased hydrostatic pressure leading to cardiogenic pulmonary edema, while TRALI occurs in the setting of increased pulmonary permeability leading to noncardiogenic pulmonary edema.
- The mainstay in management of any transfusion-related injury is to first immediately stop the transfusion. Subsequently supportive care is the hallmark of management.
- Preventive strategies are targeted to lower the incidence of TACO and TRALI.

BACKGROUND

Transfusion-associated circulatory overload (TACO) and transfusion-related acute lung injury (TRALI) are amongst the leading causes of transfusion-related morbidity and mortality. The incidence of TACO has been estimated to vary from 1% to 11%, with a higher incidence in the intensive care population; while TRALI has been reported to occur in up to a rate of 0.08% to 15.1% per patient post tranfusion.[1]

Saliently, having surgery is often associated with both TACO and TRALI, with some studies reporting up to 50% of cases being in the perioperative state.[2] Additionally, patients with hematological malignancies have been found to be at increased risk of both as well.[1] Risk factors particularly associated with development of TACO include cardiovascular disease (eg, congestive heart failure or coronary artery disease), and chronic kidney disease, while TRALI has been associated with substance abuse (eg, chronic alcohol use, tobacco use), and shock.[2]

EVIDENCE AND REVIEW

Pathophysiology

Ongoing research into the dynamic pathophysiology of TACO and TRALI is paramount in developing targeted treatments, which have yet to be established. A largely accepted two-hit model is used to explain the pathology of TACO and TRALI with the first hit being related to the patients underlying clinical condition with potentially poor baseline adaptability, following the second hit offered by the transfusion product.[1] TACO occurs in the setting of increased hydrostatic pressure leading to cardiogenic pulmonary edema with the first hit being caused by cardiac or renal dysfunction with poor adaptability to fluid overload and a second hit by the inability to manage the volume status once

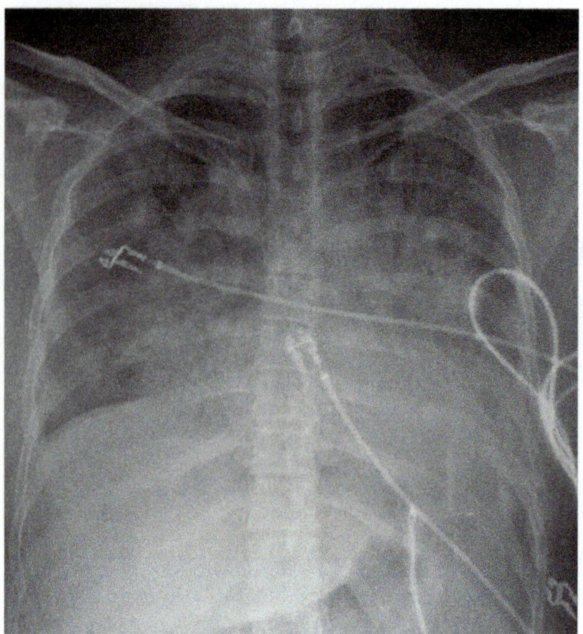

FIGURE 10–1 Plain chest radiograph demonstrating moderate, diffuse bilateral pulmonary vascular congestion and interstitial edema with infiltrates predominantly in the middle and lower lung zones consistent with pulmonary edema. In the setting of a postoperative state with large volume perioperative transfusions, this is clinically suggestive of transfusion-associated circulatory overload (TACO).

given the transfusion products.[1,3] Further, significant mediation by IL-10 has been reported to occur in TACO.[1] TRALI occurs in the setting of increased pulmonary permeability leading to noncardiogenic pulmonary edema with the first hit being caused by an inflammatory response with a second hit by certain leukocyte antibodies (eg, anti-HNA and anti-HLA antibodies).[1,3]

Clinical Presentation

Both TACO and TRALI are syndromes characterized by new onset acute respiratory distress with marked pulmonary edema that occurs within 6 hours of a blood transfusion.[1-5] TACO presents with features of circulatory overload with a positive fluid total body balance including dyspnea, tachypnea, tachycardia, jugular venous distention, increased systolic blood pressure, increased central venous pressure, and possible evidence of left heart failure with elevated B-type natriuretic peptide (BNP).[1,2,4] In contrast, TRALI is demarcated as "noncardiogenic" and presents with features of an acute inflammatory interleukin-mediated response with fever, hypotension, and tachycardia.[1,2,4] It is important to note that in the postoperative state, symptoms such as tachycardia, tachypnea, and blood pressure status may be obscured or veiled, particularly if the patient does remain intubated after surgery.

Diagnosis

TACO and TRALI are primarily clinical diagnoses, but there are multiple investigations that should be done to rule out cardiogenic and other noncardiogenic causes of acute onset respiratory distress such as pneumonia, sepsis, trauma, or acute pancreatitis. For new onset hypoxemia, a chest radiograph should be obtained. Additional testing completed, with priority based on clinical suspicion of etiology, includes complete blood count, cultures (particularly respiratory), electrocardiogram (EKG), troponin, BNP, echocardiogram, and potentially cardiac catheterization if cardiac ischemia is suspected. Severe hemolytic transfusion reactions may also present similarly to TRALI and a hematologic workup with direct antiglobulin test (DAT), haptoglobin, Lactate Dehydrogenase (LDH), urinalysis, and indirect bilirubin analyses may also be done to differentiate the two.[3] Additional testing of donor and recipient blood can be done to detect the presence of leukocyte antibodies such as anti-HLA antibodies and anti-HNA antibodies.[1,3] Finally, a unique feature to TRALI is the presence of leukopenia within the early stage of presentation; thus, it is imperative that a complete blood count is done early when it is suspected. Clinically, a diuretic challenge can also be used to differentiate the two syndromes, with benefit in clinical status to diuresis seen in TACO patients (Table 10–1).

Management

The mainstay in management of any transfusion-related injury is to first immediately stop the transfusion. Subsequently supportive care is the hallmark of management. Unfortunately, at this time there is no targeted or specific therapy used in either TACO or TRALI. For TRALI, treatments such as high-dose steroids and plasmapheresis have been attempted in the past; however, there is lack of efficacy through continued research at this time, thus these are not considered part of standard of care.[5]

When there is concern for TACO, support measures include diuresis and supplemental oxygenation which at times may require intubation.[1,4] For TRALI similarly supportive supplemental oxygenation and intubation is used; however, judicious fluid resuscitation and avoidance of diuresis is recommended.[1,4]

Future Therapies

As mentioned, current research is largely focused on the pathophysiology of both TACO and TRALI to better elucidate potential therapeutic options. Recent studies have explored multiple therapeutic approaches to TRALI, some of which include IL-10 cytokine therapy, potential downregulation of the C-Reactive Protein (CRP) pathways, inhibition of IL-8 receptors, intravenous immunoglobulin therapy, complement targeting, and have even explored the role of antiplatelet agents.[1] Further study is needed to validate these hypotheses.

Prevention

Preventive strategies are targeted to lower the incidence of TACO and TRALI. To prevent TACO, patients suspected to receive transfusions are screened for cardiac insufficiency (eg, prior to a surgery). Additionally, there is evidence that reducing the volume and rate of transfusions may also prevent TACO.[4] TRALI mitigation strategies have dramatically reduced the incidence of TRALI over the years as reported by the Food and Drug Administration;

TABLE 10–1 Distinguishing features between TACO and TRALI.[1,3]

TACO		TRALI
Increased pulmonary hydrostatic pressure	Acute onset respiratory distress within 6 hours of blood transfusion	Increased pulmonary permeability
(Pulmonary artery occlusion pressure > 18 mm Hg)	Hypoxemia (SpO_2 < 90% or PaO_2/FiO_2 < 300 mm Hg on room air)	(Pulmonary artery occlusion pressure < 18 mm Hg)
Less frequent fever	Pulmonary edema with bilateral infiltrates on chest radiograph	Fever
Hypertension	Tachypnea, dyspnea, tachycardia	Hypotension
WBC—nonspecific		WBC—transient leukopenia and thrombocytopenia
Hypervolemic		Euvolemic
Increased central venous pressure, jugular venous distension		Protein-rich edema fluid
Protein poor edema fluid		(Transudative)
(Exudative)		Normal BNP
Elevated BNP (>250 pg/mL or NT-proBNP >1,000 pg/mL)		Not responsive to diuresis
**note: BNP levels are not reliable in ICU population (ie, can be higher)*		Echocardiogram—normal to slightly decreased systolic ejection fraction
Responsive to diuresis		
Echocardiogram—decreased systolic ejection fraction < 45, no severe valvular heart; vascular pedicle width > 65 mm		

however, limitations of these mitigation strategies include shortage of appropriately screened blood products, as well as no significant 30-day mortality in those that do develop TRALI after receiving low-risk donor products.[1,4] Preventive strategies include donor HLA antibody screening (with deferral based on anti-HNA and anti-HLA antibodies), donor deferral based on pregnancy, female sex, or history of transfusion.[1,4]

AVAILABLE GUIDELINES

Unfortunately, at this time, no targeted or specific therapy or guidelines used for the diagnosis or management of either TACO or TRALI.

REFERENCES

1. Semple JW, Rebetz J, Kapur R. Transfusion-associated circulatory overload and transfusion-related acute lung injury. *Blood.* 2019;133(17):1840–1853.
2. Roubinian N. TACO and TRALI: biology, risk factors, and prevention strategies. *Hematology Am Soc Hematol Educ Program.* 2018;2018(1):585–594.
3. Kuldanek SA, Kelher M, Silliman CC. Risk factors, management and prevention of transfusion-related acute lung injury: a comprehensive update. *Expert Rev Hematol.* 2019;12(9):773–785.
4. Murphy CE, Kenny CM, Brown KF. TACO and TRALI: visualizing transfusion lung injury on plain film. *BMJ Case Rep.* 2020;13(4):e230426.
5. Nouraei SM, Wallis JP, Bolton D, Hasan A. Management of transfusion-related acute lung injury with extracorporeal cardiopulmonary support in a four-year-old child. *Br J Anaesth.* 2003;91(2):292–294.

CHAPTER

11

How Should We Manage Perioperative Vision Loss?

Yasmin Aghajan, MD & Saef Izzy, MD, MBChB

Case

A 60-year-old man presented with nasal congestion and epistaxis and was found to have a sinonasal mass with extension to the cribriform plate. He underwent endoscopic endonasal resection of an olfactory neuroblastoma. The surgery involved sinonasal and anterior skull base resection of the mass without complications. Several hours postoperatively, he developed acute onset painless bilateral vision loss. The remainder of the neurologic exam was normal. Computed tomography (CT) head showed bifrontal pneumocephalus (Figure 11–1). Dilated fundus exam was normal. Magnetic resonance imaging (MRI) of brain and orbits showed normal optic nerves and chiasm and no cerebral infarcts; magnetic resonance angiography (MRA) was unremarkable.

Key Points

- Postoperative vision loss (POVL), specifically ischemic optic neuropathy (ION), is associated with spine and cardiothoracic surgery, prone positioning, prolonged surgery, and high intraoperative blood loss.
- Differential diagnosis includes corneal injury, glaucoma, central or branch retinal artery occlusion (CRAO/BRAO), anterior or posterior ION (AION/PION), and cortical blindness. Urgent ophthalmologic evaluation and neuroimaging is essential. PION is a diagnosis of exclusion.
- Treatments of ION are without robust evidence, and include correcting hypotension and anemia, giving colloid and crystalloid, and consideration of steroids or acetazolamide.

BACKGROUND

Postoperative vision loss (POVL) is a rare but potentially devastating condition more commonly seen after spine or cardiothoracic surgery. Patients who undergo prolonged spine procedures and who have substantial blood loss are at risk for POVL.[1] Causes of POVL include ischemic optic neuropathy (ION), retinal artery occlusion, cortical blindness, acute glaucoma, or external ocular injury (Table 11–1). Urgent ophthalmologic consultation and neuroimaging should be obtained to determine the cause. Pathophysiology and treatment vary depending on etiology. Given its rarity, available evidence on treatment is based on case reports and case series in the literature. This review focuses primarily on pathophysiology, presentation, diagnosis, and management of ION.

EVIDENCE AND REVIEW

Pathophysiology

POVL is a rare temporary or permanent loss of vision associated with surgery and general anesthesia due to ION, branch or central retinal artery occlusion (BRAO, CRAO), cortical blindness, or primary ocular pathology. ION is divided into anterior ION (AION) and posterior ION (PION) based on the area of involvement of the optic nerve.

High-risk patients for ION are those undergoing spinal procedures, prone positioning, prolonged procedures, and/or experience substantial blood loss. Other risk factors include vascular risk factors such as hypertension, carotid artery disease, smoking, obesity, and diabetes.[1,2] POVL from ION is reported to occur in <0.2% of spine surgeries.[1]

The mechanism of blindness is not fully elucidated but is thought to be related to ischemic injury from decreased oxygen delivery to the optic nerve. A combination of the above risk factors, perhaps with abnormal vasoautoregulation and prothrombotic tendencies may cause optic nerve injury.

Prone positioning, including direct pressure to the eyes from the use of an intraoperative sheet roll or headrest may result in increased risk of ION or CRAO in spine surgery patients.[1,2] Intraocular pressure (IOP) is increased in the prone position which may reduce ocular perfusion pressure with decreased retinal and choroidal blood flow. However, ION has been reported

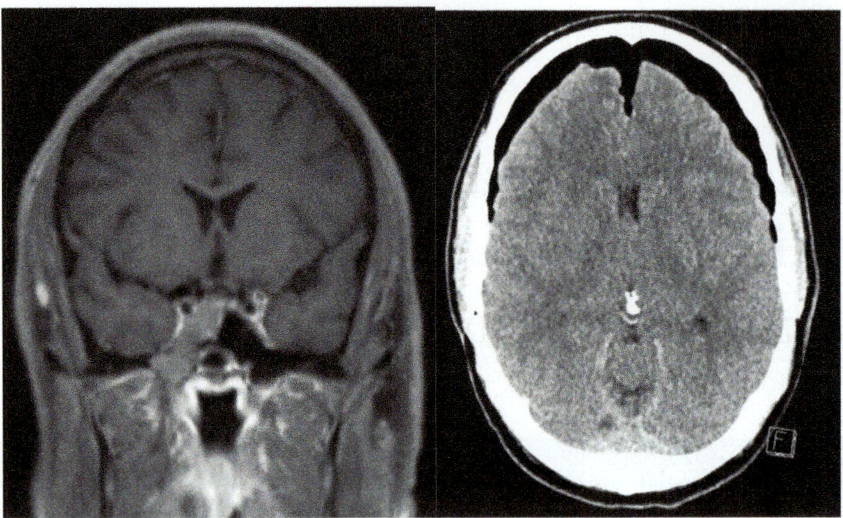

FIGURE 11–1 Postoperative noncontrast CT scan showing moderate pneumocephalus and no other acute findings.

in cases where the patient was supine and without external ocular pressure [2] as in the case presented above. Retinal venous hypertension from impaired venous drainage in jugular venous compression may be another possible etiology.[2,3] It is uncertain whether intraoperative hypotension may play a role, as it is not always present in patients who develop ION. Intraoperative blood loss, specifically large volume hemorrhage may be associated with higher risk.[1,2]

Clinical Presentation

ION presents with painless, usually bilateral severe vision loss and typically occurs within the first 24 to 48 hours postoperatively, though this can be observed upon emergence from anesthesia. Patients may have profound vision loss to the point of blindness. There may be afferent pupillary defect or decreased pupil reactivity. The clinical presentation may be distinguished from other causes of POVL, as summarized in Table 11–1.

Diagnosis

The differential diagnosis of POVL is summarized in Table 11–1. A physical examination should be done to evaluate for other neurologic deficits (in the setting of possible ischemic strokes) and assessment of visual acuity, eye movements, and visual fields. An urgent ophthalmologic evaluation is warranted to evaluate IOP and fundoscopic exam to diagnose BRAO, CRAO, AION, and other retinal pathologies. CT imaging with CT angiography of

TABLE 11–1 Differential diagnosis of POVL.

Etiology of POVL	Proposed Pathophysiology	Clinical Presentation
External ocular injury (corneal injury, abrasion)	Corneal irritation through decreased tear production, dryness, local injury	Blurry vision, tearing, redness, foreign body sensation
Ischemic optic neuropathy (AION/PION)	Ischemic injury to the optic nerve from arterial hypoperfusion, increased venous pressure, abnormal autoregulation **AION**: anterior optic nerve ischemia, prognosis is better than PION **PION**: posterior optic nerve ischemia	Painless visual loss, often bilateral, can progress to complete blindness. Most commonly associated with spine surgeries, prone position, cardiothoracic surgeries, long surgery, and massive blood loss. AION: fundus exam abnormal with optic disc edema and hemorrhages PION: fundus exam and MRI orbits may be normal
Central or branch retinal artery occlusion (CRAO/BRAO)	Emboli or direct pressure on the globe	Usually, unilateral painless vision loss if embolic. In BRAO, likely to have a superior or inferior field defect Fundus exam: ischemic retinal whitening, cherry-red spot, retinal emboli[4]
Cortical blindness	Ischemic stroke or hypoperfusion of occipital lobes	Hemianopia or complete bilateral blindness. Patients may be unaware of deficit (Anton syndrome)[4]
Acute glaucoma	Increased IOP due to abnormal aqueous humor flow. Optic nerve damage ensues from high IOP.	Painful vision loss, conjunctival erythema, poorly reactive pupil.

the head and neck should be considered to rule out hemorrhage, stroke, and evaluate carotid and ophthalmic artery patency especially if vision loss is unilateral.

In AION, a fundoscopic exam shows optic disc edema and hemorrhages. In contrast, the optic discs and fundus exam is normal in PION. There may be optic nerve enlargement or perineural enhancement suggestive of edema on MRI of the orbits. Many times, however, the immediate MRI is normal as optic atrophy develops over subsequent weeks to months. Thus, the diagnosis of PION is one of clinical *suspicion*, and ruling out other causes is critical. An initial diagnostic pathway is summarized in Figure 11–2.

Management

There is no proven treatment for perioperative ION,[1,2] though a list of suggested treatments is provided in Table 11–2 with limited evidence supporting their efficacy. Increasing blood pressure and hemoglobin to improve retinal perfusion are suggested, though data is limited to case reports. Acetazolamide may lower IOP and improve flow to the optic nerve head and retina. Steroids have not proven benefit though are considered on a case-by-case basis. If increased venous pressure is suspected, the head of bed should be kept elevated. On the contrary, if hypoperfusion is more likely, keeping the head of the bed flat may improve perfusion pressure.

TABLE 11–2 Suggested treatments for ION.

Suggested treatments for ION
Mean arterial pressure (MAP) augmentation with intravenous fluids and correction of hypotension
Colloid infusion (albumin)
Steroids (intravenous methylprednisolone or dexamethasone)
Acetazolamide
Correction of anemia
Head of bed elevated if suspect venous congestion; otherwise consider head of bed flat in case of arterial hypoperfusion

AVAILABLE GUIDELINES

Summary consensus recommendations from the American Society of Anesthesiologists Task Force[1] on reducing risk of POVL include the following:

- Patients undergoing prolonged spine procedures while prone and who have substantial blood loss are at higher risk for POVL. Inform high-risk patients of the possibility, and consider staged procedures if possible.
- Position the head higher than the heart intraoperatively and maintain neutral neck position when possible.

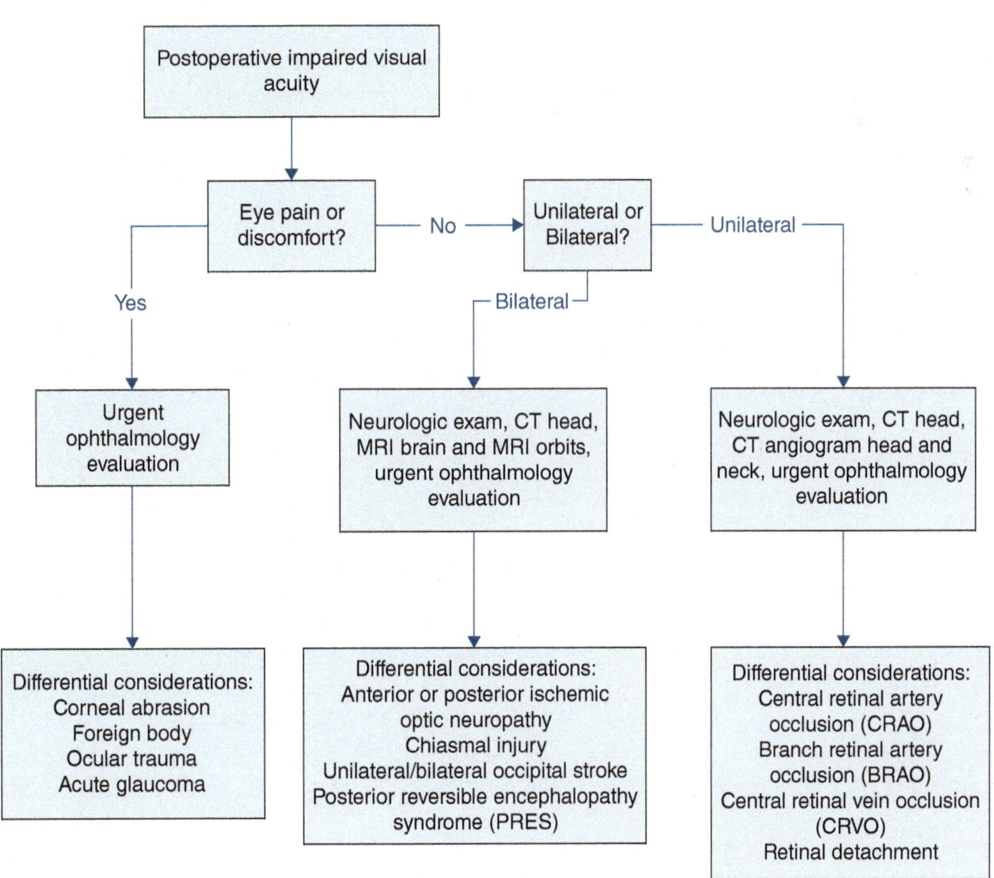

FIGURE 11–2 Initial diagnostic evaluation for POVL.

- Colloids should be used along with crystalloids to maintain intravascular volume in the setting of blood loss.
- There is no specific hematocrit or blood pressure threshold shown to reduce the risk of POVL.

REFERENCES

1. American Society of Anesthesiologists Task Force on Perioperative Blindness. Practice advisory for perioperative visual loss associated with spine surgery: a report by the American Society of Anesthesiologists Task Force on Perioperative Blindness. *Anesthesiology*. 2006;104(6):1319–1328. doi:10.1097/00000542-200606000-00027
2. Roth S. Perioperative visual loss: what do we know, what can we do? *Br J Anaesth*. 2009;103 Suppl 1(Suppl 1):i31–i40. doi:10.1093/bja/aep295
3. Mendel E, Stoicea N, Rao R, et al. Revisiting postoperative vision loss following non-ocular surgery: a short review of etiology and legal considerations. *Front Surg*. 2017;4:34. Published 2017 Jun 26. doi:10.3389/fsurg.2017.00034
4. Grover V, Jangra K. Perioperative vision loss: acomplication to watch out. *J Anaesthesiol Clin Pharmacol*. 2012;28(1):11–16. doi:10.4103/0970-9185.92427

CHAPTER

12

How Should Therapeutic Anticoagulation Be initiated in Neurologically Injured Patients?

Sherri A. Braksick, MD & Alejandro A. Rabinstein, MD

Case

A 65-year-old man with atrial fibrillation on apixaban presents after a motor vehicle accident with a small right frontal hemorrhagic contusion. He remains neurologically nonfocal and the surgical team asks the intensivist team for their opinion on the appropriate time to restart his apixaban.

Key Points

- Decisions to start therapeutic anticoagulation in patients with acute brain injury are often determined by the preference of the treatment physician given the limited availability of prospective data or society-endorsed guidelines.
- The indication for anticoagulation, estimated risk of thrombosis, and estimated risk of hemorrhage for each individual patient must be carefully considered before making the decision to provide or withhold anticoagulation.
- Patients with atrial fibrillation who develop an ischemic stroke should initiate anticoagulation between 4 and 14 days after the stroke, unless other contraindications.
- Atrial appendage closure may be considered in patients with atrial fibrillation where the risk ongoing anticoagulation is considered high.

BACKGROUND

Anticoagulation of any hospitalized patient requires a critical assessment of the risk of providing versus the risk of withholding anticoagulation. In patients with acute or subacute neurologic injury, this decision can be complex given the balance of development of new or increased intracranial hemorrhage with anticoagulation and the risk of thromboembolism when withholding therapeutic anticoagulation despite a clear indication for its administration.

EVIDENCE AND REVIEW

Therapeutic Anticoagulation in Acute Ischemic Stroke

In patients with atrial fibrillation leading to ischemic stroke, therapeutic anticoagulation is recommended 4 to 14 days after the stroke, which is titrated by the burden of ischemic stroke.[1] In a large prospective study,[2] improvement in multiple outcome measures (transient ischemic attack [TIA], stroke, intracerebral hemorrhage [ICH], extracranial bleeding) when assessed at 90 days. It is also important to note, however, that patients with higher Congestive heart failure, Hypertension, Age, Diabetes mellitus, prior Stroke or transient ischemic attack or thromboembolism, Vascular disease, Age, Sex Category score (CHADS$_2$VASC) and National Institutes of Health Stroke Scale (NIHSS) scores fared worse overall. Patients who received oral anticoagulants did better than those who received low molecular weight heparin (LMWH) followed by an oral agent or had LMWH alone. An additional prospective study[3] found that initiation of rivaroxaban within 14 days of ischemic stroke or TIA was safe, though patients in this study had mild deficits and small volumes of infarction, preventing extrapolation of the findings to patients with larger and more severe strokes.

A recent analysis of a prospective registry from Japan divided the cerebrovascular events into TIAs and strokes of three different degrees of severity and found that initiation of oral anticoagulation with a direct oral anticoagulant (DOAC) for atrial fibrillation after TIA or stroke was safe when started early (defined as 1 day prior to the actual median anticoagulation start day in each of the subgroups).[4] The findings were validated using an European registry in the same study. This proposed approach has been termed the 1-2-3-4-day rule and it is outlined in Table 12–1.[4]

TABLE 12–1 Initiating oral anticoagulation for atrial fibrillation after TIA or ischemic stroke.[4]

Severity of Ischemia	Presenting NIHSS	Timing of Anticoagulation
TIA	NA	1 day after event
Mild ischemic stroke	<8	2 days after event
Moderate ischemic stroke	8-15	3 days after event
Severe ischemic stroke	>15	4 days after event

NIHSS: National Institutes of Health Stroke Scale, TIA: transient ischemic attack.

However, it is crucial to note that the study excluded patients with high-risk factors for delayed hemorrhage (ie, large infarct volume, spontaneous hemorrhagic conversion, uncontrolled hypertension) from application of the rule. The safety of this early anticoagulation rule still needs to be confirmed in a prospective interventional study.

Therapeutic Anticoagulation after Intracranial Hemorrhage

In patients who suffer an intracranial hemorrhage with a clear indication for therapeutic anticoagulation, the decision on the timing of resumption can be complex.

In patients perceived to be at high risk of thrombosis, we often start anticoagulation with a low-intensity heparin nomogram while monitoring serial imaging and advancing the degree of anticoagulation once the patient has demonstrated clinical and radiographic stability. For other patients with lower-risk indications for anticoagulation, such as atrial fibrillation without ischemic stroke, the recommendation favors resumption of anticoagulants 7 to 8 weeks after the hemorrhage,[5] acknowledging the need to assess the individual risk/benefit balance upon considering the reintroduction of anticoagulants.

In hemorrhages that are ultimately found to be or are presumed to be due to cerebral amyloid angiopathy (CAA), the recurrence risk of intracerebral hemorrhage is much higher as compared to hemorrhages attributed to other causes.[6] Consequently, initiation of therapeutic anticoagulation in these patients may be associated with an unacceptably high risk. When a clear risk of thrombosis exists, such as a mechanical valve, a thorough discussion of the risk of providing versus withholding anticoagulation is necessary with input from the patient, their family, the neurocritical care team, and other medical providers with a vested interest in the decision, such as the cardiology or cardiac surgery services.

For patients who have suffered a subdural hematoma (SDH) and have an ongoing need for anticoagulation, the underlying cause of the SDH (spontaneous or traumatic) as well as the perceived risk of recurrence must be evaluated. Middle meningeal artery (MMA) embolization has recently become an option to reduce the risk of recurrent hemorrhage in patients presenting with chronic SDH, and can be considered in patients who need ongoing anticoagulation. A recent meta-analysis[7] found that MMA embolization was associated with substantial benefit in terms of reduction in recurrence rate, need for operative rescue, and in-hospital complications when compared to conventional management of SDH.

Therapeutic Anticoagulation after Traumatic Brain Injury

The decision to anticoagulate patients after traumatic brain injury (TBI) demands a similar evaluation to that described above for cerebrovascular events; treatment decisions should be guided by consideration to the specific intracranial pathology already present, the estimated risk of subsequent hemorrhagic complications, and the perceived risk of imminent thrombosis formation. Prospective data and guideline-based recommendations in this patient population are lacking.

Therapeutic Anticoagulation after Neurosurgical Procedures

Similar to TBI patients, randomized prospective data and guideline recommendations regarding therapeutic anticoagulation after a neurosurgical procedure are lacking. The decision to anticoagulate these patients depends on the indication for anticoagulation and risk of thrombosis, weighed against perceived risk of perioperative hemorrhage. Hemorrhage risk is estimated by the performing surgeon based on the specific procedure performed, intraoperative events, and other patient-specific patterns. Consequently, decisions to start anticoagulation in this population should always include the neurosurgical team.

AVAILABLE GUIDELINES

The American Stroke Association (ASA) guidelines in 2022[7] state that reinitiation of anticoagulation is reasonable in patients with a high risk of thromboembolism, such as those with mechanical heart valves or ventricular assist devices. In this cohort, the timing of anticoagulation depends on multiple factors, including the size and cause of the hemorrhage, perceived risk of thromboembolism, and evidence of hemorrhage stability on serial imaging. For patients with atrial fibrillation where the risk of ongoing anticoagulation is considered high risk, such as amyloid angiopathy, the ASA recommended consideration of atrial appendage closure as opposed to resumption of anticoagulation. The most recent published guideline for the management of ischemic stroke recommends initiation of anticoagulation in patients with atrial fibrillation between 4 and 14 days after the stroke.[7]

REFERENCES

1. Powers WJ, Rabinstein AA, Ackerson T, et al. Guidelines for the early management of patients with acute ischemic stroke: 2019 update to the 2018 Guidelines for the early management of acute ischemic stroke: a guideline for healthcare professionals from the American Heart Association/American Stroke Association. *Stroke.* 2019;50(12):e344–e418.
2. Paciaroni M, Agnelli G, Falocci N, et al. Early recurrence and cerebral bleeding in patients with acute ischemic stroke and atrial fibrillation: effect of anticoagulation and its timing: the RAF study. *Stroke.* 2015;46(8):2175–2182.

3. Gioia LC, Kate M, Sivakumar L, et al. Early rivaroxaban use after cardioembolic stroke may not result in hemorrhagic transformation: a prospective magnetic resonance imaging study. *Stroke*. 2016;47(7):1917–1919.
4. Kimura S, Toyoda K, Yoshimura S, et al. Practical "1-2-3-4-day" rule for starting direct oral anticoagulants after ischemic stroke with atrial fibrillation: combined hospital-based cohort study. *Stroke*. 2022;53(5):1540–1549.
5. Charidimou A, Boulouis G, Xiong L, et al. Cortical superficial siderosis and first-ever cerebral hemorrhage in cerebral amyloid angiopathy. *Neurology*. 2017;88(17):1607–1614.
6. Ironside N, Nguyen C, Do Q, et al. Middle meningeal artery embolization for chronic subdural hematoma: a systematic review and meta-analysis. *J Neurointerv Surg*. 2021; 13(10):951–957.
7. Greenberg SM, Ziai WC, Cordonnier C, et al. 2022 guideline for the management of patients with spontaneous intracerebral hemorrhage: a guideline from the American Heart Association/American Stroke Association. *Stroke*. 2022;53(7):e282–e361.

CHAPTER

13

When and How Should We Initiate Venous Thromboembolism Chemoprophylaxis in Neurosurgical Patients?

Joseph D. Burns, MD, Aya Shnawa, MD, T. Jayde Nail, MD, & David P. Lerner, MD

Case

A 63-year-old woman is admitted to the neuroICU following a craniotomy and resection of a recurrent glioblastoma. Her perioperative course has been complicated by new-onset contralateral hemiparesis related to infarct near the resection cavity. What is the appropriate plan for venous thromboembolism chemoprophylaxis in such a patient?

Key Points

- Decisions about the use of venous thromboembolism (VTE) chemoprophylaxis in patients undergoing nontrauma craniotomies and patients with traumatic brain injury (TBI) are controversial because they are high stakes, occur in a population with significant heterogeneity for risk of both VTE and intracranial hemorrhage (ICH), and are guided by suboptimal data. Nonetheless, some useful data exist.
- Patients with uncomplicated operations, good intraoperative hemostasis, and a postoperative computed tomography (CT) showing stable and nonmajor surgical bleeding can likely safely begin chemoprophylaxis 24 to 48 hours postoperatively.
- For all patients at high risk for VTE, including all malignant brain tumor patients, chemoprophylaxis should be considered beginning at 24 hours post-craniotomy.
- In TBI patients who require neurosurgical intervention, including intracranial pressure (ICP) monitor or external ventricular drainage (EVD) placement, a delay in deep vein thrombosis (DVT) chemoprophylaxis of approximately 3 days after the index cranial operation, perhaps sooner if serial CT scans separated by at least 24 hours show stability of ICH, may be appropriate.
- Higher quality data are necessary to improve VTE prophylaxis practices in neurosurgical patients.

BACKGROUND

Making decisions that optimally balance bleeding and clotting risks in cranial neurosurgery patients is a central challenge in neurocritical care that arises daily in the form of decisions regarding venous thromboembolism (VTE) prophylaxis. VTE is common in this population and, especially when it takes the form of pulmonary embolism (PE), the consequences can be devastating. However, despite being the most effective method for preventing VTE,[1] chemoprophylaxis can increase the risk of new or worsening intracranial hemorrhage (ICH) in these patients, which can also have devastating consequences. To complicate the matter further, the population of patients undergoing cranial surgery is quite heterogeneous, and the risk-to-benefit ratio of VTE chemoprophylaxis varies widely based on patient-, disease-, and operation-specific factors. Finally, as is the case in much of neurocritical care, the quality of the existing data on this topic provides few if any clear answers.[2]

The goal of this chapter is to provide useful guidance that can be applied at the bedside to answer the questions of when and how (and if) VTE chemoprophylaxis should be started in common subgroups of cranial neurosurgical patients. We first describe the problem broadly for pathophysiological and epidemiological context. Then, to account for the problem of risk-to-benefit variation due to disease- and operation-specific variables, we consider the question in two common clinical scenarios: patients undergoing cranial surgery for nontraumatic indications and patients with traumatic brain injury (TBI).

EVIDENCE AND REVIEW

Pathophysiology

Neurosurgical patients are at high risk of VTE because of derangements involving all components of Virchow's triad, many of which are unique or exaggerated compared to other surgical patients. Long duration operations (and therefore long exposure to general anesthesia) as well as prolonged postoperative immobility cause venous stasis. Endothelial injury is a particular concern in those undergoing cerebrovascular operations. Most unique to cranial neurosurgery patients, the operations themselves—by way of manipulation of the brain—as well as the underlying conditions for which the surgery is performed—especially both primary and metastatic brain tumors and TBI—are associated with significant thrombophilia.[3]

Epidemiology

The risk of deep vein thrombosis (DVT) in elective neurosurgical patients in the absence of any form of prophylaxis has been estimated to be approximately 25%.[4] Prior to contemporary prophylaxis practices, the PE rate was correspondingly high at 1% to 5%.[4,5] Importantly, the mortality rate of PE in neurosurgical patients is substantial, with an estimated range of 9% to 50%.[6-8] DVTs can also have significant long-term consequences. When severe, the postthrombotic syndrome, which develops in about 30% of patients with DVT, is associated with quality of life reductions similar to angina, cancer, or severe congestive heart failure.[9,10]

A recent analysis of over 10,000 craniotomy patients in the American College of Surgeons National Surgical Quality Improvement Project (ACS-NSQIP) found the rate of symptomatic DVT and PE in contemporary practice to be 2.4% and 1.3%, respectively.[11] In patients who undergo major orthopedic surgery, the risk of DVT with no pharmacological prophylaxis is 2.8% and that for PE 1.5%.[12] In bariatric surgery patients these risks are 2.4% and 0.3%[13]; and in intracerebral hemorrhage 2% to 4% and 1%.[14] Thus, the risk of VTE in cranial neurosurgery patients is equivalent to or exceeds that of other very high-risk populations.

Timing of Postoperative VTE

VTE risk rises in the first few days to a week postoperatively and is pathophysiologically related to immobility.[15] This is substantiated in the neurosurgical patient population by several lines of evidence. For example, Li and colleagues found that the incidence of DVT was 30.9% in neurosurgical patients who were kept in bed for more than 3 days.[16] Another study of about 6,900 patients undergoing spine surgery showed the risk of VTE rose linearly during the first 2 weeks postoperatively.[17] Finally, Khaldi and colleagues found that 84% of all DVTs occurred in the first postoperative week in a population of 555 high-risk neurosurgical patients (including all neurosurgery patients admitted to the ICU) who underwent twice weekly screening venous duplex ultrasonography.[18]

Nontraumatic craniotomy patients

The risk of clinically apparent VTE after craniotomy is estimated to be 3.2%, about one-third of which are PE and two-thirds of which are DVT.[11] The actual incidence of VTE in this population may, however, be higher, as studies of populations in whom screening ultrasound is part of routine practice have found postoperative DVT incidence rates approaching 10%. [19] Although no validated risk scores exist to guide VTE chemoprophylaxis decisions in this population, a number of studies have identified risk factors (Table 13–1).[11,19,20] Notably, within the craniotomy for tumor risk group, patients with high-grade gliomas seem to be at particularly high risk.[21]

Although intermittent pneumatic compression (IPC) devices alone clearly reduce the risk of VTE in neurosurgical patients,[19,22] there are two limitations to using them in isolation. First, the degree of effectiveness is dependent on compliance, which is consistently reported to be low, a fact that bears out in daily experience in the neuro-ICU. Second, the combination of chemoprophylaxis with IPC provides significant additional protection against VTE compared to either method alone.[4] Thus, chemoprophylaxis is frequently used in addition to IPC for post-craniotomy patients.

The potential downside of chemoprophylaxis, of course, is the possibility of an increased rate of clinically significant postoperative ICH. Many studies have examined this issue. The overall quality of these data is poor, however, thereby limiting the strength of the conclusions of various systematic reviews and meta-analyses. With these limitations in mind, the balance of existing evidence indicates, not surprisingly, that chemoprophylaxis both reduces the rate of VTE and increases the rate of postoperative ICH. The best synthesis of these data converges on a few key points:

- Overall risk of clinically apparent VTE after craniotomy is estimated to be 3.2%, about one-third of which are PE and two-thirds of which are DVT.[11]
- Absolute risk reduction for VTE with chemoprophylaxis is 1% to 3.5%.[6]
- The baseline rate of postoperative ICH without chemoprophylaxis is about 1% to 1.5%.[8,23]
- Absolute risk increase for postoperative ICH with chemoprophylaxis is 0.7% to 1%.[6,8]
- On average, ICH events are associated with more disability than VTE events, though both can be fatal.[8,13]

TABLE 13–1 Risk factors for VTE in postcraniotomy patients.

Patient	Surgical	Postoperative
Age > 60 years	Nonelective surgery	Mechanical ventilation > 48 h
Obesity	Emergency surgery	Return to OR
Dependent functional status	CNS tumor	Infection
History of VTE	Surgical time > 4 h	

- The risk of postoperative hemorrhage may be slightly higher with low molecular weight heparin (LMWH) compared to low dose unfractionated heparin (LDUH).[22]
- There is no clearly superior regimen regarding VTE prevention in this population among the various LMWH and LDUH regimens that have been studied.[6,13]
- Risk of postoperative ICH is probably higher when chemoprophylaxis is started <24 hours after surgery.[13,19,23]
- The risk of ICH is highest within the first 1 to 2 postoperative days, while the VTE risk rises more gradually over time, peaking at >1 week after operation.[13,23]

Synthesis of these facts yields the following conclusions:

- All craniotomy patients in the Neuro-ICU should receive mechanical VTE prophylaxis with IPC unless there is a significant contraindication.
- Patients with uncomplicated operations, good intraoperative hemostasis, and a postoperative CT showing stable and non-major surgical bleeding can likely safely begin chemoprophylaxis 24 to 48 hours postoperatively.
- For all patients at high risk for VTE, including all malignant brain tumor patients, chemoprophylaxis should be considered beginning at 24 hours postcraniotomy.
- LDUH may have a better associated risk-to-benefit profile than LMWH.
- Given the importance of the neurosurgeon's unique knowledge of the details of any given patient's operation, all decisions about postoperative VTE chemoprophylaxis should be made in collaboration with the operating neurosurgeon.

VTE Prophylaxis in TBI

The risk of DVT or PE may be as high as 54% in civilian TBI patients who are not treated with any prophylactic measures,[24] and the risk is highest in the first several days post injury. Menaker and colleagues[25] showed that 15% of the 94 PE events in their retrospective cohort study of over 35,000 trauma patients occurred within the first 48 hours post injury, 40% by day 4, and >50% in the first week. While retrospective studies seem to converge on the finding that early (before 72 hours post injury) initiation of chemoprophylaxis is associated with a lower risk of VTE without an increased risk of ICH progression when compared to later initiation, these studies are at risk for both significant selection bias favoring the inclusion of patients with low ICH progression rates in the early treatment groups as well as risk of being underpowered to detect significant differences in ICH rates.[26–28] For patients with early hematoma expansion within the first 24 hours, delayed chemoprophylaxis (median start time 72 hours from admission) increased the risk of delayed ICH expansion 13-fold.[29]

There are no definitive clinical trials to guide VTE chemoprophylaxis in TBI patients. In fact, the first study aimed at characterizing the risk of traumatic ICH expansion in the setting of VTE chemoprophylaxis was not published until 2002, and this was a small retrospective cohort study.[9] In the absence of high-quality empiric data, Berne, Norwood, and colleagues, based on biological plausibility and careful observation, devised a useful scheme for risk stratifying TBI patients according to their risk of spontaneous ICH expansion in an effort to identify groups of patients who could safely start early or delayed prophylaxis.[30] Phelan and colleagues at Parkland Hospital in Dallas, Texas, built on this work, creating an algorithm based on clinical and CT data that stratifies patients with low, medium, and high risk for ICH expansion.[9] In a small randomized control trial, compared to those who received placebo, patients in the low-risk arm who received LMWH chemoprophylaxis that was started 24 hours after admission did not have increased risk of ICH expansion.[31] The Parkland Protocol now forms the basis of the ACS TQIP recommendations for VTE prophylaxis in TBI and guides practice at the authors' institution[32] (Table 13–2).

TABLE 13–2 Parkland protocol for VTE chemoprophylaxis in TBI.[37,38]

Risk Group	Definition	Suggested Prophylaxis Method
Low	• Absence of moderate or high-risk criteria	Start chemoprophylaxis if CT shows stable hematoma **24 h** after injury
Moderate	• Subdural hematoma > 8 mm • Epidural hematoma > 8 mm • Contusion > 2 cm • More than one contusion per lobe • SAH with abnormal CT angiogram • Evidence of hematoma worsening on repeat CT 24 h after injury	Start chemoprophylaxis if CT shows stable hematoma **72 h** after injury
High	• Craniotomy • ICP monitor placement • EVD placement • Evidence of hematoma worsening on repeat CT 72 h after injury	• Individualized decision with a starting point of considering chemoprophylaxis on the 4th postoperative day. • Reasonable strategies might include anything from chemoprophylaxis beginning 24 h postoperatively if there is no progressive ICH on serial CT to avoidance of chemoprophylaxis for long enough to consider prophylactic, short-term IVC filter use

CT, computed tomography; EVD, external ventricular drainage; ICP, intracranial pressure; IVC, inferior vena cava; SAH, subarachnoid hemorrhage.

Despite the Parkland Protocol's utility for patients in its low- and medium-risk groups, the questions of if and when to start VTE chemoprophylaxis in TBI patients with the highest risk of spontaneous ICH expansion—those who have undergone craniotomy and/or have an ICP monitor—remain highly uncertain. This is a very heterogenous group in terms of risk for progressive ICH that includes patients with diffuse nonhemorrhagic injury and an ICP monitor at one end of the spectrum and patients with multifocal, multicompartmental traumatic ICH requiring emergent decompressive surgery at the other. Recently, Byrne and colleagues addressed this open question in a retrospective study of a cohort of nearly 5,000 patients who underwent neurosurgical intervention for TBI. Patients in this cohort were derived from 304 trauma centers and had a median Glasgow coma scale (GCS) of 7, supporting reasonable generalizability to a large population of patients with moderate and severe TBI. After adjusting for confounders, for every day that VTE chemoprophylaxis was delayed after the index neurosurgical procedure, the odds of VTE increased by 8%, while the odds of repeat neurosurgical intervention decreased by 28% per day for the first 3 days and 15% per day thereafter.[33] Taken together, these data suggest that a reasonable starting point for considerations of time to start chemoprophylaxis in the Parkland high risk group is the 4th day after any neurosurgical procedure, including insertion of an ICP monitor or external ventricular drain. Beginning on the day after surgery, to account for the large degree of heterogeneity of VTE and ICH risk in this group, the decision should be considered collaboratively by the neurointensivist and neurosurgeon, weighing the estimated degrees of risk for both ICH expansion and VTE against each other in the context of the specifics of the injury, operation, evolution of hemorrhage on serial imaging, and the presence of other VTE risk factors such as long bone or pelvic fracture, degree of immobility, and duration of mechanical ventilation. Commonly, at the authors' institutions, chemoprophylaxis after neurosurgical procedures occurs earlier than 72 hours from neurosurgical procedure if serial imaging demonstrates intracranial hemostasis.

Finally, as in nontraumatic craniotomy, the best agent and dosing schedule for chemoprophylaxis in TBI patients is unclear. Although LMWH is clearly preferred in trauma patients without TBI as it is more effective at preventing VTE without increasing risk of significant bleeding, its superiority in TBI patients is less clear.[34,35] Several studies in TBI patients have shown LMWH to be superior in terms of VTE prevention without an increased risk of ICH. Conflicting results demonstrating an increased risk of ICH with LWMH compared to LDUH, the low overall quality of the data supporting superiority of LMWH, and concerns about LMWH's longer duration of action and irreversibility, however, underlie the common use of LDUH in this group. Monitoring anti-factor Xa levels with consequent dose adjustments with the use of either agent has shown promise for better risk:benefit balance in individual patients, but this strategy lacks sufficient supporting data at present.[36]

Synthesis of these facts yields the following conclusions:

- TBI patients in the neuro-ICU are at high risk for VTE and should have mechanical VTE prophylaxis with IPC unless there is a significant contraindication.
- In patients who had early ICH expansion, there is a greater risk of additional hematoma expansion when initiating chemoprophylaxis.
- In patients who require neurosurgical intervention, including ICP monitor or EVD placement, a delay in DVT chemoprophylaxis of approximately 3 days after the index cranial operation is appropriate.
- Because of the substantial heterogeneity of progressive/recurrent ICH risk in the Parkland high risk category, individualized, carefully considered decisions are essential for patients in this group. It might be reasonable to start chemoprophylaxis at 24 to 48 hours after surgery in those at the lowest end of the ICH risk spectrum and a stable CT, while in others the delay may need to be long enough to consider short-term, prophylactic use of an IVC filter.
- Both LMWH and LDUH are reasonable agents in this group.
- All decisions about VTE chemoprophylaxis should be made collaboratively by the neurosurgeon, neurointensivist, and other involved specialists (eg, trauma surgeon, orthopedic surgeon).

REFERENCES

1. Schünemann HJ, Cushman M, Burnett AE, Kahn SR, Beyer-Westendorf J, Spencer FA, et al. American Society of Hematology 2018 guidelines for management of venous thromboembolism: prophylaxis for hospitalized and nonhospitalized medical patients. *Blood Adv*. 2018 Nov 27;2(22):3198–225.
2. Yepes-Nuñez JJ, Rajasekhar A, Rahman M, Dahm P, Anderson DR, Colunga-Lozano LE, et al. Pharmacologic thromboprophylaxis in adult patients undergoing neurosurgical interventions for preventing venous thromboembolism. *Blood Adv*. 2020 Jun 23;4(12):2798–809.
3. Ganau M, Prisco L, Cebula H, Todeschi J, Abid H, Ligarotti G, et al. Risk of deep vein thrombosis in neurosurgery: state of the art on prophylaxis protocols and best clinical practices. *J Clin Neurosci*. 2017 Nov;45:60–6.
4. Agnelli G, Piovella F, Buoncristiani P, Severi P, Pini M, D'Angelo A, et al. Enoxaparin plus compression stockings compared with compression stockings alone in the prevention of venous thromboembolism after elective neurosurgery. *N Engl J Med*. 1998 Jul 9;339(2):80–5.
5. Hamilton MG, Spetzler RF. The prospective application of a grading system for arteriovenous malformations. *Neurosurgery*. 1994 Jan;34(1):2–6; discussion 6-7.
6. Hamilton MG, Yee WH, Hull RD, Ghali WA. Venous thromboembolism prophylaxis in patients undergoing cranial neurosurgery: a systematic review and meta-analysis. *Neurosurgery*. 2011 Mar;68(3):571–81.
7. Valladares JB, Hankinson J. Incidence of lower extremity deep vein thrombosis in neurosurgical patients. *Neurosurgery*. 1980 Feb;6(2):138–41.
8. Danish SF, Burnett MG, Ong JG, Sonnad SS, Maloney-Wilensky E, Stein SC. Prophylaxis for deep venous thrombosis in craniotomy patients: a decision analysis. *Neurosurgery*. 2005 Jun;56(6):1286–92; discussion 1292-4.
9. Phelan HA. Pharmacologic venous thromboembolism prophylaxis after traumatic brain injury: a critical literature review. *J Neurotrauma*. 2012 Jul 1;29(10):1821–8.
10. Kahn SR, Partsch H, Vedantham S, Prandoni P, Kearon C; Subcommittee on Control of Anticoagulation of the Scientific and Standardization Committee of the International Society on Thrombosis and Haemostasis. Definition of post-thrombotic syndrome of the leg for use in clinical investigations:

a recommendation for standardization. *J Thromb Haemost JTH.* 2009 May;7(5):879–83.

11. Algattas H, Kimmell KT, Jahromi BS. Analysis of venous thromboembolism risk in patients undergoing craniotomy. *World Neurosurg.* 2015 Nov;84(5):1372–9.
12. Falck-Ytter Y, Francis CW, Johanson NA, Curley C, Dahl OE, Schulman S, et al. Prevention of VTE. In *Orthopedic Surgery Patients: Antithrombotic Therapy and Prevention of Thrombosis,* 9th ed, American College of Chest Physicians Evidence-Based Clinical Practice Guidelines. *Chest.* 2012 Feb 1; 141(2):e278S–e325S.
13. Gould MK, Garcia DA, Wren SM, Karanicolas PJ, Arcelus JI, Heit JA, et al. Prevention of VTE in nonorthopedic surgical patients. In *Antithrombotic Therapy and Prevention of Thrombosis,* 9th ed, American College of Chest Physicians Evidence-Based Clinical Practice Guidelines. *Chest.* 2012 Feb;141(2 Suppl):e227S–e277S.
14. Nyquist P, Bautista C, Jichici D, Burns J, Chhangani S, DeFilippis M, et al. Prophylaxis of venous thrombosis in neurocritical care patients: an evidence-based guideline: a statement for healthcare professionals from the Neurocritical Care Society. *Neurocrit Care.* 2016 Feb;24(1):47–60.
15. Arcelus JI, Monreal M, Caprini JA, Guisado JG, Soto MJ, Núñez MJ, et al. Clinical presentation and time-course of postoperative venous thromboembolism: results from the RIETE Registry. *Thromb Haemost.* 2008 Mar;99(3):546–51.
16. Li J, Ren X, Zhu X, Chen H, Lin Z, Huang M, et al. Clinical predictive factors of lower extremity deep vein thrombosis in relative high-risk patients after neurosurgery: a retrospective study. *Dis Markers.* 2020 Jun 4; 2020:5820749.
17. Cloney MB, Hopkins B, Dhillon ES, Dahdaleh NS. The timing of venous thromboembolic events after spine surgery: a single-center experience with 6869 consecutive patients. *J Neurosurg Spine.* 2018 Jan;28(1):88–95.
18. Khaldi A, Helo N, Schneck MJ, Origitano TC. Venous thromboembolism: deep venous thrombosis and pulmonary embolism in a neurosurgical population. *J Neurosurg.* 2011 Jan;114(1):40–6.
19. Faraoni D, Comes RF, Geerts W, Wiles MD; ESA VTE Guidelines Task Force. European guidelines on perioperative venous thromboembolism prophylaxis: neurosurgery. *Eur J Anaesthesiol.* 2018 Feb;35(2):90–5.
20. Kimmell KT, Jahromi BS. Clinical factors associated with venous thromboembolism risk in patients undergoing craniotomy. *J Neurosurg.* 2015 May;122(5):1004–11.
21. Chaichana KL, Pendleton C, Jackson C, Martinez-Gutierrez JC, Diaz-Stransky A, Aguayo J, et al. Deep venous thrombosis and pulmonary embolisms in adult patients undergoing craniotomy for brain tumors. *Neurol Res.* 2013 Mar;35(2):206–11.
22. Collen JF, Jackson JL, Shorr AF, Moores LK. Prevention of venous thromboembolism in neurosurgery: a metaanalysis. *Chest.* 2008 Aug 1; 134(2):237–49.
23. Senders JT, Goldhaber NH, Cote DJ, Muskens IS, Dawood HY, De Vos FYFL, et al. Venous thromboembolism and intracranial hemorrhage after craniotomy for primary malignant brain tumors: a National Surgical Quality Improvement Program analysis. *J Neurooncol.* 2018 Jan 1;136(1):135–45.
24. Geerts WH, Code KI, Jay RM, Chen E, Szalai JP. A prospective study of venous thromboembolism after major trauma. *N Engl J Med.* 1994 Dec 15;331(24):1601–6.
25. Menaker J, Stein DM, Scalea TM. Incidence of early pulmonary embolism after injury. *J Trauma.* 2007 Sep;63(3):620–4.
26. Lu VM, Alvi MA, Rovin RA, Kasper EM. Clinical outcomes following early versus late pharmacologic thromboprophylaxis in patients with traumatic intracranial hemorrhage: a systematic review and meta-analysis. *Neurosurg Rev.* 2020 Jun;43(3):861–72.
27. Hachem LD, Mansouri A, Scales DC, Geerts W, Pirouzmand F. Anticoagulant prophylaxis against venous thromboembolism following severe traumatic brain injury: a prospective observational study and systematic review of the literature. *Clin Neurol Neurosurg.* 2018 Dec;175:68–73.
28. Spano PJ, Shaikh S, Boneva D, Hai S, McKenney M, Elkbuli A. Anticoagulant chemoprophylaxis in patients with traumatic brain injuries: a systematic review. *J Trauma Acute Care Surg.* 2020 Mar;88(3):454–60.
29. Levy AS, Salottolo K, Bar-Or R, Offner P, Mains C, Sullivan M, et al. Pharmacologic thromboprophylaxis is a risk factor for hemorrhage progression in a subset of patients with traumatic brain injury. *J Trauma Inj Infect Crit Care.* 2010 Apr;68(4):886–94.
30. Norwood SH, Berne JD, Rowe SA, Villarreal DH, Ledlie JT. Early venous thromboembolism prophylaxis with enoxaparin in patients with blunt traumatic brain injury. *J Trauma.* 2008 Nov;65(5):1021–6; discussion 1026-7.
31. Phelan HA, Wolf SE, Norwood SH, Aldy K, Brakenridge SC, Eastman AL, et al. A randomized, double-blinded, placebo-controlled pilot trial of anticoagulation in low-risk traumatic brain injury: the Delayed versus Early Enoxaparin Prophylaxis I (DEEP I) study. *J Trauma Acute Care Surg.* 2012 Dec;73(6):1434–41.
32. Cryer HG, Manley GT, Adelson PD, Alali AS, Calland JF, Cipolle M, et al. ACS TQIP best practices in the management of traumatic brain injury. *J Am Coll Surg.* 2015.
33. Byrne JP, Witiw CD, Schuster JM, Pascual JL, Cannon JW, Martin ND, et al. Association of venous thromboembolism prophylaxis after neurosurgical intervention for traumatic brain injury with thromboembolic complications, repeated neurosurgery, and mortality. *JAMA Surg.* 2022 Mar 9; 157(3):e215794.
34. Ley EJ, Brown CVR, Moore EE, Sava JA, Peck K, Ciesla DJ, et al. Updated guidelines to reduce venous thromboembolism in trauma patients: a Western Trauma Association critical decisions algorithm. *J Trauma Acute Care Surg.* 2020 Nov;89(5):971–81.
35. Margolick J, Dandurand C, Duncan K, Chen W, Evans DC, Sekhon MS, et al. A systematic review of the risks and benefits of venous thromboembolism prophylaxis in traumatic brain injury. *Can J Neurol Sci J Can Sci Neurol.* 2018 Jul;45(4):432–44.
36. Rodier SG, Kim M, Moore S, Frangos SG, Tandon M, Klein MJ, et al. Early anti-Xa assay-guided low molecular weight heparin chemoprophylaxis is safe in adult patients with acute traumatic brain injury. *Am Surg.* 2020 Apr 1;86(4):369–76.
37. QIP, ACS. Best practices in the management of traumatic brain injury. *ACS Committee on Trauma.* 2015;3–23.
38. Pastorek RA, Cripps MW, Bernstein IH, Scott WW, Madden CJ, Rickert KL, et al. The Parkland protocol's modified Berne-Norwood criteria predict two tiers of risk for traumatic brain injury progression. *J Neurotrauma.* 2014 Oct 15;31(20):1737–43.

CHAPTER

14

How Do We Deal with Heparin Resistance in Therapeutic Anticoagulation?

Brooke Barlow, PharmD & Megan E. Barra, PharmD

Case

A 34-year-old man with a history of obesity (body mass index 36 kg/m^2), hypertension, and hyperlipidemia was admitted to the neurocritical care unit after presenting to the emergency department as a pedestrian struck by motor vehicle in a hit and run. On admission he was found to have multiple traumatic injuries, including diffuse multicompartment, cortical subarachnoid hemorrhage, intraventricular hemorrhage, subdural hematoma, fractures of the right anterior seventh and eighth ribs, and multiple pelvic fractures. On hospital day #8 the patient was diagnosed with bilateral upper extremity deep vein thrombosis and initiated on therapeutic anticoagulation with heparin 18 units/kg/hr titrated to aPTT 70 to 100 seconds (baseline aPTT 26 seconds). Six hours after initiation, heparin remained subtherapeutic at 30 seconds, and infusion was increased to 22 units/kg/h. Over the following 18 hours, anticoagulation with heparin remained subtherapeutic with JF's aPTT ranging from 30 to 38 seconds despite escalating heparin infusion doses to 30 units/kg/h. What are the next steps in workup and management of potential heparin resistance?

Key Points

- In patients with neurocritical illness receiving anticoagulation for the treatment of acute thromboembolisms, heparin resistance may introduce new complexity to ensure safe and effective therapeutic anticoagulation with coexisting intracranial abnormalities.
- Diagnostic workup should rule out factitious or pseudo-heparin resistance caused by access-site or laboratory error, elevated factor VIII or fibrinogen, or other etiologies to determine whether heparin anti-Xa guided monitoring may be more appropriate than aPTT-guided monitoring or if dose escalation can achieve therapeutic goals.
- While heparin is often a preferred anticoagulation choice due to its rapid-onset, low-cost, and ease of reversibility, patients with true heparin resistance in the setting of acquired or hereditary antithrombin III deficiency may require antithrombin III supplementation to maintain heparin sensitivity or switching to an alternative anticoagulant.
- Patient-specific thromboembolic and hemorrhagic risk factors, along with comorbid conditions, should guide treatment selection when managing heparin resistance in patients with neurocritical illness.

BACKGROUND

Heparin-based anticoagulation is frequently employed in the neurocritical care setting when therapeutic anticoagulation is warranted due to its rapid onset, short half-life and routine availability of protamine for rapid reversal if needed. Despite its widespread, long-standing use, heparin is fraught with challenges, notably the variability in interindividual dose-response and in some cases a complete lack of response coined "heparin resistance." Heparin resistance is characterized by the failure to achieve the desired anticoagulation target despite adequate escalation of heparin doses.[1] Heparin doses exceeding 35,000 units per day is commonly used as the threshold to suspect heparin resistance. However clinically, this threshold may be an inappropriately low threshold, as a standard heparin starting dose of 18 units/kg/h of heparin for treatment of a venous thromboembolism (VTE) in an 82-kg patient would exceed this daily threshold if maintained at this rate to achieve therapeutic goals. A weight-based threshold would confer improved sensitivity, however no such definition has yet to be defined. Reports of heparin resistance have been most commonly cited in cardiac surgery with an estimated incidence of 22%,[2] however the incidence in neurocritical care patients is limited to a few case reports, but likely underreported.[3,4] Though rare, screening at risk patients for heparin resistance is critical to mitigate risk fatal consequences.

EVIDENCE AND REVIEW

Mechanisms of Heparin Resistance

Unfractionated heparin is a large polysaccharide polymer that exerts its anticoagulant effects through binding to endogenous antithrombin III (ATIII) and potentiating its inactivation of thrombin and factor Xa by 1000-fold along with other clotting factors (Figure 14–1). Given the therapeutic effects of heparin are directly dependent its binding to endogenous ATIII, an inherited or acquired ATIII deficiency is the most common cause of heparin resistance. Acquired causes of ATIII deficiency include cirrhosis, disseminated intravascular coagulation (DIC), nephrotic syndrome, severe trauma, pregnancy complicated by eclampsia or preeclampsia, extracorporeal membrane oxygenation, and hemodialysis[5] (Figure 14–2). An estimated 20% to 70% of trauma patients have an acquired ATIII deficiency on admission, corresponding to decreased response to low-molecular weight heparin at standard doses and subsequent risk of VTE.[6] Evidence of ATIII deficiency has also been identified in acute ischemic stroke patients, with reduced ATIII and increased fibrinogen concentrations compared to controls, correlating to increased stroke severity.[7]

Non-ATIII mediated mechanisms that can contribute to heparin resistance include nonspecific binding to plasma proteins such as chemokines, extracellular matrix proteins, growth factors, glycoproteins, platelet factor 4, and lipoproteins which can lead to a significant variability in therapeutic response.[5] Neutrophil extracellular traps (NETs) are an immunologic response to infection or tissue injury that are increased in the setting of trauma or neurologic injury.[8] NETs contain highly positively charged proteins that can complex with the negatively charged heparin side chains theoretically reducing the anticoagulant effects and development of heparin resistance. Coagulation derangements such as increased factor VIII levels and hyperfibrinogenemia seen in critical illness or COVID19 can result in a phenomenon known as pseudo resistance, where activated partial thromboplastin time (aPTT) is subtherapeutic despite *in vivo* therapeutic anticoagulation. aPTT is a global coagulation assay and can be affected by various acute-phase reactants and clotting factors that may not readily reflect true heparin effects.[1,5]

Andexanet alfa is a recombinant factor Xa decoy protein that has been shown to effectively reverse the direct factor Xa inhibitors; it also possesses activity against antithrombin-dependent factor Xa inhibitors including heparin. Administration of andexanet alfa prior to heparinization for endovascular procedures has been reported to result in heparin nonresponsiveness, raising concerns regarding its use in the neurosurgical setting.[9–11] L-Asparginase, a mainstay chemotherapeutic agent for acute lymphoblastic leukemia, decreases the hepatic synthesis of endogenous anticoagulants including ATIII, carrying a heightened risk of thrombosis and subsequent heparin resistance.[12]

Diagnosis

Prompt diagnostic workup upon suspicion of heparin resistance is critical to minimize risk of thrombus propagation from subtherapeutic anticoagulant exposure or risk of bleeding from

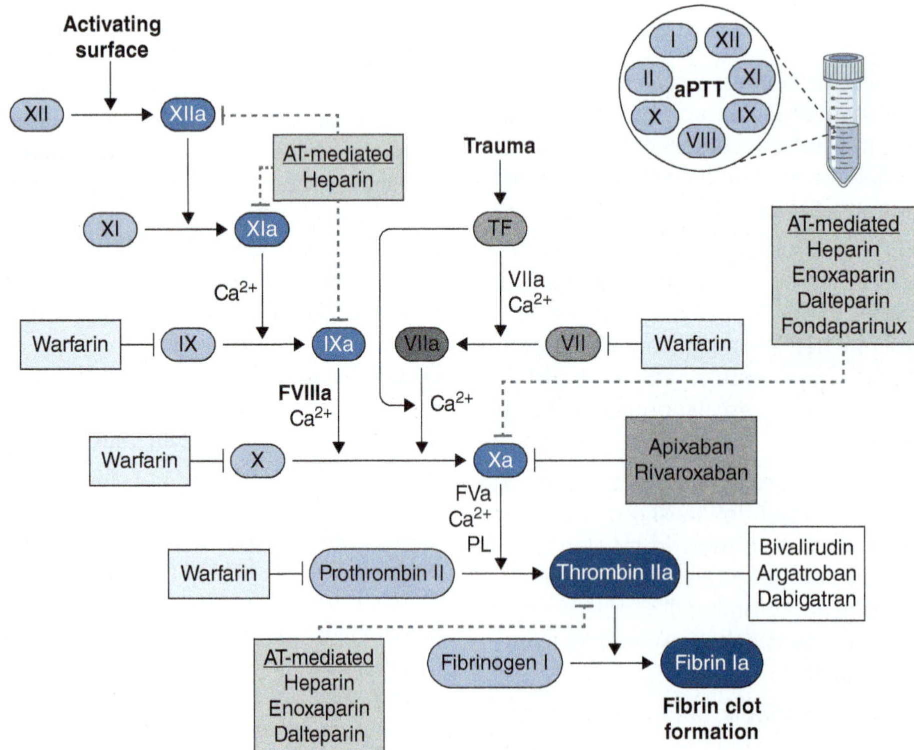

FIGURE 14–1 Coagulation cascade and site of action for anticoagulants.
Abbreviations: aPTT, activated partial thromboplastin time; AT, antithrombin III.

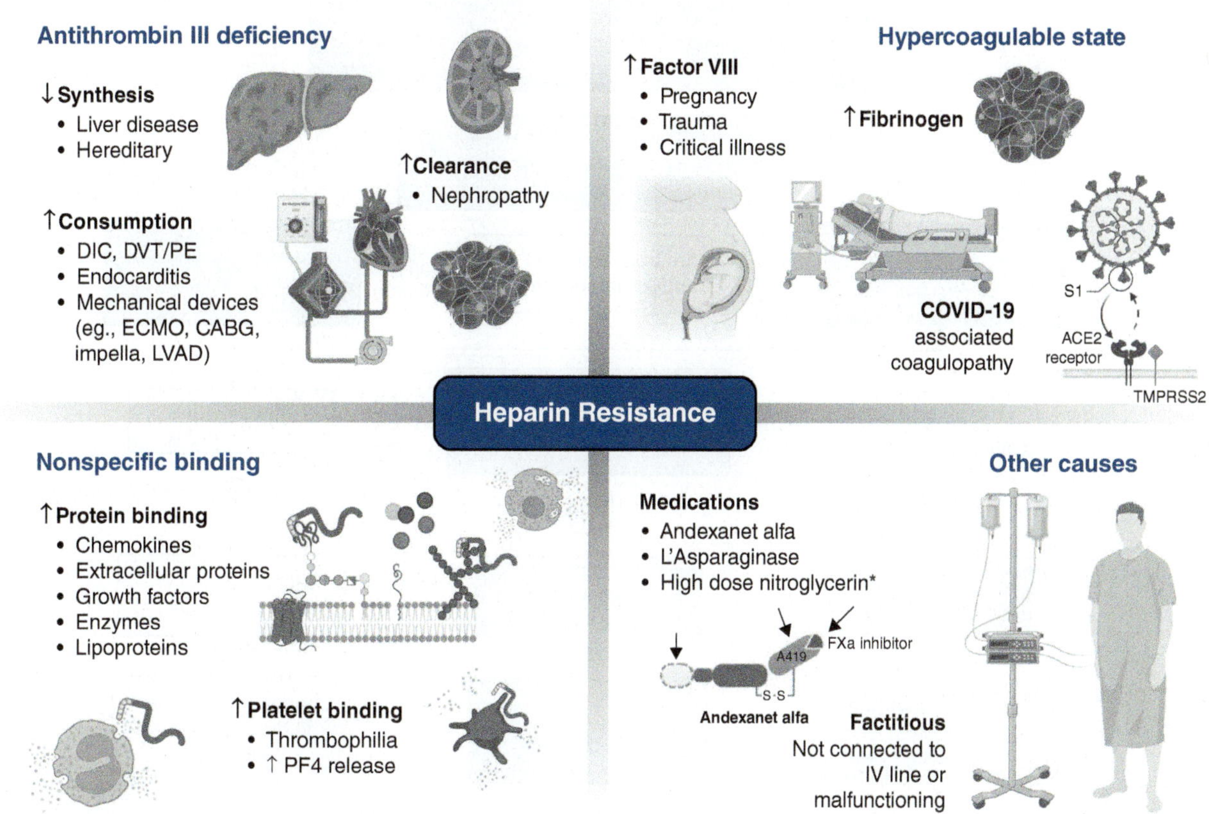

FIGURE 14–2 Mechanisms of heparin resistance.

Abbreviations: CABG, coronary artery bypass graft; DIC, disseminated intravascular coagulation; DVT/PE, deep vein thrombosis, pulmonary embolism; ECMO, extracorporeal membrane oxygenation; LVAD, left ventricular assist device; PF4, platelet factor-4.

supratherapeutic anticoagulation from escalating doses when factitious or pseudo-resistance is present (Table 14–1). First, exclusion of factitious resistance through bedside evaluation of the heparin infusion line to ensure appropriate connection between the heparin bag, the infusion tubing, and IV access site. A careful review of the medication administration record should be performed to evaluate for any potential medication-induced causes (ie, andexanet alfa, asparaginase). Initial laboratory testing should include a paired aPTT and calibrated unfractionated heparin anti-Xa level to assess for discordance.[1] If the aPTT and anti-Xa are discordant (ie, aPTT subtherapeutic, anti-Xa therapeutic), pseudo heparin resistance is the likely cause and confirmatory testing of factor VIII or fibrinogen levels can be considered. On the contrary, if aPTT and anti-Xa are concordant (ie, aPTT and anti-Xa are subtherapeutic), further testing should be targeted toward evaluation of antithrombin III deficiency. An important caveat to note is some anti-Xa assays may require supplemental antithrombin as a reagent, resulting in a falsely elevated anti-Xa in the setting of ATIII deficiency.[13] Identification of the institution-specific unfractionated heparin anti-Xa assay is critical to ensure accurate interpretation of the results to ensure timely treatment interventions are initiated (Figure 14–3).

TABLE 14–1 Coagulation laboratory parameters utilized in the diagnostic workup of heparin resistance.

Diagnostic Test	Reference Range	Heparin Resistance	Considerations
Antithrombin III functional assay	80%-130%	<80%	Some data suggest ATIII <60% portends higher risk of true heparin resistance and threshold for treatment
Chromogenic heparin anti-Xa*	0.3-0.7 IU/mL	<0.3	Some assays may contain ATIII supplementation
Factor VIII	50%-150%	>150%	ELISA test preferred over 1-step assay to reduce falsely high results[15]
Fibrinogen	200-400 mg/dL	>400 mg/dL	May be falsely low in the setting of direct thrombin inhibitor therapy[16]

*Reference range, reference range for therapeutic heparin therapy.

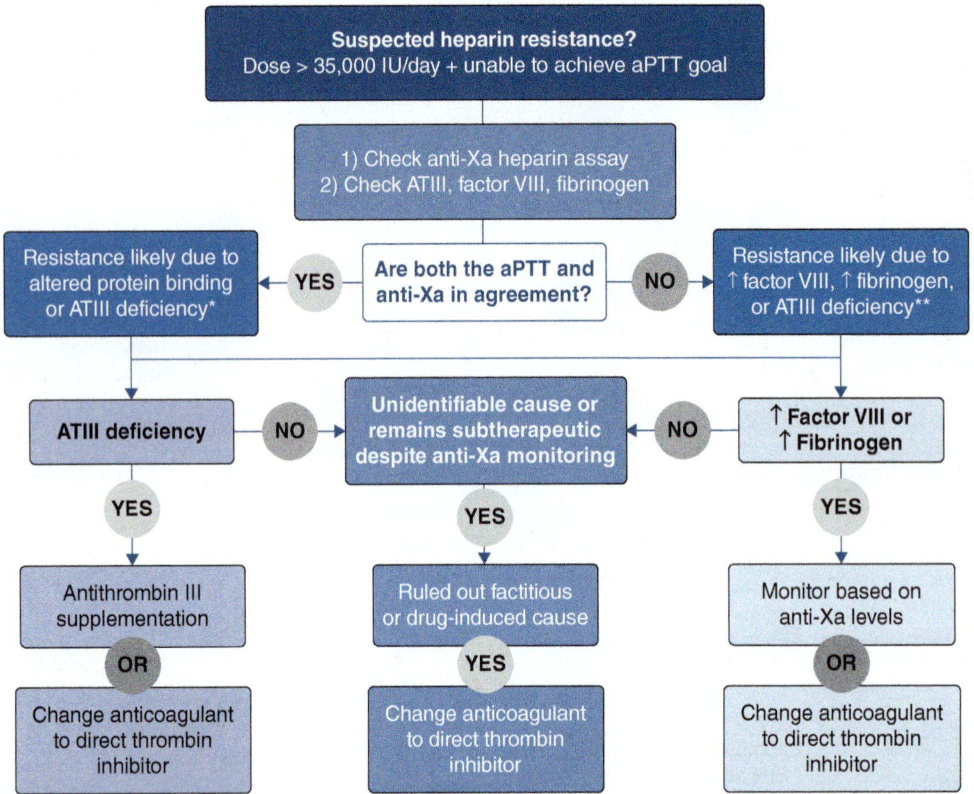

FIGURE 14–3 Heparin resistance diagnosis and treatment.

Of note, some anti-Xa assays may add antithrombin as a reagent resulting in a falsely elevated anti-Xa and may lead to a false-negative diagnosis of heparin resistance.

*If heparin anti-Xa assay does NOT contain exogenous ATIII.

**If heparin anti-Xa assay DOES contain exogenous ATIII.

Therapeutic Approach to Heparin Management

Treatment approach should be guided by underlying etiology of heparin resistance or presence of pseudo heparin resistance. Algorithmic approach to treatment is outlined in Figure 14–3.

Pseudo-Heparin Resistance: Heparin Anti-Xa versus aPTT Guided Therapy

The Anticoagulation Forum provides guidance that when heparin resistance is suspected, a paired aPTT and unfractionated heparin anti- Xa level should be drawn.[1] If aPTT is found to be unreliable and incongruent with anti-Xa levels (eg, aPTT subtherapeutic but anti-Xa therapeutic), anti-Xa guided monitoring may be utilized in place of aPTT during unfractionated heparin treatment, with a standard unfractionated heparin anti-Xa target of 0.3 to 0.7 IU/mL.[5] aPTT is a global test often utilized for monitoring during heparin therapy as it represents the ability of the heparin-antithrombin III complex to inactivate thrombin, factor Xa, and other clotting factors (Figure 14–1).[14] The heparin anti-Xa assay is another commonly used assay that measures the effect of heparin based on inhibition of activated factor X (Xa) and less vulnerable to underlying non-anticoagulation-related variables as described earlier. While there is controversy surrounding whether aPTT or anti-Xa should be utilized for monitoring of unfractionated heparin in the general patient population, anti-Xa monitoring may be more reliable in patients with inflammation, elevated fibrinogen and factor VIII, presence of antiphospholipid antibodies, and in the setting of DIC.[5]

Pseudo-Heparin Resistance: Escalating Doses of Heparin

If heparin resistance is due to elevated factor VIII and fibrinogen levels, escalating doses of heparin may be required to attain therapeutic anticoagulation. If the patient is considered stable, a heparin bolus can be considered with a repeat paired aPTT and anti-Xa checked ~60 minutes following administration. If an increase in the aPTT and/or heparin anti-Xa is observed, clinicians may opt to continue increasing heparin infusions per institutional protocol until therapeutic aPTT and/or heparin anti-Xa is achieved. Importantly, aPTT and/or anti-Xa obtained immediately post-bolus may be elevated but do not reflect whether the infusion rate is appropriate to achieve therapeutic anticoagulation given the time needed to reach steady state (~6 hours at a stable dose). Therefore, post-bolus aPTT or anti-Xa should not guide infusion rate dose modifications but instead be used to assess heparin responsiveness. If no response to the heparin bolus is seen or the aPTT and anti-Xa remain subtherapeutic despite serial dose increases, true heparin resistance may be present.[1]

Alternative Anticoagulants in Patients with Heparin Resistance or Pseudo-Heparin Resistance

Alternative anticoagulants that are not impacted by the variables that may contribute to the presence of heparin resistance or pseudo-resistance may be considered in lieu of heparin therapy for acute management. Intravenous direct thrombin inhibitors argatroban and bivalirudin directly inhibit thrombin independently of antithrombin III to elicit anticoagulant effects (Figure 14–1). The choice between argatroban and bivalirudin should be guided by patient-specific factors, such as the presence of renal and/or hepatic dysfunction (Table 14–2).[12] Limitations associated with intravenous direct thrombin inhibitors include a lack of reversal agent if a hemorrhagic complication occurs, thus use with caution in the presence of intracranial hemorrhage. It is worthwhile to note that elevated fibrinogen levels may impact the aPTT monitoring of direct thrombin inhibitors.[5] Dilute thrombin time may be an alternative for direct thrombin inhibitor monitoring, however it may not be readily available at many institutions.

Once stabilized, patients may be transitioned to oral therapy such as direct acting oral anticoagulants (apixaban, rivaroxaban, dabigatran) or vitamin K antagonists (eg, warfarin). Direct thrombin inhibitors may falsely elevate the international

TABLE 14–2 Therapeutic approach to heparin resistance management and alternative anticoagulation strategies.

	Dose	Half-life	Monitoring	Considerations
Antithrombin supplementation				
Plasma-derived ATIII (Thrombate III)	LD: 120% – baseline ATIII (%) × weight (kg) divided by 1.4% MD: LD × 0.6 every 24 h	12-24 h	ATIII 12-24 h post dose	Adjust dose every 12 h to achieve target AT level of 80%-120% followed by maintenance dosing
Recombinant ATIII (ATryn)	LD: 100 – baseline ATIII divided by 2.3 × weight (kg) MD: 100 – baseline ATIII divided by 10.2 × weight (kg) Off-label: 75 IU/kg[+]	11-17 h	ATIII 2 h post dose	Maintenance doses may be adjusted by ±30% to achieve target AT level 80%-120% Not FDA approved for treatment of thromboembolic events in hereditary AT deficiency
Fresh frozen plasma	500 IU of AT per 1 unit of FFP	4-6 h	ATIII 4-6 h post dose	Risk of transfusion associated lung injury, volume overload, infectious complications, and treatment time delay
Intravenous direct thrombin inhibitors				
Bivalirudin	0.05-0.15 mg/kg/h continuous IV infusion titrated to goal aPTT	25 min*	aPTT Renal function	Cautious use in renal impairment Impaired clearance during hypothermia May falsely increase the INR, requires specialized transition if bridging to warfarin
Argatroban	0.5-1 mcg/kg/min continuous IV infusion titrated to goal aPTT	45 min	aPTT Liver function	Avoid use in hepatic impairment Can falsely increase the INR, requires specialized transition if bridging to warfarin
Direct oral anticoagulants				
Rivaroxaban	Venous thromboembolism LD: 15 mg by mouth twice daily × 21 days MD: 20 mg by mouth once daily with food Atrial fibrillation 15 or 20 mg by mouth daily Dose adjustment required in patients with renal dysfunction.	6-9 hours	No monitoring for therapeutic effect needed	Avoid use if CrCl < 15 mL/min Avoid combined P-gp and strong CYP3A inducers or inhibitors

(Continued)

TABLE 14–2 Therapeutic approach to heparin resistance management and alternative anticoagulation strategies. (Continued)

	Dose	Half-life	Monitoring	Considerations
Apixaban	Venous thromboembolism LD: 10 mg by mouth twice daily × 7 days MD: 5 mg by mouth twice daily Atrial fibrillation 2.5 or 5 mg by mouth twice daily Dose adjustment required in select patients.	8-12 h	No monitoring for therapeutic effect needed	Considered safe for use in patients with renal impairment Avoid concurrent use of combined P-gp and strong CYP3A4 inducers. Dose adjustment required (for doses ≥5 mg) or use avoided (for doses ≤ 2.5 mg) if concurrent use of combined P-gp and strong CYP3A4 inhibitors.
Dabigatran	Venous thromboembolism 150 mg by mouth twice daily Atrial fibrillation 75 or 150 mg by mouth twice daily Dose adjustment required in patients with renal dysfunction.	12-14 h	No monitoring for therapeutic effect needed	Capsule should be taken whole, not crushed or chewed For treatment of VTE only after 5-10 days of a parenteral anticoagulant Avoid concomitant use with P-gp inducers Dose adjustment may be required in patients with concomitant P-gp inhibitors and renal impairment

Abbreviations: aPTT, activated partial thromboplastin time; ATIII, antithrombin III; CrCl, creatinine clearance; CYP, cytochrome P; FDA, Food and Drug Administration; INR, international normalized ratio; IV, intravenous; LD, loading dose; MD, maintenance dose; P-gp, P-glycoprotein; VTE, venous thromboembolism.

*Estimated bivalirudin half-life in normal renal function.

+Off-label dosing based on case reports of treatment of heparin resistance in cardiac surgery.

¯CrCl < 50 mL/min reduce rivaroxaban dose to 15 mg once daily, apixaban dose adjustment criteria for atrial fibrillation to 2.5 mg twice daily if ≥2 of the following criteria are met: age > 80 years, weight < 60 kg, or serum creatinine > 1.5, CrCl < 15-30 mL/min dose reduce dabigatran 75 mg twice daily.

normalized ratio (INR) making for a complex bridge to warfarin therapy. For patients bridged to warfarin therapy while receiving direct thrombin inhibitors therapy, chromogenic factor X monitoring should be utilized during concomitant use (a chromogenic factor X activity of 20%-40% corresponds to a usual warfarin INR of 2.0-3.0). Low molecular weight heparins and fondaparinux are antithrombin-dependent anticoagulants and should be avoided if true heparin resistance is suspected.

Heparin Resistance: Antithrombin III Repletion

In patients with known ATIII deficiency, therapeutic anticoagulation can be achieved by switching to an alternative non-ATIII-mediated anticoagulant (eg, direct thrombin inhibitors) or antithrombin III repletion with either fresh frozen plasma (FFP) or antithrombin III concentrate while continuing unfractionated heparin therapy. The normal range for ATIII is 80% to 120%, with consideration to supplementation when levels are less than 60%. Several case reports and small retrospective studies have reported increased heparin sensitivity as monitored by activated clotting time after administration of two to three units FFP.[15–17] Overall, there is a paucity of evidence to support the treatment of heparin resistance with FFP. Risks associated with FFP include immunologic and transfusion reactions, transfusion-related acute lung injury (TRALI), volume overload, and infectious complications.[18] Administration of antithrombin III concentrate has been studied more extensively, including several prospective randomized controlled trials.[19] Antithrombin III supplementation is available as recombinant antithrombin III (ATryn) and plasma-derived antithrombin III (Thrombate). Plasma-derived antithrombin III is approved by the United States Food and Drug Administration (FDA) for the treatment and prevention of thromboembolism, and prevention of perioperative and peripartum thromboembolism, in patients with hereditary antithrombin deficiency.[20] Per package insert, initial loading dose is based off of baseline antithrombin III% level and readministered every 12 to 24 hours as needed to achieve an antithrombin III level 80% to 120% of normal.[20] Recombinant antithrombin III is currently approved by the FDA for the prevention of perioperative and peripartum thromboembolic events in hereditary antithrombin-deficient patients and is not indicated for the treatment of thromboembolic events in hereditary antithrombin deficiency per package insert.[21] In patients with heparin resistance undergoing cardiac surgery, recombinant antithrombin III has been studied as a single IV bolus dose 75 IU/kg to treat heparin resistance during cardiac surgery.[19] While antithrombin III concentrate avoids many of the risks and limitations of FFP noted above, it is several-fold more expensive than FFP.[19]

It should be noted that most literature to date on this subject is in patients undergoing cardiac surgery and whether one treatment strategy is more effective and/or safer in the neurocritically ill patient population is unknown.

AVAILABLE GUIDELINES

There are no guidelines for the diagnosis and practical management of the heparin anticoagulants in the NeuroICU, and most of the literature is extrapolated from cardiovascular literature.

REFERENCES

1. Smythe MA, Priziola J, Dobesh PP, Wirth D, Cuker A, Wittkowsky AK. Guidance for the practical management of the heparin anticoagulants in the treatment of venous thromboembolism. *J Thromb Thrombolysis.* 2016;41(1):165–86. doi:10.1007/s11239-015-1315-2
2. Avidan MS, Levy JH, Scholz J, et al. A phase III, double-blind, placebo-controlled, multicenter study on the efficacy of recombinant human antithrombin in heparin-resistant patients scheduled to undergo cardiac surgery necessitating cardiopulmonary bypass. *Anesthesiology.* 2005;102(2):276–84. doi:10.1097/00000542-200502000-00007
3. Fetters L, Sirianni S. Off target: case report of heparin resistance in a neurosurgical intensive care unit patient. *Crit Care Nurse.* 2021;41(3):33–41. doi:10.4037/ccn2021303
4. Aksan N, Samaniego E, Shaban A, et al. Abstract TMP18: heparin resistance is an independent predictor of poor outcome in cerebral venous sinus thrombosis. *Stroke.* 49(Suppl_1):ATMP18–ATMP18. doi:10.1161/str.49.suppl_1.TMP18
5. Levy JH, Connors JM. Heparin resistance—clinical perspectives and management strategies. *N Engl J Med.* 2021;385(9):826–32. doi:10.1056/NEJMra2104091
6. Association of changes in antithrombin activity over time with responsiveness to enoxaparin prophylaxis and risk of trauma-related venous thromboembolism | surgery | JAMA surgery | JAMA network. Accessed November 9, 2022. https://jamanetwork.com/journals/jamasurgery/article-abstract/2793540
7. Meng R, Li ZY, Ji X, Ding Y, Meng S, Wang X. Antithrombin III associated with fibrinogen predicts the risk of cerebral ischemic stroke. *Clin Neurol Neurosurg.* 2011;113(5):380–6. doi:10.1016/j.clineuro.2010.12.016
8. Neutrophil extracellular traps exacerbate neurological deficits after traumatic brain injury. |*Sci Adv.* Accessed November 9, 2022. https://www.science.org/doi/10.1126/sciadv.aax8847
9. Müther M, Schwindt W, Mesters RM, et al. Andexanet-alfa-associated heparin resistance in the context of hemorrhagic stroke. *Neurocrit Care.* 2022;37(2):372–6. doi:10.1007/s12028-022-01573-5
10. Watson CJ, Zettervall SL, Hall MM, Ganetsky M. Difficult intraoperative heparinization following andexanet alfa administration. *Clin Pract Cases Emerg Med.* 2019;3(4):390–4. doi:10.5811/cpcem.2019.9.43650
11. Erdoes G, Birschmann I, Nagler M, Koster A. Andexanet alfa-induced heparin resistance: when anticoagulation really remains reversed. *J Cardiothorac Vasc Anesth.* 2021;35(3):908–9. doi:10.1053/j.jvca.2020.11.052
12. Goyal G, Bhatt VR. L-asparaginase and venous thromboembolism in acute lymphocytic leukemia. *Future Oncol.* 2015;11(17):2459–70. doi:10.2217/fon.15.114
13. Vera-Aguilera J, Yousef H, Beltran-Melgarejo D, et al. Clinical scenarios for discordant anti-Xa. *Adv Hematol.* 2016;2016:4054806. doi:10.1155/2016/4054806
14. Levine MN, Hirsh J, Gent M, et al. A randomized trial comparing activated thromboplastin time with heparin assay in patients with acute venous thromboembolism requiring large daily doses of heparin. *Arch Intern Med.* 1994;154(1):49–56.
15. Leong CK, Ong BC. A case report of heparin resistance due to acquired antithrombin III deficiency. *Ann Acad Med Singapore.* 1998;27(6):877–9.
16. Soloway HB, Christiansen TW. Heparin anticoagulation during cardiopulmonary bypass in an antithrombin-III deficient patient. Implications relative to the etiology of heparin rebound. *Am J Clin Pathol.* 1980;73(5):723–5. doi:10.1093/ajcp/73.5.723
17. Sabbagh AH, Chung GK, Shuttleworth P, Applegate BJ, Gabrhel W. Fresh frozen plasma: a solution to heparin resistance during cardiopulmonary bypass. *Ann Thorac Surg.* 1984;37(6):466–8. doi:10.1016/s0003-4975(10)61132-0
18. Norda R, Tynell E, Akerblom O. Cumulative risks of early fresh frozen plasma, cryoprecipitate and platelet transfusion in Europe. *J Trauma.* 2006;60(6 Suppl):S41–5. doi:10.1097/01.ta.0000199546.22925.31
19. Spiess BD. Treating heparin resistance with antithrombin or fresh frozen plasma. *Ann Thorac Surg.* 2008;85(6):2153–60. doi:10.1016/j.athoracsur.2008.02.037
20. Thrombate III [Antithrombin III (Human)] [Package Insert]. Triangle Park, NC: Grifols Therapeutics, Inc. https://Www.Fffenterprises.Com/Assets/Downloads/Product-Information/Grifols/Pi-THROMBATE-III.Pdf. January 2019.
21. Antithrombin (Recombinant) (ATryn) [Package Insert]. Framingham, MA: GTC Biotherapeutics, Inc. https://Www.Fda.Gov/Media/75529/Download. February 3, 2009.

CHAPTER

15

How Do We Differentiate ARDS from Neurogenic Pulmonary Edema?

Shaurya Taran, MD, Victoria McCredie, MBChB, PhD, & Eddy Fan, MD, PhD

Case

A 53-year-old woman presents to the emergency department with sudden-onset severe headache, loss of consciousness, and concern for possible aspiration. She is intubated for airway protection. Computed tomography reveals diffuse subarachnoid hemorrhage (SAH) with intraventricular extension; the culprit lesion is identified as a ruptured anterior communicating artery aneurysm. A bedside external ventricular drain is placed, with an opening cerebrospinal fluid pressure of 29 cm H_2O. The culprit aneurysm is endovascularly coiled without complication. On post-ictus day 1, the patient develops progressive hypoxemic respiratory failure in the intensive care unit. Bedside chest x-ray demonstrates bilateral, four-quadrant alveolar, and interstitial airspace opacities. Bloodwork is significant for elevated high-sensitivity troponin and B-type natriuretic peptide. What is the cause of this patient's respiratory decline?

Key points

- Neurogenic pulmonary edema (NPE) and acute respiratory distress syndrome (ARDS) are important pulmonary complications of devastating neurologic injury. While there is considerable overlap between the two conditions in their clinical presentation, pathophysiology, and management, there are also important differences. Proper recognition of the underlying condition can help clinicians select appropriate treatments and understand and communicate details about expected trajectory.
- NPE typically develops within minutes to hours in patients with severe brain injury and elevated intracranial pressure (ICP) and presents as hypoxemic respiratory failure in the setting of bilateral airspace opacifications. ARDS is diagnosed in the setting of hypoxemic respiratory failure not attributable to volume overload or cardiogenic pulmonary edema, occurring within 1 week of a recognized clinical insult. Chest imaging demonstrates bilateral airspace disease.
- Management of NPE and ARDS involves judicious volume management, ventilation with low tidal volumes and moderate levels of positive end-expiratory pressures (PEEP) (with careful attention to ICP), and appropriate use of sedation and/or neuromuscular blockade to facilitate safe lung ventilation. Prone position ventilation may be considered in patients with moderate-to-severe hypoxemic respiratory failure, balancing the risk of a potential increase in ICP.

BACKGROUND

Pulmonary complications are common in patients with acute neurologic injuries and are a major driver of increased morbidity and mortality.[1,2] Among the most clinically important pulmonary pathologies encountered in the neuro-intensive care unit are NPE and the ARDS.[3] Both conditions share common risk factors and pathophysiologic mechanisms. Treatment priorities involve avoidance of injurious mechanical ventilation, conservative fluid management, and (specifically relevant to neurologic patients) avoidance of extremes in partial pressure of oxygen (PaO_2) and carbon dioxide ($PaCO_2$).[4,5] However, there are also key differences in clinical presentation, overall trajectory, and occasionally underlying treatments. This chapter will provide an overview of NPE and ARDS with the goal of highlighting their similarities, differences, and management considerations.

Definitions, Pathophysiology, and Causes

NPE is defined as alveolar and interstitial edema occurring as a direct result of a central nervous system insult, and following the exclusion of other plausible causes of respiratory failure.[6,7] NPE is most commonly observed after SAH, traumatic brain injury (TBI), and intracerebral hemorrhage (ICH).[6] The incidence of NPE varies by etiology, with studies reporting a rate of up to 71% in deceased patients with SAH,[8] 50% in deceased patients with TBI,[9] and 35% in patients with ICH.[10] NPE can also occur in patients with status epilepticus, spinal cord injury and infarction, multiple sclerosis, arteriovenous malformations, and meningoencephalitis.[6] The most consistent risk factor for NPE is the severity of neurologic injury. Animal studies have shown that the risk of NPE is proportional to the level of ICP,[11] but raised ICP is not a necessary condition.[12]

NPE is thought to be mediated by a transient but massive sympathetic discharge that occurs rapidly after neurologic injury, which leads to increased pulmonary venoconstriction via local effects on the pulmonary vascular bed, increased venous return to the right heart via systemic venoconstriction, and increased left atrial pressure due to myocardial stunning or elevated left ventricular afterload.[13] These processes cause an increase in pulmonary capillary hydrostatic pressure, which causes transudation of fluid into the lung parenchyma. According to the "blast theory," the initial rapid increase in pulmonary hydrostatic pressure also promotes direct capillary damage, with subsequent leakage of an exudate containing protein and red blood cells.[14] However, it is debated whether pulmonary hypertension is a necessary precondition for NPE (studies in animal models have demonstrated NPE in its absence),[15] and it is likely that additional mechanisms are involved, including endothelial injury from inflammatory cytokines and neurologically-induced endothelial dysfunction.[16,17]

By contrast, ARDS is a complex clinical syndrome characterized by diffuse lung inflammation and alveolar damage that occurs due to direct pulmonary injury or a systemic process.[18,19] Specific causes of ARDS include sepsis, major trauma, aspiration, pneumonia, severe pancreatitis, and blood transfusions.[19,20] Whereas NPE lacks widely validated diagnostic criteria, ARDS can be diagnosed clinically using the Berlin definition.[21] By these criteria, the presence of bilateral pulmonary infiltrates occurring within 1 week of a known clinical insult, resulting in hypoxemic respiratory failure (defined as a ratio of partial pressure of oxygen to fraction of inspired oxygen concentration ($PaO_2/FiO_2 \leq 300$ mm Hg), and not fully explained by fluid overload or cardiac failure, establishes a diagnosis of ARDS.[21] The Berlin definition also enables classification of ARDS severity according to PaO_2/FiO_2 (mild, $200 < PaO_2/FiO_2 \leq 300$; moderate, $100 < PaO_2/FiO_2 \leq 200$; severe, ≤ 100).

The global burden of ARDS is high. In an observational study involving 459 intensive care units (ICUs) across 50 countries, ARDS was found to account for 10.4% of all ICU admissions and 23.4% of all patients requiring mechanical ventilation.[22] ARDS is also a common complication of brain injury, with studies demonstrating an incidence of 22% to 31% in patients with TBI, SAH, and ICH.[23-26] Among patients with TBI, ARDS is associated with longer durations of ICU admission, increased mortality, and worse neurologic outcomes.[25,27]

Similar to NPE, in which brain injury activates mechanisms that lead to downstream pulmonary injury, the development of ARDS in brain-injured patients is partly the result of a complex cross-talk between the brain and lungs.[3] Devastating brain injury primes the lungs to injury via a cascade of sympathetic and inflammatory mediators, such that a second "hit" which in other contexts would be well-tolerated, may lead to ARDS in this population.[3] However, compared to NPE, ARDS has a more complex pathophysiology that involves distinct phases. The acute, exudative phase is characterized by interstitial and alveolar edema, neutrophil and macrophage accumulation, and hyaline membrane formation. The subacute, proliferative and chronic, fibrotic phases are characterized by resolution of the neutrophilic infiltrate and progressive deposition of collagen and fibroblasts, respectively.[20]

EVIDENCE AND REVIEW

Clinical Presentation, Diagnosis, and Trajectory

Precise differentiation between NPE and ARDS is often challenging and both conditions can coexist. NPE has even been considered to represent a subtype of ARDS per the Berlin definition.[6] Nevertheless, certain features in the clinical presentation, radiographic appearance, and time course may help to differentiate NPE from ARDS.

NPE is characterized by its abrupt onset following neurologic injury, with clinical symptoms typically developing within minutes to hours of the initial insult.[28] Patients present with acute onset of dyspnea, tachypnea, hemoptysis, or pink frothy sputum and exhibit crackles to chest auscultation. Laboratory investigations may demonstrate elevations in troponin and B-type natriuretic peptide, although these are not specific to NPE.[29] Arterial blood gas analysis demonstrates hypoxemia. The electrocardiogram may be entirely normal or may show typical patterns associated with brain injury, such as deep T waves and ST segment changes.[7] Chest radiographs show bilateral, homogenous airspace opacities.[30] Transthoracic echocardiography may demonstrate impaired contractility, elevated left atrial pressure, and wall motion abnormalities, but may also be normal. Lung ultrasonography can demonstrate B-lines indicative of pulmonary edema.[31] NPE usually resolves within 48 to 72 hours of development, although it may persist in cases of ongoing severe ICP elevation.[6]

The clinical presentation of patients with ARDS is variable and relates to the underlying cause. Patients may present with tachypnea, dyspnea, tachycardia, and cyanosis. Presence of cough, sputum, and wheezing may be seen but are not consistent, and often relate to the underlying cause. Bloodwork is nonspecific and can show general signs of an inflammatory response (eg, leukocytosis with left shift) or shock (eg, elevated lactate). Arterial blood gas analysis demonstrates hypoxemia. Chest radiography demonstrates diffuse bilateral, coalescent opacities usually developing within 12 to 24 hours of the initial insult. X-rays obtained during later stages of ARDS may demonstrate an underlying reticular pattern related to progression of fibrosis.[32] Lung ultrasonography may demonstrate consolidation, pleural effusions, and B-lines.[33] Computed tomography typically shows dense consolidations in the dependent lung zones with surrounding ground-glass opacifications.[34] Clinically, ARDS evolves over a variable time course and can have manifestations lasting from days to weeks, in contrast to NPE. Additional similarities and differences are summarized in Table 15–1.

Medical Management

Key priorities in treating NPE include managing the precipitating neurologic condition and decreasing raised ICP. Halting secondary brain injury processes may attenuate the sympathetic discharge that is thought to drive NPE.[35] Neurocritical care best practices should be considered in all brain-injured patients, including head-of-bed elevation to 30° to 45°, avoidance of hyperthermia, promoting venous return from the brain by keeping the head midline and assessing fit of cervical collars, and maintaining systemic blood pressure targets (or cerebral perfusion pressure [CPP] targets in TBI). Elevated ICP should be managed with a tiered therapy approach including osmotherapy, increasing sedation, cerebrospinal fluid drainage, maintenance of $PaCO_2$ at lower end of normal, and neurosurgical evacuation of space-occupying lesions.[36] Management of pulmonary edema is achieved with judicious use of diuretics, minimizing fluid administration, and reducing left ventricular afterload. Care must be

TABLE 15–1 A comparison of NPE and ARDS.

Variable	NPE	ARDS
Etiology and risk factors	• Can occur after any devastating neurologic injury • Common causes include TBI, SAH, ICH, and status epilepticus	• Variable risk factors include trauma, aspiration, sepsis, blood transfusions, pancreatitis, and severe burns
Pathophysiology	• Neurologic injury induces a sympathetic surge with hydrostatic pressure-induced transudation of fluid into lungs; this is followed by capillary injury and fluid exudation	• Inflammatory cytokines recruit cell mediators to the lungs that cause capillary injury and diffuse alveolar damage • Capillary endothelial injury allows buildup of a protein-rich fluid into lungs • Subsequent stages involve collagen deposition and lung fibrosis
Clinical presentation and timing	• Dyspnea, tachycardia, and pink frothy sputum are common • Symptoms usually develop within minutes to hours of neurologic injury • Can occur in delayed fashion after 24-48 h	• Occurs within 7 days of inciting factor • Variable presentation includes fever, dyspnea, cough, and wheezing • Clinical signs can give a clue to the etiology (eg, productive cough may indicate pneumonia)
Laboratory and diagnostic features	• May see elevation in troponin and BNP • ECG may reveal ST changes and deep T waves • Arterial blood gases show variable degrees of hypoxemia	• Nonspecific lab abnormalities may include leukocytosis with left shift and elevated inflammatory markers • Arterial blood gases show variable degrees of hypoxemia
Radiographic features	• Chest radiographs demonstrate bilateral alveolar opacities • Echocardiographic findings may include wall motion abnormalities, stunned myocardium, and elevated left atrial pressure • Lung ultrasound may show B-lines	• Early chest radiographs indicate bilateral alveolar and interstitial opacities • After 7-10 days, radiographs demonstrate a coarse reticular pattern • Echocardiographic findings include right ventricular dysfunction and elevated right-sided pressures • Lung ultrasound may show B-lines and pleural thickening • CT scans may show dependent consolidation surrounded by areas of ground glass attenuation
Time course	• Typically resolves within 48-72 h of onset • Can persist for longer with more severe neurologic injuries • No data on long-term sequelae	• Variable time course ranging from days with mild ARDS, to weeks with severe ARDS • Multiple long-term sequelae include post-traumatic stress disorder and functional impairments

ARDS, acute respiratory distress syndrome; BNP, B-type natriuretic peptide; CT, computed tomography; ECG, electrocardiogram; ICH, intracranial hemorrhage; ICP, intracranial pressure; NPE, neurogenic pulmonary edema; SAH, subarachnoid hemorrhage; TBI, traumatic brain injury.

taken to ensure that volume management strategies do not compromise cardiac output and CPP. In patients with SAH who develop delayed cerebral ischemia, the potential risks of diuresis (eg, worsening ischemia to vulnerable brain regions) must be weighed against pulmonary benefits (eg, improving respiratory system compliance and hypoxemia). Fluid management may be guided by transpulmonary thermodilution or peripherally inserted continuous cardiac output (PiCCO) monitoring, but experience in patients with NPE is currently limited to case reports.[37,38] Inotropic agents such as dobutamine or milrinone may be used in cases where NPE is complicated by reduced left ventricular performance. Finally, sympathetic blockade with alpha antagonists such as phentolamine and chlorpromazine has been described in rat models and one human case report, with improvement reported in pulmonary edema.[39,40] The proposed mechanism is interruption of the underlying sympathetic discharge that promotes NPE.[6] Routine treatment with these agents is not currently advised given lack of good evidence for their use.

Medical management of ARDS should focus on treating the underlying precipitant. General additional supportive considerations include conservative fluid management, corticosteroids, and neuromuscular antagonists. A detailed review of these strategies is beyond the scope of this chapter but has been addressed in recent reviews.[32,41] Briefly, a conservative fluid management strategy was found in a landmark clinical trial to improve oxygenation and reduce duration of mechanical ventilation compared to a liberal fluid strategy.[42] In brain-injured patients, fluid management should be guided by additional considerations, including maintenance of CPP, and a balance must be sought between excessive diuresis (with possible compromise of CPP) and volume overload (with possible compromise of oxygenation). Corticosteroids may potentially reduce mortality from ARDS, including in ARDS resulting from COVID-19.[43] However, corticosteroids should not be administered in patients with severe TBI, given that steroid use in this context is associated with increased short- and long-term mortality.[44,45] Neuromuscular antagonists may be considered in patients with moderate to severe ARDS if required to facilitate safe ventilation, and after optimization of sedation.[46]

Ventilatory Management

Most patients with NPE or ARDS and concomitant neurologic injury will require invasive mechanical ventilation to correct hypoxemia and establish safe lung ventilation. Noninvasive ventilation (NIV) might occasionally be considered in patients with mild ARDS[47]; however, there are concerns regarding increased mortality associated with NIV in patients with moderate to severe ARDS.[48] In brain-injured patients with ARDS, low Glasgow Coma Score at presentation, ongoing brain injury, raised ICP, and the need for tight control of PaO_2 and $PaCO_2$ often make NIV a poor choice for most patients. In patients with NPE, there is no evidence for use of NIV, and use of this modality should be considered on a case-by-case basis, if at all.

The majority of high-quality data for invasive mechanical ventilation derives from studies in ARDS patients without brain injury, where there is strong evidence to maintain tidal volumes within 4 to 8 mL/kg predicted body weight and consider prone position ventilation in cases of moderate to severe hypoxemic respiratory failure.[4] Higher PEEP may be beneficial in patients with moderate to severe ARDS.[49] These three cornerstones of therapy—low tidal volume ventilation, prone positioning, and appropriate use of PEEP—are deployed to attenuate the effects of ventilator-induced lung injury (VILI), which is an important mediator of excess morbidity and mortality in ARDS.[50]

The above treatments can be applied in brain-injured patients with ARDS or NPE, but clinicians should be mindful of important instances where brain- and lung-specific priorities may come into conflict.[5] Low tidal volume ventilation can lead to $PaCO_2$ elevation, which might in turn lead to elevation of ICP via downstream cerebral vasodilation. Prone positioning may also lead to increased ICP.[51] Both maneuvers appear to be less well-tolerated in patients with baseline ICP elevation, whereas they may be safe if ICP is controlled.[5] Higher levels of PEEP may lead to reduced venous return, systemic hypotension, and reduction of CPP.[52] PEEP also has complex effects on cerebral venous drainage and may potentially elevate ICP through a Starling resistor mechanism.[53] These challenges were summarized in a recent consensus statement from the European Society of Intensive Care Medicine (ESICM) on the ventilatory management of brain-injured patients.[5]

AVAILABLE GUIDELINES

Balancing the risks and benefits, the ESICM guideline suggests that brain-injured patients with ARDS and without significant ICP elevation should receive low tidal volume ventilation, similar to general cohorts of critically ill patients.[5] In patients with significant baseline ICP elevation, evidence is lacking for a particular tidal volume strategy; a practical suggestion might therefore be to aim for the lowest safe tidal volumes with careful attention to the $PaCO_2$, ICP, and respiratory system pressures. Regarding PEEP selection in brain-injured patients with ARDS, no specific recommendations exist to guide initial settings and subsequent titration.[5] PEEP should therefore be set aiming to optimize oxygenation and while monitoring for potential perturbations to ICP and CPP. In most patients, PEEP effects on ICP can be minimized by ensuring that PEEP remains lower than ICP. Prone positioning should be considered in patients with a $PaO_2/FiO_2 \leq 150$ mm Hg provided that ICP is not elevated, similar to patients without brain injury.[5] However, in patients with baseline ICP elevation, prone positioning may worsen ICP, and decisions to proceed should be made on a case-by-case basis, balancing the improvement in hypoxemia and lung stress with the potential for ICP increase.[54] Of note, wherever ICP is a concern, insertion of monitoring devices (eg, ventricular drains or parenchymal monitors) may assist with titration of tidal volume and PEEP.

While specific evidence for the ventilatory management of patients with NPE is lacking, the same general priorities as for patients with ARDS likely still apply. Low tidal volumes should be used with careful monitoring of $PaCO_2$ and ICP. PEEP should

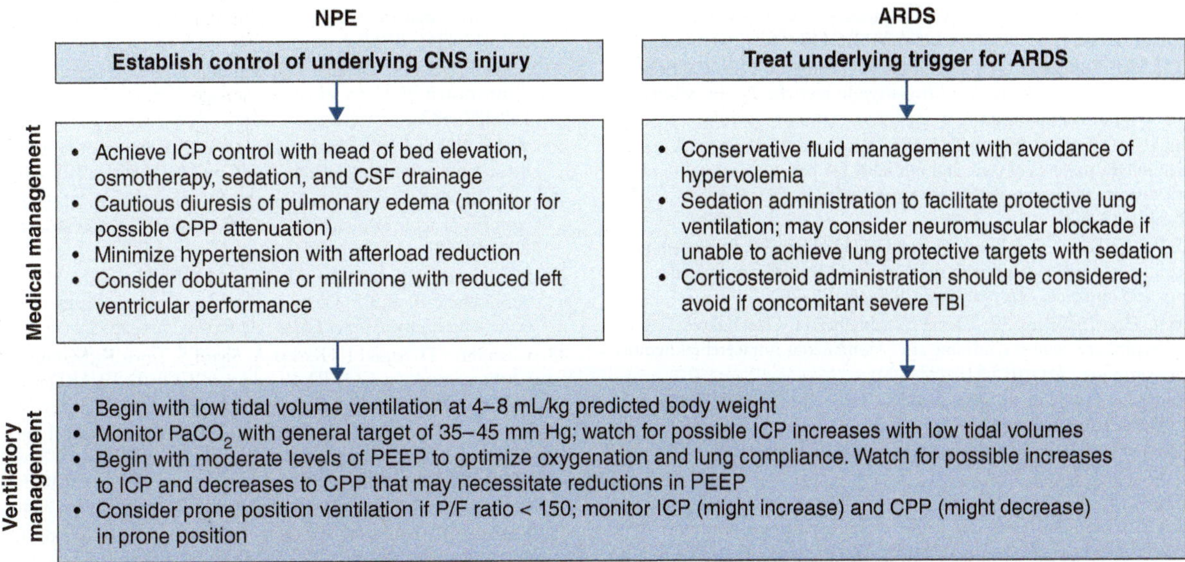

ARDS acute respiratory distress syndrome, CNS central nervous system, CPP cerebral perfusion pressure, CSF cerebrospinal fluid, ICP intracranial pressure, NPE neurogenic pulmonary edema, $PaCO_2$ arterial partial pressure of carbon dioxide, PEEP positive end expiratory pressure, TBI traumatic brain injury

FIGURE 15–1 Management algorithm for NPE and ARDS.

be applied with attention to systemic blood pressure, ICP, and CPP. Regarding prone positioning for NPE, data is currently limited to case reports.[55,56] However, there is a strong theoretical basis that prone positioning should improve hypoxemia and attenuate lung stress in NPE; it might therefore be considered in refractory cases, provided that there is no simultaneous concern for elevated ICP. These management considerations are highlighted in Figure 15–1.

CONCLUSION

NPE and ARDS are important pulmonary complications of devastating neurologic injury. While there is considerable overlap between the two conditions in their clinical presentation, pathophysiology, and management, there are also important differences. Proper recognition of the underlying condition can help clinicians select appropriate treatments and understand and communicate details about expected trajectory.

REFERENCES

1. Lee K, Rincon F. Pulmonary complications in patients with severe brain injury. *Crit Care Res Pract.* 2012;2012:207247.
2. Pelosi P, Ferguson ND, Frutos-Vivar F, Anzueto A, Putensen C, Raymondos K, et al. Management and outcome of mechanically ventilated neurologic patients. *Crit Care Med.* 2011;39:1482–1492.
3. Mrozek S, Constantin J-M, Geeraerts T. Brain-lung crosstalk: Implications for neurocritical care patients. *World J Crit Care Med.* 2015;4: 163–178.
4. Fan E, Del Sorbo L, Goligher EC, Hodgson CL, Munshi L, Walkey AJ, et al. An official American Thoracic Society/European Society of Intensive Care Medicine/Society of Critical Care Medicine Clinical Practice Guideline: mechanical ventilation in adult patients with acute respiratory distress syndrome. *Am J Respir Crit Care Med.* 2017;195:1253–1263.
5. Robba C, Poole D, McNett M, Asehnoune K, Bösel J, Bruder N, et al. Mechanical ventilation in patients with acute brain injury: recommendations of the European Society of Intensive Care Medicine consensus. *Intensive Care Med.* 2020;46:2397–2410.
6. Davison DL, Terek M, Chawla LS. Neurogenic pulmonary edema. *Crit Care.* 2012;16:212.
7. O'Leary R, McKinlay J. Neurogenic pulmonary oedema. *Continuing Education in Anaesthesia Critical Care & Pain.* 2011;11:87–92.
8. Weir BK. Pulmonary edema following fatal aneurysm rupture. *J Neurosurg.* 1978;49:502–507.
9. Rogers FB, Shackford SR, Trevisani GT, Davis JW, Mackersie RC, Hoyt DB. Neurogenic pulmonary edema in fatal and nonfatal head injuries. *J Trauma.* 1995;39:860–866; discussion 866-868.
10. Junttila E, Ala-Kokko T, Ohtonen P, Vaarala A, Karttunen A, Vuolteenaho O, et al. Neurogenic pulmonary edema in patients with nontraumatic intracerebral hemorrhage: predictors and association with outcome. *Anesth Analg.* 2013;116:855–861.
11. Gupta YK, Chugh A, Kacker V, Mehta VS, Tandon PN. Development of neurogenic pulmonary edema at different grades of intracranial pressure in cats. *Indian J Physiol Pharmacol.* 1998;42:71–80.
12. Popp AJ, Shah DM, Berman RA, Paloski WH, Newell JC, Cooper JA, et al. Delayed pulmonary dysfunction in head-injured patients. *J Neurosurg.* 1982;57:784–790.
13. Smith WS, Matthay MA. Evidence for a hydrostatic mechanism in human neurogenic pulmonary edema. *Chest.* 1997;111:1326–1333.
14. Theodore J, Robin ED. Speculations on neurogenic pulmonary edema (NPE). *Am Rev Respir Dis.* 1976;113:405–411.
15. Bowers RE, McKeen CR, Park BE, Brigham KL. Increased pulmonary vascular permeability follows intracranial hypertension in sheep. *Am Rev Respir Dis.* 1979;119:637–641.
16. Touho H, Karasawa J, Shishido H, Yamada K, Yamazaki Y. Neurogenic pulmonary edema in the acute stage of hemorrhagic cerebrovascular disease. *Neurosurgery.* 1989;25:762–768.
17. Mackersie RC, Christensen JM, Pitts LH, Lewis FR. Pulmonary extravascular fluid accumulation following intracranial injury. *J Trauma.* 1983;23:968–975.
18. Fan E, Brodie D, Slutsky AS. Acute respiratory distress syndrome: advances in diagnosis and treatment. *JAMA.* 2018;319:698–710.
19. Thompson BT, Chambers RC, Liu KD. Acute respiratory distress syndrome. *N Engl J Med.* 2017;377:562–572.

20. Matthay MA, Zemans RL. The acute respiratory distress syndrome: pathogenesis and treatment. *Annu Rev Pathol.* 2011;6:147–163.
21. Ranieri VM, Rubenfeld GD, Thompson BT, Ferguson ND, Caldwell E, Fan E, et al. Acute respiratory distress syndrome: the Berlin definition. *JAMA.* 2012;307:2526–2533.
22. Bellani G, Laffey JG, Pham T, Fan E, Brochard L, Esteban A, et al. Epidemiology, patterns of care, and mortality for patients with acute respiratory distress syndrome in intensive care units in 50 countries. *JAMA.* 2016;315:788–800.
23. Kahn JM, Caldwell EC, Deem S, Newell DW, Heckbert SR, Rubenfeld GD. Acute lung injury in patients with subarachnoid hemorrhage: incidence, risk factors, and outcome. *Crit Care Med.* 2006;34:196–202.
24. Elmer J, Hou P, Wilcox SR, Chang Y, Schreiber H, Okechukwu I, et al. Acute respiratory distress syndrome after spontaneous intracerebral hemorrhage*. *Crit Care Med.* 2013;41:1992–2001.
25. Holland MC, Mackersie RC, Morabito D, Campbell AR, Kivett VA, Patel R, et al. The development of acute lung injury is associated with worse neurologic outcome in patients with severe traumatic brain injury. *J Trauma.* 2003;55:106–111.
26. Rincon F, Ghosh S, Dey S, Maltenfort M, Vibbert M, Urtecho J, et al. Impact of acute lung injury and acute respiratory distress syndrome after traumatic brain injury in the United States. *Neurosurgery.* 2012;71:795–803.
27. Hendrickson CM, Howard BM, Kornblith LZ, Conroy AS, Nelson MF, Zhuo H, et al. The acute respiratory distress syndrome following isolated severe traumatic brain injury. *J Trauma Acute Care Surg.* 2016; 80:989–997.
28. Fontes RB, Aguiar PH, Zanetti MV, Andrade F, Mandel M, Teixeira MJ. Acute neurogenic pulmonary edema: case reports and literature review. *J Neurosurg Anesthesiol.* 2003;15:144–150.
29. Meaudre E, Polycarpe A, Pernod G, Salinier L, Cantais E, Bruder N. Contribution of the brain natriuretic peptide in neurogenic pulmonary oedema following subarachnoid haemorrhage. *Ann Fr Anesth Reanim.* 2004;23:1076–1079.
30. Gluecker T, Capasso P, Schnyder P, Gudinchet F, Schaller MD, Revelly JP, et al. Clinical and radiologic features of pulmonary edema. *Radiographics.* 1999;19:1507–1531; discussion 1532–1533.
31. Merenkov VV, Kovalev AN, Gorbunov VV. Bedside lung ultrasound: a case of neurogenic pulmonary edema. *Neurocrit Care.* 2013;18:391–394.
32. Matthay MA, Zemans RL, Zimmerman GA, Arabi YM, Beitler JR, Mercat A, et al. Acute respiratory distress syndrome. *Nat Rev Dis Primers.* 2019;5:18.
33. Chiumello D, Umbrello M, Sferrazza Papa GF, Angileri A, Gurgitano M, Formenti P, et al. Global and regional diagnostic accuracy of lung ultrasound compared to CT in patients with acute respiratory distress syndrome. *Crit Care Med.* 2019;47:1599–1606.
34. Sheard S, Rao P, Devaraj A. Imaging of acute respiratory distress syndrome. *Respir Care.* 2012;57:607–612.
35. Busl KM, Bleck TP. Neurogenic pulmonary edema. *Crit Care Med.* 2015;43:1710–1715.
36. Hawryluk GWJ, Aguilera S, Buki A, Bulger E, Citerio G, Cooper DJ, et al. A management algorithm for patients with intracranial pressure monitoring: the Seattle International Severe Traumatic Brain Injury Consensus Conference (SIBICC). *Intensive Care Med.* 2019;45:1783–1794.
37. Mutoh T, Kazumata K, Ueyama-Mutoh T, Taki Y, Ishikawa T. Transpulmonary thermodilution-based management of neurogenic pulmonary edema after subarachnoid hemorrhage. *Am J Med Sci.* 2015;350:415–419.
38. Lin X, Xu Z, Wang P, Xu Y, Zhang G. Role of PiCCO monitoring for the integrated management of neurogenic pulmonary edema following traumatic brain injury: a case report and literature review. *Exp Ther Med.* 2016;12:2341–2347.
39. Schraufnagel DE, Thakkar MB. Pulmonary venous sphincter constriction is attenuated by alpha-adrenergic antagonism. *Am Rev Respir Dis.* 1993; 148:477–482.
40. Wohns RN, Tamas L, Pierce KR, Howe JF. Chlorpromazine treatment for neurogenic pulmonary edema. *Crit Care Med* 1985;13:210–211.
41. Fernando SM, Ferreyro BL, Urner M, Munshi L, Fan E. Diagnosis and management of acute respiratory distress syndrome. *Can Med Assoc J.* 2021;193: E761–E768.
42. Wiedemann HP, Wheeler AP, Bernard GR, Thompson BT, Hayden D, deBoisblanc B, et al. Comparison of two fluid-management strategies in acute lung injury. *N Engl J Med.* 2006;354:2564–2575.
43. Chaudhuri D, Sasaki K, Karkar A, Sharif S, Lewis K, Mammen MJ, et al. Corticosteroids in COVID-19 and non-COVID-19 ARDS: a systematic review and meta-analysis. *Intensive Care Med.* 2021;47:521–537.
44. Roberts I, Yates D, Sandercock P, Farrell B, Wasserberg J, Lomas G, et al. Effect of intravenous corticosteroids on death within 14 days in 10008 adults with clinically significant head injury (MRC CRASH trial): randomised placebo-controlled trial. *Lancet.* 2004;364:1321–1328.
45. Edwards P, Arango M, Balica L, Cottingham R, El-Sayed H, Farrell B, et al. Final results of MRC CRASH, a randomised placebo-controlled trial of intravenous corticosteroid in adults with head injury-outcomes at 6 months. *Lancet.* 2005;365:1957–1959.
46. Alhazzani W, Belley-Cote E, Møller MH, Angus DC, Papazian L, Arabi YM, et al. Neuromuscular blockade in patients with ARDS: a rapid practice guideline. *Intensive Care Med.* 2020;46:1977–1986.
47. Ferguson ND, Fan E, Camporota L, Antonelli M, Anzueto A, Beale R, et al. The Berlin definition of ARDS: an expanded rationale, justification, and supplementary material. *Intensive Care Med.* 2012;38:1573–1582.
48. Bellani G, Laffey JG, Pham T, Madotto F, Fan E, Brochard L, et al. Noninvasive ventilation of patients with acute respiratory distress syndrome. Insights from the LUNG SAFE Study. *Am J Respir Crit Care Med.* 2017;195:67–77.
49. Briel M, Meade M, Mercat A, Brower RG, Talmor D, Walter SD, et al. Higher vs lower positive end-expiratory pressure in patients with acute lung injury and acute respiratory distress syndrome: systematic review and meta-analysis. *JAMA.* 2010;303:865–73.
50. Slutsky AS, Ranieri VM. Ventilator-induced lung injury. *N Engl J Med.* 2013;369:2126–2136.
51. Nekludov M, Bellander BM, Mure M. Oxygenation and cerebral perfusion pressure improved in the prone position. *Acta Anaesthesiol Scand.* 2006;50:932–936.
52. Georgiadis D, Schwarz S, Baumgartner RW, Veltkamp R, Schwab S. Influence of positive end-expiratory pressure on intracranial pressure and cerebral perfusion pressure in patients with acute stroke. *Stroke.* 2001;32:2088–2092.
53. Luce JM, Huseby JS, Kirk W, Butler J. A Starling resistor regulates cerebral venous outflow in dogs. *J Appl Physiol Respir Environ Exerc Physiol.* 1982;53:1496–1503.
54. Roth C, Ferbert A, Deinsberger W, Kleffmann J, Kästner S, Godau J, et al. Does prone positioning increase intracranial pressure? A retrospective analysis of patients with acute brain injury and acute respiratory failure. *Neurocrit Care.* 2014;21:186–191.
55. Fletcher SJ, Atkinson JD. Use of prone ventilation in neurogenic pulmonary oedema. *Br J Anaesth.* 2003;90:238–240.
56. Marshall SA, Nyquist P. A change of position for neurogenic pulmonary edema. *Neurocrit Care.* 2009;10:213–217.

CHAPTER

16

What Are Current Fluid Therapy Recommendations in Neurointensive Care Patients?

Henry Chang, MD, PhD, Salia Farrokh, PharmD, Ozan Akca, MD, & Sung-Min Cho, DO, MHS

Case

A 64-year-old man with hypertension, diabetes mellitus, and chronic kidney disease presented after roll-over motor vehicle accident and was found to have multicompartmental intracranial hemorrhages (ICHs), including a left holohemispheric subdural hematoma and bifrontal contusions. He underwent a left hemicraniectomy and placement of an intracranial pressure (ICP) monitor, with persistent ICPs > 30 mm of water. What hypertonic agents should be administered for treatment of elevated ICPs and how should this be monitored?

Key Points

- Crystalloids are the most commonly used fluids in the neurocritical care setting, while colloids further augment volume resuscitation.
- The choice of fluid should be considered in context of the patient's condition, including risk of exacerbating renal injury or systemic clotting.
- Hypertonic saline (HTS) expands systemic volume while mannitol causes diuresis to induce a hyperosmolar state, with evidence suggesting that HTS may be more effective at diminishing elevated ICP.
- Osmolar gap is preferred over serum osmolality threshold during monitoring with mannitol treatment.

BACKGROUND

Administration of intravenous fluids is a ubiquitous intervention across all pathologies encountered in the neurointensive care unit. However, data from high-quality studies to guide fluid therapy specific to these patient populations are scarce. Consequently, many common practices have been adopted from the general non-neurological intensive care unit (ICU) population, and current recommendations are often based on expert consensus rather than evidence-based medicine. This chapter reviews relevant studies for different types of fluid therapy as they apply to patients in the neurointensive care unit and highlights areas where such studies do not yet exist.

EVIDENCE AND REVIEW

General Principles

Crystalloids vs. Colloids

Crystalloid and colloid solutions are mainly differentiated by the molecular size of their components. Crystalloids, such as normal saline, lactated Ringer's solution, and plasmaLyte, are composed of small ions (Table 16–1), while colloids such as albumin, starches, dextrans, gelatins, and fresh frozen plasma contain larger molecular compounds.[1] The theoretical benefit of colloids is increased oncotic pressure promoting more effective volume expansion and resuscitation. However, a 2018 Cochrane meta-analysis of 69 studies (65 randomized controlled trials [RCTs], 4 quasi-RCTs) with 30,020 critically ill patients compared each of these colloids to crystalloids and found no difference in mortality at 30 days, 90 days, and end of follow-up.[2] An important caveat to consider is that a number of these trials excluded patients with pathologies typically encountered in the neurointensive care unit such as traumatic brain injury (TBI), stroke, ICH, and neurosurgical patients. That said, various dedicated studies in TBI,[3] acute ischemic stroke,[4] and subarachnoid hemorrhage (SAH)[5] patients have not shown conclusive benefits of albumin.

TABLE 16–1 Composition of commonly-used intravenous fluid solutions.

Fluid	Electrolytes (mEq/L)						Osmolarity (mOsm/L)	Estimated pH
	Sodium	Potassium	Chloride	Calcium	Magnesium	Buffer		
Normal saline	154	0	154	0	0	0	308	5.0-5.5
Lactated Ringers	130	4.5	109	3	0	Lactate: 28	275-280	6.50-6.75
Plasmalyte	140	5	98	0	3	Gluconate: 23 Acetate: 27	295	7.40
Albumin 5%	130-160	<2	0	0	0	0	290	7.40

In clinical practice, crystalloids are generally cheaper and more readily available, while colloids may induce allergic reactions, blood clotting disorders, and kidney injury.[2] Given these factors, and in the absence of any definitive studies showing clear superiority, crystalloids are often the fluid of choice in the ICU setting, including the neurointensive care unit. However, the use of colloids can still be justified in most neurointensive care patients—particularly at low concentration and at low doses, which seem to generally be safe. For example, the Surviving Sepsis Campaign guidelines recommend switching to albumin if crystalloids are unable to achieve mean arterial pressure (MAP) targets.[6] It is important to highlight that albumin should perhaps be avoided in TBI patients, as a subgroup analysis of 460 TBI patients in the 2004 Saline versus Albumin Fluid Evaluation (SAFE) study found that albumin was associated with higher mortality rates than normal saline (33.2% vs. 20.4% at 24 months, RR = 1.63, 95% CI = 1.17-2.26, p = .003)[3]; however, this conclusion remains somewhat controversial, as is discussed elsewhere in this chapter. The 2018 European Society of Intensive Medicine guidelines for fluid therapy recommends against colloids for resuscitation in neurointensive care patients, though the authors acknowledge this is based on low quality evidence.[7]

Balanced versus Unbalanced Crystalloids

Crystalloid solutions are usually categorized as either balanced (eg, lactated Ringer's solution and PlasmaLyte) or unbalanced (eg, normal saline). In the literature, this terminology is synonymous with buffered and unbuffered solutions. Compared to unbalanced solutions, balanced solutions contain a reduced amount of chloride ions (replaced, or "buffered," by a substitute anion such as lactate or acetate) and generally have an electrolyte composition more similar to human plasma.[8]

Mostly for historical reasons, normal saline has traditionally been the most commonly used fluid in critically ill patients.[9] Of late, due to concerns for hyperchloremia-induced metabolic acidosis[10] and acute kidney injury (AKI)[11] that may be associated with higher mortality, as well as the availability of other crystalloids, there has been much interest in the idea that balanced solutions may be preferred over unbalanced solutions.

However, the results from several large recent studies in ICU patients have been equivocal, with the Saline versus Plasma-Lyte for ICU fluid Therapy (SPLIT),[12] Balanced Solutions in Intensive Care Study (BASICS),[13] and Plasma-Lyte versus Saline Study (PLUS)[14] trials demonstrating no difference in mortality or AKI, and the Isotonic Solutions and Major Adverse Renal Events Trial (SMART)[15] showing only a modest reduction in incidence of AKI (and not mortality) with balanced solutions (Table 16–2). From a neurointensive care perspective, only two of the trials performed subgroup analysis of patients with nonspecific brain injury—the SPLIT trial, whose subgroup population sample size (n = 47) was too low to draw meaningful conclusions, and the BASICS trial, which showed an increased 90-day mortality with balanced solutions compared to unbalanced solutions (31.3% vs. 21.1%, HR = 1.48, 95% CI = 1.03-2.12, p = .02).

Hyperosmolar Therapy

Hyperosmolar therapy with either mannitol or HTS can be used for treatment of elevated intracranial pressure (ICP), though the mechanism—previously thought to be due to reduced brain volume—remains incompletely understood.[16] A pooled meta-analysis of five RCTs including a total of 112 patients showed that HTS administration was more effective than mannitol at controlling elevated ICP episodes (93% vs. 78% of episodes, RR = 1.16, 95% CI = 1.00-1.33, p = .046).[17] However, this evidence is not sufficient to make concrete conclusions about efficacy or to make strong recommendations regarding the choice of hyperosmolar agent.

At times, the hyperosmolar agent is chosen based on other physiological considerations. HTS causes systemic volume expansion while mannitol causes diuresis. In some scenarios, mannitol may induce acute renal failure,[18] while other studies suggest it acts as a free radical scavenger and inhibits programmed cell death.[19] Both brain injury and hyperosmolar therapy have been shown to disrupt the glycocalyx and cause expansion of endothelial pores.[20,21] It has been posited that colloids may leak into the parenchymal tissue and worsen ICP; in theory, larger molecular weight colloids may have lesser chance of extravasation, but this has yet to be proven in any studies.

Regardless of agent, the optimal use of hyperosmolar therapy is not well-defined. A common clinical practice is either fixed-dose mannitol injection or a serum sodium goal using a HTS infusion or bolus,[22] but this is not based on high-quality evidence. A serum osmolality threshold of 320 mOsm is frequently cited but controversial—in fact, a higher threshold

TABLE 16–2 Balanced versus unbalanced intravenous fluid studies in intensive care unit (ICU) patients.

	Entire Study Cohort				Brain injury subgroup cohort		
Study Name (year)	**Patient Population**	**Kidney Injury Outcome**	**Mortality Outcome**	**Volume Administered Median (mL) [IQR]**	**# Patients**	**Outcome**	**Limitations**
SPLIT[12] (2015)	Balanced (Plasmalyte): 1152 Unbalanced: 1110 4 medical/surgical ICUs in New Zealand 57% admitted to ICU after planned elective surgery	AKI within 90 days Balanced: 9.6% Unbalanced: 9.2% RR 1.04, 95% CI 0.80-1.36, $p = .77$	In-hospital mortality Balanced: 7.6% Unbalanced: 8.6% RR 0.88, 95% CI 0.67-1.17, $p = .40$	Day of enrollment: Balanced: 1250 [650-2500] Unbalanced: 1410 [750-2280] Over 90 days: Balanced: 2000 [1000-3500] Unbalanced: 2000 [1000-3250]	Balanced: 22 Unbalanced: 25	AKI within 90 days Balanced: 4.5% Unbalanced: 4.0% OR 1.50, 95% CI 0.09-26.00, $p = .91$	1) Lack of sample size calculations prior to trial design 2) >90% of patients received IV fluids prior to study enrollment 3) A high number of planned elective surgical admissions
SMART[15] (2018)	Balanced (lactated ringers or Plasmalyte): 7942 Unbalanced: 7860 Medical, surgical, cardiac, trauma, and neurological ICUs at Vanderbilt University Medical Center (Nashville, Tennessee)	AKI within 30 days Balanced: 14.3% Unbalanced: 15.4% OR 0.90, 95% CI 0.82-0.99, $p = .04$	30-day in-hospital mortality Balanced: 10.3% Unbalanced: 11.1% OR 0.90, 95% CI 0.80-1.01, $p = .06$	Over 30 days: Balanced: 1000 [0-3210] Unbalanced: 1020 [0-3500]	Fluid choice deferred to clinicians in patients with brain injury; no brain injury subgroup analysis	N/A	1) Investigators & clinicians not blinded to fluid choice 2) Single center study
BASICS[13] (2021)	Balanced (Plasmalyte): 5230 Unbalanced: 5290 75 ICUs in Brazil 48% admitted to ICU after planned elective surgery	AKI within 7 days Balanced: 23.6% Unbalanced: 23.5% OR 1.07, 95% CI 0.88-1.30	90-day mortality Balanced: 26.4% Unbalanced: 27.2% HR 0.97, 95% CI 0.90-1.05, $p = .47$	1st day: 1500 mL (both groups) First 3 days: 4100 mL (both groups)	Balanced: 249 Unbalanced: 237	90-day mortality Balanced: 31.3% Unbalanced: 21.1% HR 1.48, 95% CI 1.03-2.12, $p = 0.02$	A high number of planned surgical admissions may have reduced overall trial mortality
PLUS[14] (2022)	Balanced (Plasmalyte): 2515 Unbalanced : 2522 53 ICUs in Australia & New Zealand	New renal replacement therapy Balanced: 12.7% Unbalanced: 12.9% OR 0.98, 95% CI 0.83-1.16	90-day mortality Balanced: 21.8% Unbalanced: 22.0% OR 0.99, 95% CI 0.86-1.14	Balanced: 3900 [2000-6700] Unbalanced: 3700 [2000-6300]	Excluded patients with TBI or at risk for cerebral edema	N/A	1) Half of patients in balanced solutions group received >500 mL normal saline 2) Fluids given outside the ICU were not monitored

AKI, acute kidney injury; CI, confidence interval; HR, hazard ratio; ICP, intracranial pressure; ICU, intensive care unit; IQR, interquartile range; OR, odds ratio; RR, relative risk; TBI, traumatic brain injury.

(eg, 340 mOsm) may still be safe[23]—and hypernatremia to 150 to 160 mEq/L is commonly targeted, though again, not based on high-quality evidence. The 2020 NCS cerebral edema guidelines suggest using osmolar gap over a serum osmolality threshold during treatment with mannitol to monitor for the risk of AKI, but the authors caution that this is based on very low-quality evidence and they were unable to provide a recommended cutoff value for clinical use.[24] Total body fluid balance (TBB) impacts the efficacy of mannitol to achieve a change in osmolality, with each additional liter of TBB diminishing the osmolality by approximately 1.1 mOsm/L, and should be monitored in addition to the administration of hyperosmolar agents and osmolar gap (Migdady et al, 2022; PMID: 36334372).

Specific Disease Conditions

Acute Ischemic Stroke

Patients with large acute ischemic stroke may experience peri-infarct edema and elevated ICP. Although hyperosmolar therapy is commonly utilized in this setting, there is no evidence suggesting this practice improves outcomes.[24] The Albumin in Acute Ischemic Stroke (ALIAS) trial evaluated outcomes in 637 patients treated with 25% albumin at 2 g/kg compared to 638 patients treated with normal saline, and no difference was found in the number of patients with an mRS of 0 to 1 and/or NIHSS of 0 to 1 at 90 days (41% in both groups). However, the albumin group had higher rates of pulmonary edema (13% vs. 2%, RR = 7.76, 95% CI = 3.87-15.57).[4]

The 2018 European Society of Intensive Medicine guidelines for fluid therapy in neurointensive care patients recommends against the use of high-dose (20%-25%) albumin in acute ischemic stroke patients.[7] At the same time, the most recent American Heart Association guidelines for cerebral infarctions acknowledge that some practices may use mannitol or HTS for cerebral edema, but due to the lack of evidence the authors did not make any specific recommendations.[25]

Intraparenchymal Hemorrhage

There are no high-quality studies to guide fluid administration in patients with intraparenchymal hemorrhage. Similar to acute ischemic stroke, perihematoma edema may lead to elevated ICP, and this is commonly treated with hyperosmolar therapy. Guidelines from the American Heart Association and the European Stroke Organisation are based on expert consensus and state that either HTS or mannitol may be used to manage acute ICP elevations.[26,27]

Subarachnoid Hemorrhage

Intravenous fluids are often administered liberally in SAH patients to avoid hypovolemia and cerebral ischemia.[28] However, several RCTs also demonstrated that hypervolemia causes higher rates of pulmonary edema without any reduction in vasospasm risk when compared to euvolemia.[29-31] Thus, current recommendations are to target euvolemia rather than hypervolemia, though patients should receive additional fluid boluses when cerebral ischemia and/or vasospasm is suspected clinically.[32]

A 2004 retrospective study of 84 patients with SAH who required volume expansion showed that the 37 patients who received 25% albumin were more likely to have a good outcome (GOS 4-5) at 3 months compared to the 47 patients who received normal saline (68% vs. 39%, OR = 3.2, 95% CI = 1.1-11.0).[33] This was followed by 2012 Albumin in Subarachnoid Hemorrhage (ALISAH) prospective study, which found that 20 SAH patients treated with 7 days of 1.25 g/kg/day of 25% albumin had better outcomes (GOS 0-1 at 3 mo) than a population of 1000 SAH patients not treated with albumin in a prior 2005 study (IHAST[34]), though the difference was not significant (OR = 3.15, 95% CI = 0.92-10.81). Of note, the study was terminated early due to two serious adverse events (pulmonary edema and respiratory failure) in a group of seven patients treated with a higher albumin dose of 1.875 g/kg/day.[5]

Among crystalloids, normal saline or HTS is usually the recommended fluid of choice in SAH patients largely out of a desire to avoid the complications of hyponatremia, which occurs in 30% to 50% of SAH patients.[32] Hyponatremia is associated with cerebral ischemia and may be an independent risk factor for poor outcome.[35] That said, one study in 2013 randomized 36 SAH patients to either normal saline or a balanced crystalloid and did not find a significant difference in serum sodium or serum osmolality; meanwhile, balanced crystalloids caused less hyperchloremia and acidosis.[36]

Traumatic Brain Injury

A critical component of TBI management is mitigating intracranial hypertension, as it is the most frequent cause of death and secondary brain insults in these patients.[37] Thus, the usual clinical practice regarding intravenous fluids in TBI is hyperosmolar therapy with either HTS or mannitol, though there is limited high-quality evidence regarding the benefits of such a practice.

An observational study (2017) compared continuous HTS to other treatments (bolus mannitol or HTS, barbiturates, hypothermia, hypocapnia, decompressive craniectomy) in patients with TBI and elevated ICP. This study found an increased 90-day survival in 143 patients treated with continuous HTS compared to 402 patients treated without continuous HTS (HR = 1.43, 95% CI = 0.99-2.06, $p = .05$). The authors also concluded that there was no significant difference in achievement of GOS 4 to 5 between the two populations (45.2% vs. 35.8%, $p = .06$), though potentially this difference would have been statistically significant with a larger sample size.[38] Another retrospective study (2015) compared HTS versus mannitol in 48 matched ICU patients with severe TBI. This study also did not find a significant difference in 2-week mortality (OR = 0.50, 95% CI = 0.05-5.51, $p = .56$), but the HTS group had shorter ICU stays (8.5 ± 2.1 vs. 9.8 ± 0.6 days, $p = .004$) and lower ICP (0.3 ± 0.6 vs. 1.3 ± 1.3 hours/day with ICP > 25 mm Hg, $p = .001$).[39] Older studies (from 1984 to 1999) investigating hyperosmolar therapy in TBI are difficult to interpret due to lower quality of data and modern advances in general medical management.[40]

In the Brain Trauma Foundation's *Guidelines for the Management of Severe Traumatic Brain Injury* (Fourth Edition, 2016), the authors found a paucity of high-quality studies regarding fluid therapy in TBI. Ultimately, the authors concluded the following: "although hyperosmolar therapy may lower intracranial pressure, there was insufficient evidence about effects on clinical outcomes to support a specific recommendation, or to support use of any specific hyperosmolar agent, for patients with severe traumatic brain injury."[40] On the other hand, the 2020 NCS cerebral edema guidelines suggest using HTS over mannitol for the initial management of elevated ICP or cerebral edema in patients with TBI. However, the authors also noted that neither intervention should be used with the expectation for improving neurological outcomes in these patients.[24]

As mentioned previously, a subgroup analysis of 460 TBI patients in the 2004 Saline versus Albumin Fluid Evaluation (SAFE) study found that albumin was associated with higher mortality rates than normal saline (26.4% vs. 15.7% at 28 days, RR = 1.68, 95% CI = 1.16-2.43, $p = .005$).[3] Of note, however, the 4% albumin solution used in the SAFE trial was hypotonic (260 mOsm/kg) in comparison to the isotonic normal saline solution, which may render these findings inapplicable to isotonic albumin solutions.[41]

REFERENCES

1. Coppola, S., Froio, S. & Chiumello, D. Fluid resuscitation in trauma patients: what should we know? *Current Opinion in Critical Care* **20**, 444–450 (2014).
2. Lewis, S. R. *et al.* Colloids versus crystalloids for fluid resuscitation in critically ill people. *The Cochrane Database of Systematic Reviews* **8**, CD000567 (2018).
3. SAFE Study Investigators *et al.* Saline or albumin for fluid resuscitation in patients with traumatic brain injury. *The New England Journal of Medicine* **357**, 874–884 (2007).
4. Martin, R. H. *et al.* ALIAS (Albumin in Acute Ischemic Stroke) Trials: Analysis of the Combined Data from Parts 1 and 2. *Stroke* **47**, 2355–2359 (2016).
5. Suarez, J. I. *et al.* The Albumin in Subarachnoid Hemorrhage (ALISAH) multicenter pilot clinical trial: safety and neurologic outcomes. *Stroke* **43**, 683–690 (2012).
6. Rhodes, A. *et al.* Surviving Sepsis Campaign: International Guidelines for Management of Sepsis and Septic Shock: 2016. *Critical Care Medicine* **45**, 486–552 (2017).
7. Oddo, M. *et al.* Fluid therapy in neurointensive care patients: ESICM consensus and clinical practice recommendations. *Intensive Care Medicine* **44**, 449–463 (2018).
8. Langer, T. *et al.* Intravenous balanced solutions: from physiology to clinical evidence. *Anaesthesiology Intensive Therapy* **47 Spec No**, s78–s88 (2015).
9. Finfer, S. *et al.* Resuscitation fluid use in critically ill adults: an international cross-sectional study in 391 intensive care units. *Critical Care (London, England)* **14**, R185 (2010).
10. Morgan, T. J., Venkatesh, B. & Hall, J. Crystalloid strong ion difference determines metabolic acid-base change during in vitro hemodilution. *Critical Care Medicine* **30**, 157–160 (2002).
11. Suetrong, B. *et al.* Hyperchloremia and moderate increase in serum chloride are associated with acute kidney injury in severe sepsis and septic shock patients. *Critical Care (London, England)* **20**, 315 (2016).
12. Young, P. *et al.* Effect of a Buffered Crystalloid Solution vs Saline on Acute Kidney Injury Among Patients in the Intensive Care Unit: The SPLIT Randomized Clinical Trial. *JAMA* **314**, 1701–1710 (2015).
13. Zampieri, F. G. *et al.* Effect of Intravenous Fluid Treatment with a Balanced Solution vs 0.9% Saline Solution on Mortality in Critically Ill Patients: The BaSICS Randomized Clinical Trial. *JAMA* (2021). doi:10.1001/jama.2021.11684.
14. Finfer, S. *et al.* Balanced Multielectrolyte Solution versus Saline in Critically Ill Adults. *The New England Journal of Medicine* **386**, 815–826 (2022).
15. Semler, M. W. *et al.* Balanced Crystalloids versus Saline in Critically Ill Adults. *The New England Journal of Medicine* **378**, 829–839 (2018).
16. Freeman, W. D. Management of Intracranial Pressure. *Continuum (Minneapolis, Minn.)* **21**, 1299–1323 (2015).
17. Kamel, H. *et al.* Hypertonic saline versus mannitol for the treatment of elevated intracranial pressure: a meta-analysis of randomized clinical trials. *Critical Care Medicine* **39**, 554–559 (2011).
18. Visweswaran, P., Massin, E. K. & Dubose, T. D. Mannitol-induced acute renal failure. *Journal of the American Society of Nephrology* **8**, 1028–1033 (1997).
19. Diringer, M. N. & Zazulia, A. R. Osmotic therapy: fact and fiction. *Neurocritical care* **1**, 219–233 (2004).
20. Roumelioti, M.-E. *et al.* Fluid balance concepts in medicine: principles and practice. *World Journal of Nephrology* **7**, 1–28 (2018).
21. Oberleithner, H. *et al.* Salt overload damages the glycocalyx sodium barrier of vascular endothelium. *Pflugers Archiv : European Journal of Physiology* **462**, 519–528 (2011).
22. Ropper, A. H. Hyperosmolar therapy for raised intracranial pressure. *The New England Journal of Medicine* **367**, 746–752 (2012).
23. Hinson, H. E., Stein, D. & Sheth, K. N. Hypertonic saline and mannitol therapy in critical care neurology. *Journal of Intensive Care Medicine* **28**, 3–11 (2013).
24. Cook, A. M. *et al.* Guidelines for the Acute Treatment of Cerebral Edema in Neurocritical Care Patients. *Neurocritical Care* **32**, 647–666 (2020).
25. Wijdicks, E. F. M. *et al.* Recommendations for the management of cerebral and cerebellar infarction with swelling: a statement for healthcare professionals from the American Heart Association/American Stroke Association. *Stroke* **45**, 1222–1238 (2014).
26. Hemphill, J. C. *et al.* Guidelines for the Management of Spontaneous Intracerebral Hemorrhage: A Guideline for Healthcare Professionals from the American Heart Association/American Stroke Association. *Stroke* **46**, 2032–2060 (2015).
27. Steiner, T. *et al.* European Stroke Organisation (ESO) guidelines for the management of spontaneous intracerebral hemorrhage. *International Journal of Stroke: Official Journal of the International Stroke Society* **9**, 840–855 (2014).
28. Wijdicks, E. F. *et al.* Hyponatremia and cerebral infarction in patients with ruptured intracranial aneurysms: is fluid restriction harmful? *Annals of Neurology* **17**, 137–140 (1985).
29. Lennihan, L. *et al.* Effect of hypervolemic therapy on cerebral blood flow after subarachnoid hemorrhage: a randomized controlled trial. *Stroke* **31**, 383–391 (2000).
30. Egge, A. *et al.* Prophylactic hyperdynamic postoperative fluid therapy after aneurysmal subarachnoid hemorrhage: a clinical, prospective, randomized, controlled study. *Neurosurgery* **49**, 593–605; discussion 605-606 (2001).
31. Togashi, K. *et al.* Randomized pilot trial of intensive management of blood pressure or volume expansion in subarachnoid hemorrhage (IMPROVES). *Neurosurgery* **76**, 125–134; discussion 134-135; quiz 135 (2015).
32. Diringer, M. N. *et al.* Critical care management of patients following aneurysmal subarachnoid hemorrhage: recommendations from the Neurocritical Care Society's Multidisciplinary Consensus Conference. *Neurocritical Care* **15**, 211–240 (2011).
33. Suarez, J. I. *et al.* Effect of human albumin administration on clinical outcome and hospital cost in patients with subarachnoid hemorrhage. *Journal of Neurosurgery* **100**, 585–590 (2004).
34. Todd, M. M. *et al.*; Intraoperative Hypothermia for Aneurysm Surgery Trial (IHAST) Investigators. Mild intraoperative hypothermia during surgery for intracranial aneurysm. *The New England Journal of Medicine* **352**, 135–145 (2005).
35. Hasan, D., Wijdicks, E. F. & Vermeulen, M. Hyponatremia is associated with cerebral ischemia in patients with aneurysmal subarachnoid hemorrhage. *Annals of Neurology* **27**, 106–108 (1990).
36. Lehmann, L. *et al.* Randomized, double-blind trial of the effect of fluid composition on electrolyte, acid-base, and fluid homeostasis in patients early after subarachnoid hemorrhage. *Neurocritical Care* **18**, 5–12 (2013).
37. Dutton, R. P. *et al.* Trauma mortality in mature trauma systems: are we doing better? An analysis of trauma mortality patterns, 1997–2008. *The Journal of Trauma* **69**, 620–626 (2010).

38. Asehnoune, K. *et al.* Association between continuous hyperosmolar therapy and survival in patients with traumatic brain injury—a multicentre prospective cohort study and systematic review. *Critical Care (London, England)* **21**, 328 (2017).
39. Mangat, H. S. *et al.* Hypertonic saline reduces cumulative and daily intracranial pressure burdens after severe traumatic brain injury. *Journal of Neurosurgery* **122**, 202–210 (2015).
40. Carney, N. *et al. Guidelines for the Management of Severe Traumatic Brain Injury*, Fourth Edition. *Neurosurgery* **80**, 6–15 (2017).
41. Grände, P.-O. Critical evaluation of the lund concept for treatment of severe traumatic head injury, 25 years after its introduction. *Frontiers in Neurology* **8**, 315 (2017).

CHAPTER

17

What Is the Best Renal Replacement Therapy for Patients with Acute Brain Injury?

Marcey L. Osgood, DO

Case

A 68-year-old man has been admitted following a right middle cerebral artery (MCA) stroke. He has a history of chronic kidney disease, which steadily worsens over the course of his admission to the point where he becomes anuric. What is the optimal renal replacement therapy for such an individual?

Key Points

- Acute brain injury (ABI) patients are particularly susceptible to the osmotic gradients and fluid shifts occurring during renal replacement therapy (RRT) and extreme caution should be employed.
- The goal during RRT is slow removal of solutes and correction of acidosis which is most easily achieved with continuous renal replacement therapy (CRRT).
- Hypertonic saline should be used to mitigate sodium losses and counteract the shifts that will occur.
- Patients need very close monitoring of their neurologic exam as well as hemodynamic parameters to maintain mean arterial pressure (MAP) and cerebral perfusion pressure (CPP) during the RRT process.

BACKGROUND

Acute kidney injury (AKI) and RRT pose a particular challenge in the neurocritical care population. Patients with ABI have an increased susceptibility to fluid and electrolyte shifts. Shifts occurring during RRT may exacerbate brain edema and lead to increased intracranial pressure (ICP) with dire consequences. This chapter will focus on AKI in neurocritical care with special attention to the decision on RRT and mitigating the potential complications.

EVIDENCE AND REVIEW

Acute Kidney Injury in Neurocritical Care

Kidney disease improving global outcomes (KDIGO) guideline created a unifying definition for AKI that incorporates the risk, injury, failure; loss, end-stage renal disease (RIFLE) and the AKI network criteria (Table 17–1). This definition stages the kidney injury based on increase in creatinine from the baseline and degree of oliguria.[1] Based on KDIGO criteria, AKI is reported to occur in 9% to 23% of neurocritical care patients and varies widely depending on the underlying disease process.[2-5] Up to 12% of these patients will require RRT.[2-5] Development of AKI and need for RRT pertains a fivefold increase in mortality, poor functional recovery, and increased moderate to severe disability.[2,6] Those at highest risk include the extremes of age, history of chronic kidney disease and/or diabetes, increased severity of illness, and low Glasgow coma scale.[1,6] Development often occurs early in the hospital course and is associated with poor renal perfusion, contrast administration, osmotherapy, sympathetic hyperstimulation, hypernatremia and hyperchloremia making neurocritical care patients particularly susceptible.[2] It is essential to identify those at highest risk, monitor them closely with respect to electrolytes, labs and urine output along with employing a preventative strategy including avoidance of nephrotoxic agents, contrast dye, and maintenance of euvolemia and renal perfusion.

TABLE 17–1 Definition of acute kidney injury based on KDIGO.

Stage	Serum Creatinine	Urine Output
1	1.5-1.9 times baseline Or ≥ 0.3 mg/dL increase	< 0.5 mL/kg/h for 6-12 h
2	2.0-2.9 times baseline	<0.5 mL/kg/h for ≥12 h
3	3 times baseline Or ≥4 mg/dL Or Initiation of RRT	< 0.3 mL/kg/h for ≥24 h Or Anuria for ≥12 h

Indications for Renal Replacement Therapy

Decision for RRT needs to be individualized based on broad clinical context and not solely based on serum creatinine and blood urea nitrogen (BUN). Emergent RRT is recommended for those with life-threatening electrolyte disturbances (hyperkalemia), acid base abnormalities (acidemia), fluid overload (pulmonary edema), and uremic complications (bleeding, pericarditis).[1] The timing of nonemergent RRT is a complex decision and evidence suggests that accelerated early RRT is not associated with improved mortality or long-term dependence on RRT and is therefore not recommended.[7] This along with the fact that RRT has potentially negative consequences in ABI patients; it is often recommended to wait on starting RRT until absolutely necessary. However, the development of brain edema during RRT directly correlates with the level of BUN and the risk is exceptionally high when BUN is over 100 mg/dL.[8–10]

Renal Replacement Therapy and Acute Brain injury

ABI includes a variety of neurologic conditions including traumatic brain injury, hemorrhagic stroke, ischemic stroke, and subarachnoid hemorrhage. ABI patients are high risk for the development of cerebral edema and increased ICP. Management of these patients focuses on prevention of secondary brain injury through maintenance of CPP and cerebral blood flow (CBF) along with controlling ICP. ABI patients are particularly sensitive to osmotic gradients and fluid shifts and therefore RRT can have serious implications. It is critical for clinicians to be aware of how to properly manage RRT in this population.

Dialysis disequilibrium syndrome (DDS) refers to the development of cerebral edema during RRT that manifests as various neurologic symptoms from benign headaches to more severe coma, brain herniation and death.[11,12] Severe forms of DDS are described in the literature but may be underrecognized and underreported. DDS can have particularly catastrophic effects in those patients with ABI. Peterson and Swanson reported the first case of fulminant cerebral edema and brain herniation during RRT in 1964 and since that time multiple other case reports and series can be found.[13-17] Bertrand et al. went on to describe a rise in ICP seen in neurosurgery patients during RRT which has also been seen in subsequent reports.[8,9,16,17] Imaging studies with both commuted tomography and magnetic resonance imaging scans show changes in the brain following RRT that are consistent with the development of cerebral edema.[18-20] It is estimated that during RRT brain water volume increases by 3% which is equivalent to approximately 30 mL of fluid.[28] A recent review suggests that 60% of patients undergoing RRT experience an increase ICP with 20.7% developing cerebral edema on imaging, 13.8% showing clinical signs of brain herniation and 10.3% having pupillary changes.[21] Table 17–2 summarizes the literature

TABLE 17–2 All reported cases of elevated intracranial pressure, cerebral edema, brain herniation, and/or death during renal replacement therapy in patients with acute brain injury.

Author Year	N	ABI	Mode of RRT	Findings
Peterson (1964)[13]	3	TBI/SDH	IHD	Two-thirds of the cases had ABI, one had sepsis. All patients had DDS, the two ABI patients had brain herniation, cerebral edema and death.
Bertrand (1983)[8]	2	TBI	IHD	Both patients had rise in ICP during dialysis. Largest rise correlated to highest BUN.
Yoshida (1987)[17]	4	ICH/SAH	IHD	Neurosurgical patients with EVDs were noted to have rise in ICP during IHD. Signs of herniation mitigated by draining CSF.
Lin (2008)[16]	5	SDH/ICH	IHD	Neurosurgical patients with ICP monitors in place. All had rise in ICP during IHD. All patients developed brain herniation and cerebral edema. Four-fifths died and one patient survived with osmotherapy and change to CVVH
Osgood (2015)[14]	4	Stroke/TBI	IHD/CVVH	All patients had rapid brain herniation, cerebral edema, and death. One of the patients had this occur while on CVVH.
Kumar (2015)[15]	2	ICH	IHD	Both patients developed brain herniation and cerebral edema. One was reversed with osmotherapy and the other became brain dead.
Lund (2018)[9]	13	Variable	IHD/CVVH	All patients had ICP monitors in place and were receiving either IHD or CVVH. All patients regardless of mode had increase ICP during treatment correlating to the level of BUN.

ABI, acute brain injury; BUN, blood urea nitrogen; CSF, cerebrospinal fluid; CVVH, continuous venovenous hemofiltration; DDS, dialysis disequilibrium syndrome; EVD, external ventricular drain; ICH, intracerebral hemorrhage; ICP, intracranial pressure; IHD, intermittent hemodialysis; SAH, subarachnoid hemorrhage; TBI, traumatic brain injury.

surrounding development of increased ICP, cerebral edema, and brain herniation during RRT. It is important to note that the majority of these severe DDS cases occur in the setting of intermittent hemodialysis (IHD) as opposed to CRRT. It is thought that IHD results in more aggressive fluid shifts and a substantial osmotic gradient that is not as pronounced with CRRT.

The mechanism by which DDS develops is not fully elucidated, though there are three proposed mechanisms: reverse urea effect, idiogenic osmoles hypothesis, and paradoxical cerebral acidosis.[22,23] Despite ongoing debate, it is likely that all three mechanisms play a role.

Along with DDS, hemodynamic fluctuations are commonly reported during RRT, potentially resulting in decreased cerebral perfusion pressure and CBF.[8,29,30] Since its inception in 1960, IHD has been noted to result in hemodynamic instability, particularly hypotension and reduction in MAP.[31,32] Transcranial doppler monitoring has previously demonstrated drops in CBF following IHD.[33] CRRT emerged as an alternative treatment in 1977 and has been associated with improved hemodynamic stability.[31,32,34] CRRT is associated with improved MAP, cardiac output, and oxygen delivery when compared to IHD.[34] A large meta-analysis suggested that while IHD and CRRT are similar with respect to hospital mortality, hemodynamic instability and hypotension, CRRT is associated with higher MAP and reduced need for vasopressors.[32]

In critical care patients there is no established superiority of continuous or intermittent RRT with respect to mortality, morbidity, length of stay or renal recovery.[32,35] However, ABI patients require special consideration when planning RRT. As mentioned, ABI patients are highly susceptible to fluid shifts and RRT can result in dire consequences including brain edema, brain herniation, and death. Caution should be used when starting an ABI patient on RRT and clinicians should employ strategies to mitigate the potential complications. IHD very efficiently removes solute and urea from the blood, rapidly leading to an osmotic gradient which is why most cases of severe DDS, brain edema and increased ICP are seen when IHD is used. Moreover, while it has been proposed that ABI patients should preferentially undergo CRRT in an effort to prevent rapid shifts of fluid,[34,36,37] recent literature suggests that both IHD and CRRT lead to increased ICP though the effect is slower and more delayed in patients undergoing CRRT.[9] It is possible that this slower development gives the brain time to compensate and is a reason why there are fewer reports of brain edema, herniation and death are seen in CRRT patients. However, while CRRT is likely safer than IHD, increased ICP as well as brain herniation and death have been reported and patients undergoing CRRT continue to need very close monitoring.[14,38]

If feasible, CRRT is preferred and should be used when starting RRT in patients with ABI. Hemofiltration as opposed to hemodialysis is a gentler mode and should be employed.[31,37] The nephrologist and those involved in care should all be aware of the concern about rapid fluid shifts and brain edema. During CRRT, most dialysate has a standard sodium of 135 to 140 mEq/L. Infusion of 3% hypertonic saline can be used to prevent sodium falling during treatment and is recommended if the patients sodium level is higher than the amount contained in the dialysate.[36] If a patient is very high risk for cerebral edema, hypertonic saline may help to mitigate any shifts that occur during CRRT and can be used as a preventative strategy.[2]

Patients should have frequent neurologic exams to watch for signs of worsening brain edema. At our institution, we have begun to employ pupillometry on RRT patients to more closely watch for pupillary changes that may predict development of cerebral edema. It should be noted that during CRRT, increased ICP occurred 24 hours or more from the onset of RRT and patients may develop delayed edema.[9] In cases where CRRT is not available or not feasible, IHD can be used. When using IHD, we recommend a small surface area dialyzer, slow blood and dialysate flow rates with short frequent (daily) treatments to decrease the rate of solute removal and decrease the potential osmotic gradient.[2,39] Dialysate sodium should be 10 mEq higher than serum sodium to maintain appropriate serum levels throughout the dialysis process. Cooling the dialysate may also help to maintain cerebral perfusion pressure.[39] During IHD consider osmotherapy to prevent life-threatening cerebral edema.[2] If a patient develops worsening neurologic status, worsening brain edema, signs of increased ICP or herniation, RRT should be immediately stopped and osmotherapy with hypertonic saline or mannitol should be initiated. Most cases of cerebral edema associated with RRT reported in the literature were not reversible and patient mortality was high.[15,40]

REFERENCES

1. Khwaja, A. KDIGO clinical practice guidelines for acute kidney injury. *Nephron Clin Pract.* 2012;**120**(4):c179–c184.
2. Ramirez-Guerrero, G., R. Baghetti-Hernandez, and C. Ronco. Acute kidney injury at the neurocritical care unit. *Neurocrit Care.* 2022;**36**(2):640–649.
3. Saeed, F., et al. Acute renal failure is associated with higher death and disability in patients with acute ischemic stroke: analysis of nationwide inpatient sample. *Stroke.* 2014;**45**(5):1478–1480.
4. Moore, E.M., et al. The incidence of acute kidney injury in patients with traumatic brain injury. *Ren Fail.* 2010;**32**(9):1060–1065.
5. Pesonen, A., N. Ben-Hamouda, and A. Schneider. Acute kidney injury after brain injury: does it exist? *Minerva Anestesiol.* 2021;**87**(7):823–827.
6. Robba, C., et al. Acute kidney injury in traumatic brain injury patients: results from the Collaborative European NeuroTrauma Effectiveness Research in Traumatic Brain Injury Study. *Crit Care Med.* 2021;**49**(1):112–126.
7. Investigators, S.-A., et al. Timing of initiation of renal-replacement therapy in acute kidney injury. *N Engl J Med.* 2020;**383**(3):240–251.
8. Bertrand, Y.M., et al. Intracranial pressure changes in patients with head trauma during haemodialysis. *Intensive Care Med.* 1983;**9**(6):321–323.
9. Lund, A., et al. Intracranial pressure during hemodialysis in patients with acute brain injury. *Acta Anaesthesiol Scand.* 2019;**63**(4):493–499.
10. Bagshaw, S.M., et al. Dialysis disequilibrium syndrome: brain death following hemodialysis for metabolic acidosis and acute renal failure—a case report. *BMC Nephrol.* 2004;**5**:9.
11. Harris, C.P. and J.J. Townsend. Dialysis disequilibrium syndrome. *West J Med.* 1989;**151**(1):52–55.
12. Lopez-Almaraz, E. and R. Correa-Rotter. Dialysis disequilibrium syndrome and other treatment complications of extreme uremia: a rare occurrence yet not vanished. *Hemodial Int.* 2008;**12**(3):301–306.
13. Peterson, H. and A.G. Swanson. Acute encephalopathy occuring during hemodialysis. The reverse urea effect. *Arch Intern Med.* 1964;**113**:877–880.
14. Osgood, M., et al. Rapid unexpected brain herniation in association with renal replacement therapy in acute brain injury: caution in the neurocritical care unit. *Neurocrit Care.* 2015;**22**(2):176–183.

15. Kumar, A., A. Cage, and R. Dhar. Dialysis-induced worsening of cerebral edema in intracranial hemorrhage: a case series and clinical perspective. *Neurocrit Care.* 2015;**22**(2):283–287.
16. Lin, C.M., et al. Intracranial pressure fluctuation during hemodialysis in renal failure patients with intracranial hemorrhage. *Acta Neurochir Suppl.* 2008;**101**:141–144.
17. Yoshida, S., et al. Dialysis dysequilibrium syndrome in neurosurgical patients. *Neurosurgery.* 1987;**20**(5):716–721.
18. Dettori, P., et al. Changes of cerebral density in dialyzed patients. *Neuroradiology.* 1982;**23**(2):95–99.
19. La Greca, G., et al. Studies on brain density in hemodialysis and peritoneal dialysis. *Nephron.* 1982;**31**(2):146–150.
20. Chen, C.L., et al. A preliminary report of brain edema in patients with uremia at first hemodialysis: evaluation by diffusion-weighted MR imaging. *AJNR Am J Neuroradiol.* 2007;**28**(1):68–71.
21. Parsons, A.D., et al. Dialysis disequilibrium syndrome and intracranial pressure fluctuations in neurosurgical patients undergoing renal replacement therapy: systematic review and pooled analysis. *World Neurosurg.* 2022.
22. Silver, S.M., R.H. Sterns, and M.L. Halperin, brain swelling after dialysis: old urea or new osmoles? *Am J Kidney Dis.* 1996;**28**(1):1–13.
23. Arieff, A.I. Dialysis disequilibrium syndrome: current concepts on pathogenesis and prevention. *Kidney Int.* 1994;**45**(3):629–635.
24. Trinh-Trang-Tan, M.M., J.P. Cartron, and L. Bankir. Molecular basis for the dialysis disequilibrium syndrome: altered aquaporin and urea transporter expression in the brain. Nephrol Dial Transplant. 2005;**20**(9):1984–1988.
25. Arieff, A.I., et al. Brain water and electrolyte metabolism in uremia: effects of slow and rapid hemodialysis. *Kidney Int.* 1973;**4**(3):177–187.
26. Arieff, A.I., et al. Central nervous system pH in uremia and the effects of hemodialysis. *J Clin Invest.* 1976;**58**(2):306–311.
27. Kennedy, A.C., et al. The pathogenesis and prevention of cerebral dysfunction during dialysis. *Lancet.* 1964;**1**(7337):790–793.
28. Walters, R.J., et al. Haemodialysis and cerebral oedema. *Nephron.* 2001;**87**(2):143–147.
29. Davenport, A. Is there a role for continuous renal replacement therapies in patients with liver and renal failure? *Kidney Int Suppl.* 1999;(72):S62–S66.
30. Ko, S.B., et al. Pearls & oysters: the effects of renal replacement therapy on cerebral autoregulation. *Neurology.* 2012;**78**(6):e36–e38.
31. John, S. and K.U. Eckardt. Renal replacement therapy in the treatment of acute renal failure-intermittent and continuous. *Semin Dial.* 2006;**19**(6):455–464.
32. Rabindranath, K., et al. Intermittent versus continuous renal replacement therapy for acute renal failure in adults. *Cochrane Database Syst Rev.* 2007;(3):CD003773.
33. Hata, R., et al. Effects of hemodialysis on cerebral circulation evaluated by transcranial Doppler ultrasonography. *Stroke.* 1994;**25**(2):408–412.
34. Davenport, A. Renal replacement therapy in the patient with acute brain injury. *Am J Kidney Dis.* 2001;**37**(3):457–466.
35. Schefold, J.C., et al. The effect of continuous versus intermittent renal replacement therapy on the outcome of critically ill patients with acute renal failure (CONVINT): a prospective randomized controlled trial. *Crit Care.* 2014;**18**(1):R11.
36. Davenport, A. Practical guidance for dialyzing a hemodialysis patient following acute brain injury. *Hemodial Int.* 2008;**12**(3):307–312.
37. Patel, P., et al. Continuous renal replacement therapies: a brief primer for the neurointensivist. *Neurocrit Care.* 2010;**13**(2):286–294.
38. Tuchman, S., Z.P. Khademian, and K. Mistry. Dialysis disequilibrium syndrome occurring during continuous renal replacement therapy. *Clin Kidney J.* 2013;**6**(5):526–529.
39. Ghoshal, S. and A. Parikh. Dialysis-associated neurovascular injury (DANI) in acute brain injury: practical considerations for intermittent dialysis in the neuro-ICU. *Clin J Am Soc Nephrol.* 2021;**16**(7):1110–1112.
40. DiFresco, V., et al. Dialysis disequilibrium syndrome: an unusual cause of respiratory failure in the medical intensive care unit. *Intensive Care Med.* 2000;**26**(5):628–630.

SECTION III TRAUMA AND CEREBRAL EDEMA

CHAPTER

18

How Often Should We Repeat Imaging in Severe Traumatic Brain Injury?

Ronald Alvarado-Dyer, MD, Faten El Ammar, MD, & Christos Lazaridis, MD, EDIC

Case

A 20-year-old woman presents to the emergency room after a fall from a third-story window. Her Glasgow coma scale (GCS) is 8 upon initial assessment, and initial imaging reveals multifocal hemorrhagic contusions but without associated subdural or epidural hemorrhages. When should we repeat her cranial imaging?

Key Points

- No universal guidelines exist on what is the appropriate schedule for repeat imaging; however, there are imaging and clinical features that call for high vigilance and make a short (and serial thereafter) follow-up prudent.
- Although the common practice is to obtaining a follow-up computer tomography (CT) scan within 4 to 6 hours after the initial scan for routine monitoring of progression, subsequent scanning should be dictated by results of the first scan, original and follow up findings, invasive neuromonitoring data, coagulation testing, and clinical status.
- Using CREVICE guidelines, certain patient populations may require frequent monitoring, including those with decreased GCS, worsening neurologic function, or significant existing mass effect.

BACKGROUND

Fast scanning times, ease of availability, and identification of pathologies that may require acute interventions, make CT the primary imaging modality for early-stage evaluation of traumatic brain injury (TBI). Indeed, there are a number of CT classification systems for TBI including the Marshall Grade, Helsinki, Stockholm, and Rotterdam scores. The most commonly used, the Marshall score distinguishes focal from diffuse lesions and comprises part of the IMPACT score for prognostication.[1,2] In this chapter, we attempt addressing the further question of the role of repeat CT imaging, during the acute stage of the disease, to identify disease progression, and as a means of neuromonitoring. The first part reviews literature related to hemorrhagic progression of contusions (HPC), pathology crucial in monitoring via repeat radiographic evaluation. The second part offers a clinical rationale for incorporating repeat CT as a neuromonitoring modality.

EVIDENCE AND REVIEW

Lesion Progression and Repeat Imaging

In general, interpretation of CT after TBI (both initially and at repeat) should focus on addressing the following questions:

- *Is there a mass-effect producing hematoma that needs immediate surgical attention?* These most commonly refer to extra-axial collections such as subdural (SDH) and epidural (EDH) hematomas. They are often identified in the original CT and should be followed according to size, mass-effect, and overall clinical status as for example in patients under heavy sedation, where earlier radiographic follow-up is warranted.
- *Is there a focal lesion?* Either associated with petechiae or frank hemorrhagic contusions having the potential for expansion or as it is referred to "blossom." This refers to the earlier mentioned phenomenon of HPC.
- *Is this a diffuse pattern associated with generalized swelling and a high potential for intracranial hypertension (IHT)?* Brain Trauma Foundation guidelines should be followed in terms of the indications for invasive intracranial pressure (ICP) monitoring.[3]
- *Would the patient benefit from an urgent evacuation or a decompressive craniectomy (DC), or would it be more appropriate to monitor neurological status, ICP, and follow-up radiologic imaging?*
- *Is there a midline shift?* Are the basal cisterns distorted or compressed on the same side of the mass lesion? Are the basal cisterns bilaterally compressed or absent? This is a sign of IHT and coning due to the mass effect or a sequela of diffuse brain swelling.[4]
- *Is there traumatic subarachnoid hemorrhage (tSAH)?* This may be suggestive of an evolving intraparenchymal lesion; tSAH may also have independent consequences and may be linked to posttraumatic vasospasm and cerebral ischemia.[5]
- *Is there high potential for vascular injuries (arterial and venous) that should require dedicated vascular imaging?* This should take higher priority particularly with penetrating brain injury mechanisms.[6]

Contusive brain injury is invariably complicated by secondary insults due to microvascular dysfunction,[7] which worsens with time and leads to growth of the primary lesion. Microvascular dysfunction leads to: tissue ischemia due to impairment of blood flow (this can be due to direct diminution of flow, or indirectly due to impairment of pressure-flow autoregulation[8]) formation of vasogenic edema, further exacerbating tissue dysoxia; and loss of the structural integrity of surrounding microvessels, which results in expansion or progression of the hemorrhagic lesion leading to HPC.[9] Bleeding due to the original insult, in addition to HPC, and edema, lead to increasing ICP, tissue hypoperfusion, and tissue herniation.

On a CT, a contusion generally appears as a hemorrhagic lesion, although sometimes injured tissues or part of a contusive lesion can appear normal (isodense) or hypodense. A contusion is distinguished from a laceration by the fact that with a contusion, the pia mater remains intact. A contusion is distinguished from a hematoma by the fact that with a contusion, blood is intermixed with brain tissue. When head trauma results in a contusion, the hemorrhagic lesion often expands, or a new hemorrhagic lesion may develop remotely (noncontiguously) from the original contusion during the first several hours after impact.[9,10]

There has been significant interest in identifying the factors which best predict the evolution of intracranial hemorrhage in acute TBI, given that it represents a major cause of neurological deterioration and morbidity. TBI associated with cerebral contusion is a frequent cause of death and disability in trauma victims who reach the hospital alive. An important driver of considering early reimaging relates to HPC, defined as an increase in hemorrhage volume over time.[9-11] HPC, which occurs in the first few hours after head trauma, has been demonstrated in 38% to 63% of TBI patients. Studies investigating HPC have generated the following observations[9]:

- Approximately half of patients with contusions demonstrate HPC on serial CT scanning.
- HPC may involve not only the expansion of existing contusions but the delayed appearance of new and remote hemorrhagic lesions.
- HPC is equally common without surgery, after DC, and in cases with tSAH. One study found that 60% of patients with tSAH exhibited HPC on follow-up CT.[5]
- The earlier after insult the initial CT scan is obtained, the greater the likelihood that HPC will be found on a subsequent scan.
- HPC generally occurs within the first 12 hours but may occur in a delayed fashion (3-4 days after the initial impact).
- Small contusions that progress are usually clinically silent and are unlikely to require surgical decompression.
- Large contusions in patients with low initial GCS) scores are likelier to progress and often require surgical decompression (see Figure 18–1 for an example). Initial lesion volume carries a high predictive value with respect to core expansion.[10-14] In addition, patients who require contusion evacuation also tend to have an associated SDH. This suggests that patients with low GCS scores and those with extra-axial hematomas warrant more intensive vigilance; a repeat 4- to 8-hour scan should be considered of high clinical yield in patients with these characteristics, independently of clinical status.

In a retrospective review of patients with brain contusions who initially underwent nonoperative treatment, patients with significant progression were defined as those with a 30% or more increase in contusion size on CT scan (CT progression could result from expansion of the hematoma, the appearance of perihematoma hypodensity, or development of new lesions; it should be noted that there is no single definition of contusion "progression" in the literature).[10] Of 98 patients, 44 (45%) had

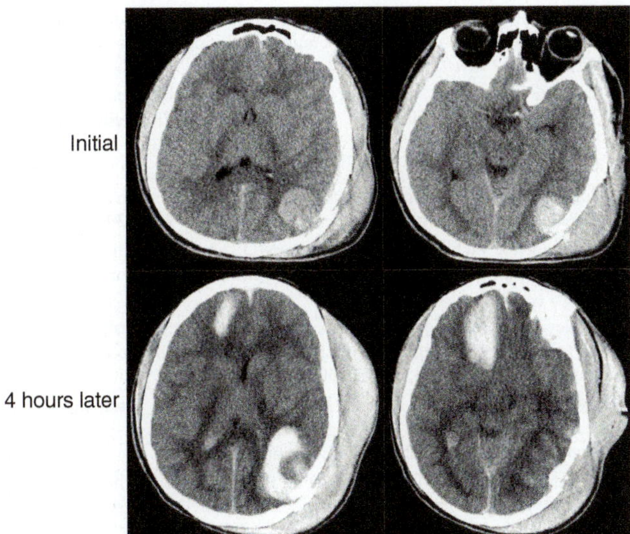

FIGURE 18–1 Young man with blunt TBI; the upper panel is from the initial CT demonstrating large left occipitoparietal scalp hematoma with underlying comminuted depressed fracture of the left parietal and occipital bones. There is an underlying left occipito-parietal hemorrhagic contusion. The lower panel shows cuts from a CT performed 4 hours from the original, and after neurologic worsening; it shows acute expansion of the left hemorrhagic contusion, new development of a right anterior, inferior frontal parenchymal hematoma, and diffuse swelling with basal cistern elimination.

significant progression on CT, and 19 (19%) required DC. They also determined that patients with large contusions and low initial GCS were at greater risk for delayed deterioration. Oertel and coworkers[13] performed a retrospective study of patients who underwent two CT scans within 24 hours of head injury. Their study examined progression of all hemorrhagic lesions, including EDH, SDH, tSAH, and intraparenchymal hemorrhages. Overall, they found that early progression of hemorrhage occurs most frequently in contusions, with a likelihood of 51%. They also observed that about half of the patients who underwent craniotomy after the first CT scan later showed evidence of hemorrhagic progression; HPC frequently continues after craniotomy, making postoperative radiographic follow-up warranted.[15-17]

CT Scanning for Neuromonitoring

In the last part we discuss the role of repeat CT imaging as a neuromonitoring modality. Severe TBI patients often have numerous confounders to reliable follow up by clinical exam alone. These may include multitrauma, heavy sedation, neuromuscular blockade, and compromised intracranial hemodynamics precluding rigorous stimulation. Saliently, clinical exam changes may represent delayed manifestations of ongoing secondary brain injury, or the end-result of unsuspected lesion development and progression as in the case of HPC discussed above. For these reasons, CT follow-up is recommended in severe TBI patients, and particularly in those with the aforementioned features.

Timing of Imaging

The timing and frequency of imaging has to be individualized according to patient characteristics. We typically obtain a routine 4 to 6-hour (from the original CT) "stability" scan in all severe TBI patients unless there are reasons to perform earlier. The 6 hours mark in terms of re-imaging is based on prior TBI retrospective studies demonstrating changes in follow-up scans performed within 12 hours after initial head injury.[15] While many studies emphasized on the importance of serial imaging,[9] their results on a low level of evidence and can't be generalized to all subtypes of TBI or other presentations of hemorrhagic strokes or lesions. In general, subsequent scanning should be dictated by results of the first scan, original and follow-up findings, invasive neuromonitoring data (ICP, cerebral perfusion pressure and in select patients partial brain tissue oxygen tension), coagulation testing, and clinical status.

AVAILABLE GUIDELINES

CT scanning is an integral part of decision-making in severe TBI both in terms of original diagnostic evaluation, and as a follow-up neuromonitoring tool. No universal guidelines exist on what is the appropriate schedule for repeat imaging, however, there are imaging and clinical features that call for high vigilance and make a short (and serial thereafter) follow-up prudent. Such clinical features include a low post-resuscitation GCS, presence of exam confounders such as intoxication or sedation, invasive neuromonitoring data (such as refractory ICP), and uncorrected coagulopathy. Imaging features include the presence of extra-axial unevacuated hematomas, larger hemorrhagic contusions, diffuse swelling, midline shift, or compressed cisterns.

In the absence of a more definitive strategy, we think it instructive to consult the so-called Imaging and Clinical Exam protocol as first used in the Benchmark Evidence from South American Trials: Treatment of Intracranial Pressure (BEST: TRIP) trial, and more recently refined in the Consensus REVised ICE algorithm (CREVICE).[18–20] These algorithms guide management of suspected IHT in the absence of invasive intracranial monitoring, based on repeated clinical examinations and CT imaging. Inspired by these algorithms, we recommend an early repeat CT, and serial scheduled scanning for patients with any of the following on the original CT:

1. Compressed cisterns (Marshall diffuse injury III);
2. Midline shift > 5 mm (Marshall diffuse injury IV);
3. Unevacuated mass lesion.

In addition, combinations of the following criteria should also trigger vigilance and repeat imaging:

1. GCS motor score ≤4;
2. Pupillary asymmetry;
3. Abnormal pupillary reactivity;
4. Marshall diffuse injury II (ie, basal cisterns are present with midline shift 0 to 5 mm and/or high or mixed-density lesion ≤ 25 mL).

Repeat CT imaging should be also performed in cases of neurologic decline as manifested in the following:

a. Decrease in the motor GCS of 1 or more points;

b. New loss of pupil reactivity;

c. Interval development of pupil asymmetry of >2 mm or bilateral mydriasis;

d. New focal motor deficit;

e. Herniation syndrome (eg, Cushing triad).

In the CREVICE algorithm it is also prescribed that if the initial CT is obtained within 4 hours of injury, a second CT is indicated within the next 12 hours. In all cases, follow-up CT imaging is recommended at 24 and 72 hours after injury, and as needed based on the clinical situation or to facilitate decision-making. We end this section with a word of caution in terms of using CT, and other noninvasive tools, as surrogates for ICP. Independent neurologic findings (pupillary dilation, posturing, decreased level of consciousness), imaging (compression of cisterns, midline shift), and noninvasive modalities such as transcranial Doppler may have poor accuracy for elevated ICP; as such, these tests should not be used independently to rule out IHT.[21] High suspicion of elevated ICP, and targeted management should be in general guided by invasive monitoring.

REFERENCES

1. Marshall LF, Marshall SB, Klauber MR, et al. The diagnosis of head injury requires a classification based on computed axial tomography. *J Neurotrauma* 1992;9 Suppl 1: S287–292.
2. Maas AI, Steyerberg EW, Butcher I, et al. Prognostic value of computerized tomography scan characteristics in traumatic brain injury: results from the IMPACT study. *J Neurotrauma* 2007;24(2):303–314.
3. Carney N, Totten AM, O'Reilly C, et al. Guidelines for the Management of Severe Traumatic Brain Injury, Fourth Edition. *Neurosurgery* 2017;80(1):6–15.
4. Miller MT, Pasquale M, Kurek S, et al. Initial head computed tomographic scan characteristics have a linear relationship with initial intracranial pressure after trauma. *J Trauma* 2004;56(5):967–972; discussion 972–973.
5. Chieregato A, Fainardi E, Morselli-Labate AM, et al. Factors associated with neurological outcome and lesion progression in traumatic subarachnoid hemorrhage patients. *Neurosurgery* 2005;56(4):671–680.
6. Loggini A, Vasenina VI, Mansour A, et al. Management of civilians with penetrating brain injury: a systematic review. *J Crit Care* 2020;56:159–166.
7. Newcombe VF, Williams GB, Outtrim JG, et al. Microstructural basis of contusion expansion in traumatic brain injury: insights from diffusion tensor imaging. *J Cereb Blood Flow Metab* 2013;33(6):855–862.
8. Mathieu F, Zeiler FA, Ercole A, et al. Relationship between Measures of Cerebrovascular Reactivity and Intracranial Lesion Progression in Acute Traumatic Brain Injury Patients: A CENTER-TBI Study. *J Neurotrauma* 2020;37(13):1556–1565.
9. Kurland D, Hong C, Aarabi B, et al. Hemorrhagic progression of a contusion after traumatic brain injury: a review. *J Neurotrauma.* 2012;29(1):19–31.
10. Alahmadi H, Vachhrajani S, Cusimano MD. The natural history of brain contusion: an analysis of radiological and clinical progression. *J Neurosurg* 2010;112:1139–1145.
11. Carnevale JA, Segar DJ, Powers AY, et al. Blossoming contusions: identifying factors contributing to the expansion of traumatic intracerebral hemorrhage. *J Neurosurg* 2018;129(5):1305–1316.
12. Chang EF, Meeker M, Holland MC. Acute traumatic intraparenchymal hemorrhage: risk factors for progression in the early post-injury period. *Neurosurgery* 2007;61:222–230; discussion, 230–231.
13. Oertel M, Kelly DF, McArthur D, et al. Progressive hemorrhage after head trauma: predictors and consequences of the evolving injury. *J Neurosurg* 2002;96:109–116.
14. Narayan RK, Maas AI, Servadei F, et al.; Traumatic Intracerebral Hemorrhage Study Group. Progression of traumatic intracerebral hemorrhage: a prospective observational study. *J Neurotrauma* 2008;25:629–639.
15. Servadei F, Nanni A, Nasi MT, et al. Evolving brain lesions in the first 12 hours after head injury: analysis of 37 comatose patients. *Neurosurgery* 1995;37(5):899–907. PMID: 28502689.
16. Aarabi B, Hesdorffer DC, Simard JM, et al. Comparative study of decompressive craniectomy after mass lesion evacuation in severe head injury. *Neurosurgery* 2009;64(5):927–940.
17. Cepeda S, Castaño-León AM, Munarriz PM, et al. Effect of decompressive craniectomy in the postoperative expansion of traumatic intracerebral hemorrhage: a propensity score-based analysis [published online ahead of print, 2019 April 26]. *J Neurosurg* 2019;1–13.
18. Chesnut RM, Temkin N, Carney N, et al. A trial of intracranial-pressure monitoring in traumatic brain injury [published correction appears in] *N Engl J Med* 2013 Dec 19;369(25):2465.
19. Chesnut RM, Temkin N, Dikmen S, et al. A method of managing severe traumatic brain injury in the absence of intracranial pressure monitoring: the imaging and clinical examination protocol. *J Neurotrauma* 2018;35(1):54–63.
20. Chesnut RM, Temkin N, Videtta W, et al. Consensus-based management protocol (CREVICE protocol) for the treatment of severe traumatic brain injury based on imaging and clinical examination for use when intracranial pressure monitoring is not employed. *J Neurotrauma* 2020;37(11):1291–1299.
21. Fernando SM, Tran A, Cheng W, et al. Diagnosis of elevated intracranial pressure in critically ill adults: systematic review and meta-analysis. *BMJ* 2019;366:l4225.

CHAPTER

19

What Are the Relative Merits of Various Hyperosmolar Agents in ICP Management?

Daniel S. Harrison, MD & Saef Izzy, MD, MBChB

Case

A 36-year-old man is brought into the emergency department by Emergency Medical Services (EMS) following a motor vehicle accident. His initial exam is pertinent for no eye opening to noxious stimuli, incoherent muttering, and profound left-sided weakness with ability to withdrawal the right arm from pain. He is intubated after becoming hypoxic in the CT scanner, which revealed large right and small left frontal contusions and 11 mm of midline shift at the septum. An intracranial pressure (ICP) monitor is placed at the bedside, which reveals ICP of 32 cm H_2O. What's the best hyperosmolar therapy agent we should start to control elevated ICP?

Key Points

- Hyperosmolar therapy may be effective in reducing ICP elevations due to cerebral edema; however, it does not clearly affect neurologic outcome in any disease state.
- There is mixed data regarding use of hypertonic saline (HTS) to target sodium level in subarachnoid hemorrhage (SAH), intracerebral hemorrhage (ICH), and acute ischemic stroke (AIS) and limited data of efficacy in hepatic encephalopathy; evidence supporting sodium targets in other disease states is lacking.
- Three percent HTS boluses may have similar efficacy to mannitol and more highly concentrated HTS for reduction of ICP.
- Mannitol may increase risk of hematoma expansion in patients with ICH; however, it is not clear that hyperosmolar therapies increase risk of hematoma expansion in patients with subdural hematoma (SDH).
- Limited available data has not shown increased risk of vasospasm or delayed cerebral ischemia (DCI) in patients with aneurysmal SAH exposed to mannitol.
- Selection of hyperosmolar agent should be individualized to patient factors including etiology of cerebral edema and patient comorbidities.

BACKGROUND

Elevated ICP may be due to an increase in intracranial volume of blood, brain parenchyma, or cerebrospinal fluid (CSF). Among other causes, cerebral edema of a variety of etiologies may increase brain volume. Hyperosmolar therapies may reduce ICP via reduction in brain volume, so long as cerebral edema is present. The primary mechanism of these agents is creation of an osmotic gradient, which pulls water from brain parenchyma into blood. This in theory requires an intact blood-brain barrier (BBB), as disruption of the BBB could result in leakage of hyperosmolar agents into brain parenchyma, reversal of the osmotic gradient, and rebound elevation in ICP. Despite this, hyperosmolar therapy is often used in disease states wherein the BBB is known to be disrupted. The pathophysiology of cerebral edema varies by underlying cause so specific agents that are effective in reducing ICP in one disease state may be less effective or ineffective in another. Here we will discuss the evidence that supports use of hyperosmolar agents for reduction of cerebral edema and elevated ICP, noting that hyperosmolar therapy has not consistently been shown to affect neurologic outcome regardless of underlying disease state.[1]

The two most commonly available hyperosmolar agents are HTS and mannitol. HTS is available in a variety of concentrations up to 23.4%. Solutions of HTS and hydroxyethyl starch (HES) are not currently available in the United States; however, these solutions have been used in clinical trials elsewhere

TABLE 19–1 General risks and benefits of selected hyperosmolar agents.

	Hypertonic Saline (More Concentrated, eg, 23.4%)	Hypertonic Saline (Less Concentrated, eg, 3%)	Mannitol
Benefits	• intravascular volume expansion • fast onset • long duration of action • robust ICP response • blood pressure augmentation (hemorrhagic shock)	• lower concern for extravasation injury • otherwise, similar benefit profile to more concentrated HTS	• n/a
Risks	• volume overload • extravasation injury* • hyperchloremic metabolic acidosis • AKI • hypotension*	• largely mixed evidence of benefit when used to target a sodium goal • otherwise, similar risk profile to more concentrated HTS	• volume depletion • AKI • theoretical increased risk of DCI (SAH) • demonstrated risk of hematoma expansion (ICH)

*More recent data has suggested that HTS use, including via peripheral administration and at faster administration rates, is low risk for acute hypotension or extravasation injury.

evaluating the efficacy of HTS. HTS is typically administered via bolus dosing for signs or symptoms of elevated ICP. It has also been evaluated as bolus or continuous infusion to target sodium level (often 145-155 mEq/L) in a variety of underlying disease states.

There are several potential general benefits and risks of HTS as indicated in Table 19–1. Relative to mannitol, HTS may have a faster onset, longer duration of action, and lead to a more robust ICP response.[2] It may augment blood pressure in hemorrhagic shock and expand intravascular volume, which could be desirable in patients who are volume depleted. It should be noted, however, that there are situations in which volume expansion may not be desirable, for example, in patients with neurogenic stress cardiomyopathy. There have been concerns that, due to direct vasodilatory effects of HTS, rapid administration could lead to hypotension; however, more recent data has suggested that HTS pushes over 2 to 5 minutes are low risk.[3] HTS is typically administered centrally given risk of extravasation injury, necessitating securement of central access for use. However, more recent data have suggested that peripheral administration is similarly low risk.[4] Finally, use of HTS is associated with risk of metabolic acidosis and acute kidney injury (AKI).

In addition to setting up an osmotic gradient, mannitol may also have a rheological effect that acts to reduce ICP. It increases red cell deformability, decreasing blood viscosity, in turn increasing cerebral blood flow and oxygen delivery, and finally leading to reflex vasoconstriction and decreased cerebral blood volume. It should be noted that this putative mechanism has not consistently been replicated in human studies.[5] In contrast to HTS, mannitol is almost exclusively administered via bolus dosing for signs or symptoms of elevated ICP. Its diuretic effect may exacerbate a volume-depleted state and use is associated with AKI in 6% to 12% of patients. The potential for vasoconstriction associated with mannitol use is theoretically worrisome in patients with SAH who are at risk for vasospasm and its use in ICH has been associated with hematoma expansion.[6] These factors should be taken into consideration when considering choice of hyperosmolar agent in these populations.

EVIDENCE AND REVIEW

Are 3% HTS boluses effective in reducing cerebral edema/ICP?

Three percent HTS bolus therapy is only studied in patients with traumatic brain injury (TBI). However, in this population, 3% HTS bolus dosing appears to be safe and effective in reducing ICP.[7] Several studies have compared 3% HTS to mannitol, and it seems to be as effective or more effective than mannitol in this regard.[8-12] There is one retrospective study directly comparing 3% HTS with 23.4% HTS that did not identify a difference in neurologic outcome between groups.[13] In contrast, authors of a recent network meta-analysis suggested that more highly concentrated HTS (10-15%) may be more effective in ICP reduction than 3% HTS.[14] Taken together, available evidence is limited but suggests that 3% HTS is a safe and effective agent for reduction of ICP and may have similar efficacy to mannitol or more highly concentrated HTS.

Is hyperosmolar therapy safe in patients with subdural hematoma (SDH)?

Reduction of brain tissue volume via use of hyperosmolar agents in patients with SDH in theory may increase the risk for hematoma expansion via reduction of pressure surrounding the hematoma. However, this has not been seen in practice. Patients receiving hyperosmolar therapies for cerebral edema have not been reported to develop spontaneous SDH. In one study of patients with TBI inclusive of SDH, 75% of all patients who received HTS experienced reversal of TTH.[15] In another, patients who received higher doses of HTS throughout their hospital courses demonstrated improved command following at 3 months.[16] In non-operative patients, early studies reported "successful treatment" of SDH with mannitol infusion.[17,18] These authors postulated that mannitol might reduce the internal pressure of the hematoma itself, reducing risk for subsequent hemorrhage. There are significant limitations of these studies including small sample sizes, lack of control groups, and dichotomization of continuous variables that limit the ability to conclude that hyperosmolar therapies truly improve ICP or neurologic outcome in this population. However, their results do not suggest that patients with SDH who received hyperosmolar therapy experienced increased risk of hematoma expansion.

Does mannitol increase risk of vasospasm and delayed cerebral ischemia (DCI) in patients with SAH?

The rheological effect of mannitol in theory leads to reduction of ICP via decrease in cerebral blood volume, which in turn is achieved by vasoconstriction. It would be reasonable then to hypothesize that patients with SAH who are already at risk for vasospasm might be put at increased risk for DCI following administration of mannitol. Limited data comparing mannitol to HTS in SAH, however, has not revealed increased rates of DCI in patients who received mannitol.[19]

Is hyperosmolar therapy effective in reducing cerebral edema in patients with SAH, TBI, ICH, and stroke?

Guidelines for the treatment of cerebral edema were published by Cook et al. in 2020.[20] Utility of hyperosmolar agents in the management of elevated ICP is largely dependent upon the etiology of cerebral edema. In patients with SAH, bolus dosing of HTS or mannitol by symptoms has consistently been shown to reduce cerebral edema. As above, the potential for vasoconstriction with mannitol raises the theoretical concern for increased risk of delayed cerebral edema, though this has not been observed in studies of patients with SAH. There is conflicting data regarding whether dosing HTS to target sodium level reduces cerebral edema in this population.

In patients with TBI, HTS and mannitol are both effective in reducing cerebral edema. Given relative frequency of volume depletion and benefit for augmenting cerebral perfusion pressure (CPP) some authors suggest using HTS preferentially over mannitol in selected patients from this population, though this is not universally accepted.[21] Data regarding use of hyperosmolar agents in patients with ICH is very limited. Potential evidence of benefit of bolus HTS in this population is derived only from data on populations of patients with cerebral edema from a variety of etiologies, among which patients with ICH are included. There is conflicting data as to whether treating to a sodium goal in this population reduces ICP. Mannitol use in patients with ICH has been linked to hematoma expansion and steroids (while not a hyperosmolar agent) for treatment of cerebral edema in this population have been associated with increased risks of infection, diabetic complications, and mortality.

In patients with AIS, both HTS and mannitol boluses are effective in reduction of cerebral edema and elevated ICP. In this population, there is data to suggest that HTS is effective in patients in whom mannitol failed. Further, prophylactic hyperosmolar therapy with mannitol in AIS may increase risk of death or disability. There is conflicting data as to whether treatment to a sodium target prevents ICP crises in this population.

Is hyperosmolar therapy effective in reducing cerebral edema in patients with meningitis and hepatic encephalopathy?

In community-acquired bacterial meningitis, ICP control may improve mortality, however, data to drive choice of ICP-lowering intervention is lacking. In this population and in patients with tuberculous meningitis, steroids do improve neurologic outcome, perhaps in part due to reduction in cerebral edema and ICP among other mechanisms. There is limited data regarding hyperosmolar therapy for elevated intracranial pressure in hepatic encephalopathy. Mannitol reduces cerebral edema and ICP in this population and 23.4% HTS has been shown to reduce brain volume in one study.[22] In a single, small, placebo-controlled study, 3% HTS boluses to target sodium 145 to 155 mEq/L did appear to decrease ICP.

Is hyperosmolar therapy effective in managing brain tumor-related cerebral edema?

Corticosteroids remain the agent of choice for treatment of acutely worsened edema and elevated ICP in this population. Evidence for osmotherapy in patients with primary or secondary brain tumors is limited. There is risk of rebound ICP elevation in patients treated with hyperosmolar therapies who have tumors that are known to cause disruption of the BBB.[23] Patients treated with HTS in one retrospective study had increased bleeding, infection, and longer ICU length of stay.[24]

Is hyperosmolar therapy effective in managing cerebral edema after cardiac arrest?

A gap in the literature exists regarding the effect of hyperosmolar agents on cerebral edema or ICP in patients with anoxic brain injury. Recent retrospective data suggests, as in other disease states, that osmolar therapy in this population does not influence neurologic outcome.[25]

REFERENCES

1. Jagannatha AT, Sriganesh K, Devi BI, Rao GSU. An equiosmolar study on early intracranial physiology and long term outcome in severe traumatic brain injury comparing mannitol and hypertonic saline. *J Clin Neurosci Off J Neurosurg Soc Australas.* 2016;27:68–73. doi:10.1016/j.jocn.2015.08.035
2. Harutjunyan L, Holz C, Rieger A, Menzel M, Grond S, Soukup J. Efficiency of 7.2% hypertonic saline hydroxyethyl starch 200/0.5 versus mannitol 15% in the treatment of increased intracranial pressure in neurosurgical patients—a randomized clinical trial [ISRCTN62699180]. *Crit Care.* 2005;9(5):R530–40. doi:10.1186/cc3767
3. O'Brien SK, Koehl JL, Demers LB, Hayes BD, Barra ME. Safety and tolerability of 23.4% hypertonic saline administered over 2 to 5 minutes for the treatment of cerebral herniation and intracranial pressure elevation. *Neurocrit Care.* Published online September 2022. doi:10.1007/s12028-022-01604-1
4. Faiver L, Hensler D, Rush SC, Kashlan O, Williamson CA, Rajajee V. Safety and efficacy of 23.4% sodium chloride administered via peripheral venous access for the treatment of cerebral herniation and intracranial pressure elevation. *Neurocrit Care.* 2021;35(3):845–852. doi:10.1007/s12028-021-01248-7
5. Diringer MN, Scalfani MT, Zazulia AR, Videen TO, Dhar R, Powers WJ. Effect of mannitol on cerebral blood volume in patients with head injury. *Neurosurgery.* 2012;70(5):1215–1218; discussion 1219. doi:10.1227/NEU.0b013e3182417bc2

6. Sun S, Li Y, Zhang H, et al. The effect of mannitol in the early stage of supratentorial hypertensive intracerebral hemorrhage: a systematic review and meta-analysis. *World Neurosurg.* Published online December 2018. doi:10.1016/j.wneu.2018.11.249
7. Huang S-J, Chang L, Han Y-Y, Lee Y-C, Tu Y-K. Efficacy and safety of hypertonic saline solutions in the treatment of severe head injury. *Surg Neurol.* 2006;65(6):539–546; discussion 546. doi:10.1016/j.surneu.2005.11.019
8. Mangat HS, Wu X, Gerber LM, et al. Hypertonic saline is superior to mannitol for the combined effect on intracranial pressure and cerebral perfusion pressure burdens in patients with severe traumatic brain injury. *Neurosurgery.* 2020;86(2):221–230. doi:10.1093/neuros/nyz046
9. Patil H, Gupta R. A comparative study of bolus dose of hypertonic saline, mannitol, and mannitol plus glycerol combination in patients with severe traumatic brain injury. *World Neurosurg.* 2019;125:e221–e228. doi:10.1016/j.wneu.2019.01.051
10. Colton K, Yang S, Hu PF, et al. Pharmacologic treatment reduces pressure times time dose and relative duration of intracranial hypertension. *J Intensive Care Med.* 2016;31(4):263–269. doi:10.1177/0885066614555692
11. Mangat HS, Chiu Y-L, Gerber LM, Alimi M, Ghajar J, Härtl R. Hypertonic saline reduces cumulative and daily intracranial pressure burdens after severe traumatic brain injury. *J Neurosurg.* 2015;122(1):202–210. doi:10.3171/2014.10.JNS132545
12. Cheng F, Xu M, Liu H, Wang W, Wang Z. A retrospective study of intracranial pressure in head-injured patients undergoing decompressive craniectomy: a comparison of hypertonic saline and mannitol. *Front Neurol.* 2018;9:631. doi:10.3389/fneur.2018.00631
13. Traficante D, Galaktionova D, Marseille U, Hochman S, Zuberi J, Madlinger R. Comparison of 3% vs. 23.4% hypertonic saline in traumatic brain injury. *J Curr Surg.* 2019;9(4):39–44.
14. Wang X, He Q, Ma L, You C. Comparison of different concentrations of hypertonic saline in patients with traumatic brain injury: evidence from direct and indirect comparisons. *Injury.* 2022;53(11):3729–3735. doi:10.1016/j.injury.2022.08.065
15. Koenig MA, Bryan M, Lewin JL 3rd, Mirski MA, Geocadin RG, Stevens RD. Reversal of transtentorial herniation with hypertonic saline. *Neurology.* 2008;70(13):1023–1029. doi:10.1212/01.wnl.0000304042.05557.60
16. Dunham CM, Malik RJ, Huang GS, Kohli CM, Brocker BP, Ugokwe KT. Hypertonic saline administration and complex traumatic brain injury outcomes: a retrospective study. *Int J Burns Trauma.* 2018;8(3):40–53.
17. Suzuki J, Takaku A. Nonsurgical treatment of chronic subdural hematoma. *J Neurosurg.* 1970;33(5):548–553. doi:10.3171/jns.1970.33.5.0548
18. Kinjo T, Mukawa J, Nakata M, Kinjo N. [Chronic subdural hematoma secondary to coagulopathy]. *No Shinkei Geka.* 1991;19(10):991–997.
19. Huang X, Yang L. [Comparison clinical efficacy of 3% hypertonic saline solution with 20% mannitol in treatment of intracranial hypertension in patients with aneurysmal subarachnoid hemorrhage]. *Zhejiang da xue xue bao Yi xue ban = J Zhejiang Univ Med Sci.* 2015;44(4):389–395. doi:10.3785/j.issn.1008-9292.2015.07.07
20. Cook AM, Morgan Jones G, Hawryluk GWJ, et al. Guidelines for the acute treatment of cerebral edema in neurocritical care patients. *Neurocrit Care.* 2020;32(3):647–666. doi:10.1007/s12028-020-00959-7
21. Quintard H, Meyfroidt G, Citerio G. Hyperosmolar agents for TBI: all are equal, but some are more equal than others? *Neurocrit Care.* 2020;33(2):613–614. doi:10.1007/s12028-020-01063-6
22. Liotta EM, Lizza BD, Romanova AL, et al. 23.4% saline decreases brain tissue volume in severe hepatic encephalopathy as assessed by a quantitative CT marker. *Crit Care Med.* 2016;44(1):171–179. doi:10.1097/CCM.0000000000001276
23. Palma L, Bruni G, Fiaschi AI, Mariottini A. Passage of mannitol into the brain around gliomas: a potential cause of rebound phenomenon. A study on 21 patients. *J Neurosurg Sci.* 2006;50(3):63–66.
24. Ally W, Hurdle A, Nesheiwat C, Finch C, Michael M, Sills A. Use of hypertonic saline in surgical patients with brain tumors to treat cerebral edema. *Crit Care Med.* 2009;37(12):A1–A542.
25. Fuller ZL, Faro JW, Callaway CW, Coppler PJ, Elmer J. Recovery among post-arrest patients with mild-to-moderate cerebral edema. *Resuscitation.* 2021;162:149–153. doi:10.1016/j.resuscitation.2021.02.033

CHAPTER

20

What Intracranial Pressure Targets Should Be Used in Severe Traumatic Brain Injury Management?

Jeffrey R. Vitt, MD, Lara L. Zimmermann, MD, Shawn Banash, MD, Kiarash Shahlaie, MD, PhD, & Ryan M. Martin, MD

Case

A 25-year-old construction worker falls from the fourth story of a construction site. Upon presentation, she is noted to have a Glasgow coma scale score of 6. Imaging reveals multifocal hemorrhage contusions, and comminuted skull fractures, but without epidural or subdural hematomas. An external ventricular drain is placed. Over the subsequent few days, her intracranial pressure (ICP) continues to spike periodically, requiring increasing sedation and hyperosmolar therapy. As this lady progresses through her post-traumatic period, what ICP should be targeted?

Key Points

- Intracranial pressure (ICP) monitoring is a foundation of severe traumatic brain injury (TBI) management and has been associated with increased therapeutic intensity, lower mortality and improved functional outcomes.
- From a practical standpoint, ICP values exceeding 20 to 22 mm Hg have been correlated in multiple studies with worse outcomes after even a short duration of time and serve as a reasonable standardized threshold to institute ICP-lowering treatments in most TBI patients.[9,12,28]
- However, ICP should not be viewed as a dichotomous variable with values below a certain threshold regarded as safe and those above considered dangerous in all patient populations.
- Moderately elevated ICP values below standard thresholds may still be harmful, particularly if sustained for long durations of time or if autoregulation is impaired, and should be viewed in context of other neurophysiologic findings including cerebral perfusion pressure (CPP), pressure reactivity (PRx), cerebral blood flow (CBF) analysis, and brain tissue oxygen tension to guide treatment decisions.
- Additionally, careful attention to ICP waveform morphology provides valuable insights into intracranial compliance and with the use of machine leaning, may eventually help forecast dangerous ICP elevations to allow for preventive rather than reactionary treatment strategies.

BACKGROUND

Over the past several decades, significant progress has been made in the management of individuals with traumatic brain injury (TBI) due to adherence to protocols focused on early targeted resuscitation and the development of centers with dedicated neurotrauma and neurocritical care expertise.[1,2] Central to the practice of neurocritical care is an emphasis on preventing secondary brain injury that results from a variety of adverse physiologic responses, including cerebral edema, neuro-inflammation, excitotoxicity, and impaired cerebral perfusion. Following the 1964 seminal publication by Lundberg on the utility of continuous ventricular-fluid pressure monitoring in head injury patients, intracranial pressure (ICP) monitoring has become a central focus of severe TBI (Glasgow coma scale 3-8) management and is strongly recommended by the Brain Trauma Foundation (BTF).[3,4]

While it is well known that elevations in ICP can lead to excess mortality and poor neurologic outcome, the precise threshold to institute treatment remains elusive.[5,6] Multiple studies have reported conflicting evidence of a safe upper limit of ICP using large TBI cohorts while the most recent BTF guidelines recommend maintaining ICP ≤ 22 mm Hg.[4,6–9] Given the substantial heterogeneity that exists in patterns of injury, patient demographics, and complex physiologic derangements following TBI, it may seem implausible that a single ICP threshold can adequately suffice to prevent neurologic deterioration in all patients. Despite these shortcomings, ICP monitoring provides critical information regarding cerebral dysfunction and remains an indispensable tool in the armamentarium of the neurointensivist. This chapter aims to review the current best practices of ICP treatment-threshold strategies with a focus toward the future of precision medicine in neurocritical care.

Pressure-Volume Relationship and ICP Waveform Analysis

Elevations in ICP are harmful to the brain due to brain compression and reduced cerebral perfusion. In severe cases, ICP may exceed the diastolic closing pressure resulting in absent or retrograde diastolic cerebral blood flow (CBF), progressing to cerebrocirculatory arrest.[10,11] In less severe cases, even moderate elevations in ICP can impair brain perfusion leading to ischemia and oligemia in vulnerable brain parenchyma.[9,12] As described in the Monroe-Kellie doctrine, an increase in any of the components of the intracranial system, namely brain, blood and cerebrospinal fluid (CSF), must be accompanied by an equivalent volumetric reduction in another constituent to maintain homeostasis.[13] Given the fixed nature of the intracranial vault, disproportionate increases in volume (such as cases of hematoma formation or acute hydrocephalus) are rapidly met with diminished compliance and the pressure-volume relationship becomes nonlinear where small alterations in volume induce large changes in ICP (Figure 20–1A).[13–15]

The compensatory reserve relationship can be mathematically portrayed by the RAP index which is a correlation coefficient (R) between ICP waveform amplitude (A) and mean ICP (P) (Figure 20–1B).[14,15] During the compensatory phase the RAP index is near 0 and indicates no synchronization between changes in volume and ICP. However, once the pressure-volume relationship shifts rightwards toward the steep portion of the curve, the RAP index approaches +1 due to impaired compliance. With further ICP increases, a critical threshold is crossed as the autoregulatory capacity is exhausted leading to passive collapse of the cerebral vasculature and a decline in ICP amplitude resulting in a negative coefficient.[14] Increased RAP values correlate with worse outcome in TBI and are strongly associated with particular imaging patterns including diffuse injury and edema.[15,16] RAP may also be used to better characterize which

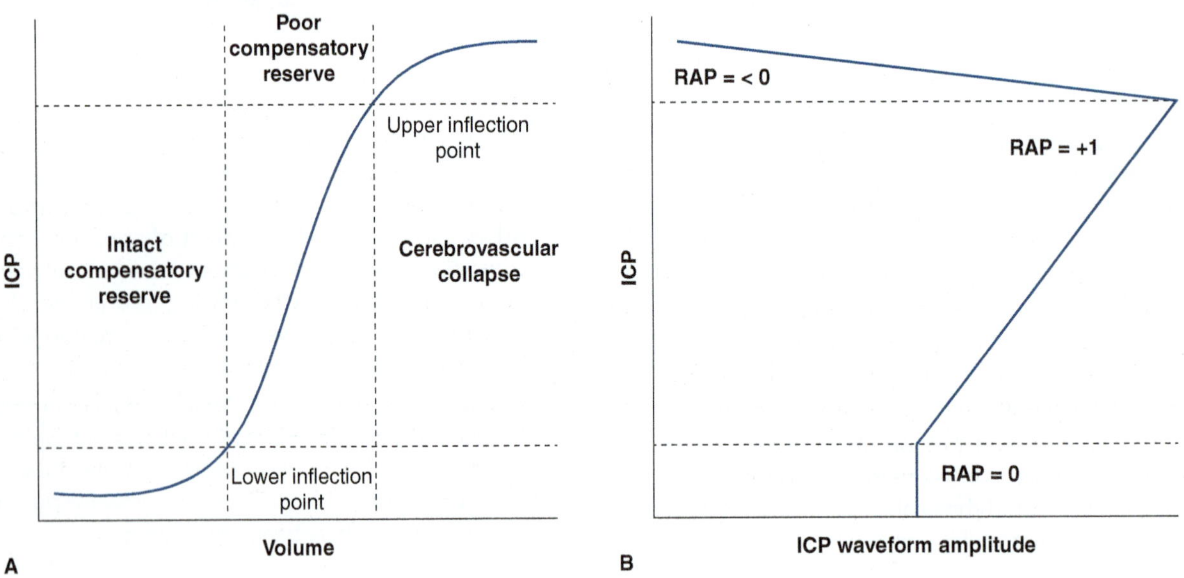

FIGURE 20–1 **(A)** The pressure-volume curve can best be represented as a sigmoid curve with three segments. In segment 1, compensatory reserve exists such that small changes in volume do not lead to significant changes in intracranial pressure (ICP). Once these compensatory reserves are exhausted in segment 2, a lower inflection point is triggered and even small volume changes result in exponential increases in ICP. Finally in segment 3, the autoregulatory capacity of the arterial system to combat declining cerebral blood flow (CBF) is overcome by elevated ICP thus leading to cerebrovascular collapse and deflection of the curve to the right. **(B)** Relationship of ICP waveform amplitude (AMP) to mean ICP. Initially there are no changes in AMP with alterations in ICP resulting in a correlation coefficient (RAP) of 0. As intracranial compliance decreases, there is an observed increase in AMP with corresponding increases in ICP, making RAP approach +1. Finally, once ICP is sufficiently elevated to impede CBF there is an inverse relationship between ICP and AMP such that further increases in ICP decrease AMP and result in a RAP < 0.

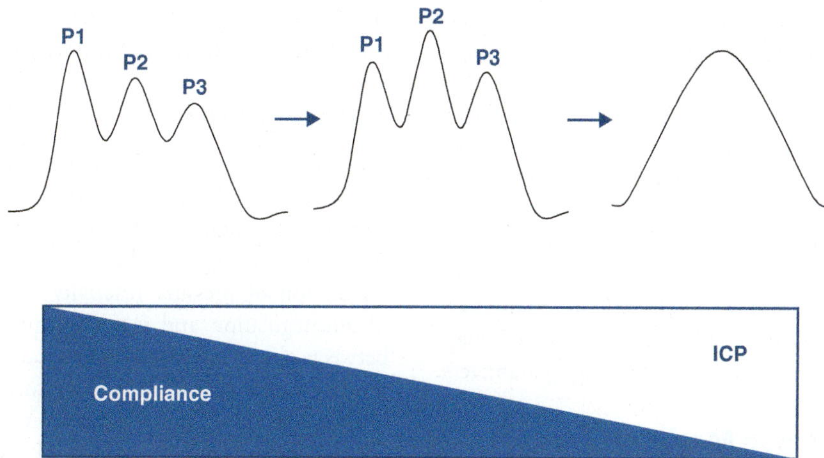

FIGURE 20–2 The ICP waveform represents oscillations of intracranial pressure (ICP) as blood flows into the brain throughout the cardiac cycle. A normal relationship is seen in which P1 (percussion wave) representing arterial pulsation is greater than P2 (tidal wave) indicating normal intracranial compliance. P3 represents the dicrotic notch. As Intracranial compliance decreases, the P2 wave becomes more prominent and exceeds P1. As compliance further decreases and ICP approaches a critical value, the ICP waveform loses its complexity and takes on a sinusoidal appearance.

episodes of ICP are pathologic with a weighted ICP calculation [ICP*(RAP-1)] aimed at magnifying the impact of ICP leading to obstructed CBF. Though this approach requires confirmation in other studies, it has been demonstrated to possess better discrimination for mortality compared to mean ICP assessment alone.[15]

While mean ICP recordings may be useful for determining the need for acute intervention, examination of the ICP waveform can provide valuable insights into intracranial compliance and risk for deterioration, even when ICP is below treatment thresholds.[17,18] In the absence of significant pathology, the ICP waveform has three notches corresponding to the systolic (P1), tidal (P2), and dicrotic waves (P3) and are of decreasing amplitude.[18] As intracranial compliance decreases, P2 and P3 begin to exceed P1 and eventually P3 disappears leaving a sinusoidal morphology (Figure 20–2).[13,18] Elevation of P2 can predict risk for subsequent ICP crisis and with advanced multiscale entropy analysis, researchers have demonstrated a reduction in ICP waveform complexity is common during periods of severely elevated ICP and outperforms mean ICP recordings and cerebrovascular reactivity as a predictor of mortality and functional outcome in TBI.[17,19]

EVIDENCE AND REVIEW

Efforts to define a treatment threshold for ICP have yielded variable results. In 1977, Miller and colleagues reported divergent mean ICP thresholds for poor outcome of >10 mm Hg and >40 mm Hg depending on whether the primary injury was diffuse or related to a mass lesion, respectively.[5] Over the next decade several small noncontrolled studies were published with optimal ICP thresholds ranging from 15 to 25 mm Hg.[6,20] **In 2000, the BTF released guidelines with a recommended ICP threshold of 20 to 25 mm Hg, and in 2007 further refined their recommendation to ≤20 mm Hg with a level II recommendation.[21]

Moving from 20 to 22 mm Hg

A retrospective study of 429 patients with severe TBI found an average ICP above 20 mm Hg was associated with a 30% absolute risk increase for mortality, though probabilistic analysis revealed an exact threshold closer to 23 mm Hg.[8] In 2011, Sorrentino et al published a single-center retrospective study of 459 severe TBI patients and by using sequential chi square analysis found an average ICP threshold of 22 mm Hg best predicted the intersection between mortality and favorable outcome and was the primary basis of evidence used by the BTF to raise the recommended ICP treatment threshold to 22 mm Hg in the 2016 guidelines.[4,22]

This most recent recommendation by the BTF has been met with significant debate, stemming from the limited number of studies available and concerns over methodologic issues and interpretation.[23-26] First, all modern studies involve patients in whom ICP is actively being managed and therefore better characterizes the impact of ICP treatment refractoriness rather than the natural history of certain ICP values themselves. Furthermore, many studies involved averaging ICP over the entire hospital stay as a static variable which is counter to the clinical reality that ICP is a dynamic parameter that frequently changes due to alterations in cerebral autoregulation and intracranial compliance.[12,27] Finally, declaring a specific treatment threshold over an entire cohort overlooks how subgroups of patients may respond differently to ICP and is an oversimplification of the complex interactions between diverse injury patterns and individual cerebral physiologic responses to changes in brain perfusion.

In the case of Sorrentino et al, while a threshold of 22 mm Hg was found to best predict outcome, the cohort was predominantly younger age men and subgroup analysis revealed a threshold of 18 mm Hg to be more appropriate for female and elderly patients.[22] Furthermore, recent analysis using high frequency measurements demonstrated that ICP values as low as 10 mm Hg may still cause harm and there is growing evidence that dynamic autoregulatory status strongly influences the range of acceptable ICPs.[7,12,28] These findings call into question the notion of a one-size-fits-all approach to establishing a safe ICP and many have argued to shift focus toward the combined impact of ICP magnitude and duration as well as individual physiologic parameters.

Using a Pressure Dose Model

Rather than focusing on static ICP thresholds to guide clinicians, a pressure-dose model has emerged, which weighs both the magnitude and duration of pathological ICP to help inform treatment options.[9,12,29] Using a threshold of 20 mm Hg, this area under the curve approach demonstrates superior predictive value for mortality and functional outcome compared to mean ICP recordings alone.[29-31] Guiza et al used high frequency ICP data and were able to model a pressure-time relationship where even ICPs ranging from 15 to 20 mm Hg could induce injury if sufficiently sustained, whereas ICP values above 20 mm Hg and 30 mm Hg correlated with worsening outcome after 37 minutes and 8 minutes, respectively.[12] Subsequent analysis has confirmed this dose relationship with evidence that short durations of high ICP appear more injurious compared to more prolonged durations of moderately elevated ICP.[9] This research has also served to provide valuable insights in the critical role cerebral autoregulation plays in the response to ICP, as small durations of elevated ICP are poorly tolerated when cerebrovascular reactivity is impaired due to critical hypoperfusion.[9,12]

Autoregulation

Autoregulation is a vital component of normal cerebral physiology and optimal perfusion and is commonly compromised in patients with moderate to severe TBI (83%-100% of patients), particularly throughout the first week after injury.[9,27] Real-time calculation of pressure reactivity (PRx) allows for estimation of autoregulation and is a continuous correlation coefficient between alterations in mean arterial pressure (MAP) and ICP; positive values denote impaired autoregulation and negative values suggest intact cerebrovascular reactivity (Figure 20–3A).[14] Several studies have demonstrated a clinical cutoff of >0.2 at which point there is significant disturbance of PRx and increased mortality.[16,28,32] The MAP range in which autoregulation is preserved is patient-specific, with elderly individuals often demonstrating a narrowed window with rightward shift that is easily disrupted in the setting of ICP elevations or worsening cerebral injury.[27,33,34] Using a CENTER TBI cohort, optimal-ICP guided by the lowest PRx was determined in nearly two-thirds of patients, ranging from 15 to 29 mm Hg, and ended up being a better predictor of outcome compared to static thresholds ICP of 20 to 22 mm Hg.[16]

Using a similar methodology, PRx can be plotted against cerebral perfusion pressure (CPP = MAP – ICP) to construct a "U-shaped" curve where the CPP value associated with the lowest PRx value is indicative of maximally preserved autoregulation (Figure 20–3B).[14] In retrospective analyses, patients experience more favorable outcomes when their mean CPP remains near the PRx derived optimal CPP (CPP_{OPT}), presumably due to

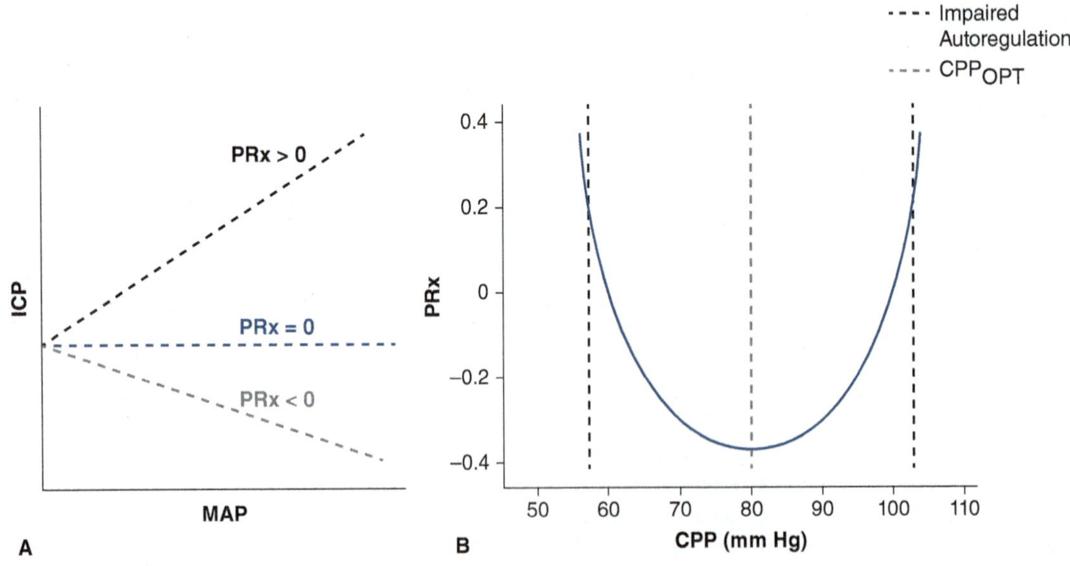

FIGURE 20–3 **(A)** Relationship of mean arterial pressure (MAP) to intracranial pressure (ICP) reflected by the pressure reactivity index (PRx). A linear relationship denoted by a PRx > 0 suggests impaired autoregulation whereas a PRx < 0 denotes intact autoregulation. **(B)** Pressure reactivity index (PRx) plotted as a function of cerebral perfusion pressure (CPP). The lowest associated PRx denotes the CPP associated with the most optimal degree of cerebral autoregulation (CPP_{OPT}). PRx values > 0.2 are a threshold for significantly impaired cerebral autoregulation.

preservation of cerebral autoregulation.[32,34] CPP is an important physiologic parameter that reflects cerebral substrate delivery, and when inappropriately low can precipitate ischemia, while excessive increases may lead to cerebral hyperemia and edema. Previous guidelines suggested targeting a CPP > 70 mm Hg based on clinical and experimental observations; however, these were later reduced to 60 to 70 mm Hg in the setting of a fivefold increase in acute respiratory distress syndrome from excessive intravenous fluids and vasopressors in the higher CPP arm with no difference in outcomes compared with lower targets.[4,35,36]

Subsequent studies have revealed that modest elevations in CPP can exert a protective effect against ICP insults, though the safe range of CPP is heavily influenced by individual physiologic parameters and autoregulatory status such that it is impossible to accurately produce fixed thresholds on a population level.[12,22,37] The COGiTATE study was a multicenter phase II trial, which aimed to evaluate the safety and feasibility of a cerebral autoregulation-guided CPP management strategy compared to a control of standard BTF recommendations of CPP 60 to 70 mm Hg.[38] The investigators found that patients in the intervention arm spent significantly less time with CPP < 60 mm Hg and an increased proportion of time with CPP > 70 mm Hg based on PRx determinations, with considerably more time with CPP near optimal CPP. While not powered to measure outcomes, fewer patients died in the intervention arm (23% vs. 44%) and there was no differences in therapeutic intensity level or reported adverse events, suggesting such a treatment strategy is safe, feasible and may improve functional recovery in TBI by ensuring optimal physiology.

REFERENCES

1. Khellaf A, Khan DZ, Helmy A. Recent advances in traumatic brain injury. *J Neurol.* 2019 Nov;266(11):2878–89.
2. Patel HC, Bouamra O, Woodford M, et al. Trends in head injury outcome from 1989 to 2003 and the effect of neurosurgical care: an observational study. *Lancet.* 2005 Oct;366(9496):1538–44.
3. Lundberg N, Troupp H, Lorin H. Continuous recording of the ventricular-fluid pressure in patients with severe acute traumatic brain injury: a preliminary report. *J Neurosurg.* 1965 Jun;22(6):581–90.
4. Carney N, Totten AM, O'Reilly C, et al. Guidelines for the management of severe traumatic brain injury, fourth edition. *Neurosurgery.* 2017 Jan 1; 80(1):6–15.
5. Miller JD, Becker DP, Ward JD, et al. Significance of intracranial hypertension in severe head injury. J Neurosurg. 1977 Oct;47(4):503–16.
6. Marmarou A, Anderson RL, Ward JD, et al. Impact of ICP instability and hypotension on outcome in patients with severe head trauma. *J Neurosurg.* 1991 Nov;75(Supplement):S59–66.
7. Hawryluk GWJ, Nielson JL, Huie JR, et al. Analysis of normal high-frequency intracranial pressure values and treatment threshold in neurocritical care patients: insights into normal values and a potential treatment threshold. *JAMA Neurol.* 2020 Sep 1;77(9):1150.
8. Balestreri M, Czosnyka M, Hutchinson P, et al. Impact of intracranial pressure and cerebral perfusion pressure on severe disability and mortality after head injury. *Neurocrit Care.* 2006;4(1):8–13.
9. Åkerlund CA, Donnelly J, Zeiler FA, et al. Impact of duration and magnitude of raised intracranial pressure on outcome after severe traumatic brain injury: a CENTER-TBI high-resolution group study. Kobeissy FH, editor. *PLOS ONE.* 2020 Dec 14;15(12):e0243427.
10. Marinoni M, Alari F, Mastronardi V, et al. The relevance of early TCD monitoring in the intensive care units for the confirming of brain death diagnosis. *Neurol Sci.* 2011 Feb 1;32(1):73–7.
11. Varsos GV, Richards HK, Kasprowicz M, et al. Cessation of diastolic cerebral blood flow velocity: the role of critical closing pressure. *Neurocrit Care.* 2014 Feb;20(1):40–8.
12. Güiza F, Depreitere B, Piper I, et al. Visualizing the pressure and time burden of intracranial hypertension in adult and paediatric traumatic brain injury. *Intensive Care Med.* 2015 Jun;41(6):1067–76.
13. Kawoos U, McCarron R, Auker C, et al. Advances in intracranial pressure monitoring and its significance in managing traumatic brain injury. *Int J Mol Sci.* 2015 Dec 4;16(12):28979–97.
14. Czosnyka M. Monitoring and interpretation of intracranial pressure. *J Neurol Neurosurg Psychiatry.* 2004 Jun 1;75(6):813–21.
15. Calviello L, Donnelly J, Cardim D, et al. Compensatory-reserve-weighted intracranial pressure and its association with outcome after traumatic brain injury. *Neurocrit Care.* 2018 Apr;28(2):212–20.
16. Zeiler FA, Kim DJ, Cabeleira M, et al. Impaired cerebral compensatory reserve is associated with admission imaging characteristics of diffuse insult in traumatic brain injury. *Acta Neurochir (Wien).* 2018 Dec;160(12):2277–87.
17. Fan JY, Kirkness C, Vicini P, et al. Intracranial pressure waveform morphology and intracranial adaptive capacity. *Am J Crit Care.* 2008 Nov 1;17(6):545–54.
18. Nucci CG, De Bonis P, Mangiola A, et al. Intracranial pressure wave morphological classification: automated analysis and clinical validation. *Acta Neurochir (Wien).* 2016 Mar;158(3):581–8.
19. Lu CW, Czosnyka M, Shieh JS, et al. Complexity of intracranial pressure correlates with outcome after traumatic brain injury. *Brain.* 2012 Aug 1; 135(8):2399–408.
20. Saul TG, Ducker TB. Effect of intracranial pressure monitoring and aggressive treatment on mortality in severe head injury. *J Neurosurg.* 1982 Apr;56(4):498–503.
21. Bratton SL, Chestnut RM, Ghajar J, et al. VIII. Intracranial pressure thresholds. *J Neurotrauma.* 2007 May;24(supplement 1):S-55–S-58.
22. Sorrentino E, Diedler J, Kasprowicz M, et al. Critical Thresholds for cerebrovascular reactivity after traumatic brain injury. *Neurocrit Care.* 2012 Apr;16(2):258–66.
23. Meyfroidt G, Bouzat P, Casaer MP, et al. Management of moderate to severe traumatic brain injury: an update for the intensivist. *Intensive Care Med.* 2022 Jun;48(6):649–66.
24. Helbok R, Meyfroidt G, Beer R. Intracranial pressure thresholds in severe traumatic brain injury: Con: The injured brain is not aware of ICP thresholds! *Intensive Care Med.* 2018 Aug;44(8):1318–20.
25. Chesnut RM, Videtta W. Situational intracranial pressure management: an argument against a fixed treatment threshold. *Crit Care Med.* 2020 Aug;48(8):1214–6.
26. Myburgh JA. Intracranial pressure thresholds in severe traumatic brain injury: Pro. *Intensive Care Med.* 2018 Aug;44(8):1315–7.
27. Sviri GE, Aaslid R, Douville CM, et al. Time course for autoregulation recovery following severe traumatic brain injury: clinical article. *J Neurosurg.* 2009 Oct;111(4):695–700.
28. Lazaridis C, DeSantis SM, Smielewski P, et al. Patient-specific thresholds of intracranial pressure in severe traumatic brain injury: clinical article. *J Neurosurg.* 2014 Apr;120(4):893–900.
29. Vik A, Nag T, Fredriksli OA, et al. Relationship of "dose" of intracranial hypertension to outcome in severe traumatic brain injury: clinical article. *J Neurosurg.* 2008 Oct;109(4):678–84.
30. Kahraman S, Dutton RP, Hu P, et al. Automated measurement of "pressure times time dose" of Intracranial hypertension best predicts outcome after severe traumatic brain injury. *J Trauma Inj Infect Crit Care.* 2010 Jul;69(1):110–8.
31. Sheth KN, Stein DM, Aarabi B, et al. Intracranial pressure dose and outcome in traumatic brain injury. *Neurocrit Care.* 2013 Feb;18(1):26–32.
32. Steiner LA, Czosnyka M, Piechnik SK, et al. Continuous monitoring of cerebrovascular pressure reactivity allows determination of optimal cerebral perfusion pressure in patients with traumatic brain injury: *Crit Care Med.* 2002 Apr;30(4):733–8.
33. Batson C, Froese L, Gomez A, et al. Impact of age and biological sex on cerebrovascular reactivity in adult moderate/severe traumatic brain injury: an exploratory analysis. *Neurotrauma Rep.* 2021 Nov 1;2(1):488–501.
34. Donnelly J, Czosnyka M, Adams H, et al. Individualizing Thresholds of cerebral perfusion pressure using estimated limits of autoregulation. *Crit Care Med.* 2017 Sep;45(9):1464–71.

35. Eker C, Asgeirsson B, Grande P, et al. Improved outcome after severe head injury with a new therapy based on principles for brain volume regulation and preserved microcirculation. *Crit Care Med.* 1998 Nov 1;26(11):1881–6.
36. Robertson C, Valadka A, Hannay H, et al. Prevention of secondary ischemic insults after severe head injury. *Crit Care Med.* 27(10):2086–95.
37. Güiza F, Meyfroidt G, Piper I, et al. Cerebral perfusion pressure insults and associations with outcome in adult traumatic brain injury. *J Neurotrauma.* 2017 Aug 15;34(16):2425–31.
38. Tas J, Beqiri E, van Kaam RC, et al. Targeting Autoregulation-Guided Cerebral Perfusion Pressure after Traumatic Brain Injury (COGiTATE): a feasibility randomized controlled clinical trial. *J Neurotrauma.* 2021 Oct 15;38(20):2790–800.

CHAPTER

21

What Is the Role of Hyperventilation in Traumatic Brain Injury?

James Tanner McMahon, MD &
Wenya Linda Bi, MD, PhD

Case

A 24-year-old man presents to the emergency department after an unhelmeted motorcycle accident. On arrival, he is hemodynamically stable, has audible gurgling with respirations, has equal and reactive pupils, and his Glasgow coma scale (GCS) is 5. He is intubated for airway protection, and an arterial blood gas reveals a partial pressure of carbon dioxide ($PaCO_2$) of 40 mm Hg. A CT scan demonstrates generalized cerebral edema, basal cistern effacement, and scattered intraparenchymal and extra-axial hemorrhage (Figure 21–1). He is started on hyperosmolar therapy and an intracranial monitor is placed, which reads 28 mm Hg. Is there a role for hyperventilation in this case? If so, what factor in the presentation most prompts the need to start this intervention? If not, what scenario would call for it?

Key Points

- Hyperventilation can reduce intracranial pressure (ICP) in the acute setting (eg, impending/ongoing herniation); however, rebound ICP is a potential negative sequelae of prolonged hyperventilation.
- Existing studies point away from the use of prophylactic hyperventilation, and away from hyperventilation for prolonged duration of time when treating refractory intracranial hypertension.
- When hyperventilation is employed, avoid $PaCO_2$ of 25 mm Hg or less.

BACKGROUND

As with many issues in the field of neurocritical care and neurosurgery, therapeutic hyperventilation in the setting of traumatic brain injury (TBI) is commonly employed but insufficiently understood. The underlying mechanisms, optimal indications, safety, and efficacy of this intervention have been investigated for decades, but answers remain complex. In this chapter, we aim to summarize the best available evidence for hyperventilation in TBI and to present a clear argument for its use in specific circumstances.

The Monro-Kelli hypothesis dictates that the contents of the cranial vault are comprised of brain parenchyma, cerebrospinal fluid (CSF), and blood, and that any increase in volume of one of these three components but necessarily be compensated for by an equal decrease in volume of the sum of the others.[1] In the setting of severe TBI, in which cerebral edema causes the volume of brain parenchyma to rise, refractory intracranial pressure (ICP) may therefore be treated with either diversion of CSF or by a decrease in the cerebral blood volume (CBV).

Autoregulation of cerebral blood flow (CBF) is directly correlated to $PaCO_2$—in fact, $PaCO_2$ is the single largest determinant of CBF, with a linear effect on CBF between $PaCO_2$ 20 and 80 mm Hg.[2] As such, induced hyperventilation (usually achieved via an increase in respiratory rate on the ventilator), with a subsequent decrease in $PaCO_2$, can result in a cerebral vasoconstriction, decreased CBF, and, hypothetically, decrease ICP.

A second hypothesis regarding the benefits of hyperventilation is that lowering of $PaCO_2$ might reverse acidosis within the brain and CSF, thereby alleviating one of the ill effects of TBI. However, prolonged hyperventilation is posited to result in loss of the inherent bicarbonate buffer within CSF, and thus prolonged hyperventilation may result in no net benefit in brain and CSF pH. The drug tromethamine (THAM), an alkalinizing agent which functions as a proton acceptor has gained interest as a possible therapy to enter the CSF and overcome the loss of buffer, and thereby allow more sustained reversal of cerebral acidosis with hyperventilation.[3]

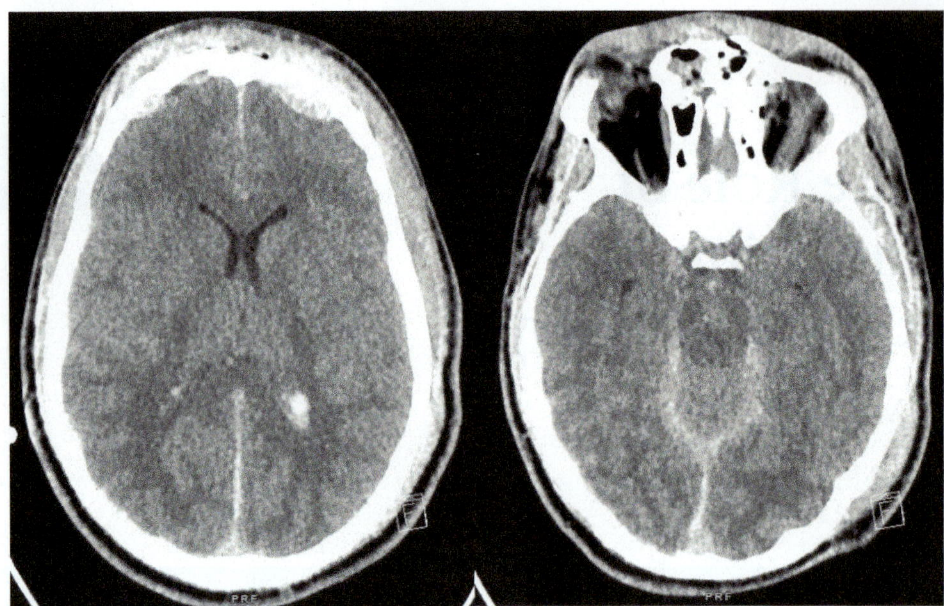

FIGURE 21–1 Axial non-contrast CT scan of the head demonstrating generalized cerebral edema, basal cistern effacement, and scatted intraparenchymal and extra-axial hemorrhage.

A concern with hyperventilation is that a decrease in CBF may deprive the brain of necessary oxygen during a time of severe stress, thereby exacerbating injury from the TBI. In fact, CBF has already been shown to be significantly decreased within at least the first 24 hours after TBI.[4–6] Further decrease in this blood supply could therefore potentially cause more harm than good. Hyperventilation also has possible non-CNS adverse effects, including barotrauma to the lungs, V/Q mismatch, increased myocardial ischemia and arrhythmias, alkalosis causing poor tissue oxygen delivery, and electrolyte disturbances.[7] Given these risks, hyperventilation should be used judiciously, in select scenarios.

EVIDENCE AND REVIEW

Two notable studies have demonstrated that hyperventilation does indeed result in a decrease in CBF and ICP. The first evaluated 186 patients with TBI, and found that a therapeutic hyperventilation to $PaCO_2$ ~30 (from ~36) resulted in decreased middle cerebral artery flow velocities (as expected) and was associated with a mean reduction in ICP from 19 to 13.[8] A second study compared effects of hyperventilation to goal $PaCO_2$ 30 versus 25 in patients with TBI, and found proportional decreases in CBF—even up to presumed ischemic levels.[9] In this study authors did note that positron emission tomography (PET) imaging of these same patients demonstrated preserved O_2 metabolism at these "ischemic" levels, thereby arguing against true injury.

The question of whether hyperventilation-induced vasoconstriction can truly lead to metabolic changes in the brain has also been investigated. Although equivocal, some studies indicate that the partial pressure of oxygen in the brain environment (PbO_2), and/or the partial pressure of oxygen in the jugular vein (SjO_2), can decrease with hyperventilation, possibly indicating inadequate O_2 supply to brain.[8,10–15] One prospective trial of 11 patients with GCS < 9 after TBI found that moderate hyperventilation resulted in significant decreases in PbO_2, but glucose, lactate, and pyruvate did not change, possibly indicating no meaningful changes in cerebral metabolic rate.[16] Other studies, however, have found increases in glutamate and lactate as well as increased lactate/pyruvate ratios.[17,18]

The most meaningful question—whether hyperventilation leads to better *clinical* outcomes in patients with severe TBI-has unfortunately undergone surprisingly little rigorous examination. Three notable retrospective studies have been published. One large example (N = 251) found improved mortality for TBI patients treated with hyperventilation ($PaCO_2$ 25-30) for a time period of 6 to 41 days, but survivors suffered worse neurological outcomes compared to normal ventilation.[19] A second retrospective of severe TBI patients in Austria found that moderate hyperventilation was associated with better ICU and 90-day outcomes, while "aggressive" hyperventilation had worse outcomes.[20] And a third, in this case in patients with *mild* TBI, found that hyperventilation was associated with worse outcomes.[21]

Two randomized controlled trials (RCTs) have been performed to further evaluate this question. One trial (N = 113) found that severe TBI patients undergoing hyperventilation to $PaCO_2$ ~25 mm Hg had worse functional outcomes (compared to normally-ventilated controls) at 3- and 6-month follow-up, but these lost significance at 1 year. Interestingly, subgroup analysis revealed that the worse outcomes were mainly derived from patients with GCS motor scores of 4 to 5, although this finding is limited by a smaller sample size. Of note, a separate group was given THAM in addition to hyperventilation, and this group had no significant difference in outcomes compared to controls.[22] A second RCT (N = 149) assigned severe TBI patients to mild hyperventilation (pCO_2 = 32 – 35) +/– THAM for 5 days. The investigators found no significant outcome difference at 3, 6, or 12 months, but patients treated with THAM had slightly better ICP control, with less time spent above ICP > 20 mm Hg.[23]

AVAILABLE GUIDELINES

In the most recent edition of the Brain Trauma Foundation guidelines, one class IIB recommendation was made: to avoid prophylactic hyperventilation to 25 mm Hg or less.[2] Hyperventilation is *reasonable as a temporizing measure in life-threatening scenarios of refractory ICPs with associated signs of impending or active herniation.*

REFERENCES

1. Mokri B. The Monro-Kellie hypothesis: applications in CSF volume depletion. *Neurology.* 2001;56(12):1746–1748.
2. Carney N, Totten AM, O'Reilly C, et al. Guidelines for the management of severe traumatic brain injury, fourth edition. *Neurosurgery.* 2017;80(1):6–15.
3. Zeiler FA, Teitelbaum J, Gillman LM, West M. THAM for control of ICP. *Neurocrit Care.* 2014;21(2):332–344.
4. Bouma GJ, Muizelaar JP, Choi SC, Newlon PG, Young HF. Cerebral circulation and metabolism after severe traumatic brain injury: the elusive role of ischemia. *J Neurosurg.* 1991;75(5):685–693.
5. Marion DW, Darby J, Yonas H. Acute regional cerebral blood flow changes caused by severe head injuries. *J Neurosurg.* 1991;74(3):407–414.
6. Sioutos PJ, Orozco JA, Carter LP, Weinand ME, Hamilton AJ, Williams FC. Continuous regional cerebral cortical blood flow monitoring in head-injured patients. *Neurosurgery.* 1995;36(5):943–949; discussion 949–950.
7. Gouvea Bogossian E, Peluso L, Creteur J, Taccone FS. Hyperventilation in adult TBI patients: how to approach it? *Front Neurol.* 2020;11:580859.
8. Rangel-Castilla L, Lara LR, Gopinath S, Swank PR, Valadka A, Robertson C. Cerebral hemodynamic effects of acute hyperoxia and hyperventilation after severe traumatic brain injury. *J Neurotrauma.* 2010;27(10):1853–1863.
9. Diringer MN, Videen TO, Yundt K, et al. Regional cerebrovascular and metabolic effects of hyperventilation after severe traumatic brain injury. *J Neurosurg.* 2002;96(1):103–108.
10. Sheinberg M, Kanter MJ, Robertson CS, Contant CF, Narayan RK, Grossman RG. Continuous monitoring of jugular venous oxygen saturation in head-injured patients. *J Neurosurg.* 1992;76(2):212–217.
11. Imberti R, Bellinzona G, Langer M. Cerebral tissue PO_2 and $SjvO_2$ changes during moderate hyperventilation in patients with severe traumatic brain injury. *J Neurosurg.* 2002;96(1):97–102.
12. Oertel M, Kelly DF, Lee JH, et al. Efficacy of hyperventilation, blood pressure elevation, and metabolic suppression therapy in controlling intracranial pressure after head injury. *J Neurosurg.* 2002;97(5):1045–1053.
13. Carmona Suazo JA, Maas AI, van den Brink WA, van Santbrink H, Steyerberg EW, Avezaat CJ. CO_2 reactivity and brain oxygen pressure monitoring in severe head injury. *Crit Care Med.* 2000;28(9):3268–3274.
14. Coles JP, Minhas PS, Fryer TD, et al. Effect of hyperventilation on cerebral blood flow in traumatic head injury: clinical relevance and monitoring correlates. *Crit Care Med.* 2002;30(9):1950–1959.
15. Svedung Wettervik T, Howells T, Hillered L, et al. Mild hyperventilation in traumatic brain injury-relation to cerebral energy metabolism, pressure autoregulation, and clinical outcome. *World Neurosurg.* 2020;133:e567–e575.
16. Brandi G, Stocchetti N, Pagnamenta A, Stretti F, Steiger P, Klinzing S. Cerebral metabolism is not affected by moderate hyperventilation in patients with traumatic brain injury. *Crit Care.* 2019;23(1):45.
17. Marion DW, Puccio A, Wisniewski SR, et al. Effect of hyperventilation on extracellular concentrations of glutamate, lactate, pyruvate, and local cerebral blood flow in patients with severe traumatic brain injury. *Crit Care Med.* 2002;30(12):2619–2625.
18. Soustiel JF, Mahamid E, Chistyakov A, Shik V, Benenson R, Zaaroor M. Comparison of moderate hyperventilation and mannitol for control of intracranial pressure control in patients with severe traumatic brain injury—a study of cerebral blood flow and metabolism. *Acta Neurochir (Wien).* 2006;148(8):845–851; discussion 851.
19. Gordon E. Controlled respiration in the management of patients with traumatic brain injuries. *Acta Anaesthesiol Scand.* 1971;15(3):193–208.
20. Mauritz W, Janciak I, Wilbacher I, Rusnak M. Severe traumatic brain injury in Austria IV: intensive care management. *Wien Klin Wochenschr.* 2007;119(1–2):46–55.
21. Tanaka C, Tagami T, Unemoto K, et al. Intracranial pressure management and neurological outcome for patients with mild traumatic brain injury who required neurosurgical intervention: a Japanese database study. *Brain Inj.* 2019;33(7):869–874.
22. Muizelaar JP, Marmarou A, Ward JD, et al. Adverse effects of prolonged hyperventilation in patients with severe head injury: a randomized clinical trial. *J Neurosurg.* 1991;75(5):731–739.
23. Wolf AL, Levi L, Marmarou A, et al. Effect of THAM upon outcome in severe head injury: a randomized prospective clinical trial. *J Neurosurg.* 1993;78(1):54–59.

CHAPTER

22

When Should We Be Performing Decompressive Craniectomies?

Mohamed A. Zaazoue, MD, MSc
& Shelly D. Timmons, MD, PhD

Case

A 29-year-old woman was found unresponsive at the bottom of a staircase. She was intubated on the scene before transporting to the emergency department (ED). Her examination showed no eye opening to pain, no motor response to pain, and she made no vocalizations prior to intubation (GCS = E1/M1/V1 = 3, now 3-I). Her pupils were dilated and unreactive bilaterally, with intact corneal reflexes bilaterally and a gag reflex. Her blood pressure was 110/80 mm Hg and her heart rate was persistently in the 50s. A noncontrast head CT showed intraparenchymal and subdural hematoma with midline shift (Figure 22–1A-B). After discussion with family, the patient was emergently for right-sided decompressive hemicraniectomy with evacuation of the hyperacute subdural hematoma and placement of an intraparenchymal intracranial pressure (ICP) monitor on the left. She was taken to the neurocritical care unit (NCC) postoperatively, with head CT showing satisfactory decompression (Figure 22–1C). On the following day, she intermittently followed commands, with pupils 2 mm, equal and reactive. ICP readings ranged between 2 and 10 mm Hg. She was extubated on postoperative day (POD) 1 and her ICP monitor was discontinued on POD#3 after no sustained ICP elevations were noted. She returned to her baseline examination within a couple of weeks, without any residual deficits. Clinic follow-up 3 months later showed resolution of intraparenchymal hematomas (Figure 22–1D), with subsequent autologous bone flap replaced shortly thereafter (Figure 22–1E).

Key Points

- Decompressive hemicraniectomy is most commonly performed in setting of elevated intracranial pressure despite medical management following severe traumatic brain injury (sTBI) or cerebral infarction.
- Leaving the bone flap off can be considered for brain swelling beyond the inner table after removal of a mass lesion or patients with contusions that are not evacuated.
- Patients with neurologic impairment felt to be attributable to elevated ICP and whose primary brain injuries are thought to be compatible with an acceptable recovery are good candidates for decompressive craniectomies.
- Decompressive craniectomy in severe TBI is associated with mortality benefit and some morbidity or neurologic function benefit; however, this is balanced with longer-term quality of life and ethical considerations.

BACKGROUND

Decompressive craniectomy (DC) involves the removal of a section of the calvarium, in addition to expansile duraplasty, to allow swollen brain tissue to expand beyond the boundaries of the native dura and skull, thereby mitigating internal compression and various forms of herniation. DC can be classified as primary versus secondary DC. Primary DC is defined as leaving the bone flap out after evacuation of a mass lesion or other emergency craniotomy. Secondary DC is decompression performed for the purposes of controlling ICP in the face of cerebral edema and herniation despite medical treatment. DC can be performed as a large "hemicraniectomy" wherein a frontotemporoparietal flap is created, or bifrontal.

The two most common indications to perform DC are severe traumatic brain injury (sTBI) and cerebral infarctions, particularly malignant middle cerebral artery (MCA) infarctions.

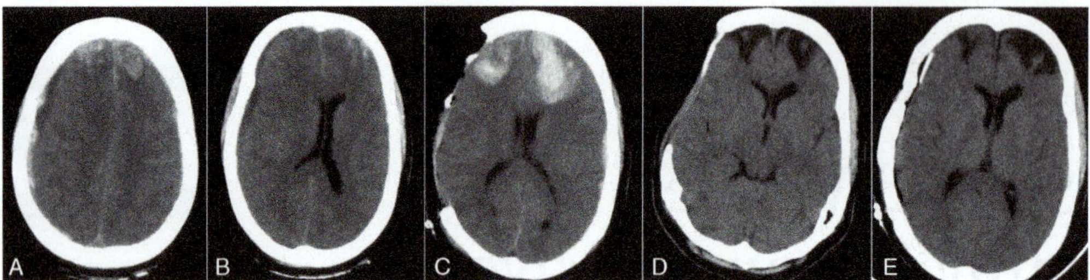

FIGURE 22–1 Noncontrast, axial CT scans of the head (**A**) showing right convexity mixed attenuation subdural hematoma (SDH), bilateral frontal contusions, and a sliver acute SDH on the left, (**B**) associated with right-to-left midline shift out of proportion to the thickness of the subdural hematoma with also partial effacement of the right lateral ventricle. (**C**) Postoperative changes after right craniectomy and right subdural hematoma evacuation with reversal of right to left midline shift. Bifrontal contusions increased with mass effect on the frontal horns, and slight increase in size of left SDH. Mild swelling of the right hemisphere out the DC defect and lack of cerebrospinal fluid (CSF) in the sulci indicative of brain edema are noted. (**D**) Resolution of hemispheric herniation through the craniectomy defect and evolution of bifrontal contusions to a state of encephalomalacia. Cisterns and sulci are noted to be patent. (**E**) CT after replacement of right calvarial bone flap (with subgaleal drain in place).

EVIDENCE AND REVIEW

Traumatic Brain Injury

Randomized controlled trials of surgical therapies for DC in trauma are challenging, particularly when compared to nonsurgical therapies, when equipoise is lacking, and with potential ethical concerns regarding withholding life-saving interventions. Additionally, severe TBI is a notoriously heterogeneous patient population with complex neurophysiology. Finally, commonly employed outcomes measures do not always capture the complexity of long-term function and must be performed at very long time-points after injury to capture maximum improvement, making research conclusions difficult. Despite the inherent challenges, two multicenter, randomized trials for DC in TBI patients have been conducted: (1) The DECRA trial: Early Decompressive Craniectomy in Patients with Severe Traumatic Brain Injury (2003-2010, published 2011) and (2) the Randomized Evaluation of Surgery with Craniectomy for Uncontrollable Elevation of Intracranial Pressure trial (RESCUEicp) (2004-2014, published 2016).

The DECRA trial[1] conducted in Australia included 155 patients aged 15 to 59 years with diffuse (ie, no mass lesions), severe TBI (Glasgow coma scale [GCS] 3-8). Patients were randomly assigned within 72 hours of injury to either surgery plus standard care or standard care alone. Patients in the surgical arm were operated with bifrontal craniectomy if they sustained early elevated ICP of >20 mm Hg for >15 minutes (continuously or intermittently) within a 1-hour period, despite first-tier medical management of ICP. First-tier therapeutic measures included sedation, normalization of $PaCO_2$, hyperosmolar therapy with mannitol or hypertonic saline, neuromuscular blockade and external ventricular drain (EVD). For the standard care group, second-tier therapeutic measures included hypothermia, barbiturates, or both. Crossover from the medical arm to the surgical arm was allowed and was performed in 18% of the standard care group as a late lifesaving measure (within protocol) and in 5% of the standard care group within 72 hours of admission (against protocol). However, the analysis was performed as an intent-to-treat analysis with these patients being analyzed in the standard treatment arm. The surgical group exhibited better ICP control (<20 mm Hg) and had shorter ICU lengths of stay. However, patients undergoing DC fared worse on the extended Glasgow outcome scale—extended (GOS-E) and had a higher risk of an unfavorable outcome (defined as upper and lower severe disability, vegetative state, or death) at 6 months, compared to the standard care group, while mortality rates at 6 months were similar between the two groups. This study faced several limitations. First, the population under study was a small subset of overall severe TBI patients, since most sTBI patients have mass lesions. The relatively short duration of ICP elevations at minimal mean elevation levels leading up to randomization called into question the appropriateness for the criteria chosen. (Median ICP for both groups during the 12 hours before randomization were at the upper range of normal [20 mm Hg].) Therefore, the generalizability of this trial to clinical practice may be limited.

RESCUEicp[2,3] was conducted in multiple countries, mostly in Europe, specifically the United Kingdom. This trial enrolled 408 patients aged 10 to 65 years with severe TBI and elevated ICP > 25 mm Hg for 1 to 12 hours despite first- and second-tier medical management. First-tier measures included head elevation, sedation, analgesia, and neuromuscular blockade (optional). Second-tier measures included hyperosmolar therapy, inotropes, hypothermia, and cerebrospinal fluid drainage via ventriculostomy. Use of barbiturates to control elevated ICP was not permitted for second-tier measures. Crossover from the medical arm to the surgical arm was allowed and was performed 37.2% of the time. Again, the surgical group showed better ICP control compared to the medical group. In the surgical group, 63% of patients underwent bifrontal DC, while 37% underwent unilateral DC, and analyses were done under intention-to-treat per study protocol, despite the high crossover rate. Of note, this trial considered upper severe disability (which includes some degree of independent function) as a good outcome in a dichotomized GOS-E analysis to more closely mirror some major stroke trial outcomes scales (modified Rankin scores [mRS]). This differed from other prior TBI studies, which had dichotomized upper severe disability as an unfavorable outcome.

At 6 months, mortality was significantly lower in the surgical arm (26.9% vs. 48.9%) and there were higher proportions of patients with good outcomes (upper severe disability, lower and upper moderate disability, and lower and upper good recovery) compared with standard treatment. However, there were also more subjects with vegetative state and lower severe disability at 6 months, which decreased at 12 and 24 months post-injury.[3] While higher rates of vegetative state, severe disability, and moderate disability were maintained at 12 and 24 months in the surgical group compared to the standard treatment group, the differences were smaller and there was an even greater proportion of patients with good outcomes (dichotomized) at 12 and 24 months in the surgical group. The mortality reductions were also sustained over time in the surgical group. Analyzed another way, the surgical group showed a greater degree of improvement over time at 24 months than the standard treatment group.

Among the patients enrolled in RESCUEicp, 18.7% of the surgical group and 24.2% of the medical group had traumatic mass lesions. However, the trial was not designed to study the effectiveness of primary DC which is performed more frequently than secondary DC. The RESCUE-ASDH is a multicenter, randomized trial that aims to compare the clinical and cost effectiveness of DC versus standard craniotomy with bone flap replacement for the management of TBI patients undergoing evacuation of an acute subdural hematoma. The study starting enrolling patients from October 2014, and enrollment was officially complete in May 2019, after randomizing 463 patients (publication pending).

Malignant Middle Cerebral Artery Infarction

Malignant MCA infarctions (stroke) occur in 1% to 10% of supratentorial strokes and are historically associated with high mortality rates approaching 80%. The malignant edema typically develops within 2 to 5 days after stroke onset; however, in some patients swelling and neurological deterioration can manifest within the first 24 hours.

Three landmark randomized controlled trials have been conducted and published addressing DC for malignant, space-occupying MCA stroke compared to conservative medical management. These were the Decompressive Craniectomy in Malignant Middle Cerebral Artery Infarcts (DECIMAL) trial (France, 2007),[4] the Decompressive Surgery for the Treatment of Malignant Infarction of the Middle Cerebral Artery (DESTINY) trial (Germany, 2007),[5] and the Hemicraniectomy after Middle Cerebral Artery Infarction with Life-Threatening Edema (HAMLET) trial (The Netherlands, 2009).[6] A planned meta-analysis of the pooled results was published in 2007.[7] Patient recruitment was interrupted in 2006 in two of the three trials (DECIMAL and DESTINY), due to efficacy, ie, significant reductions in mortality rates seen in the surgical arms.

The trials included patients aged 18 to 60 years (18-55 years in DECIMAL), with neurological deficits suggestive of MCA territory strokes, a National Institutes of Health Stroke Score (NIHSS) > 16-18, and imaging findings of an infarct involving various percentages of MCA territory on computed tomography or infarct volume > 145 cm^3 on diffusion-weighted magnetic resonance imaging, along with various other entrance criteria, including reduced or declining level of consciousness. DECIMAL included patients within 24 hours of stroke onset and surgery had to be completed within 6 hours of randomization. DESTINY included patients 12 to 36 hours from stroke onset, and surgery had to be started within 6 hours of randomization. HAMLET included patients within 96 hours of stroke onset, and surgery had to be initiated within 3 hours of randomization. For the pooled analysis, a maximum time window from stroke onset to randomization of 45 hours was adopted, ie, surgical treatment within 48 hours. Outcome measures were likewise similar but not identical between the three trials and included mRS score at either 6 or 12 months, dichotomized between favorable (either 0-3 or 0-4) and unfavorable (either 4-6 or 5-6 where 6 = death).

DECIMAL enrolled 60 patients, 30 in each group. DESTINY enrolled 32 patients, 17 in the surgery group and 15 in the medical group. HAMLET enrolled 64 patients, 32 in each group, of which 23 were included in the pooled analysis owing to the original trial's longer time window for inclusion. Pooled results showed that patients in the surgical group had better survival compared to the conservative group (78% vs. 29%), and more patients with favorable functional outcomes measured two ways: mRS ≤ 4 (75% vs. 24%), and mRS ≤ .3 (43% vs. 21%). DC was found to be beneficial in all subgroup analyses, including age (above or below 50 years), presence of aphasia, and whether surgery was done on the first or second day after stroke onset. Most deaths occurred early (within 2 weeks) and were due to transtentorial herniation.

Similar to the results of RESCUEicp in trauma, it is important to note that because of decreased mortality related to surgery, the probability of surviving in a condition that was dependent on others (mRS = 4) increased; however, the probability of severe disability (mRS = 5) was not increased.

HAMLET continued to enroll patients after the pooled analysis to assess whether or not DC would still be effective if performed within 96 hours of stroke onset. The results showed no evidence that DC improved functional outcomes if performed after 48 hours from stroke onset in that group. A follow-up study showed that beneficial results on mortality and functional outcome at 1 year were durable at 3 years.[8]

Special Patient Populations

Malignant MCA infarction age > 60 years. Since none of the previously mentioned trials for DC in malignant MCA strokes included patients >60 years of age, the effect of surgery in this age group remained uncertain. As a result, DESTINY II was conducted and published in 2014.[9] This was a multicenter, randomized, controlled trial that enrolled 112 patients, 61 years or older, with malignant MCA infarction. More patients in the surgical group survived with favorable mRS compared to the conservative group (38% vs. 18%), as a result of lower mortality rates in the surgical group (33% vs. 70%). Of note, no patients survived with an mRS score of 0 to 2 (no or mild disability), so the majority of survivors were again dependent on others for most daily needs regardless of surgical status. Therefore, this was a life-saving procedure in this age group, with overall improvements in favorable survivorship, but as expected, this was not a disability-sparing procedure given the primary pathology of MCA-distribution infarction and functional tissue loss.

Pediatric sTBI. The Guidelines for the Management of Pediatric Severe Traumatic Brain Injury (3rd edition) were published in 2019.[10] As expected, given the rigorous methodologies for evidence-based guidelines, there was insufficient evidence to support a Level I or II recommendation for DC in children. Level III evidence-based recommendations state: "Decompressive craniectomy (DC) is suggested to treat neurologic deterioration, herniation, or intracranial hypertension refractory to medical management."

ETHICAL CONSIDERATIONS AND PATIENT-CENTERED DECISION-MAKING

The results of the aforementioned trials regarding favorable and unfavorable outcomes should be interpreted with caution, for several reasons. Firstly, the outcomes measures utilized are specifically designed to compare populations of patients in a consistent and valid manner with high inter-rater reliability. They do not necessarily take into account an individual's satisfaction with their status, or even predict granular deficits within category so one category may encompass a wide range of functionality. Secondly, trial methodological limitations do not account for the specifics of a given patient's clinical situation; and thirdly, prognostication abilities remain relatively poor in the early stages of care during which these procedures must be completed in order to be effective, particularly for sTBI. The American Academy of Neurology recommends that "When discussing prognosis with caregivers of patients with a [Disorder of Consciousness (DoC)] during the first 28 days post injury, clinicians must avoid statements that suggest these patients have a universally poor prognosis."[11]

Complicating matters, decision-making in most cases is done by a family member or a legal representative, because patients are suffering from altered mental status, aphasia, or are ventilated or sedated to protect their airways and/or control ICP. Therefore, clinicians and patients/families should have clear discussions regarding patient's lifestyle and wishes if time allows, and the willingness to accept survival with various levels of disability, as well as a frank discussion regarding the limits of prognostic abilities, particularly with severe TBI. Families must also understand that in the case of malignant MCA infarctions, complete recovery is not expected, with or without surgery, due to the infarction itself. Localizing lesions to dominant and nondominant hemispheres, particular lobes and other brain structures, and associating these with anticipated deficits can be helpful and educational for families during discussion.

AVAILABLE GUIDELINES

A consensus conference of international neurotrauma experts published a number of recommendations regarding DC in 2019,[12] including that primary DC should be considered if the brain is swelling beyond the inner table at surgery after evacuating an acute attenuation subdural hematoma (SDH), and is an option for patients with contusions and mass effect when contusions are not being evacuated. For secondary DC, recommendations included consideration of the impact of underlying lesions when determining utility of DC, which was noted to be effective at reducing intracranial hypertension. ***The optimal candidate for secondary DC was noted to be a patient whose ICP elevation is thought to be the primary contributor to an eventual poor outcome and the primary brain injuries are thought to be compatible with an acceptable recovery.*** In all cases continuous ICP monitoring postoperatively was recommended. Also considered in this consensus statement were techniques, timing, patient goals, perioperative care, timing of bone flap replacement, and resource-challenged environments. Evidence-based guidelines acknowledge level IIA evidence for reduction in ICP by DC as well.[13]

DC has been shown to be effective at reducing ICP, preventing herniation, and reducing mortality for a variety of diagnoses, most especially severe traumatic brain injury and malignant MCA infarction. Proper patient selection to enhance not only survival but functional outcome demands a thorough understanding of cerebral anatomy and physiology, grasp of the technical and procedural skills necessary to optimize outcomes, compassionate discussion with family members regarding patients' premorbid status and wishes, and appreciation of the limits of prognostic abilities in disorders of consciousness within the first 4 weeks after onset.

REFERENCES

1. Cooper, D. James, et al. "Decompressive Craniectomy in Diffuse Traumatic Brain Injury." *New England Journal of Medicine*, vol. 364, no. 16, 2011, pp. 1493–1502. doi:10.1056/nejmoa1102077.
2. Hutchinson, Peter J., et al. "Trial of Decompressive Craniectomy for Traumatic Intracranial Hypertension." *New England Journal of Medicine*, vol. 375, no. 12, 2016, pp. 1119–1130. doi:10.1056/nejmoa1605215.
3. Hutchinson PJ, et al. "Consensus Statement from the International Consensus Meeting on the Role of Decompressive Craniectomy in the Management of Traumatic Brain Injury: Consensus Statement." *Acta Neurochirurgica (Wien)*. vol. 161, no. 7, 2019, pp.1261–1274. doi: 10.1007/s00701-019-03936-y. Epub 2019 May 28. PMID: 31134383; PMCID: PMC6581926.
4. Vahedi, Katayoun, et al. "Sequential-Design, Multicenter, Randomized, Controlled Trial of Early Decompressive Craniectomy in Malignant Middle Cerebral Artery Infarction (DECIMAL Trial)." *Stroke*, vol. 38, no. 9, 2007, pp. 2506–2517. doi:10.1161/strokeaha.107.485235.
5. Jüttler Eric, et al. "Decompressive Surgery for the Treatment of Malignant Infarction of the Middle Cerebral Artery (DESTINY)." *Stroke*, vol. 38, no. 9, 2007, pp. 2518–2525. doi:10.1161/strokeaha.107.485649.
6. Hofmeijer, Jeannette, et al. "Surgical Decompression for Space-Occupying Cerebral Infarction (the Hemicraniectomy after Middle Cerebral Artery

Infarction with Life-Threatening Edema Trial [HAMLET]): A Multicentre, Open, Randomised Trial." *The Lancet Neurology*, vol. 8, no. 4, 2009, pp. 326–333., doi:10.1016/s1474-4422(09)70047-x.

7. Geurts M, et al. "HAMLET Steering Committee. Surgical Decompression for Space-Occupying Cerebral Infarction: Outcomes at 3 Years in the Randomized HAMLET Trial." *Stroke*. vol. 44, no. 9, 2013, pp. 2506–2508. doi: 10.1161/STROKEAHA.113.002014. Epub 2013 Jul 18. PMID: 23868265.
8. Vahedi, Katayoun, et al. "Early Decompressive Surgery in Malignant Infarction of the Middle Cerebral Artery: A Pooled Analysis of Three Randomised Controlled Trials." *The Lancet Neurology*, vol. 6, no. 3, 2007, pp. 215–222. doi:10.1016/s1474-4422(07)70036-4.
9. Jüttler, Eric, et al. "Hemicraniectomy in Older Patients with Extensive Middle-Cerebral-Artery Stroke." *New England Journal of Medicine*, vol. 370, no. 12, 2014, pp. 1091–1100. doi:10.1056/nejmoa1311367.
10. Kochanek, Patrick M, et al. "Guidelines for the Management of Pediatric Severe Traumatic Brain Injury, Third Edition." *Pediatric Critical Care Medicine*, vol. 20, 2019. doi:10.1097/pcc.0000000000001735.
11. Joseph T. Giacino, et al. "Practice Guideline Update Recommendations Summary: Disorders of Consciousness: Report of the Guideline Development, Dissemination, and Implementation Subcommittee of the American Academy of Neurology; the American Congress of Rehabilitation Medicine; and the National Institute on Disability, Independent Living, and Rehabilitation Research." *Archives of Physical Medicine and Rehabilitation*, vol. 99, no. 9, 2018, pp. 1699–1709. ISSN 0003-9993, https://doi.org/10.1016/j.apmr.2018.07.001.
12. Kolias AG, et al. "Evaluation of Outcomes among Patients with Traumatic Intracranial Hypertension Treated with Decompressive Craniectomy vs Standard Medical Care at 24 Months: A Secondary Analysis of the RESCUEicp Randomized Clinical Trial." *JAMA Neurology*. vol. 79, no. 7, 2022, pp. 664–671. doi: 10.1001/jamaneurol.2022.1070. PMID: 35666526; PMCID: PMC9171657.
13. *Guidelines for the Management of Severe Traumatic Brain Injury*. braintrauma.org/uploads/03/12/Guidelines_for_Management_of_Severe_TBI_4th_Edition.pdf.

CHAPTER

23

When Should Barbiturate Coma Be Used to Treat Intracranial Hypertension?

Christopher M. Kyper, MD, Lauren K. Ng, MD, & William D. Freeman, MD

Case

A 35-year-old man presents after fall off a roof to the ground, found to have severe traumatic brain injury (TBI) with bilateral multicompartmental intracranial contusion. Intracranial pressure (ICP) monitoring reveals persistently elevated ICPs >35 mm H_2O despite euthermia and standing hyperosmolar therapy. When should barbiturate coma be considered and how should this be monitored?

Key Points

- Barbiturate coma may be considered for treatment of persistently elevated intracranial pressure despite increasing venous return, decreasing metabolism, hyperosmolar therapy, and perhaps surgical decompression.
- Barbiturate infusion is titrated to burst-suppression, as monitored on continuous electroencephalogram (EEG).
- The side effects of barbiturate infusion are numerous and must be closely monitored, including cardiovascular depression, ileus, cholestasis, and drug-drug interactions.

BACKGROUND

Intracranial hypertension is a commonly encountered problem in neuro-critically ill patients, and it carries high rates of both morbidity and mortality. TBI is one of the most common causes of intracranial hypertension, and in fact, intracranial hypertension is reported in 25% to 40% of all TBI cases. Other neurological causes of increased intracranial pressure (ICP) include intracranial hemorrhage, hydrocephalus, cerebral edema from cytotoxic or vasogenic sources, and status epilepticus. Systemic causes of increased ICP include fever, uncontrolled systemic hypertension, and increased intrathoracic or intra-abdominal pressures, among others.

The management of elevated ICP, or intracranial hypertension, is one of the key components of the care of all neuro-critically ill patients. This management includes both medical and surgical techniques, and often involves striking a delicate balance when factoring in the critically ill patient's other homeostatic abnormalities (eg, cardiovascular, renal, hematologic, etc.). Regardless of surgical or medical interventions required, the mainstay of intracranial hypertension management is optimization of cerebral perfusion pressure (CPP), which is defined as the mean arterial pressure (MAP) minus the ICP.

$$CPP = MAP - ICP$$

While there is some debate, many guidelines recommend an ideal CPP of 50 to 70 mmHg in neurocritical care patients. Numerous methods for achieving this goal exist and the manner in which the goal is achieved depends on patient-specific factors. These include hemodynamic stability and renal function, but nonetheless, the common objective is to increase MAP and decrease ICP, whether directly or indirectly. Surgical interventions act to directly reduce ICP and include decompressive craniectomy, external ventricular drain (EVD) placement for cerebrospinal fluid (CSF) diversion, or lumbar drain (LD) placement. Medical interventions are myriad and include vasopressors in augment MAP as well as hyperosmolar therapies (eg, mannitol and hypertonic saline solutions) to reduce ICP, all of which are discussed elsewhere in this book. Other methods of reducing ICP will focus on decreasing cerebral metabolic activity. These include targeted temperature management (TTM), fever control, and pharmacological sedation. Among these sedation techniques is the use of barbiturates to slow cerebral metabolic activity and enact a medically induced coma to optimize CPP.

Barbiturate Pharmacology

Barbiturates are a group of sedative-hypnotic medications that have a wide array of uses including treatment of seizures, insomnia, and alcohol withdrawal, as well as use in sedation, general anesthesia, and refractory intracranial hypertension. They are synthetic compounds based on barbituric acid and have been used in medical settings since the early 20th century. Phenobarbital, pentobarbital, and thiopental are some of the most used barbiturates, all of which have a common mechanism of action of enhancing activity of the inhibitory neurotransmitter γ-aminobutyric acid (GABA) by binding nonspecifically to the $GABA_A$ receptor/chloride channel to cause central nervous system (CNS) depression.

As discussed, the increased ICP translates to a potential drop in CPP which could lead to permanent widespread neuronal damage due to ischemia. Cerebral autoregulation allows for optimization of CPP along a fairly broad range of both ICPs and MAPs, but in the brain-injured patient, this autoregulation is not as effective and thus additional measures must be taken to ensure adequate CPP.

EVIDENCE AND REVIEW

Intracranial Hypertension Management—Barbiturate Coma

Early interventions in all patients with increased ICP include head of bed elevation, ensuring no impairment of jugular venous return, pain control, fever control, and avoidance of hypotension. Following this, osmotherapy can be initiated with either mannitol or hypertonic saline solutions, discussed elsewhere in this book. Intracranial hypertension that is refractory to these basic measures must be treated aggressively, and it is at this point that measures to slow the overall cerebral metabolic rate should be considered. These measures include sedation and potentially neuromuscular blockade, induced hypothermia (TTM), and the use of barbiturate coma (Figure 23–1). TTM is commonly used following cardiac arrest to slow cerebral metabolism and has a similar effect in patients with TBI or refractory intracranial hypertension. This measure is fairly resource-intensive and carries its own host of potential adverse effects which may make barbiturate infusions a more attractive option in some settings (see Table 23–1). Barbiturate coma, most commonly achieved with pentobarbital in the United States and sodium thiopental elsewhere, is often seen as a last resort along with surgical options such as decompressive hemicraniectomy, due mostly to the potential adverse effects associated with intravenous barbiturate infusions.

Pentobarbital reduces cerebral metabolic activity through enhancement of GABA activity and inhibition of the excitatory neurotransmitter glutamate. As a byproduct of this decreased metabolic rate, ICP can also be reduced. Continuous electroencephalogram (cEEG) monitoring is required when using pentobarbital to reduce ICP, as the goal will be to achieve a burst-suppression pattern on the EEG which is defined as periods of complete background suppression interspersed with bursts of cortical activity (Figure 23–2). Patients receiving sedation for

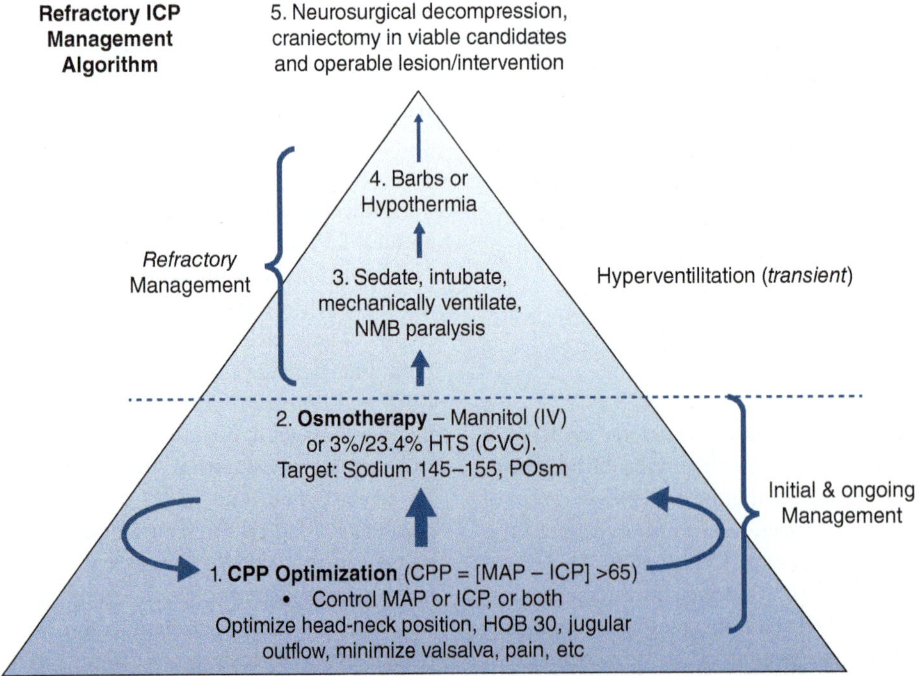

FIGURE 23–1 Pyramidal approach to ICP-CPP management. Barbs indicates barbiturates; CPP, cerebral perfusion pressure; CVC, central venous line; HOB, head of bed; HTS, hypertonic saline; ICP, intracranial pressure; IV, intravenous; MAP, mean arterial pressure; NMB, neuromuscular blockade; POsm, plasma osmolality. From: Freeman WD. How I manage ICP-CCP: a visual, yet individualized Approach. crit care. 2019 Aug27;23(1):287; Used with permission of Mayo Foundation for Medical Education and Research, all rights reserved.

TABLE 23–1 Barbituates and TTM comparision of physiological effects, side effects, and management.

	Barbiturate Coma	Targeted Temperature Management
Effect	Cerebral metabolic suppression	Cerebral metabolic suppression
Onset of effect	Rapid due to intravenous infusion	Lag due to time required to achieve goal temperature
Offset	Long half-life; "builds up in system"	Effects cease once normothermia is achieved
Adverse effects	• Cardiovascular instability • Cholestasis • Adynamic ileus • Ventilator-associated pneumonia - Metabolic acidosis - Renal failure	• Hemodynamic instability if <34°C • Peripheral vasoconstriction • Hypo-/hyperkalemia - Renal failure
Requisite Monitoring	cEEG and invasive ICP monitor	cEEG and invasive ICP monitor
Additional Management	• Vasopressors - Mechanical ventilation	• Vasopressors • Mechanical ventilation - Anti-shivering management

refractory increased ICP also require ventilatory support with endotracheal intubation and mechanical ventilation.

Once a burst-suppression pattern has been achieved on cEEG, the pentobarbital infusion can be titrated to maintain this state while adjusting vasoactive medications to maintain adequate MAP and CPP. Invasive intracranial ICP monitoring as with a subarachnoid bolt, EVD, or intraparenchymal monitor is helpful in these patients to have the most accurate assessment of CPP. From this point, it is up to the clinician to decide how long the patient will remain in burst-suppression. Often, this state is maintained for 24 to 72 hours depending on individual patient factors including the invasive ICP waveform monitoring (Figure 23–3). Once it is determined that pentobarbital weaning can begin, the patient should remain on cEEG monitoring until return of some spontaneous and continuous cortical electrical activity, ideally corresponding with return of some clinical neurological exam findings. Should there be concern for continued intracranial hypertension after cessation of the pentobarbital infusion, shared decision-making among clinicians should be undertaken regarding reinitiation of pentobarbital or other options such as therapeutic hypothermia, surgical decompression, or a combination.

Monitoring in Barbiturate Coma

Continuous pentobarbital infusion carries significant risks and requires very strict monitoring. As with all barbiturates, pentobarbital has a narrow therapeutic window. When used for managing increased ICP, the general target therapeutic level is 30 to

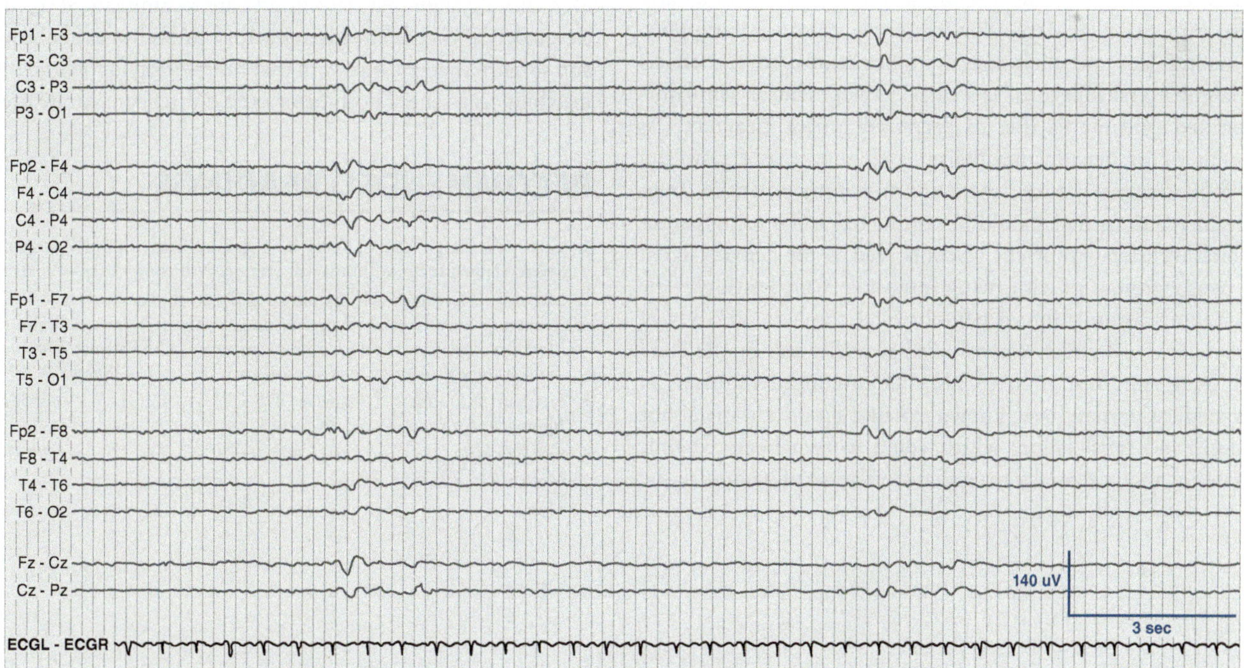

FIGURE 23–2 Standard EEG utilizing disc electrodes in the International 10-20 system of placement. In this case, the patient was in refractory status epilepticus requiring continuous pentobarbital infusion to achieve the desired "burst-suppression" pattern characterized by complete background suppression with intermittent bursts of cortical activity.

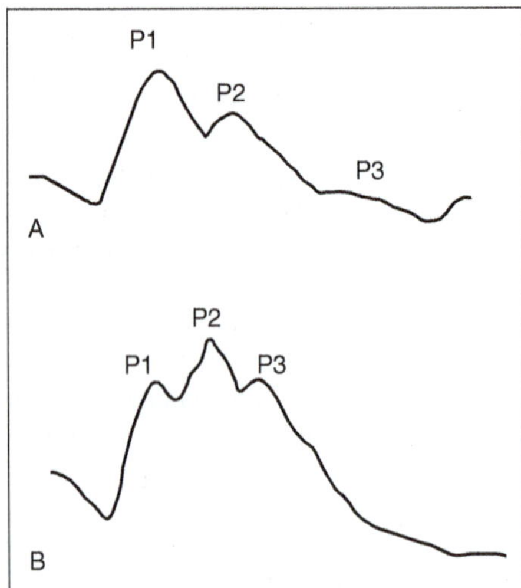

FIGURE 23–3 Invasive intracranial pressure (ICP) monitoring waveforms. Figure 23–3A represents a physiologically normal ICP waveform wherein P1 indicates cardiac systole, P2 is a measure of cerebral compliance, and P3 represents closure of the aortic valve. In Figure 23–3B, the P2 wave is a higher amplitude than the surrounding waves indicating poor cerebral compliance.

50 mcg/mL. Time to steady-state is 3 to 6 days, and the half-life for pentobarbital 35 to 50 hours. This long half-life can interfere with neurological prognostication and brain death testing in the event that it is required. In standard practice, pentobarbital level should be <5 mcg/mL before beginning proper evaluation for brain death.

In addition to CNS depression, pentobarbital will often also cause cardiovascular depression requiring vasopressor support. Adynamic ileus and cholestasis are other known adverse effects of pentobarbital infusions, as well as development of ventilator-associated pneumonia due to decreased mucus clearance. As a result of its hepatic metabolism and impact as a powerful CYP450 enzyme inducer, there are numerous potential drug-drug interactions that should be considered when using pentobarbital infusion. Propylene glycol is used as the delivery agent for pentobarbital, as with many intravenous medications. The intravenous formulation of pentobarbital contains 40% v/v of propylene glycol which is considered generally safe by the Food and Drug Administration (FDA), but prolonged infusions of this medication have been known to cause significant metabolic acidosis and renal failure which could worsen hemodynamic instability and potentially necessitate initiation of hemodialysis.

Barbiturates are a class of sedative-hypnotic medications which can be used in the management of intracranial hypertension, which is refractory to first- and second-line efforts. Often used as a last resort along with surgical decompression, barbiturate coma carries many potential adverse effects and has been shown in numerous studies to be associated with both increased morbidity and mortality. Whether this is due to the severe degree of critical illness in the selected patient population that requires intervention with continuous barbiturate infusion, or due to effects from the medications and their associated complications is unclear. TTM is another "last resort" intervention after intracranial hypertension has proven refractory to standard measures that also carries potential adverse effects and morbidity, but may be more practical in certain clinical settings. In particular, in scenarios wherein concern for neuroprognostication or brain death evaluation is raised, barbiturate coma can limit the proper evaluation due to its large volume of distribution and prohibitively long half-life. In contrast, TTM's effects are generally complete once rewarming to normothermia has been achieved, and brain death testing can be properly performed as long as core body temperature is at least 36°C. Regardless, barbiturate coma remains a powerful tool for managing intracranial hypertension that is refractory to standard measures and should be considered in most clinical scenarios that reach this stage.

AVAILABLE GUIDELINES

Current brain trauma foundation guidelines do not advocate for barbiturate use as prophylaxis against elevated ICP. However, they do state that barbiturates are recommended to control elevated ICP that is already refractory to both maximal medical and surgical therapy, but warn that monitoring for hemodynamic instability is essential both before and during barbiturate therapy.

RECOMMENDED READINGS

1. Carney N, Totten AM, O'Reilly C, et al. Guidelines for the Management of Severe Traumatic Brain Injury, 4th Edition. *Neurosurgery*. 0:1–10, 2016.
2. Marshall GT, James RF, Landman MP, et al. Pentobarbital Coma for Refractory Intra-Cranial Hypertension after Severe Traumatic Brain Injury: Mortality Predictions and One-Year Outcomes in 55 Patients. *The Journal of Trauma: Injury, Infection, and Critical Care*. 69(2):275–283, 2010.
3. Freeman WD. How I Manage ICP-CPP: A Visual, Yet Individualized Approach. *Critical Care*. 23:287, 2019.
4. Freeman WD. Management of Intracranial Pressure. *Continuum (Minneap Minn.)*. 21:1299–323, 2015.

CHAPTER

24

How Should We Manage Dysautonomia and Sympathetic Storming?

Jamie E. Podell, MD & Neeraj Badjatia, MD, MSc

Case

A 30-year old man presents after being ejected from a high-speed motor vehicle accident, found to have hemorrhagic bifrontal contusions and multifocal subarachnoid hemorrhage. He is treated with hyperosmolar agents after placement of an external ventricular drain in the intensive care unit. Starting on hospital day 6, he develops persistent fevers ranging from 101°F to 103°F, tachycardia, hypertension, and tachypnea. Physical exam is notable for high tone and rigidity throughout his extremities. Blood, urine, and respiratory cultures are negative for infective source. What workup and treatments should be enacted for this patient?

Key Points

- The paroxysmal sympathetic hyperactivity-assessment measure (PSH-AM) offers a quantification tool for diagnosis of PSH and its clinical severity.
- Abortive, maintenance, and preventative pharmacologic treatments target elements of the excitatory-inhibitor ratio model of central autonomic activity to mute sympathetic hyperactivity.
- Dysautonomia following traumatic brain injury (TBI) may be transient or persistent; early proactive treatment of sympathetic arousal benefits both populations.

BACKGROUND

Sympathetic storming, also known as paroxysmal sympathetic hyperactivity (PSH), is a clinical and physiologic syndrome of autonomic dysregulation characterized by episodes of hypertension, tachycardia, tachypnea, hyperthermia, diaphoresis, and motor rigidity.[1] It occurs in a subset of patients after acute brain injury, most commonly after moderate to severe traumatic brain injury (TBI).[2] The syndrome has been associated with worse outcomes after TBI even when controlling for other prognostic factors such as initial injury severity and age.[3,4] As such, it may represent a modifiable risk factor for poor recovery.

The most widely accepted pathophysiologic theory for PSH is the excitatory-inhibitory ratio (EIR) model. According to the EIR, PSH-inducing acute brain injury disrupts the balance between excitatory and inhibitory communication within the central autonomic network, leading to uncontrolled brainstem and spinal cord sympathetic nuclei, which become hyperexcitable and overly responsive to afferent stimuli.[1,6,14] Pharmacotherapeutic strategies simultaneously act on multiple nodes implicated in this model (Figure 24–1).

PSH tends to emerge around the second week postinjury.[4,6,15] This may, in part, be due to unmasking of symptoms from the withdrawal of sedation, analgesia, and temperature control around this time. The semiprotocolized treatment of fever and pain in acute TBI patients may be considered nonspecific universal measures in this population. While nonspecific and common after TBI, at least one study suggests that early fever is associated with later PSH.[16] We manage all critically ill febrile TBI patients without contraindications with acetaminophen, which exerts its antipyretic effect by inhibiting the enzyme cyclooxygenase (COX) and interrupting prostaglandin synthesis.[17] Prostaglandin E2 normally alters hypothalamic preoptic neurons' intrinsic firing rates to initiate the febrile response and raise the thermogenic set point. If acetaminophen is incompletely effective within the first week post-injury, we initiate surface cooling to target normothermia. Pain is also addressed universally in our TBI patients with standing acetaminophen, as needed opioids, and additional multimodal therapies such as gabapentin and baclofen, when deemed appropriate.

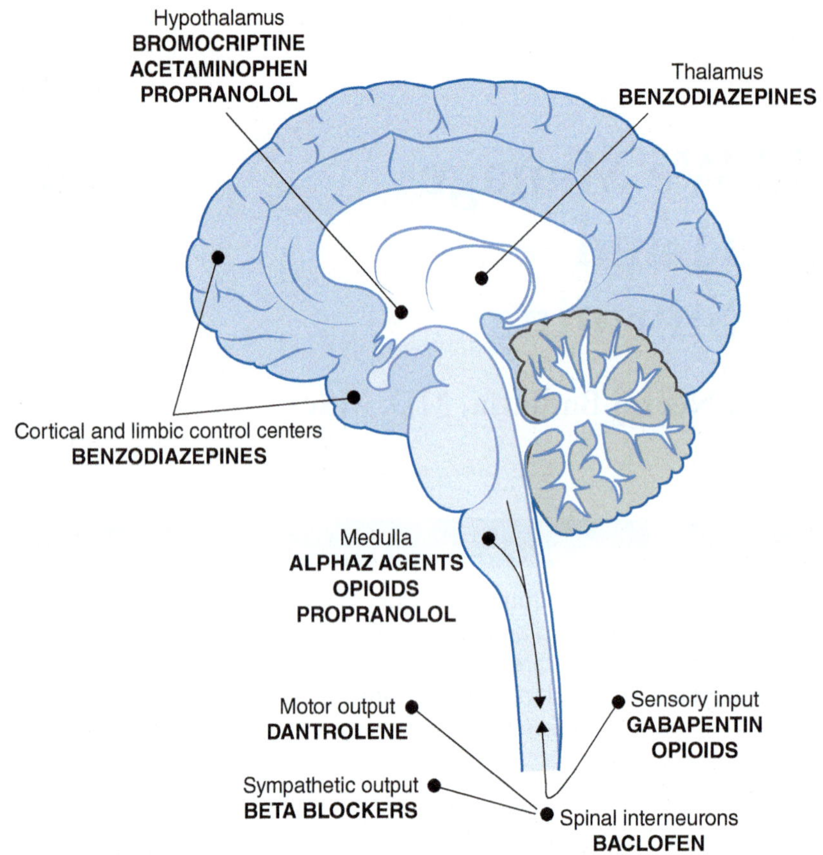

FIGURE 24–1 Schematic of paroxysmal sympathetic hyperactivity pharmacologic treatment targets.

Research and management of PSH has benefited from the publication of the PSH-assessment measure (PSH-AM),[1] an expert consensus-based tool for the standardized quantification of PSH diagnostic likelihood and clinical feature severity. PSH-AM scores may assist clinicians' decisions to escalate or wean therapies and may provide a metric to evaluate the effectiveness of various management strategies.

EVIDENCE AND REVIEW

At first recognition of a syndrome of sympathetic excess and careful consideration of differential diagnosis, calculation of the PSH-AM score can aide next steps of management, which can be integrated in the electronic medical record as a semi-automated tool (Figure 24–2). Alternative diagnoses and triggers are investigated and managed at this initial step and revisited as symptoms continue or worsen. The clinical feature severity subscore of the PSH-AM can guide decisions for treatment escalation and de-escalation.[7] We modify the clinical feature severity in the ICU to consider any patient requiring continuous infusions such as propofol, midazolam, fentanyl, or dexmedetomidine specifically to control PSH symptoms as at least moderately severe. In our experience, the PSH-AM is best tabulated during interdisciplinary rounds with engagement from bedside nurses who may provide detail beyond documented vital signs (which may miss peak paroxysmal values and do not include sweating and posturing features) to characterize clinical events.

Once it has been determined that treatment for PSH is warranted, a tiered medical approach to abortive and preventative therapy is initiated (Figure 24–2, Table 24–1). A brief summary of the evidence for these therapies follows.

Abortive Medications

We favor intravenous morphine as a fast-acting first-line abortive therapy. Morphine is the most frequently reported effective abortive medication in the literature; it may be particularly effective in reducing heart rate and respiratory rate.[5,10,18] Morphine acts primarily as a central mu opioid receptor agonist but also acts peripherally on the cardiovascular system via kappa receptors.[5] It inhibits nociceptive afferent neurons of the Peripheral Nervous System (PNS) and simultaneously activates descending central inhibitory pathways.[19] Side effects include sedation, which may impede prognosis and recovery, constipation/ileus, and dependence.

Benzodiazepines are GABA-A agonists thought to exert effects on limbic, thalamic, and hypothalamic brain regions, causing widespread neural depression.[5] Intravenous benzodiazepines

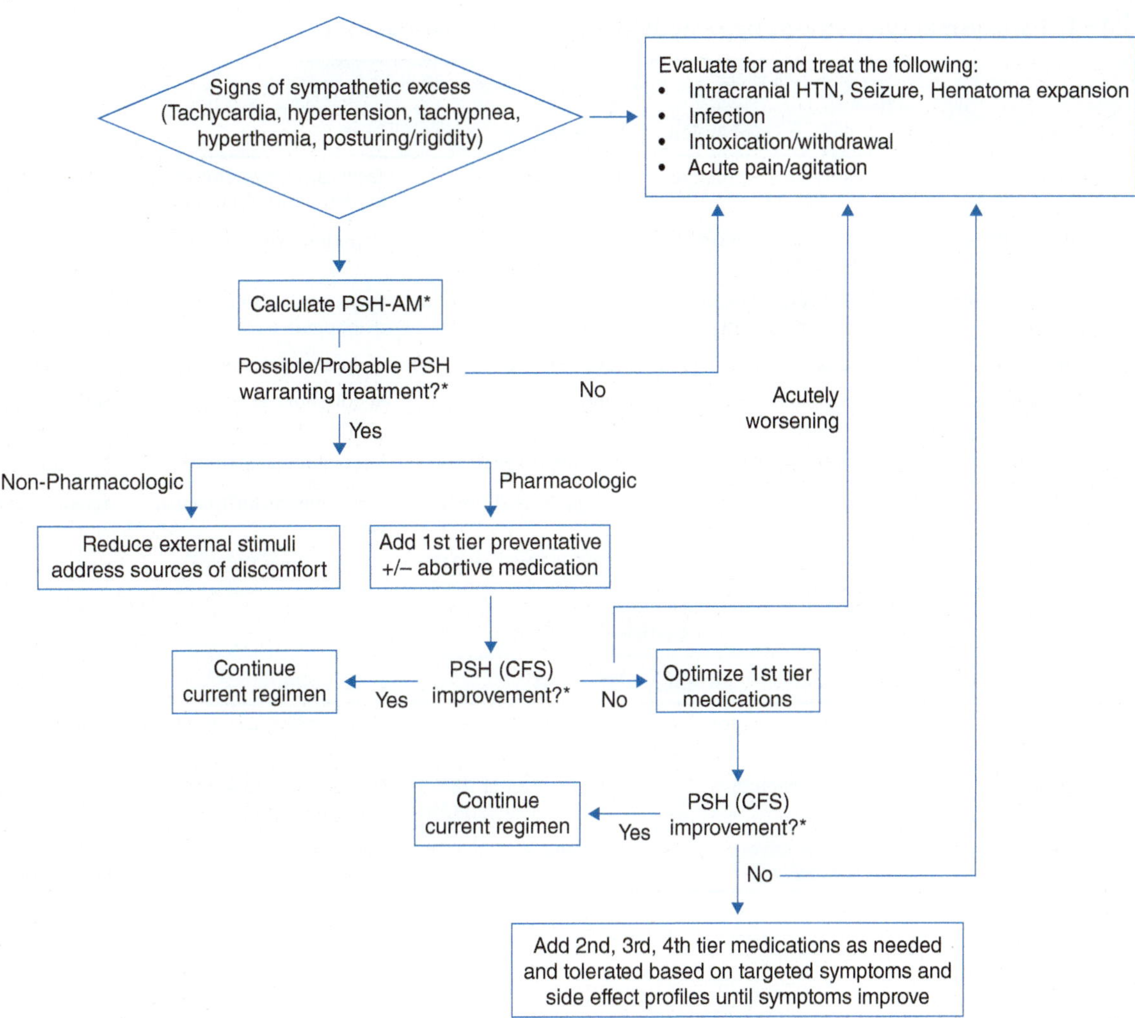

FIGURE 24–2 Paroxysmal sympathetic hyperactivity suggested treatment algorithm.

such as diazepam are also effective as abortive therapy, particularly for symptoms of tachycardia, tachypnea, and posturing/rigidity.[5,11,18] We consider diazepam a second-line abortive agent due to greater likelihood of causing delirium and lower evidence base compared to morphine.

The nonselective beta blocker labetalol, given intravenously, is an additional second-tier abortive agent that targets sympathetic outflow and is particularly useful for controlling hypertension and tachycardia associated with PSH. We consider IV labetalol second tier due to potential side effects of hypotension, decreased cerebral perfusion, and reduced efficacy as comparted to morphine.

Continuous infusions of propofol, dexmedetomidine, fentanyl, or midazolam may also be used in severe or refractory cases while uptitrating other preventative medications, particularly when the risks of storming symptoms are perceived to be greater than the side effects of sedation. For example, when tachypnea is associated with hypoxia or severe respiratory alkalosis that may provoke cerebral ischemia or when systemic hypertension provokes intracranial hypertension in the setting of autoregulation failure.

Maintenance/Preventative Medications

The nonselective beta adrenergic blocking agent propranolol has perhaps the strongest evidence base supporting its use in PSH after TBI. Both preinjury beta blocker exposure and early propranolol after TBI have been associated with improved survival.[20–22] In the TBI population, propranolol has also been associated with lower risk for venous thromboembolism (likely mediated by catecholaminergic effects on inflammation and coagulation),[23] improves agitation,[24,25] reduces fever,[26,27] and may be prescribed chronically for the management of post-traumatic headaches.[28] Animal studies have demonstrated protective effects of propranolol on cerebral autoregulation, perfusion and oxygenation, and reductions in hippocampal neuronal cell death,[29–31] but no effect on blood-brain barrier permeability.[32]

TABLE 24–1 Paroxysmal sympathetic hyperactivity suggested pharmacotherapies.

Preventative/Maintenance Pharmacotherapies					
Priority	**Drug**	**Mechanism of Action**	**Initial Dosing**	**Target Symptoms**	**Adverse Effects**
1st tier	Propranolol	Nonselective β-blocker	10-20 mg PO/NGT q6-8h	Tachycardia, hypertension, hyperthermia, diaphoresis	Bradycardia, hypotension
	Bromocriptine	Dopamine D_2 receptor agonist	2.5-5 mg PO/NGT q8h	Hyperthermia	Orthostatic hypotension
2nd tier	Dexmedetomidine or clonidine	Central α-2 adrenergic receptor agonist	0.2 mcg/kg/h IV, 0.1 mg TID, respectively	Hypertension, tachycardia, diaphoresis, agitation	Bradycardia, hypotension
	Gabapentin	Gabapentinoid	300 mg PO/NGT TID	Reduce noxious triggers	Mild sedation
3rd tier	Oxycodone	μ opioid receptor agonist	5 mg PO/NGT q6h	Reduce noxious triggers	Sedation, constipation, delirium
	Baclofen	$GABA_B$ agonist	2.5-5 mg PO/NGT q8h	Motor rigidity, spasticity	Sedation
	Clonazepam	$GABA_A$ agonist	0.5 mg PO/NGT q8-12h	Hypertension, tachycardia, rigidity	Sedation, delirium
4th tier	Dantrolene	Ryanodine receptor antagonist	25 mg PO/NGT q8-24h	Hyperthermia, rigidity	Hepatotoxicity
Abortive Pharmacotherapies					
Priority	**Drug**	**Mechanism of Action**	**Initial Dosing**	**Target Symptoms**	**Adverse Effects**
1st tier	Morphine	μ opioid receptor agonist	2-4 mg IV q2-6h PRN	Hypertension, tachycardia, tachypnea	Sedation, hypotension, constipation, delirium
2nd tier	Diazepam	$GABA_A$ agonist	5-10 mg IV q4-8h PRN	Hypertension, tachycardia, tachypnea, rigidity	Sedation, delirium
	Labetalol	Nonselective beta-blocker	10-20 mg IV q2-6h PRN	Hypertension, tachycardia, diaphoresis	Hypotension, bradycardia

Propranolol blocks catecholamine effects both centrally in hypothalamic and brainstem vasomotor centers, and peripherally in the cardiovascular system and has the advantage of reducing sympathetic effects without causing sedation. Multiple published studies have demonstrated beneficial effects of propranolol on PSH.[5] Due to its negative chronotropic and blood pressure lowering effects, hypotension and bradycardia are contraindications, and it should be used with caution in combination with analgo-sedation and alpha2 agonists.

We also favor the first-line use of the dopamine D2 agonist bromocriptine as preventative and maintenance therapy. Bromocriptine modulates dopaminergic activity within the suprachiasmatic and ventromedial nuclei of the hypothalamus.[33] important for both the coordination of thermoregulatory responses via the anterior hypothalamus and thermogenesis via dorsomedial neurons' activation of spinal sympathetic and somatic motor circuits.[34] Following acute brain injury, bromocriptine has been shown to reduce body temperature and sweating.[35] Commonly reported side effects include nausea and hypotension,[33] but we have found it to be generally well tolerated for the treatment of PSH and associated central fevers in the ICU.

Alpha-2 adrenoreceptor agonists (clonidine and dexmedetomidine) stimulate cardiovascular inhibitory neurons in the nucleus tractus solitarii and antagonize medullary sympathetic outflow centers.[5] They have antihypertensive, sedative, and analgesic properties, and several studies have reported their efficacy in treating[5,36] or preventing[37] PSH. As compared to propranolol, there is a smaller evidence base and higher incidence of bradycardia, hypotension, and sedation, leading to the recommendation that it be used as a second-, rather than first-tier therapy.

Gabapentin is a GABA analogue that is primarily used in the treatment of neuropathic pain, exerting its effects in the dorsal horns of the spinal cord via a mechanism independent of GABA B receptors (the target of baclofen). Gabapentinoids have demonstrated some efficacy in the treatment of PSH in the literature.[5,38] We consider it second-line therapy for PSH and utilize it in individuals who appear to be triggered by peripheral noxious or non-noxious stimulation.

Third-tier therapies may be no less efficacious than those listed above but are reserved for more refractory cases due to side effect profiles, particularly delirium, sedation, and dependence. In this tier, we include standing oxycodone (particularly in patients with pain triggers or for whom abortive morphine is particularly effective) and standing, longer-acting benzodiazepines (particularly in patients with significant posturing/rigidity during episodes or for whom abortive diazepam is particularly effective). The goal is to use these medications for a limited amount of time, often to aid in weaning off infusions such as propofol, fentanyl, or midazolam. The GABA-B agonist baclofen primarily targets spinal interneurons and is effective treatment for PSH mediated by hyperexcitable, disinhibited spinal circuits. Several studies have demonstrated a reduction in oral therapies required and improvement in symptoms with intrathecal baclofen.[39,40]

The muscle relaxant and ryanodine receptor antagonist dantrolene is an alternative agent that we reserve for refractory cases due to potential for hepatotoxicity, sedation, and muscle weakness. Classically, it is used in the treatment of malignant hyperthermia. While evidence for its efficacy in the treatment of PSH is more limited,[5] it is often recommended as part of multimodal therapy and may be particularly useful for motor rigidity/posturing and refractory hyperthermia.[7,9]

De-escalation and Weaning

TBI patients may develop either persistent dysautonomia or a transient sympathetic arousal state.[14] Those with persistent dysautonomia demonstrated higher magnitude and more persistent changes in heart rate and heart rate variability in response to a controlled stimulus, such as endotracheal suctioning, compared to those with transient sympathetic arousals or no dysautonomia. It is likely that the variability in PSH symptom duration relates to its heterogeneous causative structural and functional pathophysiology, and it has been suggested that more rapid recovery from PSH may be facilitated by early functional restoration of supraspinal inhibition in patients with less brainstem pathology.[6] However, in the early acute setting, it is not clear that transient sympathetic arousals should be treated any differently than those that will become more persistent; patients without significant brainstem pathology who eventually recover from clinical PSH may in fact have the most to gain from aggressive management of physiologic derangements to prevent secondary injury following a more recoverable primary injury. Given that the goal of early ICU management of acute TBI is to maintain homeostasis and prevent secondary injury, we believe that pharmacologic management of these symptoms is warranted.

These findings do, however, implicate the need for varying durations of PSH therapy. In the majority of patients with sympathetic arousals in the acute ICU phase after TBI, PSH symptoms will be self-limited, resolving or improving by day 14 of admission.[14] For this reason, we recommend attempting to wean or discontinue PSH-specific treatments by postinjury day 14 if symptoms are stable to improving at that time. Because tiers were designed with greatest risk of complications and side effects and/or lower efficacy in higher tiers, we generally advise withdrawing highest tier medications first and working backward. Exceptions can be made for continuation of medications targeting specific problematic symptoms (eg, baclofen in a patient with comorbid spasticity).

AVAILABLE GUIDELINES

At present, management of PSH remains variable across and within centers. A recent scoping review reported the published use of 48 drugs from 22 classes, but dose, route, and outcome were so inconsistently reported that no conclusions could be drawn regarding best practices.[5] Expert guidelines generally recommend a multimodal approach targeting afferent, central, and efferent autonomic pathways using a combination of both abortive and preventative medications.[5–13]

However, these guidelines are not yet evidence based. In the future, we aim to prospectively track PSH-AM scores, in order to more objectively define medication effects on PSH. A systematic approach to PSH may then enable us to test the hypothesis that PSH is an independent risk factor for poor outcome after TBI. For now, the goal of therapy is to promote recovery by maintaining physiologic homeostasis and symptomatic control of PSH.

REFERENCES

1. Baguley IJ, Perkes IE, Fernandez-Ortega JF, et al. Paroxysmal sympathetic hyperactivity after acquired brain injury: consensus on conceptual definition, nomenclature, and diagnostic criteria. *J Neurotrauma*. 2014 Sep 1; 31(17):1515–20.
2. Perkes I, Baguley IJ, Nott MT, Menon DK. A review of paroxysmal sympathetic hyperactivity after acquired brain injury. *Ann Neurol*. 2010 Aug;68(2):126–35.
3. Baguley IJ, Nicholls JL, Felmingham KL, Crooks J, Gurka JA, Wade LD. Dysautonomia after traumatic brain injury: a forgotten syndrome? *J Neurol Neurosurg Psychiatry*. 1999 Jul;67(1):39–43.
4. Podell JE, Miller SS, Jaffa MN, et al. Admission features associated with paroxysmal sympathetic hyperactivity after traumatic brain injury: a case-control study. *Crit Care Med*. 2021 Oct 1;49(10):e989–1000.
5. Tu JSY, Reeve J, Deane AM, Plummer MP. Pharmacological Management of Paroxysmal Sympathetic Hyperactivity: A Scoping Review. *J Neurotrauma*. 2021 Aug 15;38(16):2221–37.
6. Meyfroidt G, Baguley IJ, Menon DK. Paroxysmal sympathetic hyperactivity: the storm after acute brain injury. *Lancet Neurol*. 2017;16(9):721–9.
7. Marehbian J, Muehlschlegel S, Edlow BL, Hinson HE, Hwang DY. Medical management of the severe traumatic brain injury patient. *Neurocrit Care*. 2017 Dec;27(3):430–46.
8. Lump D, Moyer M. Paroxysmal sympathetic hyperactivity after severe brain injury. *Curr Neurol Neurosci Rep*. 2014 Nov;14(11):494.
9. Blackman JA, Patrick PD, Buck ML, Rust RS. Paroxysmal autonomic instability with dystonia after brain injury. *Arch Neurol*. 2004 Mar;61(3):321–8.
10. Rabinstein AA, Benarroch EE. Treatment of paroxysmal sympathetic hyperactivity. *Curr Treat Options Neurol*. 2008 Mar;10(2):151–7.
11. Samuel S, Allison TA, Lee K, Choi HA. Pharmacologic management of paroxysmal sympathetic hyperactivity after brain injury. *J Neurosci Nurs*. 2016 Apr;48(2):82–9.
12. Shald EA, Reeder J, Finnick M, et al. Pharmacological treatment for paroxysmal sympathetic hyperactivity. *Crit Care Nurse*. 2020 Jun 1;40(3):e9–16.
13. Zheng RZ, Lei ZQ, Yang RZ, Huang GH, Zhang GM. Identification and management of paroxysmal sympathetic hyperactivity after traumatic brain injury. *Front Neurol* [Internet]. 2020 Feb 25 [cited 2021 Feb 12];11. Available from: https://www.ncbi.nlm.nih.gov/pmc/articles/PMC7052349/
14. Baguley IJ, Nott MT, Slewa-Younan S, Heriseanu RE, Perkes IE. Diagnosing dysautonomia after acute traumatic brain injury: evidence for overresponsiveness to afferent stimuli. *Arch Phys Med Rehabil*. 2009 Apr;90(4):580–6.
15. Hughes JD, Rabinstein AA. Early diagnosis of paroxysmal sympathetic hyperactivity in the ICU. *Neurocrit Care*. 2014 Jun;20(3):454–9.
16. Hinson HE, Schreiber MA, Laurie AL, Baguley IJ, Bourdette D, Ling GSF. Early fever as a predictor of paroxysmal sympathetic hyperactivity in traumatic brain injury. *J Head Trauma Rehabil*. 2017;32(5):E50–4.
17. Aronoff DM, Neilson EG. Antipyretics: mechanisms of action and clinical use in fever suppression. *Am J Med*. 2001 Sep;111(4):304–15.
18. Baguley IJ, Cameron ID, Green AM, Slewa-Younan S, Marosszeky JE, Gurka JA. Pharmacological management of dysautonomia following traumatic brain injury. *Brain Inj*. 2004 May;18(5):409–17.

19. Murphy PB, Bechmann S, Barrett MJ. Morphine. In: StatPearls [Internet]. Treasure Island (FL): StatPearls Publishing; 2022 [cited 2022 Nov 2]. Available from: http://www.ncbi.nlm.nih.gov/books/NBK526115/
20. Cotton BA, Snodgrass KB, Fleming SB, et al. Beta-blocker exposure is associated with improved survival after severe traumatic brain injury. *J Trauma.* 2007 Jan;62(1):26–33; discussion 33–35.
21. Ley EJ, Leonard SD, Barmparas G, et al. Beta blockers in critically ill patients with traumatic brain injury: results from a multicenter, prospective, observational American Association for the Surgery of Trauma study. *J Trauma Acute Care Surg.* 2018;84(2):234–44.
22. Ko A, Harada MY, Barmparas G, et al. Early propranolol after traumatic brain injury is associated with lower mortality. *J Trauma Acute Care Surg.* 2016 Apr;80(4):637–42.
23. Dhillon NK, Hashim YM, Conde G, et al. Early propranolol is associated with lower risk of venous thromboembolism after traumatic brain injury. *Am Surg.* 2021 Dec;87(10):1556–60.
24. Williamson D, Frenette AJ, Burry LD, et al. Pharmacological interventions for agitated behaviours in patients with traumatic brain injury: a systematic review. *BMJ Open.* 2019 Jul 9;9(7):e029604.
25. Brooke MM, Patterson DR, Questad KA, Cardenas D, Farrel-Roberts L. The treatment of agitation during initial hospitalization after traumatic brain injury. *Arch Phys Med Rehabil.* 1992 Oct;73(10):917–21.
26. Asmar S, Bible L, Chehab M, et al. Traumatic brain injury induced temperature dysregulation: what is the role of β blockers? *J Trauma Acute Care Surg.* 2021 Jan 1;90(1):177–84.
27. Meythaler JM, Stinson AM. Fever of central origin in traumatic brain injury controlled with propranolol. *Arch Phys Med Rehabil.* 1994 Jul;75(7):816–8.
28. Evans RW. Posttraumatic headaches in civilians, soldiers, and athletes. *Neurol Clin.* 2014 May;32(2):283–303.
29. Armstead WM, Vavilala MS. Propranolol protects cerebral autoregulation and reduces hippocampal neuronal cell death through inhibition of interleukin-6 upregulation after traumatic brain injury in pigs. *Br J Anaesth.* 2019;123(5): 610–7.
30. Ley EJ, Scehnet J, Park R, et al. The in vivo effect of propranolol on cerebral perfusion and hypoxia after traumatic brain injury. *J Trauma.* 2009 Jan;66(1):154–9; discussion 159–61.
31. Zeeshan M, Hamidi M, O'Keeffe T, et al. Propranolol attenuates cognitive, learning, and memory deficits in a murine model of traumatic brain injury. *J Trauma Acute Care Surg.* 2019 Nov;87(5):1140–7.
32. Genét GF, Bentzer P, Hansen MB, Ostrowski SR, Johansson PI. Effects of propranolol and clonidine on brain edema, blood-brain barrier permeability, and endothelial glycocalyx disruption after fluid percussion brain injury in the rat. *J Trauma Acute Care Surg.* 2018 Jan;84(1):89–96.
33. Ozery M, Wadhwa R. Bromocriptine. In: StatPearls [Internet]. Treasure Island (FL): StatPearls Publishing; 2022 [cited 2022 Nov 2]. Available from: http://www.ncbi.nlm.nih.gov/books/NBK555948/
34. Pitoni S, Sinclair HL, Andrews PJD. Aspects of thermoregulation physiology. *Curr Opin Crit Care.* 2011 Apr;17(2):115–21.
35. Bullard DE. Diencephalic seizures: responsiveness to bromocriptine and morphine. *Ann Neurol.* 1987;21(6):609–11.
36. Peng Y, Zhu H, Chen H, et al. Dexmedetomidine attenuates acute paroxysmal sympathetic hyperactivity. *Oncotarget.* 2017 Sep 15;8(40):69012–9.
37. Tang Q, Wu X, Weng W, et al. The preventive effect of dexmedetomidine on paroxysmal sympathetic hyperactivity in severe traumatic brain injury patients who have undergone surgery: a retrospective study. *PeerJ.* 2017;5:e2986.
38. Baguley IJ, Heriseanu RE, Gurka JA, Nordenbo A, Cameron ID. Gabapentin in the management of dysautonomia following severe traumatic brain injury: a case series. *J Neurol Neurosurg Psychiatry.* 2007 May;78(5):539–41.
39. Pucks-Faes E, Hitzenberger G, Matzak H, Verrienti G, Schauer R, Saltuari L. Intrathecal baclofen in paroxysmal sympathetic hyperactivity: impact on oral treatment. *Brain Behav.* 2018 Nov;8(11):e01124.
40. Kim HS, Kim NY, Kim YW. Successful intrathecal baclofen therapy for intractable paroxysmal sympathetic hyperactivity in patient with pontine hemorrhage: a case report. *Clin Neuropharmacol.* 2018 Aug;41(4):138–41.

CHAPTER

25

How Can We Predict Coma Recovery in Severe Traumatic Brain Injury?

Hera A. Kamdar, MD & Samuel B. Snider, MD

Case

A 30-year-old man with no past medical history presents after being struck by a car. His Glasgow coma scale (GCS) score is 3 in the field. Over the course of the first several days his neurologic exam does not drastically improve, and his imaging demonstrates both multifocal contusions and diffuse axonal injury (DAI) (Figure 25–1). What is the prognosis for such a patient?

Key Points

- Prognostication of recovery after severe traumatic brain injury (TBI) remains a challenging process.
- International Mission for Prognosis and Analysis of Clinical Trials (IMPACT) and Corticosteroid Randomization After Significant Head Injury (CRASH) scoring systems represent some of the most well-established and validated methods for predicting outcomes after severe TBI currently.
- Structural analysis of injury patterns and functional investigations may add additional utility on a case-by-case basis.

BACKGROUND

Though many patients with severe traumatic brain injury (TBI) are comatose on arrival to the hospital, they can recover to a wide range in levels of independent function. Improvement is the rule, and persistent disorders of consciousness are rare.[1,2] It is difficult to predict early in the course whether patients will remain permanently disabled or recover independence. Accurate disability prediction is critical, since withdrawal of life sustaining therapy (WLST) based on expected prognosis, is the most common cause of death within this population.[3] Unfortunately, current clinical practice is heterogenous, with rates of WLST varying fourfold between academic institutions.[3] Advances in neuromonitoring and neuroimaging have the potential to improve neuroprognostication following severe TBI.

EVIDENCE AND REVIEW

Severity Classification and Outcome Measurement

Severity of TBI is typically classified based on the GCS score at presentation, which is an ordinal scale that quantifies the level of responsiveness based on eye-opening, verbal output, and motor responses. Mild TBI encompasses GCS score of 13 to 15, moderate as 9 to 12, and severe as ≤8.[4] While most patients with permanent disability have moderate or severe TBI, the range of outcomes for each severity strata are broad.

Disability outcomes are typically assessed with the Glasgow outcome scale-extended (GOSE) score, the only measure currently recognized by the U.S. Food and Drug Administration (FDA) for TBI clinical trials.[5,6] The GOSE is an 8-point scale based on the level of functional dependency, ranging from death to fully independent and symptom free.[7] While the scale can be used ordinally, more commonly the outcomes are binarized into "unfavorable" (typically either GOSE ≤ 3 [lower severe disability] or GOSE ≤ 4 [upper severe disability]) and "favorable" groups. Prognostic models utilizing these thresholds strive to determine the likelihood of "unfavorable outcome" at 6 months or 1 year post injury.[1,2,8]

Predicting Outcomes: Current Gold-Standard

The International Mission for Prognosis and Analysis of Clinical Trials (IMPACT) in TBI and Corticosteroid Randomization After Significant Head Injury (CRASH) studies yielded two

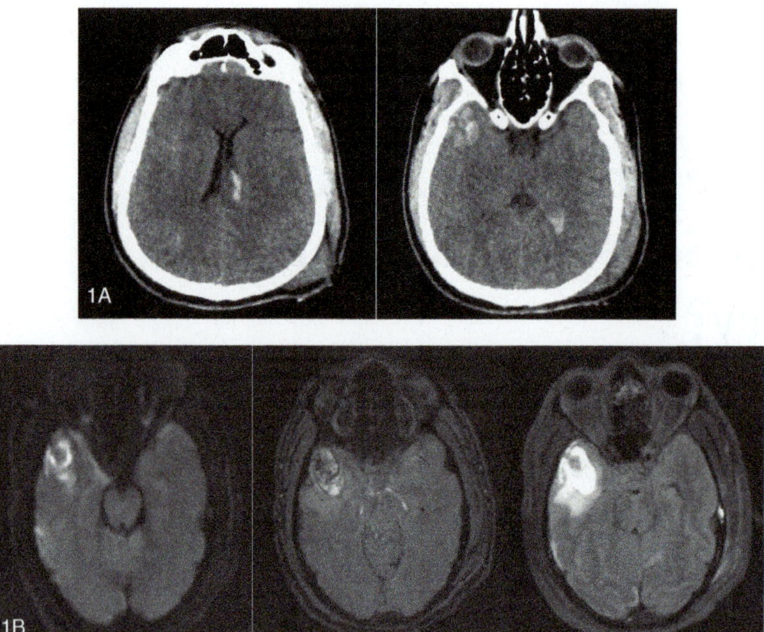

FIGURE 25–1 A CT head (**1A**) showed multifocal contusions most prominent in the right anterior temporal lobe, right greater than left traumatic subarachnoid hemorrhage, and right greater than left subdural hematomas. The patient was subsequently admitted to the neurocritical care unit, and an intracranial pressure monitor was placed. While in the neurocritical care unit, the exam improved GCS 7T (E2VTM5) and rare elevations in intracranial pressure were managed with osmotherapy. An MRI brain (**1B**) was obtained 11 days after admission and revealed grade III DAI including brainstem microhemorrhage, dominant right temporal contusion, and diffusion restriction in splenium of the corpus callosum.

well-known regression models used to predict the probability of death or unfavorable outcome 6 months after moderate or severe TBI. These models were fit with data from large observational studies and randomized controlled trials and incorporate standard clinical information on admission and summary measures from CT scans. The IMPACT (core + CT) model incorporates age, GCS motor score, pupil reactivity, CT scan-based severity classification (Marshall and Rotterdam score),[9] and presence of subarachnoid hemorrhage (SAH) on CT.[10–12] The CRASH model includes age, GCS, pupillary reactivity, and presence of major extra-cranial injury.[11,12] These models have been repeatedly validated over the last two decades across multiple datasets.[10–13] Roozenbeek et al externally validated both IMPACT and CRASH models using data from five large moderate to severe TBI studies originating in Europe, North America, and Australia.[13] While the performance varied across datasets, discrimination was always better than chance and the observed proportions of death/unfavorable outcomes matched the proportions predicted by the model.[13]

Moskowitz et al conducted a study to assess physician's perceptions and utilization of these models and found variability between providers, with up to 40% not being able to express awareness of the model.[14] Those utilizing the model, preferred to avoid the use of numerical values derived from the model due to the potential of "prognostic overconfidence in end-of-life care."[14] Other studies have also reported a lack of consistent implementation.[15]

Despite repeated validation studies, several factors have prevented these two models from achieving wider penetration into clinical practice.[14] First, while the model assigns high probability of death/unfavorable outcome to patients with extreme scores (eg, an elderly patient with two unreactive pupils, no motor responses on presentation, and diffuse injury on CT), most patients have death/unfavorable outcome probabilities in a middle range. Unfavorable outcome predictions of 40% to 60% are challenging to use clinically. Second, the performance of such models is buttressed by the inclusion of large numbers of patients who died during the hospitalization or early rehabilitation course.[16,17] This can potentially lead to a self-fulfilling prophecy, where patients without early clear behavioral signs of awareness are predicted to have unfavorable outcomes and thus are less likely to receive aggressive care.[16] Finally, these models do not incorporate detailed information about the neuroanatomic extent of the injury, nor do they incorporate advanced investigations to detect signs of awareness when absent behaviorally. Whether these additional investigations can improve model performance is an area of active investigation.

Utilizing Structural Injury Patterns for Prognosis

Severe TBI is associated with heterogenous pathology. Hemorrhagic injury occurs both inside and outside the brain parenchyma, including subdural, epidural, SAHs, and parenchymal contusions. These are well measured with CT scans. Degree of midline shift, cisternal compression, SAH, epidural hematoma, and the presence of evacuated and unevaluated mass lesions are currently incorporated by the CRASH and IMPACT score to assign probabilities of poor outcome.[9–13] However, whether the parenchymal distribution of contusive hemorrhage is related to outcome is unknown. Recent work using an unsupervised artificial intelligence model found that information from CT scans did not improve the existing IMPACT model.[18]

DAI, on the other hand, is prevalent in moderate and severe TBI and is optimally measured on MRI rather than CT scans. DAI is divided into three grades based on anatomical location: grade 1 (gray/white junction), grade 2 (callosal), and grade 3 (brainstem).[19] Early literature based on post-mortem pathology described a phenotype of patients with axonal injury throughout the brain and brainstem with persistent disorders of consciousness and dependency.[19,20] However, as MRI has enabled visualizing microscopic white matter hemorrhages anti-mortem with increasingly sensitive T2* MRI sequences, there is significant debate on the best way to measure axonal injury and on its prognostic significance. Diffusion tensor imaging can also be used to reconstruct specific white matter bundles and quantitatively measure axonal integrity. Grade 3 DAI (brainstem axonal injury) has been associated with severe disability,[21–23] but the specific location of injury within the brainstem may be prognostically important.[24] How axonal injury location interacts with known clinical and CT-based predictors is uncertain. Additional work has been done with high-angular-resolution diffusion imaging to map out disruptions in ascending arousal networks within this population to map out patterns of associated disorders of consciousness (Figure 25–2).[25]

Promising work using regional and global markers of white matter integrity, measured with diffusion tensor imaging, has demonstrated a prognostic utility superior to the IMPACT score[26] with poor-outcome specificity approaching 100%.[26,27] Confirmation of these findings in a heterogeneous cohort of severe TBI is required prior to advocating for their wider adoption.

Functional Investigations

Multiple tools have become available to detect signs of awareness when none are present behaviorally. Prior to undertaking these, the first step is a detailed and standardized behavioral assessment, to rule subtle signs of awareness. This is preferably done using a validated behavioral scale like Coma Recovery Scale-Revised (CRS-R) assessment.[28–30] These clinical assessments should be conducted in the absence of potential confounders like sedation, paralysis, limb immobilization, and auditory dysfunction.[31]

Since the phenomenon was first reported in 2006,[32] a growing area of study is evaluating for covert consciousness. Covert consciousness can be defined as the identification of evidence for awareness through analysis of EEG or functional MRI (fMRI) in patients without any clinical signs of awareness.[28] Early studies in diverse patient cohorts using EEG-signals reflecting possible awareness may be associated with better functional outcomes after injury.[33–35] Furthermore fMRI studies have identified activation patterns suggestive of covert awareness in patients with severe TBI, but the relationship to outcome is less clear.[36,37]

These techniques hold promise across a range of brain injuries; however, the clinical significance and relevance to prediction remains to be seen and validated. Limitations to these advanced techniques include extensive ancillary support with well-trained evaluators and sophisticated software, high false-negative rates, and concerns around generalizability.[31] However, as the absence of consciousness is frequently used to prompt WLST,[3] future studies are warranted.

Future Directions

The future of neuroprognostication in patients with severe TBI relies upon streamlining large amounts of multimodal data to

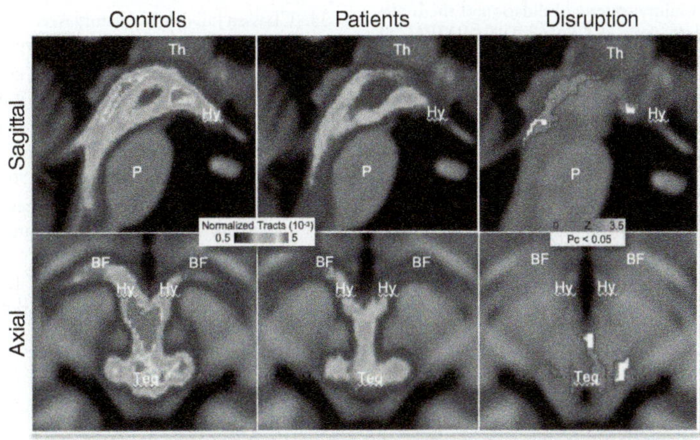

FIGURE 25–2 Adapted from Snider et al. where they performed high-angular-resolution diffusion imaging in 16 comatose patients with acute severe traumatic brain injury and compared them to 16 matched controls to show disruption of ascending arousal networks. The right column shows peak differences between groups. Adapted Snider SB, Bodien YG, Bianciardi M, Brown EN, Wu O, Edlow BL. Disruption of the ascending arousal network in acute traumatic disorders of consciousness. Neurology. 2019;93(13):e1281-e1287.

identify independent and generalizable predictors of functional recovery. Large international and national consortiums (eg, CENTER-TBI, TRACK-TBI) have been enrolling patients over the last 10 years and will insights in the years to come.

REFERENCES

1. Kowalski RG, Hammond FM, Weintraub AH, et al. Recovery of consciousness and functional outcome in moderate and severe traumatic brain injury. *JAMA Neurol.* 2021;78(5):548–557.
2. McCrea MA, Giacino JT, Barber J, et al. Functional outcomes over the first year after moderate to severe traumatic brain injury in the prospective, longitudinal TRACK-TBI Study. *JAMA Neurol.* 2021;78(8):982–992.
3. Turgeon AF, Lauzier F, Simard JF, et al. Mortality associated with withdrawal of life-sustaining therapy for patients with severe traumatic brain injury: a Canadian multicentre cohort study. *CMAJ.* 2011;183(14):1581–1588.
4. Maas AI, Stocchetti N, Bullock R. Moderate and severe traumatic brain injury in adults. *Lancet Neurol.* 2008;7(8):728–741.
5. Bagiella E, Novack TA, Ansel B, et al. Measuring outcome in traumatic brain injury treatment trials: recommendations from the traumatic brain injury clinical trials network. *J Head Trauma Rehabil.* 2010;25(5): 375–382.
6. Wilde EA, Whiteneck GG, Bogner J, et al. Recommendations for the use of common outcome measures in traumatic brain injury research. *Arch Phys Med Rehabil.* 2010;91(11):1650–1660.e17.
7. Wilson L, Boase K, Nelson LD, et al. A manual for the Glasgow outcome Scale-extended interview. *J Neurotrauma.* 2021;38(17):2435–2446.
8. Yuh EL, Jain S, Sun X, et al. Pathological computed tomography features associated with adverse outcomes after mild traumatic brain injury: a TRACK-TBI study with external validation in CENTER-TBI. *JAMA Neurol.* 2021;78(9):1137–1148.
9. Elkbuli A, Shaikh S, McKenney K, Shanahan H, McKenney M, McKenney K. Utility of the Marshall & Rotterdam classification scores in predicting outcomes in trauma patients. *J Surg Res.* 2021;264:194–198.
10. Maas AI, Marmarou A, Murray GD, Teasdale SG, Steyerberg EW. Prognosis and clinical trial design in traumatic brain injury: the IMPACT study. *J Neurotrauma.* 2007;24(2):232–238.
11. MRC CRASH trial collaborators, Perel P, Arango M, et al. Predicting outcome after traumatic brain injury: practical prognostic models based on large cohort of international patients. *BMJ.* 2008;336(7641):425–429.
12. Majdan M, Lingsma HF, Nieboer D, Mauritz W, Rusnak M, Steyerberg EW. Performance of IMPACT, CRASH and Nijmegen models in predicting six month outcome of patients with severe or moderate TBI: an external validation study. *Scand J Trauma Resusc Emerg Med.* 2014;22:68. Published 2014 Nov 19.
13. Roozenbeek B, Lingsma HF, Lecky FE, et al. Prediction of outcome after moderate and severe traumatic brain injury: external validation of the International Mission on Prognosis and Analysis of Clinical Trials (IMPACT) and Corticoid Randomisation After Significant Head injury (CRASH) prognostic models. *Crit Care Med.* 2012;40(5):1609–1617.
14. Moskowitz J, Quinn T, Khan MW, et al. Should we use the IMPACT-model for the outcome prognostication of TBI patients? A qualitative study assessing physicians' perceptions. *MDM Policy Pract.* 2018;3(1):2381468318757987.
15. Hallen SA, Hootsmans NA, Blaisdell L, Gutheil CM, Han PK. Physicians' perceptions of the value of prognostic models: the benefits and risks of prognostic confidence. *Health Expect.* 2015;18(6):2266–2277.
16. Izzy S, Compton R, Carandang R, Hall W, Muehlschlegel S. Self-fulfilling prophecies through withdrawal of care: do they exist in traumatic brain injury, too? *Neurocrit Care.* 2013;19(3):347–363.
17. Xie Q, Ni X, Yu R, Li Y, Huang R. Chronic disorders of consciousness. *Exp Ther Med.* 2017;14(2):1277–1283.
18. Pease M, Arefan D, Barber J, et al. Outcome prediction in patients with severe traumatic brain injury using deep learning from head CT scans. *Radiology.* 2022;304(2):385–394.
19. Adams, J H, Doyle D, Ford I, et al. Diffuse axonal injury in head injury: definition, diagnosis and grading. *Histopathology.* 1989;49–59.
20. Johnson VE, Stewart W, Smith DH. Axonal pathology in traumatic brain injury. *Exp Neurol.* 2013;246:35–43.
21. Chelly H, Chaari A, Daoud E, et al. Diffuse axonal injury in patients with head injuries: an epidemiologic and prognosis study of 124 cases. *J Trauma.* 2011;71(4):838–846.
22. Skandsen T, Kvistad KA, Solheim O, Lydersen S, Strand IH, Vik A. Prognostic value of magnetic resonance imaging in moderate and severe head injury: a prospective study of early MRI findings and one-year outcome. *J Neurotrauma.* 2011;28(5):691–699.
23. Janas AM, Qin F, Hamilton S, et al. Diffuse axonal injury grade on early MRI is associated with worse outcome in children with moderate-severe traumatic brain injury. *Neurocrit Care.* 2022;36(2):492–503.
24. Izzy S, Mazwi NL, Martinez S, et al. Revisiting grade 3 diffuse axonal injury: not all brainstem microbleeds are prognostically equal. *Neurocrit Care.* 2017;27(2):199–207.
25. Snider SB, Bodien YG, Bianciardi M, Brown EN, Wu O, Edlow BL. Disruption of the ascending arousal network in acute traumatic disorders of consciousness. *Neurology.* 2019;93(13):e1281–e1287.
26. Galanaud D, Perlbarg V, Gupta R, et al. Assessment of white matter injury and outcome in severe brain trauma: a prospective multicenter cohort. *Anesthesiology.* 2012;117(6):1300–1310.
27. Puybasset L, Perlbarg V, Unrug J, et al. Prognostic value of global deep white matter DTI metrics for 1-year outcome prediction in ICU traumatic brain injury patients: an MRI-COMA and CENTER-TBI combined study. *Intensive Care Med.* 2022;48(2):201–212.
28. Edlow BL, Fins JJ. Assessment of covert consciousness in the intensive care unit: clinical and ethical considerations. *J Head Trauma Rehabil.* 2018;33(6):424–434.
29. Giacino JT, Kalmar K, Whyte J. The JFK coma recovery scale-revised: measurement characteristics and diagnostic utility. *Arch Phys Med Rehabil.* 2004;85(12):2020–2029.
30. American Congress of Rehabilitation Medicine, Brain Injury-Interdisciplinary Special Interest Group, Disorders of Consciousness Task Force, Seel RT, Sherer M, et al. Assessment scales for disorders of consciousness: evidence-based recommendations for clinical practice and research. *Arch Phys Med Rehabil.* 2010;91(12):1795–1813.
31. Edlow BL, Naccache L. Unmasking covert language processing in the intensive care unit with electroencephalography. *Ann Neurol.* 2021;89(4):643–645.
32. Owen AM, Coleman MR, Boly M, Davis MH, Laureys S, Pickard JD. Detecting awareness in the vegetative state. *Science.* 2006;313(5792):1402.
33. Claassen J, Doyle K, Matory A, et al. Detection of brain activation in unresponsive patients with acute brain injury. *N Engl J Med.* 2019;380(26):2497–2505.
34. Sokoliuk R, Degano G, Banellis L, et al. Covert speech comprehension predicts recovery from acute unresponsive states. *Ann Neurol.* 2021;89(4):646–656.
35. Egbebike J, Shen Q, Doyle K, et al. Cognitive-motor dissociation, and time to functional recovery in patients with acute brain injury in the USA: a prospective observational cohort study. *Lancet Neurology.* 2022;704–713.
36. Edlow BL, Chatelle C, Spencer CA, et al. Early detection of consciousness in patients with acute severe traumatic brain injury. *Brain.* 2017;140(9):2399–2414
37. Norton L, Kazazian K, Gofton T, et al. Functional Neuroimaging as an assessment tool in critically ill patients. *Ann Neurol.* 2023;93(1):131–141.

CHAPTER

26

What Is the Role of Neurostimulants in Recovery After Severe Traumatic Brain Injury?

Kelly D. Nahum, DO & Brett M. Tracy, MD

Case

A 31-year-old male patient who presented with a severe traumatic brain injury after being in a motorcycle accident without wearing a helmet. His intensive care unit (ICU) course was complicated by refractory intracranial pressure, which was treated with sedation and hyperosmolar therapy. MRI brain on day 12 showed right frontal/temporal and parietal contusion and signs of corpus callosum and brainstem microbleeds. On day 15, the patient is minimally responsive (Glasgow Coma Scale [GCS] score was 5T), with bilaterally reactive pupils. Should we start a neurostimulant?

Key Points

- Amantadine and methylphenidate may accelerate the rate of cognitive recovery.
- Concomitant administration of methylphenidate and amantadine may provide therapeutic synergy during the immediate hospitalization phase following a severe TBI.
- Several retrospective studies that studied the NS utilization rates and adverse drug event in patients with acute disorders of consciousness (DoC) showed reasonable tolerance and safety profile.
- Randomized control trials with larger sample sizes and more homogenous cognitive outcome variables are needed prior to widespread implementation of NSs.

BACKGROUND

Nearly 1.7 million people in the United States sustain a traumatic brain injury (TBI) each year.[1] While most injuries are mild and resolve without consequence, approximately 1% to 2% of patients with a severe TBI will experience some form of impairment in their level of consciousness and/or cognitive function.[1,2] The exact neurobiology of this alteration is uncertain but likely occurs due to extensive downregulation of the excitatory neural pathways after trauma-induced deafferentation of neurons in the corticothalamic system.[3,4]

The clinical manifestation of neurological impairment often falls along a behavioral spectrum commonly referred to as disorders of consciousness (DoC). The continuum of DoC includes coma, vegetative state, or minimally conscious state, and each category can be differentiated by certain behavioral features (Table 26–1).[3] Unfortunately, at one-year postinjury, 50% of patients in a vegetative state fail to regain consciousness and 50% of patients in a minimally conscious state remain disabled.[5] These findings illuminate the need for novel treatment strategies that augment neurorecovery following a TBI.

Neurostimulants (NSs) are an emerging therapeutic option to treat neurological impairment following a severe TBI.[1,3] There are five general types of NS: central nervous system stimulants, dopaminergic agents, acetylcholinesterase inhibitors, selective serotonin reuptake inhibitors, and gamma-aminobutyric acid (GABA) agonists.[6] The cognitive effect of each of these medications has been examined, and many of the studies assess different domains using noninterchangeable cognitive measurement scales.[6] Selected scales are summarized in (Table 26–2), and an understanding of them is helpful to appreciate how NSs may impact neurorecovery. Cognition incorporates multiple domains like sensory-perceptual-motor skills, attention, memory, executive function, language, and visuo-spatial and constructional abilities.[3] No singular measurement scale can adequately and accurately capture an individual's cognitive function status.[7]

TABLE 26–1 Behavioral features associated with disorders of consciousness.

State	Arousal/Attention	Cognition	Language	Visual Perception	Motor
Coma	No sleep-wake cycles	None	None	None	Primitive reflexes only
Vegetative	Intermittent wakefulness	None	None	Visual startle (inconsistent)	Involuntary movements only
Minimally conscious	Intermittent wakefulness periods	Inconsistent self- or environmental awareness	Single words or short phrases	Object recognition	Object manipulation; localization

Source: Adapted from "Disorders of consciousness after acquired brain injury: the state of the science," by Giacino JT, Fins JJ, Laureys S, Schiff ND, *Nature Reviews Neurology*, 2014;10(2), p. 101. (doi:10.1038/nrneurol.2013.279). Copyright 2014 by Macmillan Publishers Limited.[3]

EVIDENCE AND REVIEW

Amantadine

Amantadine is the most frequently prescribed medication used to treat patients with a DoC due to a TBI.[5,8] The drug is believed to work by increasing extracellular dopamine levels through blocking reuptake and facilitating synthesis.[9,10] It is also an N-methyl-D-aspartate receptor antagonist, which may provide downstream neuroprotection through inhibition of proteolysis and neurofilament compaction.[9,11,12]

One of the first studies to explore amantadine's role in neurologic recovery following TBI was by Meythaler et al in 2002. They performed a double-blind, randomized, crossover trial among 35 patients with an acute diffuse axonal injury. During the first 6 weeks following injury, 15 patients (group 1) received amantadine and 20 patients (group 2) received placebo. After 6 weeks, group 2 patients began a 6-week course of amantadine and Group 1 received placebo. During the first 6 weeks of the study, there were significant improvements in group 1's Disability Rate Scale (DRS), Glasgow Outcome Scale (GOS), and Functional Independence Measure-Cognitive (FIM-Cog) scores. However, when transitioned to placebo in the following 6 weeks, there was no continued improvement. During the first 6 weeks for group 2, there were spontaneous and significant improvements in cognition while on placebo. During the next 6 weeks when group 2 was treated with amantadine, there were additional improvements in DRS and FIM-Cog scores.[13] At the end of the 12-week study, both groups had similar levels of cognitive recovery. These findings suggest that the cognitive response from amantadine is drug-dependent and that clinical improvement may occur when amantadine is given at any point within 3 months of injury.[13]

TABLE 26–2 Selected outcome measures.

Outcome Scale	Range	Items Assessed
Disability rating scale (DRS)[a]	0-29	Eye opening, motor response, communication ability, feeding, toileting, grooming, level of functioning, and employability
Full Outline of UnResponsiveness (FOUR)	0-16	Eye response, motor response, brainstem reflexes, and respirations
Functional independence measure—cognitive (FIM-Cog)	5-35	Communication (comprehension and expression) and social cognition (social interaction, problem solving, and memory)
Glasgow Coma Scale (GCS)	3-15	Eye, motor, and verbal responses
Glasgow Outcome Scale (GOS)	1-5	Consciousness, daily dependence (mental and physical), and employability
Mini-mental state exam (MMSE)	0-30	Orientation (temporal and spatial), memory (registration and recall), attention and calculation, language (verbal and written), and visuospatial function

[a]For all outcome scales, higher scores reflect better performance except for DRS.

Further evidence to support amantadine in the TBI population was provided by Giacino et al in their 2012 landmark study.[5] They performed a multicenter, prospective, double-blind, randomized, placebo-controlled trial among 184 rehabilitation inpatients who were either in a vegetative state or minimally conscious state 4 to 16 weeks postinjury. Patients were randomized to receive amantadine or placebo for 4 weeks, followed by a 2-week drug washout period. Among the 87 patients in the amantadine group, the rate of improvement on the DRS was significantly faster during the 4-week treatment period. In addition, the overall cognitive improvement seen in the amantadine group was maintained after treatment discontinuation and a smaller proportion of patients in the amantadine group remained in a vegetative state (18% vs. 31%).[5] However, the improvement rate decreased during the 2-week drug washout period and was slower than the placebo group. The researchers concluded that the rate of cognitive improvement is accelerated by amantadine and is drug-dependent.[5]

In contrast to these positive discoveries, Ghalaenovi et al found no cognitive benefit associated with amantadine for patients with an acute, moderate-severe TBI.[14] The investigators performed a double-blind, randomized controlled trial among patients with a Glasgow Coma Scale (GCS) score ≤ 9 on hospital admission. Patients received 6 weeks of amantadine (n = 19) or placebo (n = 21) and the GCS and Full Outline of UnResponsiveness (FOUR) scores were assessed on the 1st, 3rd, and 7th day of treatment. The only significant finding was the change in GCS scores between days 1 and 7, which was greater in the amantadine group (4 vs. 2, P = .04). There were no other differences in mini-mental state exam (MMSE), GOS, or DRS scores at 6-month follow-up between groups. Based on these findings, the authors suggested that amantadine has no meaningful effect on cognition or consciousness in patients with a moderate-severe TBI.[14]

Hammond et al likewise found no cognitive benefit associated with amantadine in patients with a chronic TBI (>6 months postinjury).[15] The researchers performed a parallel-group, randomized, double-blind, placebo-controlled trial of amantadine 100 mg twice daily for 60 days on 119 individuals. After 28 days of treatment, the placebo group had a significantly greater improvement in memory, attention, and processing speed compared to the amantadine group. At day 60, no significant difference in cognitive function was detected between groups. The authors surmised that amantadine does not enhance cognitive function and may transiently impair cognition within the first 28 days of treatment.[15]

Given the heterogeneity of results from these studies and several others, Mohamed et al performed a meta-analysis of 26 studies investigating amantadine's effect on TBI.[16] They noted a significant improvement in cognition when amantadine was given within the first week of injury and when prescribed for less than a month. On meta-regression that included timing of treatment onset, patient age, and TBI severity, an earlier administration of amantadine had the strongest association with the cognitive effect of amantadine.[16] On subgroup analysis, cognitive improvements were significantly better for patients <18 years of age and among patients with a moderate TBI. Furthermore, they found no difference in hospital length of stay or adverse events when comparing amantadine to placebo. The authors submit that compared to placebo, there is moderate evidence to support that amantadine improves cognitive function in patients with a TBI.[16]

Methylphenidate

Methylphenidate inhibits dopamine and norepinephrine transport and reuptake, which possibly enhances consciousness and cognition in patients with a TBI.[7,17–19] While methylphenidate has not been studied as extensively as amantadine, it does have a larger body of literature compared to the other NSs. In 1996, Plenger et al conducted a randomized, double-blind, placebo-controlled trial among 23 patients with moderate-severe TBI. Patients received either methylphenidate .3 mg/kg/dose twice daily or placebo for 30 consecutive days during a subacute recovery phase.[20] The methylphenidate group had significantly better DRS scores as well as improved motor and attention performance at 30 days. However, there was no difference between groups at 90 days. The authors concluded that methylphenidate may accelerate the rate of cognitive recovery but does not impact the final level of recovery attained.[20]

In 2004, Whyte et al conducted a double-blind, placebo-controlled, repeated crossover study among 34 adults with a severe TBI during the postacute recovery phase.[21] Patients either received methylphenidate .3 mg/kg/dose twice daily or placebo for 6 weeks. The researchers noted that methylphenidate significantly improved cognitive processing speeds but had no effect on sustained attention or dual task performance.[21] Similar results were obtained by Willmott and Ponsford in their 2008 randomized, crossover, double-blind, placebo-controlled trial of methylphenidate .3 mg/kg/dose twice daily among 40 rehabilitation inpatients with a moderate-severe TBI.[22] Over a 2-week period, patients receiving methylphenidate had significantly improved cognitive processing speeds. In addition, patients with worse GCS scores and slower baseline processing speeds demonstrated the greatest cognitive response to methylphenidate.[22]

Considering the potential cognitive amelioration associated with NSs, Herrold et al retrospectively compared rehabilitation inpatients with a severe TBI who received one NS (n = 31) versus multiple NSs (n = 84). While more than two-thirds of the cohort received multiple NSs, there was no difference in recovery of full consciousness or improved behavior between groups.[23] Another study with similar purpose was performed by Tracy et al in 2021. They retrospectively examined the effect of amantadine (monotherapy) versus amantadine and methylphenidate (dual therapy) on return to consciousness among 76 patients with an acute, severe TBI. Patients receiving dual therapy (n = 49) had significantly improved neurorecovery (measured by GCS scores), and dual therapy increased the likelihood of neurorecovery. The researchers suggested that concomitant administration of methylphenidate and amantadine may provide therapeutic synergy during the immediate hospitalization phase following a severe TBI.[24]

Are Neurostimulants Safe to Use in the NeuroICU?

The "off-label" use of pharmacological stimulant therapy for the treatment of DoC following severe TBI has been increasing. Over the last few years, several studies have examined NS utilization rates and adverse drug events in patients with acute DoC and showed reasonable tolerance and safety profiles. More studies that focus on evaluating the optimal dose, duration, and efficacy are still warranted. Other areas needing further analysis include the effect of NSs when introduced at different times, when prescribed for distinct time intervals, or when given to patients with different TBI pathologies and severities. Until these issues are addressed, it seems unlikely that a scientific organization will fully endorse or provide guidelines on NS use in the TBI population. Nevertheless, any intervention that could conceivably accelerate return to consciousness or improve cognition for patients with a TBI deserves thorough examination and thoughtful consideration.

REFERENCES

1. Rabinowitz AR, Watanabe TK. Pharmacotherapy for Treatment of Cognitive and Neuropsychiatric Symptoms After mTBI. *Journal of Head Trauma Rehabilitation*. 2020;35(1):76–83. doi:10.1097/HTR.0000000000000537
2. Løvstad M, Andelic N, Knoph R, et al. Rate of disorders of consciousness in a prospective population-based study of adults with traumatic brain injury. *Journal of Head Trauma Rehabilitation*. Published online 2014. doi:10.1097/HTR.0000000000000017
3. Giacino JT, Fins JJ, Laureys S, et al. Disorders of consciousness after acquired brain injury: the state of the science. *Nature Reviews Neurology*. 2014;10(2):99–114. doi:10.1038/nrneurol.2013.279
4. Edlow BL, Claassen J, Schiff ND, Greer DM. Recovery from disorders of consciousness: mechanisms, prognosis and emerging therapies. *Nature Reviews Neurology*. 2021;17(3):135–156. doi:10.1038/s41582-020-00428-x

5. Giacino JT, Whyte J, Bagiella E, et al. Placebo-controlled trial of amantadine for severe traumatic brain injury. *New England Journal of Medicine.* 2012;366(9):819–826. doi:10.1056/NEJMoa1102609
6. Kakehi S, Tompkins DM. A review of pharmacologic neurostimulant use during rehabilitation and recovery after brain injury. *Annals of Pharmacotherapy.* 2021;55(10):1254–1266. doi:10.1177/1060028020983607
7. Whyte J, Vaccaro M, Grieb-Neff P, Hart T. Psychostimulant use in the rehabilitation of individuals with traumatic brain injury. *Journal of Head Trauma Rehabilitation.* 2002;17(4):284–299. doi:10.1097/00001199-200208000-00003
8. Barra ME, Izzy S, Sarro-Schwartz A, Hirschberg RE, Mazwi N, Edlow BL. Stimulant therapy in acute traumatic brain injury: prescribing patterns and adverse event rates at 2 level 1 trauma centers. *Journal of Intensive Care Medicine.* 2020;35(11):1196–1202. doi:10.1177/0885066619841603
9. Kochanek P, Jackson T, Ferguson N, et al. Emerging therapies in traumatic brain injury. *Seminars in Neurology.* 2015;35(01):83–100. doi:10.1055/s-0035-1544237
10. Jenkins PO, de Simoni S, Bourke NJ, et al. Dopaminergic abnormalities following traumatic brain injury. *Brain.* 2018;141(3):797–810. doi:10.1093/brain/awx357
11. Al-Sarraj S. The pathology of traumatic brain injury (TBI): a practical approach. *Diagnostic Histopathology.* 2016;22(9):318–326. doi:10.1016/j.mpdhp.2016.08.005
12. Meythaler JM, Peduzzi JD, Eleftheriou E, Novack TA. Current concepts: diffuse axonal injury–associated traumatic brain injury. *Archives of Physical Medicine and Rehabilitation.* 2001;82(10):1461–1471. doi:10.1053/apmr.2001.25137
13. Meythaler JM, Brunner RC, Johnson A, Novack TA. Amantadine to improve neurorecovery in traumatic brain injury–associated diffuse axonal injury. *Journal of Head Trauma Rehabilitation.* 2002;17(4):300–313. doi: 10.1097/00001199-200208000-00004
14. Ghalaenovi H, Fattahi A, Koohpayehzadeh J, et al. The effects of amantadine on traumatic brain injury outcome: a double-blind, randomized, controlled, clinical trial. *Brain Injury.* Published online 2018. doi:10.1080/02699052.2018.1476733
15. Hammond FM, Sherer M, Malec JF, et al. Amantadine did not positively impact cognition in chronic traumatic brain injury: a multi-site, randomized, controlled trial. *Journal of Neurotrauma.* 2018;35(19):2298–2305. doi:10.1089/neu.2018.5767
16. Mohamed MS, el Sayed I, Zaki A, Abdelmonem S. Assessment of the effect of amantadine in patients with traumatic brain injury: a meta-analysis. *Journal of Trauma and Acute Care Surgery.* 2022;92(3):605–614. doi:10.1097/TA.0000000000003363
17. Bhatnagar S, Iaccarino MA, Zafonte R. Pharmacotherapy in rehabilitation of post-acute traumatic brain injury. *Brain Research.* 2016;1640:164–179. doi:10.1016/j.brainres.2016.01.021
18. Arnsten AFT, Li BM. Neurobiology of executive functions: catecholamine influences on prefrontal cortical functions. *Biological Psychiatry.* 2005;57(11):1377–1384. doi:10.1016/j.biopsych.2004.08.019
19. Husson I, Mesplès B, Medja F, Leroux P, Kosofsky B, Gressens P. Methylphenidate and MK-801, an N-methyl-d-aspartate receptor antagonist: shared biological properties. *Neuroscience.* 2004;125(1):163–170. doi:10.1016/j.neuroscience.2004.01.010
20. Plenger PM, Dixon CE, Castillo RM, Frankowski RF, Yablon SA, Levin HS. Subacute methylphenidate treatment for moderate to moderately severe traumatic brain injury: a preliminary double-blind placebo-controlled study. *Archives of Physical Medicine and Rehabilitation.* 1996;77(6):536–540. doi:10.1016/S0003-9993(96)90291-9
21. Whyte J, Hart T, Vaccaro M, et al. Effects of methylphenidate on attention deficits after traumatic brain injury. *American Journal of Physical Medicine & Rehabilitation.* 2004;83(6):401–420. doi:10.1097/01.PHM.0000128789.75375.D3
22. Willmott C, Ponsford J. Efficacy of methylphenidate in the rehabilitation of attention following traumatic brain injury: a randomised, crossover, double blind, placebo controlled inpatient trial. *Journal of Neurology, Neurosurgery & Psychiatry.* 2009;80(5):552–557. doi:10.1136/jnnp.2008.159632
23. Herrold AA, Pape TLB, Guernon A, Mallinson T, Collins E, Jordan. Prescribing multiple neurostimulants during rehabilitation for severe brain injury. *The Scientific World Journal.* Published online 2014:1–7. doi:10.1155/2014/964578
24. Tracy BM, Silverman ME, Cordero-Caballero C, Durr EA, Gelbard RB. Dual neurostimulant therapy may optimize acute neurorecovery for severe traumatic brain injuries. *Journal of Surgical Research.* 2021;268:546–551. doi:10.1016/j.jss.2021.07.037

CHAPTER

27

How Do We Decrease the Risk of Recurrence in Non-Acute Subdural Hematomas?

Casey Jarvis, MD & Wenya Linda Bi, MD, PhD

Case

A 63-year-old right-handed man, not on any anticoagulation or antiplatelet agents, presented a month after a fall off of his bike with progressively severe headaches and word-finding difficulties. He was diagnosed with bilateral left greater than right subdural hematomas and treated with bilateral mini-craniotomies for evacuation, with resolution of his symptoms. Two months later, he returned with new left-sided weakness and found to have a significant right holohemispheric recurrent subacute subdural hematoma (Figure 27-1). What strategies might decrease subdural hematoma recurrence for this patient?

Key Points

- Medical management of chronic subdural hematoma (cSDH), including atorvastatin and tranexamic acid (TXA), may play a role.
- Increased risks and adverse events associated with dexamethasone usage likely do not outweigh the benefits.
- Burr holes or mini-craniotomy is associated with lower risk of complications compared to a large craniotomy; however, operative treatment should be tailored to the individual patient's needs and risk factors.
- Stripping of subdural membranes does not significantly improve outcomes in a majority of cases.
- Subgaleal or subdural drains after cSDH evacuation reduce recurrence risk.
- Adjunctive strategies such as subdural evacuating port system (SEPS) drainage, aspiration of pneumocephalus, and middle meningioma embolization expand surgical treatment options for select patients.

BACKGROUND

Chronic subdural hematoma (cSDH) is a common affliction, predominantly affecting the elderly population, with an incidence of approximately 58 per 100,000 people over the age of 65 per year.[1,2] cSDH is a particularly onerous neurosurgical issue due to the relatively high rate of recurrence, ranging from 10% to 30% in the literature.[1,2] Recurrence is highly morbid for patients and can lead to poor outcomes such as decreased functional status, return to operating room (OR), and death. Despite the prevalence of this condition, there is a lack of consensus on the most effective treatment option to decrease the likelihood of recurrence. Numerous treatment options exist, ranging from medical management to operative intervention, including twist drill drainage (<5 mm in diameter), typically done at the bedside, burr holes or what some refer to as a "mini-craniotomy" (5-30 mm), or craniotomy (>30 mm). No randomized controlled studies exist to date comparing the efficacy of these surgical approaches.

Evidence and Review

Medical Management

cSDH recurrence is believed to occur secondary to a combination of rebleeding from immature, fragile vessels in the membrane that develop around a hematoma, which are prone to leakage, and an inflammatory response that may further undermine vascular structures and inhibit proper coagulation.[3,4,5] Medical management strategies have arisen to target these hypotheses, including the utilization of steroids as well as statins, which, aside from reducing cholesterol levels, have also been shown to reduce inflammation within the vascular wall and promote vascular repair.[3] Data on these medical management options remain mixed. In a 2018 randomized controlled trial of 254 patients with cSDH, atorvastatin was suggested to

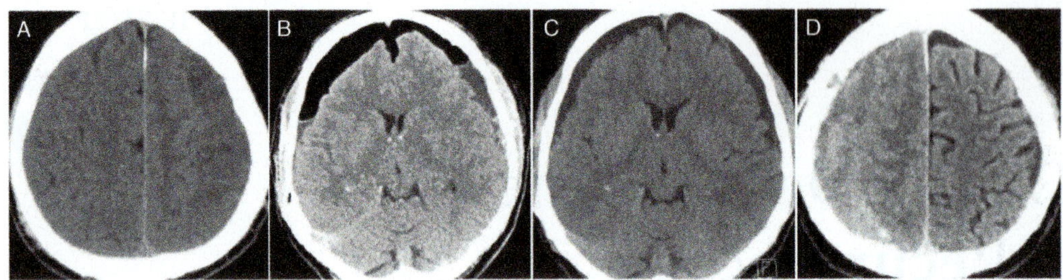

FIGURE 27–1 Non-contrast head computed tomography (CT) scan demonstrating (**A**) large left holohemispheric subacute subdural hematoma with resultant mass effect and midline shift with smaller right holohemispheric subacute subdural hematoma, (**B**) improved mass effect after evacuation on immediate postoperative scan, (**C**) improved pneumocephalus and subdural hygromas at 1-month follow-up, and (**D**) new recurrence of a right holohemispheric subdural hematoma at 2 months after the initial operation.

effectively reduce radiographic hematoma volume as well as clinically improve neurologic function.[3] The literature on dexamethasone usage is more controversial, with some studies reporting that dexamethasone in conjunction with surgery increases morbidity with no benefit in outcomes,[6] while others note that it may aid in reducing recurrence when coupled with surgery.[7] A randomized controlled trial in 748 patients demonstrated that while treatment of cSDH patients with dexamethasone resulted in less frequent return to OR, it was also associated with fewer favorable outcomes and an increase in adverse events.[8] Dexamethasone has also been suggested to enhance the efficacy of atorvastatin in the medical management of cSDH.[9]

Operative Evacuation Strategies

Operative interventions are often favored over medical management for large or symptomatic cSDH. Burr holes or mini-craniotomy are often considered to have a better safety profile as compared to a large open craniotomy, with acceptable recurrence rates.[5,10,11,12] An initial dilemma centered on handling of the membrane encapsulating subacute to cSDHs. A landmark paper by Svien and Gelety in 1964 demonstrated that open craniotomy for cSDH evacuation resulted in increased risk of recurrence and decreased functional status compared to burr holes for drainage without manipulation of the subdural membranes, although these findings were not statistically significant.[11] A systematic review by Weigel et al in 2003 supported this opinion, finding that burr hole was more effective than bedside twist drill evacuation, and both more effective and safer than craniotomy.[12] However, a more recent meta-analysis in 2010 reported that while open craniotomy carries a higher risk of morbidity and mortality, it confers the lowest recurrence rate as compared to burr holes or twist drill evacuation.[10] Twist drill evacuation is reported to carry a similar efficacy and safety profile compared to burr holes or mini-craniotomy,[6,12] while also having the added benefit of being a bedside procedure and avoiding general anesthesia.[6] Patient-specific factors may influence choice of specific treatment decisions.

Drain Placement

Placement of drains are found to reduce cSDH recurrence across the literature. In a randomized controlled trial of 269 patients, drains left after burr holes for cSDH reduced recurrence by 14.7% and decreased mortality at 6 months by about 10%.[2] A subsequent meta-analysis further supported this finding, demonstrating a relative risk of .46 for recurrence of cSDH when drains were inserted.[6] While there is strong evidence that leaving a drain reduces the recurrence risk of cSDH, debate remains regarding timing of drainage, drain location, and active versus passive drainage. In a Danish study of cSDH recurrence, they found that 48 hours of drainage time had a lower morbidity than 96 hours with no difference in recurrence rates, and passive subdural drainage resulted in a lower recurrence rate than passive subgaleal drainage.[1] The 2019 cSDH-Drain Trial conversely demonstrated that subperiosteal drains led to less recurrence, fewer adverse events, and improved outcomes and mortality compared to subdural drains.[13] This study similarly employed passive drainage and maintained the drains for 48 hours.

Other innovative methods for reducing cSDH recurrence have emerged in recent years. One notable example is the subdural evacuating port system (SEPS), which combines bedside twist drill access with port drainage to access the subdural space and applies suction to evacuate the SDH. This differs from traditional subdural drain placement in that no catheter is left within the intracranial space, theoretically reducing complication risks. In preliminary studies, the efficacy of evacuation with SEPS method was found to be about 74%, similar to that of burr holes.[14] Failure, as defined by recurrence or need for secondary procedure, was associated with radiographic appearance of mixed density blood, likely indicative of septations.[15]

Pneumocephalus Aspiration

Another concept to reduce cSDH accumulation is the subdural pneumocephalus aspiration technique.[16] This method postulates that pneumocephalus hinders cerebral re-expansion and is a risk factor for cSDH recurrence. In this technique, patients undergo a routine mini-craniotomy for SDH evacuation, with placement of a subdural drain. Following scalp closure, post-procedural pneumocephalus is gently aspirated from a syringe attached to the drain until fluid returns. The drain is clamped and later removed in an airtight fashion. The authors observed that patients who underwent the pneumocephalus aspiration technique had less reaccumulation and a lower rate of recurrence requiring operative intervention at 1 month as compared to historical controls who underwent standard cSDH evacuation with postoperative drain placement.[16]

Middle Meningeal Artery Embolization

Middle meningeal artery (MMA) embolization is a promising endovascular technique used either alone or in conjunction with conventional surgical treatment methods to treat and prevent cSDH recurrence. MMA embolization is believed to prevent recurrence by inhibiting blood flow to the capillary feeders of the dura thought to contribute to hematoma reaccumulation.[4,17] Studies have shown that MMA embolization can reduce cSDH recurrence requiring operative intervention by 10%.[18] A meta-analysis including double- and single-armed studies found that recurrence rates after MMA embolization average at approximately 2% to 4% as compared to an average of 27% with conventional surgical treatment methods, with no significant increase in complications.[17] While large randomized controlled trials are pending, a pilot study of 46 patients randomized to either surgical treatment of cSDH or surgical treatment with MMA embolization found that the patients who underwent both surgical treatment and MMA embolization had a smaller volume of hematoma remaining at 3 months follow-up compared to the surgical treatment alone group.[4] In patients on anticoagulation or other medical comorbidities, MMA embolization may prove a particularly attractive option.

Available Guidelines

While no official societal guidelines exist on the treatment of cSDH, a 2010 Chronic Subdural Haematoma Review put out by the Congress of Neurological Surgeons asserted that burr holes or mini-craniotomies (5-30 mm in diameter) may be the most efficient cSDH treatment choice to balance risk of recurrence and mortality/morbidity (class II evidence) and that leaving a drain decreases reaccumulation risk (class I evidence).[5]

REFERENCES

1. Andersen-Ranberg NC, Debrabant B, Poulsen FR, Bergholt B, Hundsholt T, Fugleholm K. The Danish chronic subdural hematoma study-predicting recurrence of chronic subdural hematoma. *Acta Neurochir (Wien)* 161: 885–894, 2019.
2. Santarius T, Kirkpatrick PJ, Ganesan D, et al. Use of drains versus no drains after burr-hole evacuation of chronic subdural haematoma: a randomised controlled trial. *Lancet* 374:1067–1073, 2009.
3. Jiang R, Zhao S, Wang R, et al. Safety and efficacy of atorvastatin for chronic subdural hematoma in Chinese patients: a randomized clinical trial. *JAMA Neurol* 75:1338–1346, 2018.
4. Ng S, Derraz I, Boetto J, et al. Middle meningeal artery embolization as an adjuvant treatment to surgery for symptomatic chronic subdural hematoma: a pilot study assessing hematoma volume resorption. *J Neurointerv Surg* 12:695–699, 2020.
5. Santarius T, Kirkpatrick PJ, Kolias AG, Hutchinson PJ. Working toward rational and evidence-based treatment of chronic subdural hematoma. *Clin Neurosurg* 57:112–122, 2010.
6. Almenawer SA, Farrokhyar F, Hong C, et al. Chronic subdural hematoma management: a systematic review and meta-analysis of 34,829 patients. *Ann Surg* 259:449–457, 2014.
7. Yao Z, Hu X, Ma L, You C. Dexamethasone for chronic subdural haematoma: a systematic review and meta-analysis. *Acta Neurochir (Wien)* 159: 2037–2044, 2017.
8. Hutchinson PJ, Edlmann E, Bulters D, et al. Trial of dexamethasone for chronic subdural hematoma. *N Engl J Med* 383:2616–2627, 2020.
9. Wang D, Gao C, Xu X, et al. Treatment of chronic subdural hematoma with atorvastatin combined with low-dose dexamethasone: phase II randomized proof-of-concept clinical trial. *J Neurosurg* 1–9, 2020.
10. Lega BC, Danish SF, Malhotra NR, Sonnad SS, Stein SC. Choosing the best operation for chronic subdural hematoma: a decision analysis. *J Neurosurg* 113:615–621, 2010.
11. Svien HJ, Gelety JE. On the surgical management of encapsulated subdural hematoma. A comparison of the results of membranectomy and simple evacuation. *J Neurosurg* 21:172–177, 1964.
12. Weigel R, Schmiedek P, Krauss JK. Outcome of contemporary surgery for chronic subdural haematoma: evidence based review. *J Neurol Neurosurg Psychiatry* 74:937–943, 2003.
13. Soleman J, Lutz K, Schaedelin S, et al. Subperiosteal vs subdural drain after burr-hole drainage of chronic subdural hematoma: a randomized clinical trial (cSDH-Drain-Trial). *Neurosurgery* 85:E825–E834, 2019.
14. Rughani AI, Lin C, Dumont TM, Penar PL, Horgan MA, Tranmer BI. A case-comparison study of the subdural evacuating port system in treating chronic subdural hematomas. *J Neurosurg* 113:609–614, 2010.
15. Kenning TJ, Dalfino JC, German JW, Drazin D, Adamo MA. Analysis of the subdural evacuating port system for the treatment of subacute and chronic subdural hematomas. *J Neurosurg* 113:1004–1010, 2010.
16. Chavakula V, Yan SC, Huang KT, et al. Subdural pneumocephalus aspiration reduces recurrence of chronic subdural hematoma. *Oper Neurosurg (Hagerstown)* 18:391–397, 2020.
17. Srivatsan A, Mohanty A, Nascimento FA, et al. Middle meningeal artery embolization for chronic subdural hematoma: meta-analysis and systematic review. *World Neurosurg* 122:613–619, 2019.
18. Shotar E, Meyblum L, Premat K, et al. Middle meningeal artery embolization reduces the post-operative recurrence rate of at-risk chronic subdural hematoma. *J Neurointerv Surg* 12:1209–1213, 2020.

CHAPTER

28

How Should We Treat Postoperative Pneumocephalus?

Ulrick S. Kanmounye, MD, MSc, Kent R. Richter, MD, & Clemens M. Schirmer, MD, PhD

Case

A 55-year-old woman undergoes a bifrontal craniotomy for meningioma resection. She has a delayed recovery of neurologic status afterwards. Serial computed tomography (CT) scans demonstrate significant bilateral pneumocephalus. How should we think about and manage this situation?

Key Points

- Serial noncontrast head computed tomography (CT) scans can promptly detect pneumocephalus progression, and the association of intracranial hypertension signs with imaging confirms tension pneumocephalus.
- While risk factors associated with tension pneumocephalus are known, few high-quality studies have evaluated its prevention and management.
- The indications and superiority of pneumocephalus evacuation techniques tend to be influenced by surgical and institutional preference/expertise and are yet to be evaluated prospectively or in a meta-analysis.
- There is a need for significant multicenter double-blinded (ie, study subjects and outcome assessors blinded) randomized controlled trials (RCTs) to rigorously define and test the benefit of therapeutic and preventative strategies.

BACKGROUND

Pneumocephalus (pneumatocele or intracranial aerocele) is the presence of air in the extracerebral, intracerebral, or intravascular space.[1,2] Thomas first described this entity in 1866.[3] Pneumocephalus is classified based on lesional age (ie, acute if they are less than 72 hours old or delayed if they are more than 72 hours old) and severity (ie, simple or tension; tension is characterized by significant mass effect and high intracranial pressure).[1] Tension pneumocephalus following cranial surgery is a rare emergency (2.5%), and subdural air collections cause the majority.[4]

EVIDENCE AND REVIEW

Although pneumocephalus is rare and most cases can be treated conservatively, neurosurgeons should be on the lookout for signs indicative of tension pneumocephalus. This represents a neurosurgical emergency with significant potential to impact patient outcomes adversely.[5] The increased morbidity and mortality rates associated with tension pneumocephalus warrant this chapter. The prompt recognition of tension pneumocephalus, especially in high-risk surgical patients, is paramount. This goal can be achieved by meticulously analyzing postoperative head computed tomography (CT) scans to identify radiologic signs such as widening interhemispheric space and air presence in multiple cisterns of the subarachnoid spaces.[6] However, surgeons should look for false positives like fat grafts that seal dural breaches following skull base surgery.[7] Fat (−30 to −70 Hounsfield units) can be mistaken for air (−1,000 Hounsfield Unit) because both appear dark and are common following endoscopic skull base surgery.[8]

Pathophysiology

Two proposed mechanisms contribute to the formation of pneumocephalus. Walter E. Dandy described the first mechanism in May 1926 (ball valve theory), and M. Horowitz described the second in 1964 (inverted-soda-bottle effect).[9,10] Dandy proposed pneumocephalus resulting from unidirectional air movement from the extracranial to the intracranial space.[9] In contrast, Horowitz argued that the negative pressure from cerebrospinal fluid (CSF) loss traps air in the cranium.[10]

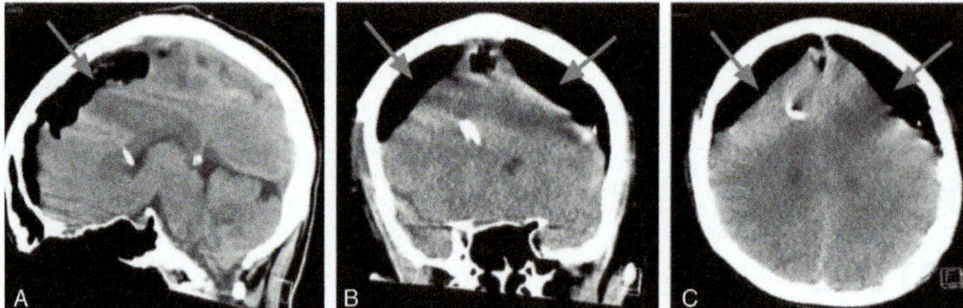

FIGURE 28–1 Plain sagittal (**A**), coronal (**B**), and axial (**C**) head computed tomography showing subdural air accumulation (Mount Fuji sign)—arrows.

Causes and Risk Factors

Pneumocephalus can be congenital, infectious, neoplastic, spontaneous, traumatic, or iatrogenic.[1] Iatrogenic causes include cranial surgeries, spine surgeries, ventriculostomies, and lumbar punctures.[1] Some amount of pneumocephalus is inevitable after cranial surgery and spinal surgeries that breach the dura; however, the volume of trapped air is increased by intraoperative administration of mannitol, prolonged operative time, nitrous oxide anesthesia, hydrocephalus, ventriculoperitoneal shunting, and semi-/seating position during posterior fossa surgery.[2] Pneumocephalus following posterior fossa surgery can be as large as 179 mL, and the semi-seating place increases the mean air volume by 39.5 mL ($p < .001$).[11]

Prevention

Head position during surgery and closure is a significant contributor to tension pneumocephalus. The surgeon should opt for a different position or take precautions to minimize subdural air accumulation. Some authors have suggested prepping both sides of the head before bilateral subdural hematoma evacuation to "allow rapid turning of the head after completion of drainage on one side."[7] Also, the head position during the closure should place the remaining dural defect at the highest point of the cranial cavity, so subdural air drains naturally.[7] Other methods include flushing the intradural space with the irrigation fluid.[7]

In the only prospective, single-blind randomized controlled trial (RCT) examining strategies for preventing postoperative pneumocephalus, Sandhu et al[12] found that the use of pure oxygen for intraoperative ventilation does not prevent postoperative pneumocephalus in craniotomy patients.[12] A systematic look at the spectrum of described strategies for pneumocephalus management as reported in case reports and case series since Sandhu et al[12] suggest variable or relatively minimal adoption of their findings and recommendations with continued and widespread use of legacy strategies without evidentiary basis. The variations in institutional protocols 5 years after this article was published indicate possible equipoise or lack of rigorous testing of hypotheses in this space. A larger multicenter RCT with blinding of the patients and outcome assessors may help resolve this equipoise. A multicenter RCT will have the benefit of increasing buy-in and sample size, which in turn should help standardize patient management and answer secondary outcome questions definitively. Finally, a multicenter RCT will open the doors to alternative trial designs, such as cluster randomization, allowing comparison of the significant prevention protocols used in everyday practice.

Diagnosis

Normal pneumocephalus is noted on CT scan up to 3 weeks post-cranial surgery with a prevalence of 100% during the 1st week and 26% during the 3rd week.[4,6] The less dense air rises to the higher subdural space and accumulates opposite the frontal lobes when a patient is placed in a decubitus position. The appearance of peaking frontal lobes surrounded by air collections is referred to as the Mt. Fuji sign (Figure 28–1— arrows), and air bubbles can be found in the subarachnoid cisterns (Figure 28–2—black arrow).

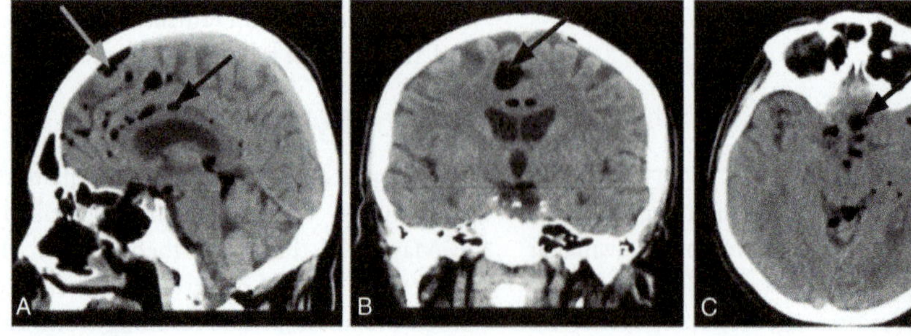

FIGURE 28–2 Plain sagittal (**A**), coronal (**B**), and axial (**C**) head computed tomography showing subdural (Mount Fuji sign)—Gray arrow—and subarachnoid air accumulations (air bubble sign)—Black arrows.

Cisternal air bubbles result from the passage of air from the subdural space to the subarachnoid space via a tear in the arachnoid membrane. As the subdural tension increases, the pressurized air compresses the arachnoid membrane until it finds a weak spot to breach.

Conservative Management

Most pneumocephalus are asymptomatic and are treated conservatively because the trapped air is absorbed.[2] Conservative treatment involves placing the patient in the semi-Fowler position at 30° and preventing Valsalva maneuvers or fever.[13] Supplemental O_2, with a nonrebreather facemask, in patients with >30 mL can help with postoperative pneumocephalus, and reduce the gas volume by 34% more than with room air alone (P = .009).[14] In an RCT of normobaric hyperoxia versus room air, Hong et al[15] found higher mean pneumocephalus volume changes (P = .001) and air resorption rates (P = .002) among patients treated with normobaric hyperoxia. The normobaric hyperoxia protocol used in this trial included 100% FiO_2 administered over an endotracheal tube for 3 hours.[15] Hyperbaric O_2 therapy is recommended if the pneumocephalus is caused by nitrous oxide anesthesia.[16]

Similar to postoperative pneumocephalus prevention, most evidence about pneumocephalus management has been from observational studies. Also, postoperative pneumocephalus management RCTs have had limited sample sizes and unblinded outcome assessors.[15,17] However, unlike postoperative pneumocephalus prevention, there seems to be a broader consensus on some treatment strategies. For example, conservative treatment is widely accepted, including bed rest, head elevation, supplemental oxygen, minimization of positive pressure, pain control, and frequent neurologic monitoring.[1,7,13,18] Other protocols include using the minimum required flow rate or pressure in patients who do not require invasive respiratory support.[19] Similarly, high ventilation pressure and volumes are avoided in patients requiring invasive respiratory support.[19] Finally, postoperative lumbar punctures are done carefully and only when necessary to minimize air entry in the meningeal spaces.

Surgical Intervention

Tension pneumocephalus can cause delayed postoperative awakening, coma, and death. Surgical intervention, which includes burr holes, needle aspiration, and closure of the dural defect, is warranted when tension pneumocephalus causes intracranial hypertension or rapid deterioration in patients. The symptoms are delayed because air accumulates in the intracranial space when the intracranial volume has been reduced (induced hypocapnia, increased venous drainage, and CSF loss), so the intracranial pressure rises gradually postoperatively as the intracranial volume increases.[20]

For the most part, the surgical treatment of postoperative pneumocephalus is that of CSF leaks.[7] Some interventions target subdural air evacuation specifically. These include burr holes, needle or controlled decompression, ventriculostomy if air accumulates in the ventricles, and decompressive craniectomy.[7,18]

Recently, subdural evacuating port systems (SEPS), traditionally indicated for subdural hematoma drainage, have been used to treat tension pneumocephalus.[19] Proponents of this modality justify its use because the procedure can be done expediently and at the bedside. Also, the equipment is low-cost and readily available, and the technique does not require irrigation, aspiration, or a catheter.[19] In addition, SEPS proponents point to its high safety profile in subdural hematoma evacuations as a reason for its adoption.[19]

REFERENCES

1. M Das J, Bajaj J. Pneumocephalus. In: *StatPearls*. StatPearls Publishing; 2022. Accessed May 2, 2022. http://www.ncbi.nlm.nih.gov/books/NBK535412/
2. Jhaveri MD, Salzman KL, Ross JS, Moore KR, Osborn AG, Ho CY. *ExpertDDx: Brain and Spine*. Elsevier—Health Sciences Division; 2017.
3. Thomas AL. Du pneumatocele du crane—Google Scholar. Accessed June 12, 2022. https://scholar.google.com/scholar_lookup?title=Du%20pneumatocele%20du%20crane&journal=Arch%20Gen%20Med%20%28Paris%29&volume=1&pages=34-55&publication_year=1866&author=Thomas%2CL
4. Reasoner DK, Todd MM, Scamman FL, Warner DS. The Incidence of pneumocephalus after supratentorial craniotomy: observations on the disappearance of intracranial air. *Anesthesiology*. 1994;80(5):1008–1012. doi:10.1097/00000542-199405000-00009
5. You CG, Zheng XS. Postoperative pneumocephalus increases the recurrence rate of chronic subdural hematoma. *Clin Neurol Neurosurg*. 2018;166:56–60. doi:10.1016/j.clineuro.2018.01.029
6. Ishiwata Y, Fujitsu K, Sekino T, et al. Subdural tension pneumocephalus following surgery for chronic subdural hematoma. *J Neurosurg*. 1988;68(1):58–61. doi:10.3171/jns.1988.68.1.0058
7. Schirmer CM, Heilman CB, Bhardwaj A. Pneumocephalus: case illustrations and review. *Neurocrit Care*. 2010;13(1):152–158. doi:10.1007/s12028-010-9363-0
8. Brain mapping: the methods—2nd edition. Accessed June 12, 2022. https://www.elsevier.com/books/brain-mapping-the-methods/toga/978-0-12-693019-1
9. Dandy WE. Pneumocephalus (Intracranial pneumatocele or aerocele). *Arch Surg*. 1926;12(5):949–982. doi:10.1001/archsurg.1926.01130050003001
10. Horowitz M. Intracranial pneumocoele. An unusual complication following mastoid surgery. *J Laryngol Otol*. 1964;78:128–134. doi:10.1017/s0022215100061910
11. Machetanz K, Leuze F, Mounts K, et al. Occurrence and management of postoperative pneumocephalus using the semi-sitting position in vestibular schwannoma surgery. *Acta Neurochir (Wien)*. 2020;162(11):2629–2636. doi:10.1007/s00701-020-04504-5
12. Sandhu G, Gonzalez-Zacarias A, Fiorda-Diaz J, et al. A prospective randomized clinical trial to evaluate the impact of intraoperative ventilation with high oxygen content on the extent of postoperative pneumocephalus in patients undergoing craniotomies. *Br J Neurosurg*. 2019;33(2):119–124. doi:10.1080/02688697.2018.1562031
13. Karavelioglu E, Eser O, Haktanir A. Pneumocephalus and pneumorrhachis after spinal surgery: case report and review of the literature. *Neurol Med Chir (Tokyo)*. 2014;54(5):405–407. doi:10.2176/nmc.cr2013-0118
14. Gore PA, Maan H, Chang S, Pitt AM, Spetzler RF, Nakaji P. Normobaric oxygen therapy strategies in the treatment of postcraniotomy pneumocephalus. *J Neurosurg*. 2008;108(5):926–929. doi:10.3171/JNS/2008/108/5/0926
15. Hong B, Biertz F, Raab P, et al. Normobaric hyperoxia for treatment of pneumocephalus after posterior fossa surgery in the semisitting position: a prospective randomized controlled trial. *PloS One*. 2015;10(5):e0125710. doi:10.1371/journal.pone.0125710
16. Paiva WS, de Andrade AF, Figueiredo EG, Amorim RL, Prudente M, Teixeira MJ. Effects of hyperbaric oxygenation therapy on symptomatic pneumocephalus. *Ther Clin Risk Manag*. 2014;10:769–773. doi:10.2147/TCRM.S45220

17. CHAN DDYC. High concentration of inspired oxygen for pneumocephalus after evacuation of chronic subdural haematoma: a randomized controlled trial (HOPE study). clinicaltrials.gov; 2022. Accessed November 27, 2022. https://clinicaltrials.gov/ct2/show/NCT04725851
18. Wankhade BS, Beniamein MMK, Alrais ZF, Mathew JI, Alrais GZ. What should an intensivist know about pneumocephalus and tension pneumocephalus? *Acute Crit Care.* Published online April 13, 2022. doi:10.4266/acc.2021.01102
19. Doron O, Schneider JR, Ellis JA. Application of the subdural evacuating port system for the drainage of postoperative tension pneumocephalus: a technical note. *Surg Neurol Int.* 2022;13:204. doi:10.25259/SNI_120_2022
20. Lemkuil BP, Drummond JC, Patel PM, Lam A. Anesthesia for neurologic surgery and neurointerventions - ClinicalKey. Accessed May 2, 2022. https://www.clinicalkey.com/#!/content/book/3-s2.0-B9780323596046000572

CHAPTER

29

How Should We Manage Postoperative and Traumatic CSF Leaks?

David D. Liu, MD & Wenya Linda Bi, MD, PhD

Case

A 28-year-old man is in the trauma intensive care unit (ICU) after high-speed motor vehicle trauma. On hospital day 3, he is noted by his nurse to have intermittent low-volume clear nasal leakage. Computed tomography (CT) head shows a nondisplaced fracture through the cribriform plate and frontal sinus without pneumocephalus. He is intubated and heavily sedated due to recent laparotomy and thoracotomy. The patient is afebrile, hemodynamically stable, and does not have leukocytosis. How should his cerebrospinal fluid (CSF) leak be treated, including nonoperative and operative considerations?

Key Points

- Evidence for the use of prophylactic antibiotics to prevent meningitis in the setting of a cerebrospinal fluid (CSF) leak is mixed.
- Traumatic CSF leaks from basilar skull fractures most often respond to nonoperative interventions, including CSF diversion with lumbar drain placement.
- If CSF leak persists after 5 to 7 days of diversion from a lumbar drain, operative repair should be considered.
- The response of postoperative CSF leaks to conservative interventions depends on the timing of the leak after the initial operation, extent of the formed fistula, and flow rate.
- For high-flow or persistent CSF leaks prompting operative repair, vascularized tissue offers the most durable repair, when available.

BACKGROUND

Cranial cerebrospinal fluid (CSF) leaks are most commonly observed following trauma or prior operative interventions. Initial workup is guided by symptoms such as intermittent rhinorrhea or positional headache. However, these symptoms may be obscured if the clinical exam is limited by mental status. Up to 80% of cranial CSF leaks are caused by trauma, and another 15% occur in the postoperative setting, especially after skull base procedures.[1] Less commonly, CSF leaks can occur spontaneously in the setting of idiopathic intracranial hypertension,[2] which is outside of the intensive care unit (ICU) setting. Many CSF leaks present in a delayed fashion, and sometimes only present after meningitis, which can complicate up to 20% of untreated cases.[3]

When suspected, evaluation includes laboratory evaluation (beta2-transferrin assay of collected fluid, which may take days to result), high-resolution computed tomography (CT) imaging with inspection of the bone window, and in difficult-to-localize lesions, with direct visualization aided by dyes such as fluorescein. For anterior skull base defects, radionucleotide "pledget" studies can help confirm the presence of a CSF leak while CT myelogram may further pinpoint the location of the leak. Notably, glucose levels and "halo sign" of suspected CSF are neither sensitive nor specific due to admixture with other fluids.[4] Treatment consists of conservative management, including acetazolamide, lumbar drainage for CSF diversion, and possibly antibiotics; if these fail, endoscopic or open repair is pursued. No randomized controlled studies comparing these modalities exist.

EVIDENCE AND REVIEW

Prophylactic Antibiotics

By definition, a CSF leak implies the existence of a direct fistula from the intracranial compartment to the extracranial space. Thus, one of the most serious consequences of persistent CSF leak is meningitis. Prophylactic antibiotics such as cephalosporins at meningitis dosing can be considered in addition to default conservative management such as sinus precautions (avoiding coughing, sneezing, nose blowing, straining, stool softeners, elevation of head, and bed rest). The use of prophylactic antibiotics is controversial since broad-spectrum antibiotics breed virulence, and these drug-resistant organisms have been shown to increase mortality in neurological ICUs.[5]

A meta-analysis reviewing cases between 1970 and 1995 suggested that prophylactic antibiotics lowered infection rates, with 6/237 (2.5%) patients who received antibiotics developing meningitis versus 9/87 (10.3%) with those who did not receive antibiotics.[6] Conversely, another meta-analysis reviewing cases between 1970 and 1996 reported an odds ratio of 1.15, in favor of antibiotics reducing meningitis; however, this was not statistically significant (95% CI 0.68-1.94, ± 0.678).[7] A 2015 Cochrane review examined five clinical trials with a total of 208 patients and concluded that prophylactic antibiotics did not appear to impact rates of meningitis.[8] The limitations in the sample and quality of evidence are shown in Figure 29–1.

The risk for meningitis may depend on the duration of the leak and formation of a fixed fistula as well as underlying patient characteristics. One study suggests that patients with CSF lasting greater than 24 hours are at elevated risk for persistent leakage and eventual surgical repair and that this group of patients would benefit from prophylactic antibiotics.[9] However, traumatic leaks can present in a delayed manner, and it is often difficult to know precisely when the leak began. Further studies and large clinical trials are required to determine whether prophylactic meningitis antibiotics are indicated in the setting of known CSF leak and, if so, which subgroups of patients would benefit the most from prophylactic antibiotics.

Conservative Management

Management of CSF leaks depends on the flow rate, timing of observed leak, and presumed mechanism of leak. For very scant intermittent drainage with a low-risk mechanism, oral acetazolamide may help reduce the volume of CSF production sufficiently to allow spontaneous healing at the leak site.[10] For intermittent low-volume leaks, reducing CSF egress with lumbar drainage can promote healing of intracranial CSF fistulas without additional operative intervention. CSF leak from traumatic basilar skull fractures is often more receptive to such conservative measures than postoperative defects. For high-volume leaks, especially if in the early postoperative setting suggestive of inadequate repair or with overtly displaced craniofacial fractures causing an open defect, consideration should be given for more proactive fix of the underlying defect.

Numerous case series have demonstrated high success rates for lumbar drainage, but no clinical trials delineate the optimal amount or length of drainage. Success rates for lumbar drainage vary between 40% and 90% in the literature, with a

Antibiotic prophylaxis compared with placebo for preventing meningitis in BSF

Patient or population: patients with a recent BSF independent of the presence or severity of CSF leakage

Settings: in-hospital care

Intervention: antibiotic prophylaxis

Comparison: placebo

Outcomes	Relative effect (95% CI)	No. of participants (studies)	Quality of the evidence (GRADE)	Comments
Frequency of meningitis	**OR 0.69 (0.29 to 1.61)**	208 (4)	⊕⊕⊕⊖ moderate[1]	
All-cause mortality	**OR 1.68 (0.41 to 6.95)**	208 (4)	⊕⊕⊕⊖ moderate[1]	
Meningitis-related mortality	**OR 1.03 (0.14 to 7.40)**	208 (4)	⊕⊕⊕⊖ moderate[1]	
Need for surgical correction in patients with CSF leakage	Not estimable	109 (1)	⊕⊕⊖⊖ low[2]	
Non-CNS infection	**OR 0.61 (0.15 to 2.46)**	52 (1)	⊕⊕⊕⊕ High	

BSF: basilar skull fracture; **CI:** confidence interval; **CNS:** central nervous system; **CSF:** cerebrospinal fluid; **OR:** odds ratio

FIGURE 29–1 Evidence summary from Ratilal 2015 Cochrane review. (Reproduced with permission from Bernardo O Ratilal, João Costa, Lia Pappamikail, et al. Antibiotic prophylaxis for preventing meningitis in patients with basilar skull fractures: Cochrane Database of Systematic Reviews. John Wiley and Sons; 2015.)

higher rate of resolution with longer therapy. For example, one series showed a 39.5% resolution rate with 3 days of drainage, whereas other series achieved 70% to 90% resolution with an average of 6.5 days of drainage, and a low subsequent rate of recurrence.[11,12] The probability of success may vary with anatomical location: one study demonstrated that lumbar drainage resolved temporal bone leaks 60% of the time versus 26% in anterior skull base leaks.[13,14] Lumbar drain placement and prolonged drainage also associate with numerous risks, ranging from positional headaches to subdural hygroma or hematoma and in rare circumstances, acute visual loss (from traction on the optic nerves) or herniation from overdrainage. The decision for placement of lumbar drain should be balanced with the potential risks of drainage and the incurred length of hospitalization.

Surgical Repair

When surgical repair is required, the choice of approach depends on the location of defect (anterior skull base, lateral skull base, or posterior fossa fistula), the need for and availability of vascularized versus nonvascularized tissue options, the comorbidities of the patient, and the surgeon's experience. In a systematic review, both endoscopic and open repair achieved a ~90% success rate.[15] However, compared with open approaches, the endoscopic group had lower rates of meningitis (3.9% vs. 1.1%), abscess/wound infection (6.8% vs. 0.7%), sepsis (3.8% vs. 0%), and perioperative mortality (0% vs. 1.4%). A randomized trial demonstrated that lumbar drainage can be used in the perioperative period with surgical repair to improve the probability of successful repair.[16]

AVAILABLE GUIDELINES

No official guidelines exist for the usage of prophylactic antibiotics in CSF leak. There is Level III evidence from a 2015 Cochrane review that antibiotics reduce the frequency of meningitis but do not reduce mortality, although these conclusions are not statistically significant.

No official guidelines exist on the necessity or timing of operative repair for CSF leak. Level III evidence suggests up to 1 week of lumbar drainage as initial management followed by endoscopic repair may minimize morbidity. When surgical repair is required, the choice of approach depends on the location of defect, the need for vascularized versus nonvascularized tissue, the comorbidities of the patient, and the surgeon's experience.

REFERENCES

1. Zlab MK, Moore GF, Daly DT, Yonkers AJ. Cerebrospinal fluid rhinorrhea: a review of the literature. *Ear Nose Throat J* 1992;71(7):314–317. (In English).
2. Schievink WI. Spontaneous spinal cerebrospinal fluid leaks and intracranial hypotension. *JAMA* 2006;295(19):2286–2296. DOI: 10.1001/jama.295.19.2286.
3. Daudia A, Biswas D, Jones NS. Risk of meningitis with cerebrospinal fluid rhinorrhea. *Ann Otol Rhinol Laryngol* 2007;116(12):902–905. (In English). DOI: 10.1177/000348940711601206.
4. Ray AM. Halo sign is neither sensitive nor specific for cerebrospinal fluid leak. *Ann Emerg Med* 2009;53(2):288. DOI: 10.1016/j.annemergmed.2008.06.474.
5. Price DJ, Sleigh JD. Control of infection due to Klebsiella aerogenes in a neurosurgical unit by withdrawal of all antibiotics. *Lancet* 1970;2(7685):1213–1215. (In English). DOI: 10.1016/s0140-6736(70)92179-3.
6. Brodie HA. Prophylactic antibiotics for posttraumatic cerebrospinal fluid fistulae. A meta-analysis. *Arch Otolaryngol Head Neck Surg* 1997;123(7):749–752. (In English). DOI: 10.1001/archotol.1997.01900070093016.
7. Villalobos T, Arango C, Kubilis P, Rathore M. Antibiotic prophylaxis after basilar skull fractures: a meta-analysis. *Clin Infect Dis* 1998;27(2):364–369. (In English). DOI: 10.1086/514666.
8. Ratilal BO, Costa J, Pappamikail L, Sampaio C, Antibiotic prophylaxis for preventing meningitis in patients with basilar skull fractures. *Cochrane Database Syst Rev* 2015;2015(4). DOI: 10.1002/14651858.CD004884.pub4.
9. Friedman JA, Ebersold MJ, Quast LM. Persistent posttraumatic cerebrospinal fluid leakage. *Neurosurg Focus* 2000;9(1):e1. (In English). DOI: 10.3171/foc.2000.9.1.1.
10. Van Berkel MA, Elefritz JL. Evaluating off-label uses of acetazolamide. *Am J Health Syst Pharm* 2018;75(8):524–531. DOI: 10.2146/ajhp170279.
11. Lemole Jr GM, Henn JS, Zabramski JM, Sonntag, VKH. The management of cranial and spinal CSF leaks. *Barrow Quarterly* 2001;17(4).
12. Brodie HA, Thompson TC. Management of complications from 820 temporal bone fractures. *Am J Otol* 1997;18(2):188–197. (In English).
13. Loew F, Pertuiset B, Chaumier EE, Jaksche H. Traumatic, spontaneous and postoperative CSF rhinorrhea. *Adv Tech Stand Neurosurg* 1984;11:169–207. (In English). DOI: 10.1007/978-3-7091-7015-1_6.
14. Yilmazlar S, Arslan E, Kocaeli H, et al. Cerebrospinal fluid leakage complicating skull base fractures: analysis of 81 cases. *Neurosurg Rev* 2006;29(1):64–71. (In English). DOI: 10.1007/s10143-005-0396-3.
15. Komotar RJ, Starke RM, Raper DM, Anand VK, Schwartz TH. Endoscopic endonasal versus open repair of anterior skull base CSF leak, meningocele, and encephalocele: a systematic review of outcomes. *J Neurol Surg A Cent Eur Neurosurg* 2013;74(4):239–250. (In English). DOI: 10.1055/s-0032-1325636.
16. Zwagerman NT, Wang EW, Shin SS, et al. Does lumbar drainage reduce postoperative cerebrospinal fluid leak after endoscopic endonasal skull base surgery? A prospective, randomized controlled trial. *J Neurosurg* 2019;131(4):1172–1178. (In English). DOI: 10.3171/2018.4.Jns172447.

CHAPTER

30

How Do We Avoid Complications After Decompressive Hemicraniectomy?

Sean Lyne, MD & Wenya Linda Bi, MD, PhD

Case

A 37-year-old man on aspirin for prophylactic heart health presented after a fall down 12 steps. Initial head computed tomography (CT) revealed a right frontal intraparenchymal hemorrhagic contusion over overlying fracture (Figure 30–1A). After initial measures proved insufficient to control his elevated intracranial pressure (ICP), he underwent a right hemicraniectomy and hematoma evacuation (Figure 30–1B). Two weeks postoperatively, the patient was noted to have clear fluid draining from his incision, consistent with cerebrospinal fluid (CSF; Figure 30–1C). He returned to the operating theater for wound revision and washout, but as he continued to leak CSF afterward, required a subsequent lumbar drain to promote incisional healing. However, several days later, he developed waxing and waning mental status in the setting of a sunken flap, prompting a cranioplasty (Figure 30–1D). Following cranioplasty, he once again developed progressive ventriculomegaly and an enlarging extra-axial fluid collection, consistent with communicating hydrocephalus (Figure 30–1E). How can we best avoid the many postoperative complications associated with decompressive hemicraniectomies?

Key Points

- Decompressive hemicraniectomy can be fraught with numerous complications, each with distinct complications for prevention.
- Avoiding revision surgery for inadequate decompression is a key modifiable risk factor.
- Patients should be routinely assessed for early replacement of the bone flap to help restore intracranial CSF dynamics.

BACKGROUND

Hemicraniectomy is a life-saving neurosurgical procedure that is often performed in the setting of increased intracranial pressure (ICP) following intracerebral hemorrhage, cerebral infarction with malignant edema, or severe traumatic brain injury (TBI), especially in the setting of elevated ICP not responsive to medical management. Beyond the intraoperative risks, a variety of complications are associated with the sequelae of hemicraniectomy, both immediate and longer term. These range from acute complications such as inadequate decompression with persistent herniation or hemorrhagic transformation of underlying brain injury to more delayed complications including infection, communicating hydrocephalus, craniectomy associated progressive extra-axial fluid collections with treated hydrocephalus (CAPECTH), and the syndrome of the trephined (sunken flap syndrome). While each one of these conditions is recognized clinically, the literature surrounding their prevalence, diagnosis, and management is relatively sparse as randomized clinical trials largely examine functional outcomes and mortality following decompressive craniectomy and less so complications thereof.

EVIDENCE

Reoperation Following Inadequate Decompression

One of the more common complications following a decompressive craniectomy is inadequate decompression, with persistent mass effect causing herniation, and possible need to return to the operating room to remove additional bone.[1] Risk factors associated with reoperation for further decompression include

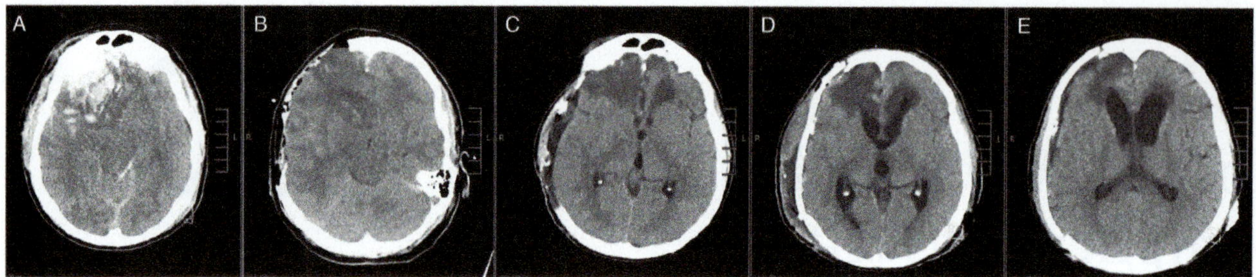

FIGURE 30–1 Axial computed tomography (CT) head following (**A**) preop, (**B**) status-post decompression, (**C**) syndrome of trephined, (**D**) status-post cranioplasty, and (**E**) hydrocephalus.

higher Glasgow coma scale, smaller hemorrhage, and increased extent of midline shift.[1] Those undergoing repeat surgery experience a 20-fold increased likelihood of major complications, threefold increase in in-hospital mortality, and are two and a half times more likely to be either dead or dependent at 6 months.

Blossoming of a known contusion or development of a new hemorrhage after initial decompression may also further prompt reoperation.[2] New or enlarging hemorrhages are postulated to ensue following loss of the tamponade effect by the overlying bone after initial decompression. This is supported by the evidence that most new hemorrhages that occur after decompressive hemicraniectomy occur ipsilateral to the craniectomy defect. The rates of delayed hematoma formation range from 20% to 50%[1,2] and should be identified with early postoperative computed tomography (CT) imaging and close monitoring of clinical status.[3]

The guidelines for decompressive hemicraniectomy in severe TBI recommend a craniectomy measuring 12 by 15 cm at minimum to allow for adequate decompression, although this is tailored to the individual patient condition.[2,4–6] In addition to making a large absolute size of craniectomy, adequate removal of bone toward the middle fossa floor near the inferior temporal bone is particularly important, as that allows for maximum decompression at the level of the uncus and therefore becomes a targeted therapy to prevent uncal herniation in the setting of elevated ICP.

Infection and Wound Healing Complications

In decompressive hemicraniectomy, the risk of wound infection is augmented by the generally immobile nature of the patient population, suboptimal nutrition status, and relatively large incision whose vascular supply might be compromised by the emergent setting, especially near the posterior edge of the commonly employed question-mark-shaped incision. A recent systematic review identified an approximately 10% rate of superficial incisional infection with deeper infections including epidural and subdural empyema occurring in up to 4.8% of patients after decompressive hemicraniectomy.[7] Additionally, replacement of the native or synthetic bone flap confers another 5.4% risk for infection.

Complication avoidance should be targeted to these common causes. Operative technique should include the preservation of available temporal arterial blood supply if at all possible as well as meticulous incisional closure. Early and adequate nutrition is critical to promote wound healing, and consultation with institutional dieticians is critical to maximize the surgical wound healing substrate. Moreover, pressure offloading is critical to maximize adequate local tissue blood flow.

Perturbed CSF Dynamics and Hydrocephalus

The rigid convinces of the cranial vault are thought to play an important role in cerebrospinal fluid (CSF) dynamics, facilitating physiologic conduction of fluid pressure waves. The reported complication rate of hydrocephalus following hemicraniectomy, although with varying definitions, has been estimated in the literature to range from 1% to 86%.[8] Hydrocephalus can manifest as ventriculomegaly with communicating hydrocephalus or the development of external fluid collections underneath the scalp flap, which may further compromise incisional healing. The development of hydrocephalus portends a poorer outcome,[9] and one modifiable factor that may minimize the risk of hydrocephalus is the timing of cranioplasty.[10] A retrospective review of over 90,000 pediatric patients with TBI reported that cranioplasty within 30 days associated with a lower likelihood of developing hydrocephalus compared to patients who underwent a more delayed cranioplasty.

The formation of extra-axial fluid collection (EAC) is often considered "external hydrocephalus," referring to the accumulation of excess fluid compartment outside of the ventricles, either with or without replacement of the bone flap. However, these fluid collections may also be observed despite CSF shunting.[11] In one retrospective review of 21 patients with EACs after decompressive craniectomy, 18 of 21 developed collections despite CSF diversion. Therefore, it has been posited that extra-axial collections may not always reflect external hydrocephalus and may be more appropriately termed CAPECTH and can be effectively reversed with cranioplasty.[11] Another retrospective review of 12 consecutive hemicraniectomy patients documented that three patients developed EACs (25%) ranging from 3 to 55 days,[12] and all resolved spontaneously without CSF diversion or earlier cranioplasty. One analysis of 96 patients with EACs (as described by the authors) distinguished two phenotypes of EACs: complicated and uncomplicated.[13] Complicated EACs were those requiring multiple methods of drainage and where conservative management was not an option, while uncomplicated EACs were managed with observation or resolved after a single intervention for drainage. Notably, in these studies, the only factor that was documented as significantly impacting resolution of EACs was replacement of the bone flap (cranioplasty), likely as it restores CSF dynamics.

Syndrome of the Trephined

Persistent defects of the cranial vault can also lead to symptomatic development of headaches, nausea, emesis, altered mental status, and neuropsychiatric symptoms termed the syndrome of the trephined. The prevalence of this syndrome following hemicraniectomy is estimated at approximately 10% and may be more common in men.[3,14] The postulated mechanism attributes this syndrome to a decrease in ICP following hemicraniectomy and possibly a drop of ICP to negative values with loss of intracranial postural ICP control and pulse wave amplitude.[15] Early identification of symptoms, with observation of the sinking scalp flap, and consequently the underlying brain, should prompt immediate cranioplasty and often leads to improvement of symptoms in days.[14]

REFERENCES

1. Lan M, Dambrino RJ, Youssef A, et al. Repeat surgery after decompressive craniectomy for traumatic intracranial hemorrhage: outcomes and predictors. *World Neurosurg.* 2020;133:e757–e766. doi:10.1016/j.wneu.2019.09.148
2. Qiu W, Guo C, Shen H, et al. Effects of unilateral decompressive craniectomy on patients with unilateral acute post-traumatic brain swelling after severe traumatic brain Injury. *Crit Care Lond Engl.* 2009;13(6):R185. doi:10.1186/cc8178
3. Gopalakrishnan MS, Shanbhag NC, Shukla DP, Konar SK, Bhat DI, Devi BI. Complications of decompressive craniectomy. *Front Neurol.* 2018;9:977. doi:10.3389/fneur.2018.00977
4. Hawryluk GWJ, Rubiano AM, Totten AM, et al. Guidelines for the management of severe traumatic brain injury: 2020 update of the decompressive craniectomy recommendations. *Neurosurgery.* 2020;87(3):427–434. doi:10.1093/neuros/nyaa278
5. Cooper DJ, Rosenfeld JV, Murray L, et al. Patient outcomes at twelve months after early decompressive craniectomy for diffuse traumatic brain injury in the randomized DECRA clinical trial. *J Neurotrauma.* 2020;37(5):810–816. doi:10.1089/neu.2019.6869
6. Jiang JY, Xu W, Li WP, et al. Efficacy of standard trauma craniectomy for refractory intracranial hypertension with severe traumatic brain injury: a multicenter, prospective, randomized controlled study. *J Neurotrauma.* 2005;22(6):623–628. doi:10.1089/neu.2005.22.623
7. Kurland DB, Khaladj-Ghom A, Stokum JA, et al. Complications associated with decompressive craniectomy: a systematic review. *Neurocrit Care.* 2015;23(2):292304. doi:10.1007/s12028-015-0144-7
8. De Bonis P, Sturiale CL, Anile C, et al. Decompressive craniectomy, interhemispheric hygroma and hydrocephalus: a timeline of events? *Clin Neurol Neurosurg.* 2013;115(8):1308–1312. doi:10.1016/j.clineuro.2012.12.011
9. Honeybul S, Ho KM. Decompressive craniectomy for severe traumatic brain injury: the relationship between surgical complications and the prediction of an unfavourable outcome. *Injury.* 2014;45(9):1332–1339. doi:10.1016/j.injury.2014.03.007
10. Bonow RH, Oron AP, Hanak BW, et al. Post-traumatic hydrocephalus in children: a retrospective study in 42 pediatric hospitals using the pediatric health information system. *Neurosurgery.* 2018;83(4):732–739. doi:10.1093/neuros/nyx470
11. Nalbach SV, Ropper AE, Dunn IF, Gormley WB. Craniectomy-associated progressive extra-axial collections with treated hydrocephalus (CAPECTH): redefining a common complication of decompressive craniectomy. *J Clin Neurosci Off J Neurosurg Soc Australas.* 2012;19(9):1222–1227. doi:10.1016/j.jocn.2012.01.016
12. Ropper AE, Nalbach SV, Lin N, Dunn IF, Gormley WB. Resolution of extra-axial collections after decompressive craniectomy for ischemic stroke. *J Clin Neurosci Off J Neurosurg Soc Australas.* 2012;19(2):231–234. doi:10.1016/j.jocn.2011.08.004
13. DiRisio AC, Stopa BM, Pompeu YA, et al. Extra-axial fluid collections after decompressive craniectomy: management, outcomes, and treatment algorithm. *World Neurosurg.* 2021;149:e188–e196. doi:10.1016/j.wneu.2021.02.052
14. Ashayeri K, Jackson EM, Huang J, Brem H, Gordon CR. Syndrome of the trephined: a systematic review. *Neurosurgery.* 2016;79(4):525–534. doi:10.1227/NEU.0000000000001366
15. Lilja-Cyron A, Andresen M, Kelsen J, Andreasen TH, Fugleholm K, Juhler M. Long-term effect of decompressive craniectomy on intracranial pressure and possible implications for intracranial fluid movements. *Neurosurgery.* 2020;86(2):231–240. doi:10.1093/neuros/nyz049

CHAPTER

31

What Is the Benefit of Antibiotic Prophylaxis for Ventricular, Subdural, and Subgaleal Drains?

Nora C. Kim, MD, Donato Pacione, MD, & Ariane Lewis, MD

Case

A 73-year-old woman is admitted to the neurologic intensive care unit (neuroICU) following a spontaneous intraparenchymal hemorrhage with intraventricular extension and associated hydrocephalus. An external ventricular drain is placed and is expected to remain in place for several days. Does she need prolonged prophylactic systemic antibiotics until the drain is removed?

Key Points

- While the use of prophylactic systemic antibiotics for patients with neurosurgical drains may seem like a means to reduce the risk of surgical site infections (SSIs) and drain-related infections (DRIs), data do not suggest prolonged prophylactic systemic antibiotics (PPSA) use is beneficial. In fact, it can potentially lead to complications like nosocomial infections.
- Acknowledging that literature on this topic is limited, in accordance with the Neurocritical Care Society (NCS) recommendation, we recommend prophylactic systemic antibiotic use be limited to preprocedural single-dose administration for patients with external ventricular drain (EVDs), subdural drains, or subgaleal drains.

BACKGROUND

Drain placement can increase the risk of surgical site infection (SSI).[1] Drain-related infections (DRIs) after neurosurgical procedures lead to postprocedural morbidity and mortality and prolong the length of hospitalization. Neurosurgeons and neurointensivists employ different tactics to minimize the risk of DRI, including administration of prophylactic systemic antibiotics to patients who have neurosurgical drains.[2,3] While the intent of this practice is to minimize risk of complications, this can actually increase morbidity and mortality due to Clostridium difficile infection (CDI) and growth of multidrug-resistant organisms (MDRO). Because of this, administration of prophylactic systemic antibiotics to patients with neurosurgical drains remains controversial and practice varies across institutions.

A 2015 survey of members of the Neurocritical Care Society (NCS) demonstrated that opinions vary about the use of prolonged prophylactic systemic antibiotics (PPSA) to prevent DRI for patients with neurosurgical drains or devices (Table 31–1).[4] The highest percentage of respondents believed there was a need for PPSA in patients with Jackson-Pratt spinal drains with instrumentation (35%), while the lowest percentage supported the need for PPSA for patients with subgaleal drains (19%).[4] Less than one-third of respondents (29%) believed PPSA should *not* be used for *any* patients with neurosurgical drains or devices.[4]

In this chapter, we explore the literature regarding the benefit of antibiotic prophylaxis for ventricular, subdural, and subgaleal drains.

EVIDENCE AND REVIEW

Ventricular Drains

Cerebrospinal fluid (CSF) diversion with an external ventricular drain (EVD) is a common strategy to relieve and measure elevated intracranial pressure. The incidence of ventriculostomy-related infection (VRI), a serious complication of EVD

TABLE 31–1 The percentage of respondents who agreed/strongly agreed with the need for prolonged prophylactic systemic antibiotics (PPSA) for each type of drain/device.[4,5]

Type of Drain	Percentage of Agreement
Spinal drain with instrumentation	35
Conventional EVD catheter	25
Subdural drain	25
Spinal drain without instrumentation	19
Subgaleal drain	19
Antibiotic-impregnated EVD catheter	16
Intraparenchymal monitor	16
Silver-impregnated EVD catheter	14
Lumbar drain	11

EVD, external ventricular drain.

placement, is 6% to 23%.[6] VRI can lead to 8 to 19 excess days of hospitalization,[7,8] with an average increase in cost of over US $35,000.[7]

Timing and Duration of Prophylactic Systemic Antibiotics

The standard of care for the use of prophylactic systemic antibiotics for VRI prevention varies across institutions. While some hospitals do not use any prophylactic systemic antibiotics, others administer (1) a single dose of preprocedural antibiotics, (2) periprocedural antibiotics for 24 hours, or (3) PPSA from placement until EVD removal.[5,8] Cinibulak et al found that 55% of 99 neurosurgical units in Germany regularly used single-dose antibiotic prophylaxis and 15% regularly administered PPSA to patients with EVDs.[9] Contrastingly, in a survey of 52 members of the NCS, who were predominantly from the United States, 55% of respondents reported their institution used PPSA for patients with EVDs.[5]

Although some studies have demonstrated PPSA was associated with a lower incidence of VRI, they did not evaluate other outcomes.[6,10] However, several studies have demonstrated that discontinuation of PPSA for patients with EVDs was associated with reduction in CDI and other nosocomial infections, while there was no change in the rate of VRI.[3,5,11] Similarly, some studies showed that the use of preinsertion systemic antibiotic prophylaxis did not impact the rate of VRI, while others found that a single preprocedural dose of antibiotics decreased the rate of VRI.[11–14]

Other Infection Prevention Strategies

In addition to the use of prophylactic systemic antibiotics to prevent VRIs, there are numerous other infection prevention measures (Table 31–2). For example, multiple studies have shown the use of antibiotic-impregnated EVDs can decrease the rate of VRI.[3,5,6,10,13] The use of conventional EVD catheters with daily intrathecal vancomycin administration from Day 4 until

TABLE 31–2 Strategies to prevent infections in patients with ventricular or subdural/subgaleal drains.

Type of Drain	Strategies
Ventricular	• Antibiotic-impregnated catheters[3,5,6,10,13] • Conventional EVD with daily intrathecal vancomycin administration from day 4 to removal[15] • Minimize duration of EVD[7,12] • Minimize frequency of CSF sampling[5,12]
Subdural/subgaleal	• Topical vancomycin powder sprinkled over bone flap[16]

CSF, cerebrospinal fluid; EVD, external ventricular drain.

catheter removal also lowered rates of VRI (11.9% vs. 2.7%, $P < .01$).[15] Some studies have suggested that increased CSF sampling frequency may increase the rate of VRI.[5,12] Minimizing the duration of EVD placement is also an important means to prevent VRI.[7,12]

There are other strategies, many of which are often bundled together to reduce VRI, whose impact is indeterminate. VRI prevention protocols sometimes include specific guidance on the location of the procedure, incision size, type of aseptic technique, amount of hair removal, type of dressing, and method to secure the catheter.[5,12,13] Whyte et al found that there was no significant difference in the rate of VRI after creation of a bundle that included an insertion checklist, maintenance worksheet, dressing change procedure, and changes in CSF sampling (7.8% prebundle vs. 8.6% postbundle, $P = 1$).[14]

Subdural/Subgaleal Drains

Subdural and subgaleal drains are often left in place postoperatively after a craniotomy or craniectomy. As is the case with EVDs, placement of these drains can increase the risk of postoperative infection.[17] Consequently, there are ongoing efforts to determine and employ the optimal strategies to prevent infection.[1]

Timing and Duration of Prophylactic Systemic Antibiotics

There is scant literature on infection prevention strategies for patients with subdural and subgaleal drains. This is likely due to the fact that with the exception of subdural evacuating port system placement (ie, SEPS), subdural and subgaleal drain placement is usually part of a craniotomy or craniectomy, so infection prevention practices are considered in that context. Soleman et al surveyed 144 neurosurgeons who were predominantly from Europe on their practices related to subdural drain placement and found that 77% of respondents used prophylactic systemic antibiotics; 32% administered PPSA until removal of the drain.[18] Use of PPSA for patients with subdural drains may be higher in the United States, as the aforementioned survey of members of the NCS (who were predominantly from the United States) demonstrated that 48% of respondents reported PPSA use for this patient population (29% reported PPSA use for patients with subgaleal drains).[4]

Lewis et al demonstrated that an institutional initiative to discontinue PPSA for patients with subdural or subgaleal drains did not increase the frequency of SSI.[19] Of 105 patients who were given PPSA before the initiative, 1 (1%) developed a deep SSI and 1 (1%) developed a superficial SSI. Of the 80 patients who were not given PPSA, 0 developed a deep SSI and 1 (1%) developed a superficial SSI. There were two (2%) patients who were given PPSA who developed CDI, while zero patients who were not given PPSA developed CDI. There were three (3%) patients who were given PPSA who had growth of a resistant organism in their blood/sputum/urine; zero patients who were not given PPSA had growth of a resistant organism.

Other Infection Prevention Strategies

Studies on other infection prevention strategies for patients with subdural or subgaleal drains are limited. Abdullah et al reported that topical vancomycin powder sprinkled over the bone flap significantly decreases the rate of SSI when subgaleal drains are left in place following a craniotomy.[16] Whyte et al observed a nonsignificant reduction in VRI when the aforementioned EVD bundle was applied to patients with subdural or subgaleal drains (1 (3%) vs. 0).[14]

AVAILABLE GUIDELINES

In 2016, the NCS issued a statement for healthcare professionals on the management of EVDs which included a conditional recommendation (based on low-quality evidence) for one dose of antibiotics prior to EVD insertion and a strong recommendation against the use of antibiotics for the duration of EVD placement.[20] Although these recommendations are specific to EVD management, they have also been applied to patients with subdural and subgaleal drains.[14]

REFERENCES

1. Abu Hamdeh S, Lytsy B, Ronne-Engström E. Surgical site infections in standard neurosurgery procedures—a study of incidence, impact and potential risk factors. *British Journal of Neurosurgery.* 2014;28(2):270–275. doi:10.3109/02688697.2013.835376
2. Flibotte JJ, Lee KE, Koroshetz WJ, Rosand J, McDonald CT. Continuous antibiotic prophylaxis and cerebral spinal fluid infection in patients with intracranial pressure monitors. *Neurocritical Care.* 2004;1(1):61–68. doi:10.1385/ncc:1:1:61
3. Murphy RKJ, Liu B, Srinath A, et al. No additional protection against ventriculitis with prolonged systemic antibiotic prophylaxis for patients treated with antibiotic-coated external ventricular drains. *Journal of Neurosurgery.* 2015;122(5):1120–1126. doi:10.3171/2014.9.jns132882
4. Lewis A, Czeisler BM, Lord AS. Prolonged prophylactic antibiotics with neurosurgical drains and devices: Are we using them? Do we need them? *American Journal of Infection Control.* Dec 1 2016;44(12):1757–1758. doi:10.1016/j.ajic.2016.06.039
5. Lewis A, Czeisler BM, Lord AS. Variations in strategies to prevent ventriculostomy-related infections: a practice survey. *Neurohospitalist.* Jan 2017;7(1):15–23. doi:10.1177/1941874416663281
6. Sonabend AM, Korenfeld Y, Crisman C, Badjatia N, Mayer SA, Connolly ES, Jr. Prevention of ventriculostomy-related infections with prophylactic antibiotics and antibiotic-coated external ventricular drains: a systematic review. *Neurosurgery.* Apr 2011;68(4):996–1005. doi:10.1227/NEU.0b013e3182096d84
7. Lyke KE, Obasanjo OO, Williams MA, O'Brien M, Chotani R, Perl TM. Ventriculitis complicating use of intraventricular catheters in adult neurosurgical patients. *Clinical Infectious Diseases.* 2001;33(12):2028–2033. doi:10.1086/324492
8. Camacho EF, Boszczowski Í, Basso M, et al. Infection rate and risk factors associated with infections related to external ventricular drain. *Infection.* 2011;39(1):47–51. doi:10.1007/s15010-010-0073-5
9. Cinibulak Z, Aschoff A, Apedjinou A, Kaminsky J, Trost HA, Krauss JK. Current practice of external ventricular drainage: a survey among neurosurgical departments in Germany. *Acta Neurochirurgica.* 2016;158(5):847–853. doi:10.1007/s00701-016-2747-y
10. Sheppard JP, Ong V, Lagman C, et al. Systemic antimicrobial prophylaxis and antimicrobial-coated external ventricular drain catheters for preventing ventriculostomy-related infections: a meta-analysis of 5242 cases. *Neurosurgery.* Jan 1 2020;86(1):19–29. doi:10.1093/neuros/nyy522
11. Dellit TH, Chan JD, Fulton C, et al. Reduction in *Clostridium difficile* infections among neurosurgical patients associated with discontinuation of antimicrobial prophylaxis for the duration of external ventricular drain placement. *Infection Control & Hospital Epidemiology.* 2014;35(5):589–590. doi:10.1086/675828
12. Dakson A, Kameda-Smith M, Staudt MD, et al. A nationwide prospective multicenter study of external ventricular drainage: accuracy, safety, and related complications. *Journal of Neurosurgery.* 2022;137(1):249257. doi:10.3171/2021.7.jns21421
13. Hepburn-Smith M, Dynkevich I, Spektor M, Lord A, Czeisler B, Lewis A. Establishment of an external ventricular drain best practice guideline: the quest for a comprehensive, universal standard for external ventricular drain care. *Journal of Neuroscience Nursing.* Feb 2016;48(1):54–65. doi:10.1097/JNN.0000000000000174
14. Whyte C, Alhasani H, Caplan R, Tully AP. Impact of an external ventricular drain bundle and limited duration antibiotic prophylaxis on drain-related infections and antibiotic resistance. *Clinical Neurology Neurosurgery.* Mar 2020;190:105641. doi:10.1016/j.clineuro.2019.105641
15. Fu RZ, Anwar DR, Laban JT, Maratos EC, Minhas PS, Martin AJ. Pre-emptive intrathecal vancomycin therapy reduces external ventricular drain infection: a single centre retrospective case-control study. *British Journal of Neurosurgery.* 2017;31(1):16–20. doi:10.1080/02688697.2016.1229741
16. Mallela AN, Abdullah KG, Brandon C, Richardson AG, Lucas TH. Topical vancomycin reduces surgical-site infections after craniotomy: a prospective, controlled study. *Neurosurgery.* Oct 1, 2018;83(4):761–767. doi:10.1093/neuros/nyx559
17. Bratzler DW, Dellinger EP, Olsen KM, et al. Clinical practice guidelines for antimicrobial prophylaxis in surgery. *Surgical Infections.* 2013;14(1):73–156. doi:10.1089/sur.2013.9999
18. Soleman J, Kamenova M, Lutz K, Guzman R, Fandino J, Mariani L. Drain insertion in chronic subdural hematoma: an international survey of practice. *World Neurosurgery.* Aug 2017;104:528–536. doi:10.1016/j.wneu.2017.04.134
19. Lewis A, Sen R, Hill TC, et al. Antibiotic prophylaxis for subdural and subgaleal drains. *Journal of Neurosurgery.* Mar 2017;126(3):908–912. doi:10.3171/2016.4.JNS16275
20. Fried HI, Nathan BR, Rowe AS, et al. The insertion and management of external ventricular drains: an evidence-based consensus statement. *Neurocritical Care.* 2016;24(1):61–81. doi:10.1007/s12028-015-0224-8

SECTION IV CEREBROVASCULAR AND INTRACRANIAL HEMORRHAGE

CHAPTER

32

What Are the Noninvasive Options to Monitor for Vasospasm After Aneurysmal Subarachnoid Hemorrhage?

Victor Lopez-Rivera, MD, Anna Cervantes-Arslanian, MD, & Hormuzdiyar Dasenbrock, MD, MPH

Case

A 52-year-old woman is in the ICU 6 days after suffering a subarachnoid hemorrhage from a ruptured posterior communicating artery aneurysm. Hunt-Hess grade was 3 upon presentation with a score of 3 on the modified Fisher scale. The aneurysm has since been secured with endovascular coiling. What noninvasive options exist for monitoring such a patient for cerebral vasospasm?

Key Points

- Despite the current variability in clinical practice, neurological exam remains the best tool to assess for cerebral vasospasm (CVS), with noninvasive imaging providing additional information to guide the need for more advanced imaging (eg, computed tomography angiogram [CTA] and computed tomography perfusion [CTP]) as well as indication for aggressive medical management or endovascular therapy when indicated.
- Centers should also take into consideration their resources regarding staff and advanced neuroimaging availability to decide on whether routine surveillance is technically feasible.

BACKGROUND

Management of aneurysmal subarachnoid hemorrhage (aSAH) is directed toward decreasing the morbidity and mortality that result from secondary complications. Cerebral vasospasm (CVS), the narrowing of intracranial arteries that can potentially lead to hypoperfusion and ischemic deficits, is one of the most feared complications from aSAH.[1] CVS can be classified as radiographic, when there is no associated neurological deficit, or symptomatic, which often leads to delayed cerebral ischemia (DCI), a new focal neurologic deficit or change in consciousness and radiographic evidence of a new infarction.[2,3] CVS and DCI are a substantial cause for the poor outcomes following aSAH.[4] Early risk stratification to identify the most vulnerable patients is crucial. Physicians must recognize clinical and radiographic markers of CVS at the earliest timepoint in order to deliver timely intervention and avoid DCI. Several noninvasive options exist to screen and monitor for CVS, which combined with proper surveillance protocols can improve outcomes.

EVIDENCE AND REVIEW

Risk Stratification

In order to provide opportune and effective treatment for aSAH patients, one should assess the individualized risk of CVS. Studies have identified certain baseline characteristics that represent a higher likelihood of aSAH patient to go into CVS, including younger age, female gender, rebleeding from the ruptured aneurysm, cigarette smoking, alcoholism, prior heart disease, diabetes mellitus, and body mass index (BMI).[5] Besides clinical characteristics, radiographic markers can aid in guiding risk stratification and need for treatment. The Fisher and modified Fisher scales are well-validated tools for predicting the risk of CVS, but several other grading scores have been developed including VASOGRADE,[6] subarachnoid hemorrhage early brain edema score (SEBES),[7] global cerebral edema (GCE),[8] and HAIR (HH, Age, IVH, Rebleed).[9] These tools can aid in deciding type and intensity of monitoring and potential complication of such against the patient's risk of CVS and other forms of neurologic deterioration.

Clinical Monitoring

aSAH patients admitted to a neurologic intensive care unit (neuroICU) should undergo neurological checks every hour for 48 to 72 hours following ictus.[2,6,10] Based on clinical judgment, neurological and vital signs assessments can be lowered; however, the physician should weigh the patient's risk of developing CVS. When deciding on frequency of neurological checks, it is also relevant to consider conditions which may influence the risk of vasospasm, in particular those that are modifiable. For instance, fever, hyponatremia, hypovolemia, hypotension, and hypercapnia/hypocapnia have shown to contribute to worsening CVS.[4,11-14] Additionally, the importance of a proper sleep cycle should be taken into account, as poor sleep hygiene may confound a patient's neurological exam.[10]

As CVS most frequently leads to distal vessel hypoperfusion, it is crucial that neurological checks include components testing cortical signs.[15] Although the site of aneurysm rupture and pattern of aSAH can guide the examiner to focus on specific deficits, neurological exam should be thorough in order to identify early signs of CVS, as patients may only experience subtle changes in mentation/attention/behavior (anterior cerebral artery [ACA]), speech and/or motor function (middle cerebral artery [MCA]), or visual acuity (posterior cerebral artery [PCA]) based on the territory affected.[16] The neurological exam remains the most dependable tool to monitor patients at risk for CVS in aSAH patients when logistically feasible.[17] However in patients who are intubated or deeply sedated, the neurological assessment may be limited.[6] In this scenario, imaging modalities may provide additional information when CVS is suspected (Table 32–1).

Transcranial Doppler (TCD)

TCD sonography is a frequently employed surveillance tool for monitoring the development of vasospasm by trending the blood flow velocities of proximal intracranial vessels.[18] The most frequently insonated intracranial vessel in clinical practice is the MCA, as it is easily insonated through the temporal window.[19] In the anterior circulation, a mean flow velocity > 120 cm/s or an increase of >50 cm/s in 24 hours suggests vasospasm.[18,20] CVS can then be classified by the mean flow velocity into mild vasospasm 120 to 149 cm/s, moderate vasospasm 150 to 199 cm/s, and severe vasospasm > 200 cm/s.[21] However, elevated mean flow velocities may be related to other conditions, such as a hyperdynamic state.

The Lindegaard ratio (LR) aids in differentiating hyperemia from true vasospasm, calculated by dividing the mean flow velocity of the vessel of interest (eg, MCA) by the mean flow

TABLE 32–1 Noninvasive and invasive imaging modalities for cerebral vasospasm screening.

Modality	Parameter	Interpretation	Advantage	Disadvantage
TCD	Mean flow velocity, Lindegaard ratio (LR)	↑mean flow velocity, LR > 3	Noninvasive, cost-effective	High variability, limited exam by bone windows
CTA	Vessel caliber	↓ vessel diameter	Noninvasive, cost-effective, available, quick acquisition	Contrast nephropathy, radiation, artifacts
CTP/MRP	Cerebral blood volume (CBV), cerebral blood flow (CBF), mean transit time (MTT)	↓ CBV and CBF, ↑ MTT	Identifies tissue at risk, assesses extent of infarct, reliable, available	Needs expert interpretation, variability on results based on imaging acquisition
cEEG	Alpha-delta ratio (ADR)	↓ ADR	Readily available, continuous monitoring	Needs expert interpretation
NIRS	Regional cerebral oxygen saturation (rSO_2)	12% decrease in rSO_2	Continuous monitoring, indirect measurement of oxygen delivery, available with other invasive monitoring	Poor consensus regarding parameter cut-off

cEEG, continuous electroencephalography; CTA, computed tomography angiogram; CTP, computed tomography perfusion; MRP, magnetic resonance perfusion; NIRS, near-infrared spectroscopy; TCD, transcranial doppler.

velocity of the ipsilateral more proximal vessel (eg, extracranial internal carotid artery).[22] An LR > 3 is highly suspicious of true vasospasm, with an LR of 3 to 5 suggesting mild-moderate vasospasm, and an LR > 6 indicating severe vasospasm.[18] Data supporting the use of TCD and normal reference ranges are less well studied in the posterior circulation. However, mean velocities of >70 cm/s in the basilar or >110 cm/s in the PCA suggest CVS.[18,19,21] When assessing the posterior circulation, the LR is instead calculated by the mean flow velocity of the basilar artery by the velocity of the vertebral artery (BA/VA). An LR BA/VA ratio > 2.5 is indicative of CVS.[23]

Although TCD is a simple, noninvasive screening tool, limitations exist. TCDs are more reliable when assessing for vasospasm of the MCA with a positive predictive value (PPV) of 83% to 100%, but lower PPV is observed for the anterior cerebral artery (PPV 41%-100%) and the BA (PPV 63%), with the lowest PPV for the posterior cerebral artery (PPV 37%).[22] This is due to the limited transorbital and transforaminal windows for assessment of the anterior cerebral artery and BA, respectively, as these are less reliably insonated compared to the transtemporal window when evaluating the MCA.[21] Moreover, the reliability of TCDs may be compromised by the operator's experience, the equipment utilized, and other factors that limit the exam (eg, cervical collar, surgical dressings, and poor bone windows).

Computed tomography (CT)

Computed tomography angiogram (CTA) provides another noninvasive modality to assess for CVS.[24,25] In identifying moderate-severe CVS, CTA provides an accuracy of 87% to 97.5% and a negative predictive value (NPV) of 95% to 99.5% compared to catheter angiogram (Digital subtraction angiography [DSA]).[22] Furthermore, CTA avoids the risks associated with DSA (eg, stroke and vascular injury) and is a quicker and less expensive imaging modality, although still it poses a risk for contrast-induced nephropathy and exposes the patient to radiation. CTA may be limited in the evaluation of more distal cerebral arteries, as their small diameter (2-3 mm) significantly limits the depiction of changes in vessel diameter.[26] Motion artifact and technique for dye administration may also limit quality of images. Additionally, the restricted spatial resolution of CTA impedes observers from reliably identifying changes of <30% in diameter narrowing, and thus, it is said that CTA has higher accuracy in the diagnosis of moderate-severe than of mild CVS.[27] Moreover, observers may use different methods to assess for CVS with CTA, with some practitioners using the admission (ie, baseline) imaging compared to the most recent imaging, while others may use the contralateral unaffected vasculature. CTA findings should be correlated to the patient's clinical status, as patients may only experience radiographic CVS that may not warrant treatment. Contrarily, in high-risk aSAH patients (eg, Hunt-Hess grades 4-5) with a neurological deficit that is highly suspicious of CVS, the use of CTA may be bypassed, given the higher likelihood of CVS.

CT perfusion (CTP) allows a noninvasive evaluation of the perfusion dynamics of the brain tissue, with this modality being easily incorporated into the standard CT/CTA protocol performed for aSAH patients at some centers.[28] Given that CVS leads to decreased cerebral blood flow (CBF) and cerebral blood volume (CBV) of brain tissue that is typically in a higher metabolic demand given the ongoing inflammatory process secondary to aSAH, CTP can be utilized to identify hypoperfused territory and estimate the extent of angiographic vasospasm.[24,29] CBF and CBV parameters have been routinely used to identify tissue at risk for DCI, although more recent studies have proven the superiority of other markers, such as mean transit time (MTT) and time to drain (TTD) with a significantly higher correlation with angiographic findings. When compared to CTA, CTP has a similar sensitivity (74.1% CTP vs. 79.6% CTA) and specificity (93% CTP vs. 93.1% CTA) for diagnosis of CVS.[25] Nonetheless, the technical nuances of this imaging modality may hinder its accuracy for screening of CVS.

Magnetic Resonance Imaging

Magnetic resonance perfusion (MRP) may be another imaging modality available at stroke centers. Benefits of using MRP include avoidance of radiation, less coil artifact, and detection of blood-brain barrier disruption that might suggest risk for ischemia, prior visible changes in vessel diameter, or hypoperfusion deficits.[30] However, its implementation may be restricted by its cost, as well as time and technical requirements, especially for mechanically ventilated patients and those with elevated intracranial pressure who may not tolerate lying flat for longer study durations.

Continuous Electroencephalography

Several studies have identified patterns on continuous electroencephalography (cEEG) that may emerge as a response to a disequilibrium in the blood supply and demand, with decreasing alpha-delta ratio (ADR) and relative alpha variability (RAV) being the most common parameters.[31,32] Other criteria include isolated alpha suppression and increasing epileptiform abnormalities, such as lateralized rhythmic delta activity (LRDA), lateralized periodic discharges (LPD), or generalized periodic discharges (GPD).[31] A recent systematic review found that cEEG had a low sensitivity (18.8%) but a high specificity (94.4%) in detection of angiographic-proven CVS.[32] There is some variability in the reported sensitivities of cEEG in the literature due to different definitions of electrographic parameters, with some authors defining a decrease of 30% ADR in a single reading, while others used a higher cut-off (eg, 50%). The accuracy of cEEG to detect CVS is higher when used in combination with other modalities, such as TCDs.[31]

Near-Infrared Spectroscopy

Near-infrared spectroscopy (NIRS) offers a continuous, indirect measurement of oxygen delivery and utilization in a given area, described as regional cerebral oxygen saturation (rSO_2). This modality was initially used during cardiac surgery, and its use has now been adopted in monitoring of CVS.[38] Most studies have defined a decrease of >12% in rSO_2 compared to baseline as highly suggestive of CVS; however, a normal range of cerebral

rSO_2 is not well defined and there remains no consensus on the cut-off value for rSO_2 to guide intervention for CVS.[33]

Surveillance Protocols for Vasospasm

Some stroke centers may perform noninvasive and invasive imaging routinely to tailor medical management of aSAH patients and to risk-stratify those who would benefit from prompt intervention, particularly in patients with a limited neurological exam.[34] The most widely available and easily accessible tool for assessing CVS in the neuroICU is the TCD,[18] with most centers performing them routinely every day between days 3 and 21 after aSAH to guide the need for other imaging modalities.[3] CTA with or without CTP may be routinely performed on days 3 to 5 and days 7 to 10, with subsequent CTA/CTP performed if there's presence of CVS, if there were changes in medical therapy, or patients received endovascular treatment.[35] Additionally, centers may perform a standardized acquisition of DSA on days 7 to 10 for identification of radiographic vasospasm.[36,37] Although this may allow early identification of CVS, this may also lead to treatment of asymptomatic vasospasm.

REFERENCES

1. Vespa PM, Nuwer MR, Juhász C, et al. Early detection of vasospasm after acute subarachnoid hemorrhage using continuous EEG ICU monitoring. *Electroencephalogr Clin Neurophysiol.* 1997;103(6):607–615. doi:10.1016/S0013-4694(97)00071-0
2. Macdonald RL. Delayed neurological deterioration after subarachnoid haemorrhage. *Nat Rev Neurol.* 2014;10(1):44–58. doi:10.1038/nrneurol.2013.246
3. Kistka H, Dewan MC, Mocco J. Evidence-based cerebral vasospasm surveillance. *Neurol Res Int.* 2013;2013:1–6. doi:10.1155/2013/256713
4. Connolly ES, Rabinstein AA, Carhuapoma JR, et al. Guidelines for the management of aneurysmal subarachnoid hemorrhage: a guideline for healthcare professionals from the American Heart Association/American Stroke Association. *Stroke.* 2012;43(6):1711–1737. doi:10.1161/STR.0b013e3182587839
5. Rumalla K, Lin M, Ding L, et al. Risk factors for cerebral vasospasm in aneurysmal subarachnoid hemorrhage: a population-based study of 8346 patients. *World Neurosurg.* 2021;145:e233–e241. doi:10.1016/j.wneu.2020.10.008
6. de Oliveira Manoel AL, Jaja BN, Germans MR, et al. The VASOGRADE: a simple grading scale for prediction of delayed cerebral ischemia after subarachnoid hemorrhage. *Stroke.* 2015;46(7):1826–1831. doi:10.1161/STROKEAHA.115.008728
7. Ahn SH, Savarraj JP, Pervez M, et al. The subarachnoid hemorrhage early brain edema score predicts delayed cerebral ischemia and clinical outcomes. *Neurosurgery.* 2018;83(1):137–145. doi:10.1093/neuros/nyx364
8. Claassen J, Carhuapoma JR, Kreiter KT, et al. Global cerebral edema after subarachnoid hemorrhage. *Stroke.* 2002;33(5):1225–1232. doi:10.1161/01.STR.0000015624.29071.1F
9. Lee VH, Ouyang B, John S, et al. Risk stratification for the in-hospital mortality in subarachnoid hemorrhage: the HAIR score. *Neurocrit Care.* 2014;21(1):14–19. doi:10.1007/s12028-013-9952-9
10. Kishore K, Cusimano MD. The fundamental need for sleep in neurocritical care units: time for a paradigm shift. *Front Neurol.* 2021;12:637250. doi:10.3389/fneur.2021.637250
11. Oliveira-Filho J, Ezzeddine MA, Segal AZ, et al. Fever in subarachnoid hemorrhage: relationship to vasospasm and outcome. *Neurology.* 2001;56(10):1299–1304. doi:10.1212/wnl.56.10.1299
12. Alabbas F, Hadhiah K, Al-Jehani H, et al. Hyponatremia as predictor of symptomatic vasospasm in aneurysmal subarachnoid hemorrhage. *Interdiscip Neurosurg.* 2020;22:100843. doi:10.1016/j.inat.2020.100843
13. Foreman P, Griessenauer CJ, Shoja MM, et al. Hypocapnia as a poor prognostic factor in aneurysmal subarachnoid hemorrhage. *Med Gas Res.* 2013;3(1):25. doi:10.1186/2045-9912-3-25
14. Reiff T, Barthel O, Schönenberger S, et al. High-normal PaCO2 values might be associated with worse outcome in patients with subarachnoid hemorrhage – a retrospective cohort study. *BMC Neurol.* 2020;20(1):31. doi:10.1186/s12883-020-1603-0
15. Mahajan C, Gupta N. Chapter 13 - Vasospasm. In: Prabhakar H, ed. *Complications in Neuroanesthesia.* Academic Press; 2016:103–109. doi:10.1016/B978-0-12-804075-1.00013-4
16. Claassen J, Bernardini GL, Kreiter K, et al. Effect of cisternal and ventricular blood on risk of delayed cerebral ischemia after subarachnoid hemorrhage: *Stroke.* 2001;32(9):2012–2020. doi:10.1161/hs0901.095677
17. Diringer MN, Bleck TP, Claude Hemphill J, et al. Critical care management of patients following aneurysmal subarachnoid hemorrhage: recommendations from the Neurocritical Care Society's Multidisciplinary Consensus Conference. *Neurocrit Care.* 2011;15(2):211. doi:10.1007/s12028-011-9605-9
18. Lau VI, Arntfield RT. Point-of-care transcranial Doppler by intensivists. *Crit Ultrasound J.* 2017;9(1):21. doi:10.1186/s13089-017-0077-9
19. D'Andrea A, Conte M, Scarafile R, et al. Transcranial Doppler ultrasound: physical principles and principal applications in neurocritical care unit. *J Cardiovasc Echography.* 2016;26(2):28. doi:10.4103/2211-4122.183746
20. Harders AG, Gilsbach JM. Time course of blood velocity changes related to vasospasm in the circle of Willis measured by transcranial Doppler ultrasound. *J Neurosurg.* 1987;66(5):718–728. doi:10.3171/jns.1987.66.5.0718
21. Samagh N, Bhagat H, Jangra K. Monitoring cerebral vasospasm: How much can we rely on transcranial Doppler. *J Anaesthesiol Clin Pharmacol.* 2019;35(1):12. doi:10.4103/joacp.JOACP_192_17
22. Greenberg M. Vasospasm. In: Greenberg M, ed. *Handbook of Neurosurgery.* 9th ed.; New York: Thieme; 2019: 1237.
23. Sviri GE, Ghodke B, Britz GW, et al. Transcranial Doppler grading criteria for basilar artery vasospasm. *Neurosurgery.* 2006;59(2):360–366; discussion 360-366. doi:10.1227/01.NEU.0000223502.93013.6E
24. Binaghi S, Colleoni ML, Maeder P, et al. CT Angiography and perfusion CT in cerebral vasospasm after subarachnoid hemorrhage. *Am J Neuroradiol.* 2007;28(4):750–758.
25. Greenberg ED, Gold R, Reichman M, et al. Diagnostic accuracy of CT angiography and CT perfusion for cerebral vasospasm: a meta-analysis. *Am J Neuroradiol.* 2010;31(10):1853–1860. doi:10.3174/ajnr.A2246
26. Anderson GB, Ashforth R, Steinke DE, et al. CT angiography for the detection of cerebral vasospasm in patients with acute subarachnoid hemorrhage. *AJNR Am J Neuroradiol.* 2000;21(6):1011–1015.
27. Letourneau-Guillon L, Farzin B, Darsaut TE, et al. Reliability of CT angiography in cerebral vasospasm: a systematic review of the literature and an inter- and intraobserver study. *Am J Neuroradiol.* 2020;41(4):612–618. doi:10.3174/ajnr.A6462
28. Omoto K, Nakagawa I, Nishimura F, Yamada S, Motoyama Y, Nakase H. Computed tomography perfusion imaging after aneurysmal subarachnoid hemorrhage can detect cerebral vasospasm and predict delayed cerebral ischemia after endovascular treatment. *Surg Neurol Int.* 2020;11:233. doi:10.25259/SNI_14_2020
29. Killeen RP, Gupta A, Delaney H, et al. Appropriate use of CT perfusion following aneurysmal subarachnoid hemorrhage: a Bayesian analysis approach. *Am J Neuroradiol.* 2014;35(3):459–465. doi:10.3174/ajnr.A3767
30. Lanzman B, Heit JJ. Advanced MRI measures of cerebral perfusion and their clinical applications. *Top Magn Reson Imaging.* 2017;26(2):83–90. doi:10.1097/RMR.0000000000000120
31. Rosenthal ES, Biswal S, Zafar SF, et al. Continuous electroencephalography predicts delayed cerebral ischemia after subarachnoid hemorrhage: a prospective study of diagnostic accuracy: EEG Accurately Predicts DCI. *Ann Neurol.* 2018;83(5):958–969. doi:10.1002/ana.25232
32. Scherschinski L, Catapano JS, Karahalios K, et al. Electroencephalography for detection of vasospasm and delayed cerebral ischemia in aneurysmal subarachnoid hemorrhage: a retrospective analysis and systematic review. *Neurosurg Focus.* 2022;52(3):E3. doi:10.3171/2021.12.FOCUS21656
33. Francoeur CL, Lauzier F, Brassard P, et al. Near infrared spectroscopy for poor grade aneurysmal subarachnoid hemorrhage—a concise review. *Front Neurol.* 2022;13:874393. doi:10.3389/fneur.2022.874393
34. Bulsara KR, Günel M, Amin-Hanjani S, et al. Results of a national cerebrovascular neurosurgery survey on the management of cerebral vasospasm/

delayed cerebral ischemia. *J NeuroInterventional Surg.* 2015;7(6):408–411. doi:10.1136/neurintsurg-2014-011223

35. Ascanio LC, Dmytriw AA, Chida K, et al. Evaluation of the utility of early routine computed tomography angiography in subarachnoid hemorrhage patient outcomes. *J Clin Neurosci.* 2021;89:133–138. doi:10.1016/j.jocn.2021.04.003
36. Winslow N, Ehsan M, Klopfenstein J. Delayed ischemic neurologic deficit with vasospasm in aneurysmal subarachnoid hemorrhage after negative post-bleed day 7 angiography. *Clin Neurol Neurosurg.* 2022;220:107353. doi:10.1016/j.clineuro.2022.107353
37. Arias EJ, Vajapey S, Reynolds MR, et al. Utility of screening for cerebral vasospasm using digital subtraction angiography. *Stroke.* 2015;46(11): 3137–3141. doi:10.1161/STROKEAHA.115.010081
38. Labak C, Shammassian BH, Zhou X, et al. Multimodality monitoring for delayed cerebral ischemia in subarachnoid hemorrhage: a mini review. *Front Neurol.* 2022;13:869107. doi:10.3389/fneur.2022.869107

CHAPTER

33

What Are the Invasive Options to Monitor for Vasospasm After Aneurysmal Subarachnoid Hemorrhage?

Rahul A. Sastry, MD & Michael Reznik, MD

Case

A 52-year-old woman is in the ICU 6 days after suffering a subarachnoid hemorrhage from a ruptured posterior communicating artery aneurysm. Hunt-Hess grade was 3 upon presentation with a score of 3 on the modified Fisher scale. The aneurysm has since been secured with endovascular coiling. What invasive options exist for monitoring such a patient for cerebral vasospasm?

Key Points

- Once delayed cerebral ischemia has been identified, the need for enhanced monitoring to prevent recurrent neurologic deterioration is critical.
- Intracranial pressure and cerebral perfusion pressure, as derived from invasive intracranial monitoring, remain imprecise tools that can detect some conditions for global ischemia but are not sensitive enough for focal vasospasm.
- Limited data suggest that lactate/pyruvate ratios can help titrate optimal tissue oxygenation parameters.
- There is likely an emerging role for brain tissue oxygenation, cerebral blood flow, and cerebral microdialysis. However, given the small sample size and available studies, much further work is needed to establish their clinical utility on a more widespread basis.

BACKGROUND

Delayed cerebral ischemia (DCI) is a major cause of poor neurologic outcomes after aneurysmal subarachnoid hemorrhage (aSAH) and particularly after high-grade aSAH.[1–3] The development of DCI is most often correlated with the presence of angiographic vasospasm from sustained arterial smooth muscle contraction and diminished cerebral blood flow (CBF) to brain parenchyma.[4–6] However, it is also well established that not all patients with DCI have angiographic vasospasm and that not all patients with angiographic vasospasm develop DCI.[4,7–9] It is likely that there are other contributory pathophysiologic mechanisms, such as a loss of local cerebral autoregulation, microthrombosis, and cortical spreading depolarizations.

A variety of methods have been employed to identify impending DCI in the neurocritical care setting. The gold-standard indicator remains the neurologic exam, and changes in exam should raise suspicion for DCI and trigger additional diagnostic workup. However, patients with high-grade aSAH often have relatively poor neurologic exams and are at high risk of clinically silent DCI,[8] as a change in neurologic exam may not be readily apparent. As such, the detection of vasospasm or DCI in these patients can be a major clinical challenge. While a number of noninvasive options exist and are an important part of a clinician's vasospasm detection toolbox, invasive modalities can provide more direct information that may be especially valuable for the care of patients with high-grade aSAH.

EVIDENCE AND REVIEW

Invasive neuro-monitoring is used at many institutions for the detection of vasospasm and DCI in aSAH, including specific probes for intracranial pressure (ICP), brain tissue oxygenation ($PbtO_2$), CBF, and cerebral microdialysis. However, high-quality evidence to support their use is currently limited. Additionally, their measurements should be interpreted in a local context as they provide only a regional assessment of hypoxia, CBF, and metabolic derangement. As such, these intracranial monitors cannot provide information about other brain regions that may also be at risk for DCI.

Intracranial Pressure

ICP monitors are commonly used in patients with high-grade aSAH due to concomitant concerns of intracranial hypertension. However, ICP measurements are also useful to calculate global cerebral perfusion pressure (CPP) in the setting of impending DCI or vasospasm. Although low CPP is associated with an increased risk of brain tissue hypoxia, it remains imprecise. While the specificity for low CPP and high ICP to detect hypoxic states is high (>90% in some studies when correlated with $PbtO_2$), the sensitivity remains poor (<20%).[10,11]

Options for ICP monitoring include intraparenchymal probes and external ventricular drains (EVDs). EVDs are placed in the intraventricular space and have the added advantages of cerebrospinal fluid diversion for the management of hydrocephalus or intracranial hypertension and potential for intraventricular medication administration. Intraparenchymal probes are microtransducers that are placed in peripheral brain parenchyma, often as part of a "bundle" of intracranial monitors. Intraparenchymal probes are commonly used in the context of traumatic brain injury and offer the advantages of ICP monitoring with relatively lower risk of intraparenchymal hemorrhage and/or infection than EVDs.[12] As such, clinicians should weigh the risks and benefits of each type of monitor for a given patient.

Brain Tissue Oxygen

BOOST-2 was a phase 2 trial in patients with traumatic brain injury (TBI) designed to assess whether a management protocol informed by $PbtO_2$ and ICP values would reduce the total burden of brain hypoxia. Results from the trial suggest that aggressive measures to avoid local and global cerebral hypoxia (as defined by the maintenance of $PbtO_2$ > 20 mm Hg) may indeed play a role in the prevention of ischemia and adverse neurologic/functional outcomes.[13] In aSAH, data suggest that the identification of periods of localized cerebral hypoxia is associated with impaired vasoreactivity, anaerobic metabolism, DCI, and adverse neurologic outcomes.[10,11,14,15] Although attempts at $PbtO_2$-based optimization after aSAH have thus far yielded mixed results, evidence from the BOOST-2 trial will likely encourage further research.[16,17] Importantly, appropriate identification of at-risk vascular territories is necessary to guide probe placement, a consideration that should be further addressed as part of future studies of optimal monitoring protocols.

Cerebral Blood Flow

Although noninvasive assessment of CBF with xenon computed tomography (CT) has been correlated with the development of vasospasm and DCI in aSAH, the lack of continuous data acquisition limits its utility.[18–20] On the other hand, intraparenchymal CBF monitors utilize thermal diffusion techniques to directly assess impairments in cerebral autoregulation and vasoreactivity in real time. These monitors have been successfully applied in severe TBI to identify optimal CPP thresholds and guide interventions to augment mean arterial pressure (MAP).[17,18,20] In aSAH, small patient series have demonstrated a correlation between declining CBF and the development of symptomatic vasospasm.[21] In a study of 14 patients with aSAH, bedside monitoring with thermal-diffusion flowmetry showed differential estimates of CBF based on vasospasm status (25 ± 4 mL/100 g/min vs. 21 ± 4 mL/100 g/min). However, given the small scale of these studies, further work is needed to establish clinical utility.

Cerebral Microdialysis

Cerebral microdialysis samples low-molecular-weight compounds from the extracellular fluid surrounding local brain parenchyma and allows for direct assessment of cerebral metabolism, with certain changes in metabolite concentrations potentially signaling impending ischemia.[22] In a prospective study of aSAH patients, cerebral microdialysis from a high-risk vascular territory corresponding to each patient's culprit aneurysm resulted in the early detection of alterations in glutamate, glucose, and pyruvate metabolism that preceded DCI, with a higher sensitivity and specificity than both Transcranial Dopplers (TCDs) and angiography (Table 33–1).[23] In another prospective trial of 42 patients

TABLE 33–1 A comparison of various invasive monitoring modalities for vasopasm after aneurysmal subarachnoid hemorrhage.

Modality	Pros	Cons
Angiography	• Gold standard sensitivity/specificity • Can treat identified vasospasm with intra-arterial therapy	• Time and cost-intensive • Stroke is a risk of procedure • Limited data about use for screening in absence of clinical correlate
ICP monitoring	• Allows for calculation of CPP • Can monitor continuously	• Monitors are invasive and have associated procedural risks • Data are obtained from region of brain in which monitor is placed • CPP may be poor surrogate of local brain ischemia
Brain tissue oxygenation monitoring	• Early evidence suggests brain tissue oxygenation may be superior to CPP	• Monitors are invasive • Data must be obtained from vascular territory in question
Cerebral blood flow monitoring	• Can measure CBF directly	• Monitors are invasive • Limited evidence specifically in aSAH patients
Cerebral microdialysis	• Can directly measure metabolic markers of brain tissue ischemia • Can monitor semicontinuously	• Monitors are invasive

aSAH, aneurysmal subarachnoid hemorrhage; CBF, cerebral blood flow; CPP, cerebral perfusion pressure; ICP, intracranial pressure.

with aSAH, alterations in lactate/glucose and lactate/pyruvate ratios (LPR) in high-risk vascular territories preceded DCI and predicted its development with high sensitivity and specificity.[24] A retrospective analysis of combined microdialysis and $PbtO_2$ monitoring in 19 patients with aSAH found that, although 86% of instances of decreased $PbtO_2$ were associated with elevated LPR (>40, a common threshold[25]), many instances of elevated LPR were also not associated with decreased $PbtO_2$, suggesting relatively low specificity.[10]

AVAILABLE GUIDELINES

Given the limited state of the available literature, few guidelines exist on the use of invasive measures for the early detection and monitoring of vasospasm after aSAH.

REFERENCES

1. Macdonald RL, Hunsche E, Schüler R, Wlodarczyk J, Mayer SA. Quality of life and healthcare resource use associated with angiographic vasospasm after aneurysmal subarachnoid hemorrhage. *Stroke*. 2012;43(4):1082-1088. doi:10.1161/STROKEAHA.111.634071
2. Rosengart Axel J., Schultheiss Kim E., Tolentino Jocelyn, Macdonald R. Loch. Prognostic Factors for Outcome in Patients With Aneurysmal Subarachnoid Hemorrhage. *Stroke*. 2007;38(8):2315-2321. doi:10.1161/STROKEAHA.107.484360
3. Helbok R, Kofler M, Schiefecker AJ, et al. Clinical Use of Cerebral Microdialysis in Patients with Aneurysmal Subarachnoid Hemorrhage-State of the Art. *Front Neurol*. 2017;8:565. doi:10.3389/fneur.2017.00565
4. Crowley R. Webster, Medel R., Dumont Aaron S., et al. Angiographic Vasospasm Is Strongly Correlated With Cerebral Infarction After Subarachnoid Hemorrhage. *Stroke*. 2011;42(4):919-923. doi:10.1161/STROKEAHA.110.597005
5. Suwatcharangkoon Sureerat, De Marchis Gian Marco, Witsch Jens, et al. Medical Treatment Failure for Symptomatic Vasospasm After Subarachnoid Hemorrhage Threatens Long-Term Outcome. *Stroke*. 2019;50(7):1696-1702. doi:10.1161/STROKEAHA.118.022536
6. Li K, Barras CD, Chandra RV, et al. A Review of the Management of Cerebral Vasospasm After Aneurysmal Subarachnoid Hemorrhage. *World Neurosurg*. 2019;126:513-527. doi:10.1016/j.wneu.2019.03.083
7. Vergouwen MDI, Ilodigwe D, Macdonald RL. Cerebral infarction after subarachnoid hemorrhage contributes to poor outcome by vasospasm-dependent and -independent effects. *Stroke*. 2011;42(4):924-929. doi:10.1161/STROKEAHA.110.597914
8. Francoeur CL, Mayer SA. Management of delayed cerebral ischemia after subarachnoid hemorrhage. *Crit Care*. 2016;20. doi:10.1186/s13054-016-1447-6
9. Pluta RM, Hansen-Schwartz J, Dreier J, et al. Cerebral vasospasm following subarachnoid hemorrhage: time for a new world of thought. *Neurol Res*. 2009;31(2):151-158. doi:10.1179/174313209X393564
10. Chen HI, Stiefel MF, Oddo M, et al. Detection of cerebral compromise with multimodality monitoring in patients with subarachnoid hemorrhage. *Neurosurgery*. 2011;69(1):53–63. doi:10.1227/NEU.0b013e3182191451
11. Schmidt JM, Ko S-B, Helbok R, et al. Cerebral perfusion pressure thresholds for brain tissue hypoxia and metabolic crisis after poor-grade subarachnoid hemorrhage. *Stroke J Cereb Circ*. 2011;42(5):1351–1356. doi:10.1161/STROKEAHA.110.596874
12. Tavakoli S, Peitz G, Ares W, Hafeez S, Grandhi R. Complications of invasive intracranial pressure monitoring devices in neurocritical care. *Neurosurg Focus*. 2017;43(5):E6. doi:10.3171/2017.8.FOCUS17450
13. Okonkwo DO, Shutter LA, Moore C, et al. Brain oxygen optimization in severe traumatic brain injury phase-II: a phase II randomized trial. *Crit Care Med*. 2017;45(11):1907–1914. doi:10.1097/CCM.0000000000002619
14. Jaeger M, Schuhmann MU, Soehle M, Nagel C, Meixensberger J. Continuous monitoring of cerebrovascular autoregulation after subarachnoid hemorrhage by brain tissue oxygen pressure reactivity and its relation to delayed cerebral infarction. *Stroke*. 2007;38(3):981–986. doi:10.1161/01.STR.0000257964.65743.99
15. Bohman L-E, Pisapia JM, Sanborn MR, et al. Response of brain oxygen to therapy correlates with long-term outcome after subarachnoid hemorrhage. *Neurocrit Care*. 2013;19(3):320–328. doi:10.1007/s12028-013-9890-6
16. Rass V, Solari D, Ianosi B, et al. Protocolized brain oxygen optimization in subarachnoid hemorrhage. *Neurocrit Care*. 2019;31(2):263–272. doi:10.1007/s12028-019-00753-0
17. Tackla R, Hinzman JM, Foreman B, Magner M, Andaluz N, Hartings JA. Assessment of cerebrovascular autoregulation using regional cerebral blood flow in surgically managed brain trauma patients. *Neurocrit Care*. 2015;23(3):339–346. doi:10.1007/s12028-015-0146-5
18. Rosenthal G, Sanchez-Mejia RO, Phan N, Hemphill JC, Martin C, Manley GT. Incorporating a parenchymal thermal diffusion cerebral blood flow probe in bedside assessment of cerebral autoregulation and vasoreactivity in patients with severe traumatic brain injury: clinical article. *J Neurosurg*. 2011;114(1):62–70. doi:10.3171/2010.6.JNS091360
19. Rostami E, Engquist H, Howells T, et al. Early low cerebral blood flow and high cerebral lactate: prediction of delayed cerebral ischemia in subarachnoid hemorrhage. *J Neurosurg*. 2017;128(6):1762–1770. doi:10.3171/2016.11.JNS161140
20. Le Roux P, Menon DK, Citerio G, et al. Consensus summary statement of the international multidisciplinary consensus conference on multimodality monitoring in neurocritical care. *Neurocrit Care*. 2014;21(2):1–26. doi:10.1007/s12028-014-0041-5
21. Vajkoczy P, Horn P, Thome C, Munch E, Schmiedek P. Regional cerebral blood flow monitoring in the diagnosis of delayed ischemia following aneurysmal subarachnoid hemorrhage. *J Neurosurg*. 2003;98(6):1227–1234. doi:10.3171/jns.2003.98.6.1227
22. Zhou T, Kalanuria A. Cerebral Microdialysis in Neurocritical Care. *Curr Neurol Neurosci Rep*. 2018;18(12):101. doi:10.1007/s11910-018-0915-6
23. Unterberg AW, Sakowitz OW, Sarrafzadeh AS, Benndorf G, Lanksch WR. Role of bedside microdialysis in the diagnosis of cerebral vasospasm following aneurysmal subarachnoid hemorrhage. *J Neurosurg*. 2001;94(5):740–749. doi:10.3171/jns.2001.94.5.0740
24. Skjøth-Rasmussen J, Schulz M, Kristensen SR, Bjerre P. Delayed neurological deficits detected by an ischemic pattern in the extracellular cerebral metabolites in patients with aneurysmal subarachnoid hemorrhage. *J Neurosurg*. 2004;100(1):8–15. doi:10.3171/jns.2004.100.1.0008
25. Sánchez-Guerrero A, Mur-Bonet G, Vidal-Jorge M, et al. Reappraisal of the reference levels for energy metabolites in the extracellular fluid of the human brain. *J Cereb Blood Flow Metab*. 2017;37(8):2742–2755. doi:10.1177/0271678X16674222

CHAPTER

34

What Are the Optimal Blood Pressure Parameters for Postoperative Vascular Neurosurgery Patients?

Max Shutran, MD & Carlos David, MD

Case

A 56-year-old woman with a history of hypertension and smoking presents to the hospital after being found unresponsive at home. On admission she is responsive only to noxious stimulation and shows abnormal motor posturing on the right side. Her imaging demonstrates a large left frontal intracerebral hemorrhage (ICH) and a left pericallosal artery aneurysm. She undergoes emergency left frontal craniotomy for hematoma evacuation and aneurysm clipping. What are the considerations in managing her blood pressures postoperatively?

Key Points

- Blood pressure management is an important facet of postoperative care in multiple neurosurgical conditions.
- Although there are few high-quality data to provide guidance for postoperative blood pressure control, it is possible to use the existing data to reach a reasonable set of recommendations.

BACKGROUND

The importance of blood pressure in neurosurgical disease has a long history dating back to Dr. Harvey Cushing, who in 1901 described the reflex hypertension that accompanies a rise in intracranial pressure and in 1903 advocated for the use of intraoperative blood pressure monitoring as a standard of care in neurosurgery. It is well known that extremes of blood pressure, either hypotension or hypertension, can be deleterious in the neurosurgical patient. Hypotension can reduce cerebral perfusion to critical levels in states of cerebrovascular insufficiency or in diseases with elevated intracranial pressure and loss of autoregulation, such as traumatic brain injury. Hypertension, conversely, can cause ICH in postoperative neurosurgical patients and can lead to other systemic and central nervous system complications.

In cerebrovascular neurosurgery, there are several unique considerations that guide blood pressure management postoperatively. In aneurysm surgery, there is a distinction between ruptured and unruptured cases, as patients with ruptured aneurysms may experience vasospasm postoperatively that necessitates augmentation of the blood pressure to avoid cerebral ischemia. Patients with unruptured aneurysms generally do not have this requirement and can be managed within a relatively normal blood pressure range. In intracranial bypass, there are several factors that may necessitate keeping blood pressure within a very close range. Postoperative hypotension following carotid endarterectomy is a well-known issue that is attributed to the manipulation of the carotid sinus and is easily treated postoperatively, but attention needs to also be played to avoid postoperative hypertension following the recanalization of a severely stenotic carotid artery to avoid hyperperfusion syndrome.

EVIDENCE AND REVIEW

Optimal Postoperative Blood Pressure Target

There are few high-quality studies specifically examining the optimal blood pressure goals for postoperative cerebrovascular neurosurgery patients. However, guidelines can be extrapolated by examining studies of postoperative ICH as well as spontaneous ICH, ischemic stroke, and other diseases.

In a case control study of craniotomies performed at a single center from 1976 to 1992 with a 1:2 matching scheme, the overall incidence of postoperative clinically significant ICH recorded

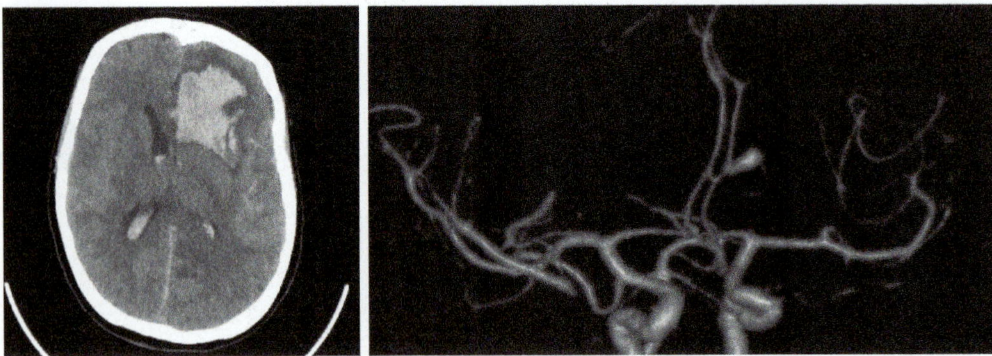

FIGURE 34–1 **Left:** Axial computed tomography scan demonstrating a left frontal intraparenchymal hemorrhage with intraventricular extension. **Right:** Subsequent 3D reconstructed angiogram demonstrating an associated pericollosal artery aneurysm.

in this study was 0.77% (86 out of 11,214 patients).[1] Such incidence may be lower than expected because the inclusion mechanism required a neurological deterioration that prompted the discovery of ICH. The analyzable population included 69 patients who experienced postoperative ICH and 138 matched control patients without ICH. The major finding of the study was that patients with postoperative ICH were significantly more likely to have had postoperative hypertension (defined as systolic blood pressure [SBP] > 160 mm Hg or diastolic blood pressure > 90 mm Hg), with an odds ratio of 24.[1] There are several possible reasons for this besides a direct correlation between postoperative hypertension and ICH, such as the fact that hypertension can be seen as a response to ICH. However, it seems reasonable to infer that postoperative blood pressure should be maintained below 160/90 mm Hg when feasible to reduce the risk of ICH.

Blood Pressure Targets in Ischemic and Hemorrhagic Strokes

An analysis of 17,398 ischemic stroke patients from the International Stroke Trial examined the relationship to SBP recorded immediately prior to randomization and early and late outcomes.[2] It showed a U-shaped relationship between baseline SBP and outcomes, with early death (within 14 days) increasing by 17.9% for every 10 mm Hg below 150 mm Hg and increasing by 3.8% for every 10 mm Hg above 150 mm Hg. These data suggest that 150 mm Hg may be an optimal SBP target in cerebral ischemia and that deviations either below or above this can have deleterious consequences.

In terms of hemorrhagic strokes, there are several studies that investigate the optimal blood pressure target including INTERACT-2 and ATACH-2 which were published in 2013 and 2016, respectively, and are already reviewed in detail in another chapter of this book.[3,4] They each studied the effect of a blood pressure goal of <140 mm Hg systolic on hemorrhage expansion in patients with spontaneous nonlesional ICH. Both studies found that the stricter blood pressure goal reduced hematoma expansion as compared to a more liberal guideline-driven systolic goal of 180 mm Hg. However, in the ATACH-2 trial, there was no significant difference in functional outcome and it reported an increased risk of adverse renal events in the intensive treatment arm. Although these studies are not directly applicable to postoperative craniotomy patients, their results provide a rationale for strict blood pressure control in patients who may be at risk of postoperative ICH.

Blood Pressure Target After Clipping of Unruptured Aneurysm

The primary goal of blood pressure control following surgery for clipping of an unruptured intracranial aneurysm is to decrease the risk of intracranial hemorrhage. Patients with unruptured aneurysms should not have any significant autoregulatory impairment and should be able to tolerate a SBP range of approximately 100 to 150 mm Hg without undue consequence. For hypertensive patients, maintaining this goal requires the use of as-needed IV antihypertensive agents such as a continuous nicardipine or clevidipine infusion or intermittent IV labetalol. Although the optimal duration of blood pressure control following elective aneurysm clipping is unknown, it is reasonable to maintain for at least 24 hours after surgery, given that most postoperative hemorrhages seem to occur within 12 to 24 hours.[5] We would recommend that patients undergoing a craniotomy for clipping of an unruptured aneurysm have the SBP controlled to <150 mm Hg for at least 24 hours.

Blood Pressure Target After Clipping of Ruptured Aneurysm

For patients with ruptured aneurysms, the postoperative blood pressure goals depend on the presence or absence of cerebral vasospasm. Although most patients will not develop significant vasospasm or delayed cerebral ischemia in the first few days after aneurysm rupture, there are patients who present late after a ruptured aneurysm and those who display evidence of early vasospasm on presentation. The management of cerebral vasospasm and delayed cerebral ischemia is outside the scope of this chapter, but permissive and induced hypertension are important adjuncts in treating vasospasm and preventing cerebral infarction. For a patient who presents with a ruptured aneurysm without evidence of early vasospasm and undergoes surgery for clipping, it is reasonable to keep the SBP < 150 mm Hg for about 24 hours after surgery. After this time period, caution should be used in actively treating hypertension in the patient with subarachnoid hemorrhage, as hypertension may represent a physiological response to cerebral vasospasm that should not be suppressed once the culprit aneurysm has been occluded.

Blood Pressure Target After Carotid Endarterectomy

Carotid endarterectomy remains an important and evidence-based surgical intervention to reduce the risk of stroke in patients with both symptomatic and asymptomatic carotid stenosis. Patients who undergo carotid endarterectomy are known to have wide variability in heart rate and blood pressure postoperatively, which is attributed to direct manipulation of the carotid sinus. The most serious complication of carotid endarterectomy is stroke, which can be either ischemic or hemorrhagic. The prevention of ischemic stroke relies mainly on good surgical technique to ensure that the endarterectomized vessel surface is clean and regular without protruding intimal flaps, sutures, or other irregularities which can lead to vessel thrombosis. Hemorrhagic strokes are attributed to cerebral hyperperfusion. It is thought that hyperperfusion can occur after recanalization of a significantly chronically narrowed carotid artery because the intracranial vessels have become maximally dilated with time and are subjected to an abrupt increase in flow after surgery. Hyperperfusion syndrome can present as severe headaches, seizures, or neurological deficits and can lead to ICH ipsilateral to the side of surgery.

A recent paper analyzed 36 studies of cerebral hyperperfusion syndrome (CHS) after carotid endarterectomy and found that elevated postoperative SBP was significantly associated with this potentially serious complication.[6] The authors found that CHS was rare with 1% total incidence and that ICH had 0.5% incidence. The definition of CHS was slightly variable between different studies, but all included studies used either a combination of severe headache and evidence of hyperperfusion on imaging (edema, elevated cerebral blood volume, and hemorrhage) or multiple clinical characteristics including seizures and focal deficit in the absence of ischemia. The median time from surgery to presentation with CHS was 5 days. There was a significant increase in the incidence of CHS with postoperative blood pressures greater than 150 mm Hg. The authors suggest targeting a postoperative SBP of 140 to 160 mm Hg or lower if the baseline preoperative SBP was lower.

Blood Pressure Target After Intracranial Bypass

The indications for extracranial-intracranial bypass include giant or fusiform aneurysms that require trapping and flow replacement, and some ischemic conditions that require flow augmentation (Moyamoya syndrome, chronic carotid, or middle cerebral artery occlusion). A review of the evolution of these indications over time is beyond the scope of this chapter. The bypass vessel is most commonly either the superficial temporal artery (for flow augmentation) or an artery or vein interposition graft from the cervical carotid artery (for flow replacement).

One of the most disappointing complications that can be seen is early occlusion of a bypass graft. Depending on the pathology being treated, the manifestations of early graft failure can range from asymptomatic to fully fledged strokes. Although early graft occlusion can reflect a technical problem with the bypass such as kinking, excessive tension, or redundant tissue in the lumen, it is also possible for inadequate flow through the bypass to lead to thrombosis. Vein grafts are the most prone to this type of graft failure. Sundt et al had previously estimated that a mean flow of 40 mL/min is required to maintain flow in a vein graft bypass.[7] Sia et al combined measurement of graft velocities in 12 patients with computational fluid dynamic models and inferred that a minimum mean arterial pressure (MAP) of 60 mm Hg would be required to maintain 40 mL/min of flow and thus recommended this as a minimum postoperative MAP threshold.[3]

As is the case in carotid endarterectomy, extracranial-intracranial bypass for ischemic conditions can result in CHS with the risk of neurological deficit or ICH. This is less well studied in bypass than in carotid endarterectomy. Yamaguchi et al studied this phenomenon in 50 patients undergoing bypass for atherosclerotic occlusive cerebrovascular disease and found that the only important predictor of postoperative hyperperfusion was presence of the steal phenomenon on preoperative xenon computed tomography (CT) perfusion.[8] The steal phenomenon is said to occur when the regional cerebral blood flow in the ischemic territory paradoxically decreases after administration of acetazolamide due to the vascular territory in question already having achieved maximal vasodilation and blood being shunted to other areas of the brain where the vessels dilate in response to acetazolamide. Blood pressure was not found to be an important predictor in their study. However, based on the data in carotid endarterectomy, it seems reasonable to control the SBP to <160 mm Hg postoperatively in cases in which the steal phenomenon was present preoperatively.

AVAILABLE GUIDELINES

Although no high-quality evidence for specific postoperative blood pressure goals in cerebrovascular neurosurgery exists, some recommendations can be made based on knowledge of pathophysiology and on trials carried out on the effects of blood pressure in neurological disease processes mentioned above.

REFERENCES

1. Basali A, Mascha EJ, Kalfas I, Schubert A. Relation between perioperative hypertension and intracranial hemorrhage after craniotomy. *Anesthesiology* 2000;93(1):48–54.
2. Leonardi-Bee J, Bath PM, Phillips SJ, Sandercock PA, Group ISTC. Blood pressure and clinical outcomes in the International Stroke Trial. *Stroke* 2002;33(5):1315–1320.
3. Anderson CS, Heeley E, Huang Y, et al. Rapid blood-pressure lowering in patients with acute intracerebral hemorrhage. *N Engl J Med* 2013;368(25):2355–2365.

4. Qureshi AI, Palesch YY, Barsan WG, et al. Intensive blood-pressure lowering in patients with acute cerebral hemorrhage. *N Engl J Med* 2016;375(11):1033–1043.
5. Kalfas IH, Little JR. Postoperative hemorrhage: a survey of 4992 intracranial procedures. *Neurosurgery* 1988;23(3):343–347.
6. Bouri S, Thapar A, Shalhoub J, et al. Hypertension and the post-carotid endarterectomy cerebral hyperperfusion syndrome. *Eur J Vasc Endovasc Surg* 2011;41(2):229–237.
7. Sundt TM, 3rd, Sundt TM, Jr. Principles of preparation of vein bypass grafts to maximize patency. *J Neurosurg* 1987;66(2):172–180.
8. Yamaguchi K, Kawamata T, Kawashima A, Hori T, Okada Y. Incidence and predictive factors of cerebral hyperperfusion after extracranial-intracranial bypass for occlusive cerebrovascular diseases. *Neurosurgery* 2010;67(6): 1548–1554; discussion 1554.

CHAPTER

35

How Should Blood Pressure Be Managed After Spontaneous Intraparenchymal Hemorrhage?

David P. Lerner, MD

Case

A 68-year-old man with hypertension and hyperlipidemia presented to the emergency department for evaluation of acute onset left-sided weakness. His initial examination demonstrated weakness in the left face, arm, and leg and hypesthesia in the same distribution. His vitals on arrival to the emergency department were pertinent for noninvasive blood pressure of 198/108 mm Hg. A noncontrast head CT was obtained (Figure 35–1). What is the most appropriate blood pressure goal for this patient?

Key Point

- Systolic blood pressure control to <140 mm Hg improves functional and mortality outcomes in patients with intraparenchymal hemorrhages, although a stepwise improvement can be observed with lowering of systolic blood pressure < 180 mm Hg.

BACKGROUND

Hypertension is a major risk factor for spontaneous intraparenchymal hemorrhage. It is also associated with hematoma expansion and poor neurologic outcome.[1] Commonly, patients will present with acute hypertension in the setting of intraparenchymal hemorrhage, as seen in the case above. Although initially thought to be a monophasic disease process, it is now known there can be ongoing hemorrhage even after ictus. Because of this, there has been focus on attempts to minimize hematoma expansion with blood pressure control.[2] Animal and human studies show early blood pressure lowing prevents hematoma expansion. However, that correlates to improved clinical outcomes remain unclear.

EVIDENCE AND REVIEW

Multiple trials have evaluated the ideal blood pressure goal in spontaneous supratentorial intraparenchymal hemorrhage and their correlation with outcome. There are mixed results for changes in mortality and functional outcome as well as complications of blood pressure management.

Blood pressure management in acute intracerebral hemorrhage can decrease hematoma expansion. However, the degree, or absolute value, of blood pressure control is not without risk and may not improve mortality or functional outcome. Notably, the Intensive Blood Pressure Reduction in Acute Cerebral Haemorrhage Trial 2 (INTERACT-2) and Antihypertensive Treatment of Acute Cerebral Hemorrhage 2 (ATACH-2) trials, published in 2013 and 2016, both corroborated a reduction in hematoma expansion with strict blood pressure control but differ in adverse event rate as well as functional outcome.[3,4]

INTERACT-2 studied patients over 18 years of age with a spontaneous supratentorial intracerebral hemorrhage with an elevated blood pressure between 150 mm Hg and 220 mm Hg. The treatment arm was to obtain and sustain a systolic blood pressure (SBP) of <140 mm Hg while the control group was to follow standard of care at the time in which SBP was <180 mm Hg. The primary outcome of the study was death or major disability

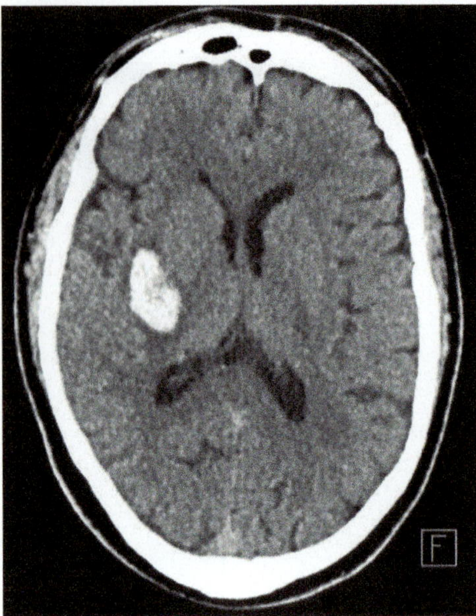

FIGURE 35–1 Noncontrast axial head CT at the level of the thalami with right basal ganglia intraparenchymal hemorrhage typical of hypertensive etiologies.

(defined as modified Rankin score (mRS) of 3-5) at 90 days. The secondary outcomes studied were all-cause mortality and cause-specific mortality, five dimensions of health-related quality of life, safety outcome of early neurologic deterioration, severe hypotension, and hematoma expansion.

INTERACT-2 demonstrated:

- Intensive blood pressure group achieved blood pressure goal at 6 hours from randomization.
- Those in the intensive blood pressure group more commonly required two or more antihypertensive medications (26.6% vs. 8.1%).
- There was no difference in medical or surgical treatments in the first 7 days from randomization except for decision to withdrawal active treatment and care (5.4% vs. 3.3%).
- There was no difference in hematoma expansion over 24 hours in the intensive or guideline blood pressure groups.
- There was no difference between the intensive and guideline-based blood pressure groups for nonfatal serious adverse events.

Despite being a large, randomized, multicenter control trial, there were a number of limitations to the INTERACT-2 trial. Two significant criticisms of the study are the time from randomization to target blood pressure—for the intensive blood pressure population, the average time to goal was 6 hours. Lack of standardization for medication administration in the intensive blood pressure group introduced complexity in assessing efficacy of interventions. Additionally, when evaluating the actual blood pressures achieved, both the intensive treatment and guideline arms reached significantly lower blood pressure than target.

The ATACH-2 trial was followed as a multicenter, international, open-label randomized trial evaluating intensive blood pressure (<140 mm Hg) versus guideline-driven protocol (<180 mm Hg). Specific exclusion criteria included potential surgical candidates, with large hemorrhages over 60 mL, infratentorial primary hemorrhage, considerable intraventricular extension, moderate thrombocytopenia, and coagulopathy. The primary endpoint of the study was death or disability (defined as mRS of 4–5) at 90 days with secondary outcomes being quality-of-life measures at 90 days, hematoma expansion, and treatment-related adverse side effects.

One thousand patients enrolled in the trial, with no difference in death or major disability at 90 days between the two arms: 38.7% intensive versus 37.7% guideline. There was also no difference in hematoma expansion, death, or serious adverse events. There was an increase in adverse renal events in the intensive treatment arm, but there is lack of definition of this result. Despite the lack of treatment effect, there were appropriate changes in blood pressure. Like INTERACT-2, the blood pressure control exceeded expectation: for the intensive blood pressure control group, the average SBP was 128.9 while for the guideline group, the average SBP was 141.1 (Table 35–1).

Nearly half of the patients enrolled in the trial were of Asian descent, and the large majority of hemorrhages were deep structure hemorrhages (basal ganglia and thalamus) with consequent underrepresentation of lobar/cortical hemorrhages. These two distinct hemorrhages have distinct pathophysiologic etiologies and may have different responses to blood pressure management. Also, there was a large treatment failure rate in the intensive treatment arm as compared to the guideline-based treatment (12.2% vs. 0.8%, respectively). This high failure rate, despite having a lower SBP, may have masked any outcome differences.

Notably, a preplanned pooled analysis of INTERACT-2 and ATACH-2 examined a combined 3,809 patients (20 were excluded due to insufficient blood pressure data)[5] and observed that achieving SBP control was continuously associated with better functional outcomes, including higher chance of a shift to a favorable mRS outcome (OR 0.90 per 10 mm Hg higher SBP achieved), as well as improvements in chance of good outcome at 90 days as measured by mRS, functional independence at 90 days,

TABLE 35–1 ATACH-2 outcome and safety data.

	Intensive Treatment	Standard Treatment
Mean SBP first 2 hours	128.9 ± 16	141.1 ± 14.8
Death or disability	38.7%	37.7%
Hematoma expansion	18.9%	24.4%
Death	6.6%	6.8%
Treatment-related serious adverse event	1.6%	1.2%
Any serious adverse event within 3 months	25.6%	20.0% (P = .06)
Renal adverse events within 7 days	9.0%	4.0% (P = .002)

SBP, systolic blood pressure.

lower chances of death at 90 days, and lower chances of hematoma expansion or neurologic deterioration within 24 hours.

Taken altogether, results of INTERACT-2 and ATACH-2 support the notion that early aggressive blood pressure lowering to targets of <140 mm Hg is achievable and safe in many patients. The efficacy of doing this in terms of patient benefit was not borne out in primary results of the trials, but preplanned pooled analysis of the two trials did show benefits in all major outcome categories.

AVAILABLE GUIDELINES

A recent blood pressure management guideline[6,7] from the AHA and American Stroke Association summarized their guidelines as such:

> "For ICH patients presenting with SBP between 150 and 220 mm Hg and without contraindication to acute BP treatment, acute lowering of SBP to 140 mm Hg is safe (Class I; Level of Evidence A) and can be effective for improving functional outcome (Class IIa; Level of Evidence B)."

REFERENCES

1. Anderson CS, Huang Y, Arima H, et al. Effects of early intensive blood pressure-lowering treatment on the growth of hematoma and perihematomal edema in acute intracerebral hemorrhage: the Intensive Blood Pressure Reduction in Acute Cerebral Haemorrhage Trial (INTERACT). *Stroke.* 2010;41:307–312.
2. Antihypertensive Treatment of Acute Cerebral Hemorrhage (ATACH) Investigators. Antihypertensive treatment of acute cerebral hemorrhage. *Crit Care Med.* 2010;38:637–648.
3. The INTERACT2 Investigators. Rapid blood-pressure lowering in patients with acute intracerebral hemorrhage. *N Engl J Med.* 2013;386:2355–2365.
4. The ATACH-2 Trial Investigators. Intensive blood-pressure lowering in patients with cerebral hemorrhage. *N Engl J Med.* 2016;375:1033–1043.
5. Moullaali TJ, Wang X, Martin RH, et al. Blood pressure control and clinical outcomes in acute intracerebral haemorrhage: a preplanned pooled analysis of individual participant data. *Lancet Neurology.* 2019;18(9):857–864.
6. Hemphill JC 3rd, Greenberg SM, Anderson CS, et al. Guidelines for the management of spontaneous intracerebral hemorrhage: a guideline for healthcare professionals from the American Heart Association/American Stroke Association. *Stroke.* 2015;46:2032–2060.
7. Greenberg SM, Ziai WC, Cordonnier C, et al. "2022 Guideline for the management of patients with spontaneous intracerebral hemorrhage: A guideline from the American Heart Association/Americal Stroke Association." *Stroke.* 2022;53:e282-361.

CHAPTER

36

Is There a Role for Invasive Hemodynamic Monitoring in Spontaneous Subarachnoid Hemorrhage?

Fawaz Philip Tarzi, MD &
May Kim-Tenser, MD, MHA, FAHA

Case

A 60-year-old man is admitted following a spontaneous subarachnoid hemorrhage (SAH) from a rupture posterior communicating artery aneurysms. Notably, he has a history of coronary artery disease, heart failure with preserved ejection fraction, and moderate aortic stenosis. What type of hemodynamic monitoring should be considered in such a patient?

Key Points

- Current evidence that supports the use of invasive hemodynamic monitoring tools in patients diagnosed with spontaneous subarachnoid hemorrhage (SAH) is of limited quality.
- Hemodynamic derangements and management of the SAH patient is important in a neurocritical care unit, and the utility of invasive monitoring should be considered and assessed on a case-by-case basis.
- In certain patients with complicated hemodynamic and volume status management, the additional information from invasive monitoring may outweigh the risks.

BACKGROUND

SAH is a common diagnosis among patients in neurocritical care units which can lead to high rates of mortality and permanent disability. The overall prognosis of this disease has improved significantly, an observation that has been largely attributed to recent advances in medical and surgical management.[1] Most cases of spontaneous SAH are aneurysmal subarachnoid hemorrhages (aSAHs) which can lead to injury of many organs in addition to the brain. Up to 80% of patients diagnosed with SAH develop medical complications, including cardiac, pulmonary, renal, hepatic, hematological, metabolic, and endocrine dysfunction. The most common complications of SAH are myocardial dysfunction and pulmonary edema.[2]

Early identification of these complications can lead to early treatment and improved outcomes. Thus, many critical care clinicians attempt to monitor these complications with both invasive and noninvasive techniques. This chapter will review some of the more familiar invasive and noninvasive techniques that have been used to monitor patients diagnosed with spontaneous aSAH.[3,4]

EVIDENCE AND REVIEW

Arterial Lines and Central Venous Catheters

Arterial lines are used for continuous measurement of arterial blood pressure and its associated waveform. Arterial lines can also provide continuous measurements of mean arterial pressure (MAP) which can be used to measure continuous cerebral perfusion pressures in patients managed with intracranial pressure monitoring.[5] This procedure was first discovered in 1847 and was later modified upon the introduction of the Seldinger technique which involved the placement of a catheter into the lumen of the artery.[6]

Central venous catheters (CVCs) were first described in 1929 and are typically placed to provide access to a central vein and to maintain central venous pressure (CVP) monitoring. CVP measurements <8 cm H_2O suggest hypervolemia.[7] The results of a recent study published by Maissen et al[8] revealed that elevated CVPs correlated with increased intracranial pressure, notably in patients with hypervolemia. While the insertion procedure was initially modified to utilize the Seldinger technique, more recent modifications include the use of ultrasound guidance.

Arterial lines and CVCs are considered to be among the cornerstones of management and monitoring protocols for patients in critical care units. Many patients diagnosed with SAH are monitored with one or both of these devices, which represent the basis of several invasive techniques to be discussed in this chapter.

The Swan-Ganz Pulmonary Artery Catheter

The Swan-Ganz pulmonary artery catheter (PAC) was first introduced in the 1970s by Drs. Jeremy Swan and William Ganz as an alternative method for right heart catheterization that could be used to monitor patients in critical care settings.[9] The introduction of this device led to the increased use of invasive hemodynamic monitoring in critical care units worldwide, as it could be used to assess and monitor shock and circulatory dysfunction that might develop in response to any one of several etiologies. In 2000, it was estimated that 1.5 million PACs were sold in the United States alone. PACs were in wide use to monitor patients undergoing cardiac surgery as well as patients in cardiac, surgical, and medical intensive care units.[10] The device is inserted into a central vein and then advanced through the right side of the heart into the pulmonary artery. The tip of the catheter is placed in the main pulmonary artery; at this site, the balloon can be inflated and deflated to facilitate measurements of intrapulmonary pressure. The balloon is inflated to provide pulmonary capillary wedge pressures (PCWPs) that provide an indirect measurement of the left-sided cardiac filling pressures. The PAC also provides measurements of cardiac output (CO) via the thermodilution method. This method involves an injection of cold or room temperature fluid into the right atrium followed by an evaluation of the temperature change in the PAC. This measurement can identify CO as the volume of blood in circulation per unit of time.[11]

PACs have been in widespread use from 1980 through the early 2000s in multiple critical care settings and have been used frequently to monitor patients diagnosed with SAH. In one earlier study, Finn et al[12] reported on the outcomes of 32 patients diagnosed with aSAH who were maintained on a specific hemodynamic regimen. While 14 patients of the 32 aSAH patients developed neurological complications, improvements in PCWP led to the resolution of these deficits in several cases.

In another more recent study, 453 patients diagnosed with aSAH were divided into two groups. The first group included patients diagnosed with hypervolemia based on CVP and hypertension, while the second group received treatment to achieve normovolemia as defined by PCWP. The patients in the second group developed significantly fewer complications such as pulmonary edema and sepsis as well as decreased mortality. However, one limitation of this study was the lack of clarity as to whether euvolemia or simply the act of PAC monitoring was the reason for the observed reduction in complications.[13]

An article published in 1995 in *Neurosurgery* focused on the complications associated with Swan-Ganz catheterization performed for hemodynamic monitoring of patients diagnosed with SAH. As part of this study, Rosenwasser et al[14] found that 13% of the SAH patients developed catheter-related sepsis, 2% had congestive heart failure, 1.3% developed subclavian vein thrombosis, and 1% developed pneumothorax. The high rate of catheter-associated infection was attributed in part to the duration of the catheterization, which ranged from 7 to 19 days. This was substantially longer than the 48- to 72-hour duration of catheterization reported for the general critical care population. Other sources of infection were concurrent illnesses, for example, urinary tract infections or pneumonia.

Trends regarding the use of pulmonary artery catheterization for the aSAH population were evaluated based on data from the US National Inpatient Sample collected between 2000 and 2010. The overall trends included an overall decrease in the use of PAC over time among patients in this cohort. This trend correlates with the general decline in the use of PACs in critical care, given the lack of support for their use from large randomized controlled trials (RCTs)[15] as well as the emergence of less invasive and in some cases fully noninvasive monitoring devices.

Pulse Index Continuous Cardiac Output (PiCCO) Monitors

The device utilizes both arterial lines and CVCs to monitor a wide range of hemodynamic variables. This technology emerged in the early 1990s as the first calibrated arterial pressure wave analyzer. These devices have been modified since that time and are currently available as PiCCO plus and PiCCO2.[16] The device works by measuring CO based on the temperature change over time after injection of 10 to 15 mL of cold saline through a CVC via an arterial line with a thermistor device at its tip. The CO is calculated using the Stewart-Hamilton thermodilution equation. The device is capable of measuring stroke volume (SV) via a modified Wesseling equation (ie, SV = systolic area over impedance). Other hemodynamic values that can be measured by this device include stroke volume variation (SVV), cardiac index (CI), and pulse pressure variation (PVV)[16]

A recent study that focused on the importance of hemodynamic monitoring in patients with SAH and vasospasm enrolled 116 patients with aSAH and compared PiCCO monitoring against conventional management with either pulmonary artery catheterization or measurement of CVP. The results revealed that patients monitored by transpulmonary thermodilution using the PiCCO system were less likely to develop vasospasm (50% with PiCCO guidance vs. 66% with standard therapy). These patients also developed fewer cardiopulmonary complications secondary to medical therapy, such as pulmonary edema, arrhythmia, and vasogenic edema.[17]

PiCCO can also be used to calculate the pulmonary vascular permeability index (PVPI) which is the ratio of the extravascular lung water to pulmonary blood volume. Results from several studies have revealed that higher values of PVPI are associated with increased permeability of alveolocapillary walls, which is a finding that correlates with an increased incidence of pulmonary edema.[18]

Pulmonary edema develops in 10% to 29% of patients diagnosed with SAH and is a critical complication that significantly increases the risk of substantial morbidity and mortality.[19] The results of a study that enrolled 204 SAH patients in a multicenter cohort analysis revealed that the 52 patients who developed pulmonary edema were those with a higher mean extravascular lung water index (ELWI). Furthermore, the subset of patients who developed pulmonary edema group exhibited biphasic changes in PVPI (increased on day 6 and day 10 post-SAH), CI (decreased on day 2 and day 10 post-SAH), and global end-diastolic volume (GEDV) index (increased on days 6-14 post-SAH). These changes reflect our current understanding of the pathophysiology of pulmonary edema in this patient cohort. Specifically, patients diagnosed with SAH can develop early pulmonary edema secondary to cardiac failure as well as a later response that is more inflammatory in nature.[20]

Another study focused on the use of PiCCO to identify postoperative hemodynamic differences that develop in SAH patients who underwent either coiling or clipping of their SAH lesions. The results of this study revealed that while hemodynamics were similar during the early period postprocedure, during the vasospasm period, the group treated with a clipping procedure had an elevated PVPI and pulmonary edema compared to the group that underwent coiling. Additionally, the clipping group exhibited a higher average EVLWI compared to the coiling group, with a noted gradual improvement of the initial site of SAH.[21]

TABLE 36–1 Overview of subarachnoid hemorrhage invasive hemodynamic monitoring devices.

Device	Measurements Provided	Potential Use in SAH Patients
Arterial line	MAP	Continuous blood pressure monitoring; information used to facilitate continuous cerebral perfusion
Central venous catheter	CVP	Diagnosis of hypervolemia
FloTrac	CO, SV, SVV, PPV	Volume status for early goal-directed therapy
Pulse Index Continuous Cardiac Output (PiCCO)	CO, GEDV, SVV, CVP, PPV	Use decreases the incidence of complications related to pulmonary edema
Swan-Ganz pulmonary artery catheter	CO, RVEDV, CVP, PAP, PCWP	Used for hemodynamic monitoring during vasospasms and to prevent complications related to pulmonary edema and sepsis

CO, cardiac output; CVP, central venous pressure; GEDV, global end-diastolic volume; MAP, mean arterial pressure; PAP, pulmonary artery pressure; PCWP, pulmonary capillary wedge pressure; PPV, pulse pressure variation; RVEDV, right ventricular end-diastolic volume; SV, stroke volume; SVV, stroke volume variation.

The FloTrac System

The FloTrac system is a minimally invasive monitoring device that includes a sensor unit. It was developed in the early 2000s as a minimally invasive method that might be used instead of pulmonary artery catheterization or PiCCO.[22] The FloTrac system utilizes a pulse wave analysis technique to estimate blood flow and CO in a continuous fashion. It does not require external calibration but relies instead on individual demographic data, including weight, height, age, and sex. The direct relationship between arterial pulsatility, SV, and heart rate is used to calculate CO with adjustments made to arterial compliance based on demographic data. These monitoring devices are capable of calculating CO and SVV; if CVP is available, it will also provide values for systemic vascular resistance (SVR). These devices have been evaluated many times in cardiac surgery and intensive care units with varying results, albeit with a generally acceptable level of agreement with findings obtained using the more invasive monitoring techniques.[23]

An earlier study explored the role of FloTrac in perioperative hemodynamic monitoring in 16 patients who underwent surgical clipping to treat a SAH. The hemodynamic values obtained from the FloTrac were compared with findings obtained using the PiCCO system and CVP within 12 hours after surgery. Although the study enrolled only a few patients, the results revealed that the FloTrac system underestimated CI by 39.5% during surgery and by 30.6% among patients in the intensive care unit (ICU). Despite these somewhat discouraging results, SVV obtained using this system was found to be a useful predictor in patients with hypovolemia who were maintained on mechanical ventilation.[24] Another study assessed the use of FloTrac in a pilot RCT to assess the efficacy of early goal-directed therapy during endovascular repair of an aSAH. The study included 40 patients who were randomized to early goal-directed therapy using FloTrac data with a predetermined algorithm *versus* the control group. The results of this study revealed that patients were more likely to undergo early correction of hemodynamic derangements when FloTrac-based therapy was employed compared to the control group.

However, one limitation of this study was that patients were treated with the FloTrac system in the immediate reoperative period and that this modality has been validated only in intubated patients with a tidal volume of at least 8 mL/kg.[25]

Nonetheless, this minimally invasive method can be deployed rapidly, is easy to use, and requires no manual calibration. Based on findings in the current literature, we conclude that FloTrac provides additional information that might be used to assess volume status in mechanically ventilated aSAH patients (Table 36–1).

AVAILABLE GUIDELINES

Current American Heart Association guidelines for the management of SAH do offer a Class IIA recommendation for the monitoring of volume status in "certain patients" with SAH by "some combination of central venous pressure, pulmonary wedge pressure, and fluid balance."[26] However, they do not specify guidelines as to how these measurements should be obtained or which patients may be best candidates for invasive monitoring.

In parallel, the 2011 Neurocritical Care Society's Multidisciplinary Consensus Conference statement does state that "[m]onitoring of volume status may be beneficial" but that "[c]entral venous lines should not be placed solely to obtain CVP measures" and "[u]se of [pulmonary artery catheters (PACs)] incurs risk and lacks evidence of benefit. Routine use of PACS is not recommended."[27] They do note, however, that invasive monitoring technologies are available and that "no specific modality can be recommended over clinical assessment".

REFERENCES

1. Mackey J, Khoury JC, Alwell K, et al. Stable incidence but declining case-fatality rates of subarachnoid hemorrhage in a population. *Neurology*. 2016 Nov 22;87(21):2192–2197.
2. Rabinstein AA. Critical care of aneurysmal subarachnoid hemorrhage: state of the art. *Acta Neurochirurgica Supplement*. 2015;120:239–242.
3. Zaroff JG, Rordorf GA, Ogilvy CS, Picard MH. Regional patterns of left ventricular systolic dysfunction after subarachnoid hemorrhage: evidence for neurally mediated cardiac injury. *Journal of the American Society of Echocardiography*. 2000 Aug;13(8):774–779.
4. Muroi C, Keller M, Pangalu A, Fortunati M, Yonekawa Y, Keller E. Neurogenic pulmonary edema in patients with subarachnoid hemorrhage. *Journal of Neurosurgical Anesthesiology*. 2008 Jul;20(3):188–192.
5. Tse B, Burbridge MA, Jaffe RA, Brock-Utne J. Inaccurate blood pressure readings in the intensive care unit: an observational study. *Cureus*. 2018 Dec 11;10(12):e3716.
6. Pierre L, Pasrija D, Keenaghan M. Arterial Lines. In: StatPearls [Internet]. Treasure Island (FL): StatPearls Publishing; 2023 Jan.
7. Suarez JI, Shannon L, Zaidat OO, et al.: Effect of human albumin administration on clinical outcome and hospital cost in patients with subarachnoid hemorrhage. *Journal of Neurosurgery*. 2004 Apr;100(4):585–590.
8. Maissen G, Narula G, Strässle C, Willms J, Muroi C, Keller E. Functional relationship of arterial blood pressure, central venous pressure, and intracranial pressure in the early phase after subarachnoid hemorrhage. *Technology and Health Care*. 2022 May 12;30(3):591–604.
9. Thakkar AB, Desai SP. (2018) 'Swan, Ganz, and their catheter: Its evolution over the past half century', *Annals of Internal Medicine*, 169(9), p. 636. doi:10.7326/m17-2145.
10. Bernard GR, Sopko G, Cerra F, et al. Pulmonary artery catheterization and clinical outcomes. *JAMA*. 2000 May 17;283(19):2568.
11. Argueta EE, Paniagua D. Thermodilution cardiac output. *Cardiology in Review*. 2019 May;27(3):138–144.
12. Finn SS, Stephensen SA, Miller CA, Drobnich L, Hunt We. Observations on the perioperative management of aneurysmal subarachnoid hemorrhage. *Journal of Neurosurgery*. 1986 Jul;65(1):48–62.
13. Kim DH, Haney CL, van Ginhoven G. Reduction of pulmonary edema after SAH with a pulmonary artery catheter-guided hemodynamic management protocol. *Neurocritical Care*. 2005;3(1):11–15.
14. Rosenwasser RH, Jallo JI, Getch CC, Liebman KE. Complications of Swan-Ganz catheterization for hemodynamic monitoring in patients with subarachnoid hemorrhage. *Neurosurgery*. 1995 Nov 1;37(5):872–875.
15. Inouye S, Jin D, Cen S, et al. Trends in the use of pulmonary artery catheterization in the aneurysmal subarachnoid hemorrhage population. *Journal of Clinical Neuroscience*. 2016 Sep;31:133–136.
16. Hendy A, Bubenek S. Pulse waveform hemodynamic monitoring devices: recent advances and the place in goal-directed therapy in cardiac surgical patients. *Romanian Journal of Anaesthesia and Intensive Care*. 2016 Apr 1; 23(1):55–58.
17. Mutoh T, Kazumata K, Ishikawa T, Terasaka S. Performance of bedside transpulmonary thermodilution monitoring for goal-directed hemodynamic management after subarachnoid hemorrhage. *Stroke*. 2009 Jul;40(7):2368–2374.
18. Monnet X, Anguel N, Osman D, Hamzaoui O, Richard C, Teboul JL. Assessing pulmonary permeability by transpulmonary thermodilution allows differentiation of hydrostatic pulmonary edema from ALI/ARDS. *Intensive Care Medicine*. 2007 Feb 26;33(3):448–453.
19. Hoff RG, Rinkel GJ, Verweij BH, Algra A, Kalkman CJ. Pulmonary edema and blood volume after aneurysmal subarachnoid hemorrhage: a prospective observational study. *Critical Care*. 2010;14(2): R43.
20. Obata Y, Takeda J, Sato Y, Ishikura H, Matsui T, Isotani E. A multicenter prospective cohort study of volume management after subarachnoid hemorrhage: circulatory characteristics of pulmonary edema after subarachnoid hemorrhage. *Journal of Neurosurgery*. 2016 Aug;125(2):254–263.
21. Horie N, Iwaasa M, Isotani E, Ishizaka S, Inoue T, Nagata I. Impact of clipping versus coiling on postoperative hemodynamics and pulmonary edema after subarachnoid hemorrhage. *BioMed Research International*. 2014;2014:1–9.
22. Button D, Weibel L, Reuthebuch O, Genoni M, Zollinger A, Hofer CK. Clinical evaluation of the FloTrac/VigileoTM system and two established continuous cardiac output monitoring devices in patients undergoing cardiac surgery. *British Journal of Anaesthesia*. 2007 Sep;99(3):329–336.
23. Slagt C, Malagon I, Groeneveld ABJ. Systematic review of uncalibrated arterial pressure waveform analysis to determine cardiac output and stroke volume variation. *British Journal of Anaesthesia*. 2014 Apr;112(4):626–637.
24. Mutoh T, Ishikawa T, Nishino K, et al.: Evaluation of the FloTrac uncalibrated continuous cardiac output system for perioperative hemodynamic monitoring after subarachnoid hemorrhage. *Journal of Neurosurgical Anesthesiology*. 2009 Jul;21(3):218–225.
25. Chui J, Craen R, Dy-Valdez C, Alamri R, Boulton M, Pandey S, et al. Early goal-directed therapy during endovascular coiling procedures following aneurysmal subarachnoid hemorrhage: a pilot prospective randomized controlled study. *Journal of Neurosurgical Anesthesiology*. 2022 Jan;34(1):35–43.
26. Connolly ES, Rabinstein AA, Carhuapoma JR, Derdyn CP, Dion J, et al. Guidelines for the management of aneurysmal subarachnoid hemorrhage. *Stroke*. 2012 May;43:1711–1737.
27. Diringer MN, Bleck TP, Hemphill JC, et al.: Critical care management of patients following aneurysmal subarachnoid hemorrhage: recommendations from the Neurocritical Care Society's Multidisciplinary Consensus Conference. *Neurocritical Care*. 2011;15:211–240.

CHAPTER

37

What Is the Role of Albumin in Managing Aneurysmal Subarachnoid Hemorrhage?

Mariyam Humayun, MBBS, Jose I. Suarez, MD, & Rohan Mathur, MD, MPA

Case

A 57-year-old woman with a Hunt and Hess grade 2, modified Fisher grade 3 aneurysmal subarachnoid hemorrhage (aSAH) with a now secured anterior communicating artery aneurysm. On day 7 of her intensive care unit (ICU) care, she started to develop worsening confusion and left-side weakness. Patient's transcranial doppler reported increase in velocities in right internal carotid artery (ICA) and anterior cerebral artery (ACAs), and repeat computed tomography angiogram (CTA) head and neck showed moderate worsening of right anterior cerebral artery (RACA) vasospasm. She is clinically hypovolemic, and the ICU has started hydration with normal saline but it has resulted in worsening pulmonary edema. Should we start standing albumin to improve this patient's clinical outcome?

Key Points

- While data for the neuroprotective role of 25% human albumin in aneurysmal subarachnoid hemorrhage (aSAH) remain inconclusive, it is likely safe to use in specific scenarios.
- It can be used in conjunction with saline to maintain euvolemia in patients at risk of delayed cerebral ischemia where there is a concern for volume overload.
- Further research will help clarify if routine use of 25% human albumin is indicated in this patient population.

BACKGROUND

aSAH is a rare disease with an incidence of 6.1 per 100,000 person years.[1] It is associated with high mortality and morbidity despite advancements in critical care. Current treatment focuses on urgent securement of aneurysm and subsequent prevention of secondary brain injury such as rebleeding and delayed cerebral ischemia (DCI). This chapter provides an overview of the use and role of albumin in maintaining volume status in aSAH.

Albumin is one of the major proteins in the human body and has a multitude of beneficial properties at a molecular level. It exerts a potent antioxidant effect and can trap free radical species, preventing oxidative damage to tissues. With its ligand-binding abilities, it also helps in removing toxic products from plasma.[2] It is known to have anti-inflammatory and antiapoptotic properties which help in protecting the microvasculature and decrease vascular leakage.[3]

Volume status in aSAH is often a point of contention. Triple H therapy, once advocated for in aSAH, included hypervolemia as one of its components to prevent the development of cerebral vasospasm and DCI. Saline and human albumin were used in conjunction to achieve hypervolemia and higher central venous pressure goals.[4] Modern neurocritical care has shifted the paradigm toward euvolemia, given lack of benefit and possible adverse cardiopulmonary effects associated with hypervolemia.[5] Hypovolemia remains a risk factor for vasospasm, and DCI and should be avoided. Natriuresis, often associated with cerebral salt wasting common in aSAH, can increase risk for vasospasm and DCI.[6] Given the concern for hypovolemia and electrolyte disturbances, fluids are often necessary to prevent complications in aSAH. While crystalloids have become the mainstay for volume resuscitation in aSAH, human albumin can still be helpful in certain cases.

EVIDENCE AND REVIEW

Albumin in Critical Care

Use of human albumin in critical care is controversial. The SAFE study, a randomized clinical trial of ICU patients, showed that there was no mortality difference between use of 4% human albumin and normal saline.[7] A post-hoc analysis of the SAFE dataset investigated a subset of severe traumatic brain injury patients. There was an association between administration of 4% human albumin, choice of resuscitation fluid, and increased mortality.[8] In patients with sepsis, there have been no significantly different outcomes with either fluid type, although a trend toward improved mortality was seen in the human albumin group.[9]

Certain situations in intensive care may benefit from human albumin use. Albumin contributes to the majority of the intravascular oncotic pressure in the body. Given its colloid osmotic pressure, it is thought to have a higher likelihood to stay in the intravascular compartment compared to crystalloids. Thus, the volume of fluids being administered can be reduced with colloid use, which can be helpful in patients with concern about fluid status or underlying cardiopulmonary function.[10] Hypoalbuminemia is common in critically ill patients and has been associated with poor outcomes.[11] While data regarding albumin replacement leading to improved clinical outcomes remain inconclusive, it is often used in selective populations. It is used to increase efficacy of diuretics in patients with low albumin levels. Albumin is also used in liver disease for volume expansion after large volume paracentesis and in spontaneous bacterial peritonitis.[10]

Neuroprotective Effects of Albumin

With its abundant antioxidant and anti-inflammatory properties, human albumin has been explored as a neuroprotective agent. Preclinical studies have shown that albumin prevents oxidant-driven neuronal injury and reduces DNA damage and cell death in cultured neurons.[12] It may play a role in neuronal differentiation, cell signaling, and activation of inflammatory pathways.[12] Initial studies in ischemic stroke models produced promising results with use of 25% human albumin. Animal ischemic stroke models demonstrated improvement in neurological scores, brain swelling, and reduction in infract volume.[13] A phase 3 randomized, placebo-controlled trial tested the superiority of 25% human albumin over isotonic saline in acute ischemic stroke patients. It did not show any benefit in the 90-day primary, functional outcome between the two groups.[14] Patients in the human albumin group did have higher rates of pulmonary edema, congestive heart failure, and symptomatic intracranial hemorrhage.[14] Human albumin is also being investigated for its therapeutic role in Alzheimer's disease, given it can bind and prevent polymerization of amyloid-beta protein. Further clinical studies are needed to see if this translates into clinical benefit.[12]

Therapeutic Role of Human Albumin in aSAH

DCI is one of the most dreaded complications in aSAH. Thus, after the initial promising results with ischemic stroke studies, 25% human albumin was also assessed for a possible neuroprotective benefit in aSAH.

A retrospective study with 164 patients evaluated use of 25% human albumin in aSAH patients with particular focus on functional outcomes and hospital cost; 25% human albumin and/or saline were used to achieve hypervolemia with goal central venous pressure of >8 mm Hg. A subgroup analysis, strictly comparing 25% human albumin to the nonalbumin group, showed a trend toward improved mortality and significantly improved 3-month functional outcomes (Odds Ratio [OR] 3.2, 95% confidence interval 1.10-11) in the albumin group. The study concluded that 25% human albumin administration likely improved mortality and reduced inpatient hospital cost associated with aSAH. Authors were able to debunk some negative associations with human albumin, though it is to keep in mind that this was an observational study and definitive conclusions cannot be made.[4]

The albumin in subarachnoid hemorrhage (ALISAH) was a multicenter pilot trial to assess the safety and tolerability of 25% human albumin in this disease process.[15] Forty-eight patients were enrolled in a multitier dose escalation protocol; 25% human albumin doses < 1.25 g/kg/day for 7 consecutive days were found to be safe to use in aSAH. Higher doses were associated with adverse cardiovascular effects including volume overload and pulmonary edema. Authors also noted a trend toward improved functional outcome with 25% human albumin use. Patients who received 1.25 g/kg/day of 25% human albumin did have a dose-dependent response, and better functional scores were noted at 3 months when compared to other doses of albumin administered in the study.[15] Given the results from this study, a phase II randomized clinical trial, ALISAH II, has been designed. This ongoing study will help to delineate potential effects of 25% human albumin on DCI, cerebral edema, and long-term outcomes in aSAH. ALISAH II also will afford the opportunity to study potential biomarkers associated with potential mechanisms of action of 25% human albumin and inform future studies and strengthen the scientific premise. Of particular interest will be the effect of 25% human albumin on the integrity of the endothelial glycocalyx and the neurovascular unit. If the results of ALISAH II demonstrate salutary effects of 25% human albumin, then a definitive phase III clinical trial to investigate its efficacy will be undertaken (Table 37–1).

TABLE 37–1 Major studies looking at the efficacy of human albumin in neurocritical care patient populations of interest.

Author (year)	Study Design (*n*)	Population	Conclusion
Finfer et al (2004)	Randomized clinical trial (RCT)	General ICU	No difference in mortality with 4% albumin
Myburgh et al (2007)[8]	Post hoc follow-up RCT	Traumatic brain injury (TBI)	Higher mortality rates with albumin
Suarez et al (2004)	Retrospective observational (164)	aSAH	Improved clinical outcome, reduced cost with albumin
Suarez et al (2012)	Phase 1, pilot study (47)	aSAH	Albumin dose up to 1.25 g/kg/day was safe to use
Ginsberg et al (2013)	Phase III randomized controlled trial	Ischemic stroke	No clinical benefit of 25% albumin over normal saline (stopped early due to futility)

Hypoalbuminemia in critically sick patients has been associated with higher rates of infectious complications. Hospital course for aSAH is often complicated by nosocomial infections. An observational cohort study in aSAH reported that patients with low albumin levels on admission or with decreasing albumin levels in the first 3 days had higher rates of hospital-acquired infections.[16] The investigators of the ALISAH II study will be collecting information on adverse effects including nosocomial infections to determine whether their rate is higher in the 25% human albumin group compared to the saline group.

AVAILABLE GUIDELINES

No existing guidelines to use albumin in SAH. Existing literature for 25% human albumin use in aSAH has shown some promising results with potential to possibly help in particular complications of SAH. It may be worthwhile for future studies to also evaluate specific ICU outcomes including renal and infectious complications.

REFERENCES

1. Etminan N, Chang HS, Hackenberg K, et al.: Worldwide incidence of aneurysmal subarachnoid hemorrhage according to region, time period, blood pressure, and smoking prevalence in the population: a systematic review and meta-analysis.*JAMA Neurol.* 2019;76(5):588–597. doi:10.1001/jamaneurol.2019.0006
2. Roche M, Rondeau P, Singh NR, et al.: The antioxidant properties of serum albumin.*FEBS Lett.* 2008;582(13):1783–1787. doi:10.1016/j.febslet.2008.04.057
3. Vincent JL, Russell JA, Jacob M, et al.: Albumin administration in the acutely ill: what is new and where next? [published correction appears in Crit Care. 2014;18(6):630. Roca, Ricard Ferrer [corrected to Ferrer, Ricard]]. *Crit Care.* 2014;18(4):231. Published 2014 Jul 16. doi:10.1186/cc13991
4. Suarez JI, Shannon L, Zaidat OO, et al.: Effect of human albumin administration on clinical outcome and hospital cost in patients with subarachnoid hemorrhage.*J Neurosurg.* 2004;100(4):585–590. doi:10.3171/jns.2004.100.4.0585
5. Keyrouz SG, Diringer MN. Clinical review: Prevention and therapy of vasospasm in subarachnoid hemorrhage. *Crit Care.* 2007;11(4):220. doi:10.1186/cc5958
6. Brown RJ, Epling BP, Staff I, et al.: Polyuria and cerebral vasospasm after aneurysmal subarachnoid hemorrhage. *BMC Neurol.* 2015;15:201. Published 2015 Oct 13. doi:10.1186/s12883-015-0446-6
7. Finfer S, Bellomo R, Boyce N, et al.: A comparison of albumin and saline for fluid resuscitation in the intensive care unit. *N Engl J Med.* 2004;350(22):2247–2256. doi:10.1056/NEJMoa040232
8. SAFE Study Investigators, Australian and New Zealand Intensive Care Society Clinical Trials Group, Australian Red Cross Blood Service. Saline or albumin for fluid resuscitation in patients with traumatic brain injury. *N Engl J Med.* 2007;357(9):874–884. doi:10.1056/NEJMoa067514
9. SAFE Study Investigators, Finfer S, McEvoy S, et al.: Impact of albumin compared to saline on organ function and mortality of patients with severe sepsis. *Intensive Care Med.* 2011;37(1):86–96. doi:10.1007/s00134-010-2039-6
10. Melia D, Post B. Human albumin solutions in intensive care: A review. *J Intensive Care Soc.* 2021;22(3):248–254. doi:10.1177/1751143720961245
11. Vincent JL, Dubois MJ, Navickis RJ, et al.: Hypoalbuminemia in acute illness: is there a rationale for intervention? A meta-analysis of cohort studies and controlled trials. *Ann Surg.* 2003;237(3):319–334. doi:10.1097/01.SLA.0000055547.93484.87
12. Prajapati KD, Sharma SS, Roy N. Current perspectives on potential role of albumin in neuroprotection. *Rev Neurosci.* 2011;22(3):355–363. doi:10.1515/RNS.2011.028
13. Belayev L, Liu Y, Zhao W, et al.: Human albumin therapy of acute ischemic stroke: marked neuroprotective efficacy at moderate doses and with a broad therapeutic window. *Stroke.* 2001;32(2):553–560. doi:10.1161/01.str.32.2.553
14. Ginsberg MD, Palesch YY, Hill MD, et al.: High-dose albumin treatment for acute ischaemic stroke (ALIAS) Part 2: a randomised, double-blind, phase 3, placebo-controlled trial. *Lancet Neurol.* 2013;12(11):1049–1058. doi:10.1016/S1474-4422(13)70223-0
15. Suarez JI, Martin RH, Calvillo E, et al.: The Albumin in Subarachnoid Hemorrhage (ALISAH) multicenter pilot clinical trial: safety and neurologic outcomes. *Stroke.* 2012;43(3):683–690. doi:10.1161/STROKEAHA.111.633958
16. Wang P, Zhang Y, Wang X, et al.: Association between serum albumin and hospital-acquired infections after aneurysmal subarachnoid hemorrhage [published online ahead of print, 2021 Dec 30]. *Neurocrit Care.* 2021;10.1007/s12028-021-01421-y. doi:10.1007/s12028-021-01421-y

CHAPTER

38

What Is the Role of Mechanical and Chemical Thrombectomy in Venous Sinus Thrombosis?

Daniel M. S. Raper, MBBS

Case

A 55-year-old woman with history of factor 5 leiden, hypertension (HTN), and diabetes mellitus (DM) presented with 5 days of worsening headache and nausea. Capillary transit time heterogeneity (CTH) showed right parietal cortical bleed. Clinical target volume (CTV) showed right transverse sinus thrombosis. She was started on therapeutic Lovenox, however, continued to have headache, and 2 days later started to have left-side weakness. Repeat CTV on day 5 showed worsening of right transverse sinus thrombosis with extension to jugular view. When should we consider endovascular intervention for patients with cerebral venous sinus thrombosis (CVST)?

Key Points

- There are two situations where endovascular thrombectomy (EVT) is reasonable. First, if the patient is in extremis—usually comatose, potentially with elevated intracranial pressure or with a large burden of venous infarction. Second, if the patient fails to improve neurologically or worsens within the first few days after initiation of anticoagulation.
- Performing EVT safely for these patients may provide a reasonable risk-to-benefit ratio and promote revascularization of an occluded sinus earlier than anticoagulation alone.
- Mechanical thrombectomy alone, usually with stent retriever in addition to suction with a large bore catheter, and with the addition of intrasinus infusion of thrombolytic are both reasonable options.
- Unfortunately, due to the relative rarity of severe cerebral venous sinus thrombosis (CVST) cases and the paucity of high-level evidence guiding intervention, the exact target population, timing, and techniques that will result in the optimal outcomes for refractory CVST patients are likely to remain neurologic intensive care unit (neuroICU) dilemmas for some time.

BACKGROUND

Although many patients with CVST remain neurologically intact, a minority of cases can lead to significant management dilemmas for the intensivist and neurosurgeon or neurointerventionalist. Current guidelines from the European Stroke Organization leave endovascular intervention out of their treatment algorithm,[1] and U.S. recommendations suggest that endovascular therapy should be considered only for patients who are comatose or who deteriorate despite first-line anticoagulation.[2,3] Let's dig into this idea in a little more detail to understand how to identify a refractory case.

Common symptoms associated with CVST include headache, which becomes progressively more severe, followed by seizures and ischemic or hemorrhagic stroke.[4] Seizures can be focal or generalized and occurred in 34% of patients in a large study within a week after thrombosis.[5] Localizing neurological deficits usually follow hours to days after the initial headache.[4] Papilledema can develop over the course of days to weeks after CVST (Table 38–1). The difficulty with these symptoms, when it comes to decision-making for patients, is that they develop slowly and unpredictably. The normal time course for the evolution of symptoms in CVST is hours to days, but progression may extend over the course of weeks in some cases.[4] Most practitioners therefore wait until after progression occurs, or after a patient deteriorates with new symptoms, before considering interventional options.

TABLE 38–1 Cerebral venous sinus thrombosis symptoms associated with poor outcome.

Endovascular intervention may be considered in these cases
Altered mental state
Seizure
Deep venous sinus thrombus
Long segment superior sagittal sinus thrombus
Coma
ICH

ICH, intracranial hemorrhage.

EVIDENCE AND REVIEW

Despite the presence of intracranial hemorrhage (ICH), the best initial treatment is anticoagulation. For most patients, anticoagulation is safe even with mild or moderate burden of subarachnoid hemorrhage (SAH) or ICH. A review article on CVST published in 2021 in the *New England Journal of Medicine* summarized the balance of evidence for anticoagulation in the treatment of CVST.[4] It turns out that evidence of anticoagulation is not strong, and a Cochrane review on the topic concluded that heparin can be safe, but the evidence supporting its efficacy in treating established thrombus within a cerebral venous sinus is rather weak.[6] Treatment in the acute phase is primarily with low-molecular-weight heparin, in preference to unfractionated heparin.[7] In the chronic phase, direct oral anticoagulants are probably a better choice than warfarin due to a better safety profile.[8–10] With modern medical therapy, about a third of comatose CVST patients can have a full recovery.[11] The key to successful clinical outcome appears to be achieving recanalization of the venous sinuses. Both warfarin and dabigatran were associated with good rates of recanalization (about two-thirds of cases),[8] but predicting which patients are going to respond well is still a challenge. Of course, identifying and treating any underlying causes for CVST are an essential part of the management of this condition.

How Long Should You Wait Before You Say that Medical Treatment Has Failed?

There is no consensus on this point. It is reasonable to consider endovascular thrombectomy (EVT) for patients who deteriorate within 24 to 48 hours from the initiation of anticoagulation. For patients who present *in extremis*, it is reasonable to consider EVT after lifesaving measures such as decompressive hemicraniectomy or CSF drainage have been performed.

Is Endovascular Thrombectomy Safe? Is It Effective?

A few review articles have summarized the literature on EVT for CVST. Earlier review articles emphasize that mechanical thrombectomy (MT) should be reserved for patients with "a very severe presentation or rapidly declining neurological symptoms despite appropriate anticoagulant therapy."[12] But as the tools we have at our disposal have dramatically improved, more interventionalists are willing to attempt MT earlier in the course for these patients. Reported rates of near to complete recanalization, in a systematic review of studies conducted between 1995 and 2004, were almost 75%, and despite 47% of patients being in a stuporous or comatose state prior to intervention, good outcome was achieved in 85% of patients after intervention.[5] Most cases (70%) utilized intrasinus thrombolysis in addition to the MT.

On the other hand, an analysis of the Nationwide Inpatient Sample from 2004 to 2014 suggested that patients who received EVT had higher mortality, with an odds ratio of 1.96, after adjustment for age and other complications.[13]

More recently, a randomized trial has attempted to provide a higher level of evidence to guide the use of EVT in CVST patients. The TO-ACT (Thrombolysis or Anticoagulation for Cerebral Venous Thrombosis) trial was a multicenter, open-label, blinded endpoint RCT conducted in the Netherlands, China, and Portugal and reported in *JAMA Neurology* in 2020.[14] Patients with at least one risk factor for a poor outcome (including altered mental status, ICH, or deep venous system thrombosis) were randomized to either EVT or anticoagulation only. EVT included MT, intravenous thrombolysis, or both. The primary outcome was the proportion of patients with a good outcome, defined as modified Rankin Scale (mRS) of 0 to 1 at 12 months, and there were no significant differences between the groups (about 70% of patients reached the good outcome in both groups), and in fact the trial was stopped early because of no difference in the primary outcome.

In contrast to this negative result, a more modern literature review of 235 patients from 17 studies reported better outcomes with EVT.[15] Forty percent of patients were in a coma or had severe encephalopathy before they were taken for EVT, a large majority of cases (88%) included thrombolysis, and complete radiographic resolution was achieved in 70% of patients.[15]

The dramatic increase in the use of endovascular treatments for acute stroke has brought with it an explosion of new devices and techniques, from large bore catheters that are designed for navigating into the distal intracranial vessels to stent retrievers and balloons that are safer and more compliant. These devices mean that EVT can be attempted safely in CVST, even if the evidence from older studies and large trials has not supported its widespread use yet.

Is EVT Safe in Patients with Large Intracranial Hemorrhage (ICH)?

EVT appears to be equally safe and effective in CVST patients regardless of the presence of ICH. Of course, large ICH should prompt evaluation for surgical decompression.[16] However, the presence of ICH in and of itself is not a contraindication to endovascular therapy.

Should Endovascular Thrombolysis Be Attempted Before, Instead of, or Together with Mechanical Thrombectomy?

There is no good modern comparison in the literature on this topic, so different interventionalists will have different practices and a variety of approaches are reasonable. Nonrandomized attempts to compare intrasinus thrombolysis with MT have not been able to show differences in outcomes.[17,18] Most of the series that report outcomes after EVT include patients treated with both MT alone as well as MT with intrasinus thrombolysis, often in most cases.[19] Some surgeons will wait for failure of MT first before trying intra-sinus thrombolytic infusion, potentially avoiding an increased bleeding risk. A systematic review of earlier literature from over a decade ago suggested that thrombolysis was associated with a significant increase in major bleeding.[20] Newer endovascular techniques in which more thrombolytic medication is infused either through a microcatheter within the clot or via a larger bore aspiration catheter at the clot face may have a better safety profile, but evidence for this is purely anecdotal.

How Do You Judge a Successful Mechanical Thrombectomy in Venous Sinus Thrombosis? Are There Any Other Endovascular Techniques that Can Be Useful?

CVST can be challenging and unrewarding to attack endovascularly. Clots are typically large in diameter and extend for long segments of the intracranial sinuses. Often, a contiguous clot will extend from the mid-superior sagittal sinus all the way down to the jugular bulb! Attempting to remove all of this clot is a fool's errand, and typically multiple passes of a stent retriever designed for removal of thromboemboli from intracranial arteries result in fragments of thrombus at each pass. Achieving a channel through the clot is a victory, even if it seems narrow. Other endovascular techniques have been described, such as dragging a compliant balloon from distal to proximal into a large bore aspiration catheter.[21] These remain the realm of case reports, but they may be useful to consider in refractory cases.

Does Mechanical Thrombectomy Improve Intracranial Pressure?

Endovascular therapy aims at recanalizing the sinus and is therefore an indirect treatment for ICP. Although it may lower intracranial pressure over time, it should not replace decompressive hemicraniectomy in patients with refractory ICP issues or concern for herniation. Decompressive hemicraniectomy is an effective treatment for elevated ICP and, in those cases in which herniation is imminent, is lifesaving.

What About CVST Associated with Hypercoagulable States like Heparin-induced Thrombocytopenia (HIT)?

Thankfully, this is extremely rare. In these cases, heparin and platelet infusions are contraindicated. Medical treatment consists of intravenous immune globulin (IVIg) or plasma exchange along with a nonheparin anticoagulant like fondaparinux, argatroban, rivaroxaban, or apixaban.[22] EVT is not contraindicated and may be considered earlier in the treatment paradigm than for other cases.

AVAILABLE GUIDELINES

Current guidelines from the European Stroke Organization leave endovascular intervention out of their treatment algorithm,[1] and U.S. American Heart Association/American Stroke Association and Society of NeuroInterventional Surgery recommendations suggest that endovascular therapy should be considered only for patients who are comatose or who deteriorate despite first-line anticoagulation.[2,3]

REFERENCES

1. Ferro JM, Bousser M-G, Canhao P, et al. European Stroke Organization guideline for the diagnosis and treatment of cerebral venous thrombosis—endorsed by the European Academy of Neurology. *Eur J Neurol* 2017;24: 1203–1213.
2. Saposnik G, Barinagarrementeria F, Brown RD Jr, et al. Diagnosis and management of cerebral venous thrombosis: a statement for healthcare professionals from the American Heart Association/American Stroke Association. *Stroke* 2011;42:1158–1192.
3. Lee SK, Mokin M, Hetts SW, et al. Current endovascular strategies for cerebral venous thrombosis: report of the SNIS Standards and Guidelines Committee. *J Neurointerv Surg* 2018;10:803–810.
4. Ropper AH, Klein JP. Cerebral venous thrombosis. *N Engl J Med* 2021;385: 59–64.
5. Lindgren E, Silvis SM, Hiltunen S, et al. Acute symptomatic seizures in cerebral venous thrombosis. *Neurology* 2020;95(12):e1706–e1715.
6. Coutinho J, de Bruijn SF, Deveber G, Stam J. Anticoagulation for cerebral venous sinus thrombosis. *Cochrane Database Syst Rev* 2011;8:CD002005.
7. Misra UK, Kalita J, Chandra S, et al. Low molecular weight heparin versus unfractionated heparin in cerebral venous sinus thrombosis: a randomized controlled trial. *Eur J Neurol* 2012;19:1030–1036.
8. Ferro JM, Coutinho JM, Dentali F, et al. Safety and efficacy of dabigatran etexilate vs dose-adjusted warfarin in patients with cerebral venous thrombosis: a randomized clinical trial. *JAMA Neurol* 2019;76:1457–1465.
9. Yaghi S, Shu L, Bakradze E, et al. Direct oral anticoagulants versus warfarin in the treatment of cerebral venous thrombosis (ACTION-CVT): a multicenter international study. *Stroke* 2022;53:728–738.
10. Giles JA, Balasetti VKS, Zazulia AR. Non-vitamin K antagonist oral anticoagulants for the treatment of cerebral venous sinus thrombosis: a retrospective, matched cohort analysis. *Neurocrit Care* 2021;35:783–788.
11. Ferro JM, Aguiar de Sousa D. Cerebral venous thrombosis: an update. *Curr Neurol Neurosci Rep* 2019;19:74.
12. Capecchi M, Abbattista M, Martinelli I. Cerebral venous sinus thrombosis. *J Thromb Haemost* 2018;16:1918–1931.
13. Siddiqui FM, Weber MW, Dandapat S, et al. Endovascular thrombolysis or thrombectomy for cerebral venous thrombosis: study of Nationwide Inpatient Sample 2004-2014. *J Stroke Cerebrovasc Dis* 2019;28(6):1440–1447.
14. Coutinho JM, Zuurbier SM, Bousser MG, et al. Effect of endovascular treatment with medical management vs standard care on severe cerebral venous thrombosis: the TO-ACT randomized clinical trial. *JAMA Neurol* 2020;77:966–973.

15. Ilyas A, Chen C-J, Raper DM, et al. Endovascular mechanical thrombectomy for cerebral venous sinus thrombosis: a systematic review. *J Neurointerv Surg* 2017;9:1086–1092.
16. Hemphill JC 3rd, Greenberg SM, Anderson CS, Becker K, Bendok BR, Cushman M, et al. Guidelines for the management of spontaneous intracerebral hemorrhage: a guideline for healthcare professionals from the American Heart Association/American Stroke Association. *Stroke* 2015;46: 2032–2060.
17. Stam J, Majoie CBLM, van Delden OM, et al. Endovascular thrombectomy and thrombolysis for severe cerebral sinus thrombosis. A prospective study. *Stroke* 2008;39:1487–1490.
18. Siddiqui FM, Banerjee C, Zuurbier M, et al. Mechanical thrombectomy versus intrasinus thrombolysis for cerebral venous sinus thrombosis: a nonrandomized comparison. *Intervent Neuroradiol* 2014:20:336–344.
19. Siddiqui FM, Dandapat S, Banerjee C, et al. Mechanical thrombectomy in cerebral venous thrombosis: systematic review of 185 cases. *Stroke* 2015;46:1263–1268.
20. Dentali F, Squizzato A, Gianni M, et al. Safety of thrombolysis in cerebral venous thrombosis. A systematic review of the literature. *Thromb Haemost* 2010;104(5):1055–1062.
21. Kojima D, Akamatsu Y, Yoshida J, et al. Drag-out technique using a large balloon fixed with an aspiration catheter for retrieving residual thrombus on the wall of the superior sagittal sinus: illustrative case. *J Neurosurg Case Lessons* 2022;3(21):CASE22116.
22. Greinacher A, Selleng K, Warkentin TE. Autoimmune heparin-induced thrombocytopenia. *J Thromb Haemost* 2017;15:2099–2114.

CHAPTER

39

How Do We Manage Postoperative Venous Sinus Thrombosis?

Turki Elarjani, MD, Michael Silva, MD, & Carolina G. Benjamin, MD, FAANS

Case

A 45-year-old woman underwent a suboccipital approach for a right posterior fossa tumor. Postop day 5, she started to complain of worsening headaches and nausea. Computerized tomography of the head (CTH) showed expected postoperative changes with signs of worsening cerebellar edema and a small right cerebellar bleed. Cerebral venous thrombosis (CVT) was done and showed right transverse sinus thrombosis. How should we best manage postoperative CVT?

Key Points

- Postoperative cerebral venous thrombosis (CVT) is more frequent than previously thought and is often undetected due to the lack of symptoms and dedicated imaging.
- In case CVT involves dominant sinuses, there is a high risk of cerebrospinal fluid leak that may require permanent diversion.
- There is a growing body of literature that supports that anticoagulation is unnecessary unless patients present with signs and symptoms of venous infarction, involvement of the superior sagittal sinus, dominant transverse sinus with poor collaterals, deep venous system, or elevated intracranial pressure.

BACKGROUND

Spontaneous CVT is a rare disease that predominantly affects women (76%) with an estimated incidence of 3/1,000,000.[1] When compared to arterial stroke, venous ischemia and infarction constitute up to 1% of strokes.[2] Risk factors include hypercoagulable state, pregnancy, oral contraceptives, cancer, postpartum, and surgery.[3] Signs and symptoms are attributed to venous congestion, and in turn, elevated intracranial pressure (ICP) that can range from headache, nausea/vomiting, and papilledema to intracerebral hemorrhage (ICH). Treatment for spontaneous CVT is to initiate anticoagulation regardless of ICH.[3] Postoperative CVT can occur after surgery surrounding any dural venous sinus and is commonly seen after posterior fossa surgeries adjacent to the transverse-sigmoid sinuses.[4] In contrast to spontaneous CVT, there is no particular preponderance in gender or age group.[5–7] Previously, the incidence of postoperative CVT was thought to be 6% to 11%; however, recent prospective studies have documented that the incidence can be as high as 39%.[6,7] There seems to be a tendency to develop CVT most commonly after the translabyrinthine approach followed by the retrosigmoid approach, which could be attributed to extensive sinus exposure, sinus desiccation, and thermal conduction of the microscope lamp or drill.[5,7,8] Interestingly, rates of CVT are not dependent on the duration of operation or pathology encountered.[6,8]

EVIDENCE AND REVIEW

Which Cerebral Sinus Is Most Commonly Involved?

Postoperative CVT most commonly occurs on the ipsilateral side of surgery, especially on the nondominant sinus.[6,7] It can be speculated that the nondominant sinus is amenable for thrombosis, given the smaller caliber, less collateral flow, and slow venous flow with stagnation risk. Less commonly, postoperative CVT can involve the superior sagittal sinus or deep venous systems such as the internal cerebral veins. In three studies, CVT was incidentally diagnosed or symptoms were attributed to headache, vomiting, and cerebrospinal fluid (CSF) leak; all patients were scanned within 5 days of surgery.[9–11] Studies

TABLE 39–1 Summary of the current literature.

Author (Year)	Study Type	Number of Patients with CVT	Sinus Involved	Dominance	Symptoms	Treatment	Outcome
Moore et al (2014)	Retrospective	5/43 (11.6%)	Right: Transverse (4), sigmoid (1), internal jugular (1) Left: Transverse (1)	Right (4)	Asymptomatic (4) Ataxia and incoordination (1)	Anticoagulation (5)	No hemorrhage or infarct (4), improved ataxia (1)
Apra et al (2017)	Retrospective	12/180 (6.7%)	No laterality mentioned; transverse (8) and sigmoid (11)	NA	Asymptomatic (12)	Anticoagulation (7) Conservative (5)	No hemorrhage or infarct (12), recanalization of patients treated (7); no recanalization of conservative management (5)
Abou-Al-Shaar (2018)	Retrospective	7/116 (6%)	Right: Transverse (3), sigmoid (3), and internal jugular (2) Left: Transverse (3), sigmoid (4), internal jugular (1)	Right (2)	Asymptomatic (7)	Anticoagulation (7)	ICH, Intraventricular, and subdural hemorrhage (1), no hemorrhage or infarct (6)
Benjamin et al (2018)	Prospective	24/74 (32.4%)	NA	NA	Asymptomatic (24)	Conservative (24)	No hemorrhage or infarct (24)
Guazzo et al (2020)	Prospective	21/54 (38.9%)	No laterality, transverse (8); sigmoid (20), internal jugular (10)	No laterality; dominant (17)	Asymptomatic (21)	Conservative (21)	No hemorrhage or infarct (21)
Kow et al (2020)	Retrospective	20/126 (15.8%)	NA	No laterality, dominant (10)	Asymptomatic (17), confusion (2), decreased level of consciousness (1)	Conservative (16), anticoagulation (4)	Death (1), no hemorrhage or infarction (19)

CVT, cerebral venous thrombosis; ICH, intracerebral hemorrhage.

showed that CSF leak is associated with postoperative CVT especially in a dominant sinus, and the need for a ventriculoperitoneal shunt is more likely in a dominant sinus thrombosis.[6,7] Despite a higher than anticipated incidence, postoperative CVTs are mostly asymptomatic and are found incidentally on postoperative imaging studies.[9–11] Overall, postoperative CVTs are higher than previously thought and often undetected due to the lack of symptoms and dedicated imaging modalities such as computed tomography (CT) venograms, MR venograms, or formal diagnostic angiograms are not regularly ordered.

Should I Start Anticoagulation to Treat Postoperative CVT?

Treatment of postoperative CVT is a more controversial topic, as the supporting literature is limited. There is a potential risk of stroke and edema if CVT left untreated versus potentially catastrophic hemorrhage if fully anticoagulated. Moore et al reported their results with no increased risk of bleeding after having anticoagulated their postoperative CVT patients with fractionated heparin bridged with warfarin.[12] There have been other studies demonstrating that anticoagulation for postoperative CVT does not alter the rates of sinus recanalization.[4,5,7] Furthermore, one study reported a hemorrhagic complication with an epidural and intracerebral hematoma with intraventricular extension from anticoagulation, thus highlighting the potential risks.[5] Given the potential risks of anticoagulation, other studies have recommended observation and intravenous hydration. Benjamin et al studied 74 patients who underwent retrosigmoid, middle fossa, and translabyrinthine approach and found 24 patients (32.4%) with CVT. Furthermore, 23/24 of patients with CVT were managed conservatively with prophylactic anticoagulation dose without adverse events while one patient was started on intravenous hydration based on the physician's preference.[6] Similarly, Kow et al performed postoperative scan within 1 week to 6 months in patients who experienced a decline in mental status and managed their patients with occlusive thrombosis conservatively, started anticoagulation in 4/20 patients, and only 1 mortality related to occlusive CVT was reported.[8] Guazzo et al presented 21 patients with postoperative CVT, and all were treated conservatively and remained asymptomatic.[7] Further, they recommended anticoagulation treatment only when patients demonstrate symptoms of elevated ICP or venous infarction.[7] Thus, postoperative CVT of the transverse sinus has a more benign course of what was thought of previously and aggressive management may carry higher risks than benefits unless progressive symptoms are experienced warranting anticoagulation.

Nondominant transverse sinus thromboses are usually asymptomatic with good outcomes; however, thromboses in dominant transverse sinus, the superior sagittal sinus, or deep venous system are poor. For example, Chang et al presented their case of a patient who underwent transsphenoidal resection of a craniopharyngioma that was diagnosed with a 4-week postoperative CVT at the superior sagittal sinus and right transverse sinus after episodes of vomiting.[9] The patient was managed with anticoagulation, transvenous thrombolysis, and mechanical thrombectomy yet passed away after 4 days despite aggressive management. Similarly, Tan et al reported a case of a pediatric patient who underwent craniotomy and resection of a pineal germ cell tumor that subsequently developed a right-sided internal cerebral vein thrombosis.[11] The patient did not have predisposing factors for hypercoagulation; however, possible causes of the thrombosis could pertain to surgical manipulation of internal cerebral veins. The child was managed conservatively, and upon discharge, there is minimal residual weakness of the left side. The patient developed visual field deficits, seizures, and left hemiplegia; however, the authors treated the patient conservatively with subsequent improvement in symptoms except impairment in memory and behavior.[11] The improvement in neurological status is likely related to the patient's age.[11] Liu et al reported a case of right transverse sinus thrombosis after an elective tonsillectomy.[10] The patient was treated with a transvenous thrombolysis followed by anticoagulation due to progressive headaches with partial resolution of thrombus and symptoms improvement at follow-up. Hence, postoperative thromboses of the dominant transverse, superior sagittal sinus, and deep venous system have a different natural history and worse outcomes if left untreated. Pediatric population may have a better outcome; however, literature in pediatric CVT is lacking (Table 39–1).

REFERENCES

1. Pizzi MA, Alejos DA, Siegel JL, Kim BY, Miller DA, Freeman WD. Cerebral venous thrombosis associated with intracranial hemorrhage and timing of anticoagulation after hemicraniectomy. *J Stroke Cerebrovasc Dis.* 2016;25(9):2312–2316.
2. Stam J. Thrombosis of the cerebral veins and sinuses. *N Engl J Med.* 2005;352:1791–1798.
3. Saposnik G, Barinagarrementeria F, Brown RD Jr, et al. Diagnosis and management of cerebral venous thrombosis: a statement for healthcare professionals from the American Heart Association/American Stroke Association. *Stroke.* 2011;42:1158–1192.
4. Apra C, Kotbi O, Turc G, et al. Presentation and management of lateral sinus thrombosis following posterior fossa surgery. *J Neurosurg.* 2017;126:8–16.
5. Abou-Al-Shaar H, Gozal YM, Alzhrani G, Karsy M, Shelton C, Couldwell WT. Cerebral venous sinus thrombosis after vestibular schwannoma surgery: a call for evidence-based management guidelines. *Neurosurg Focus.* 2018;45(1):E4.
6. Benjamin CG, Sen RD, Golfinos JG, et al. Postoperative cerebral venous sinus thrombosis in the setting of surgery adjacent to the major dural venous sinuses. *J Neurosurg.* 2018:1–7.
7. Guazzo E, Panizza B, Lomas A, et al. Cerebral venous sinus thrombosis after translabyrinthine vestibular schwannoma—a prospective study and suggested management paradigm. *Otol Neurotol.* 2020;41(2):e273–e279.
8. Kow CY, Caldwell J, McHugh F, Sillars H, Bok A. Dural venous sinus thrombosis after cerebellopontine angle surgery: should it be treated? *J Clin Neurosci.* 2020;75:157–162.
9. Chang T, Yang YL, Gao L, Li LH. Cerebral venous sinus thrombosis following transsphenoidal surgery for craniopharyngioma: a case report. *World J Clin Cases.* 2020;8(6):1158–1163.
10. Liu Y, Zhao J, Zhu M, Wu Y, Ma H. Cerebral venous sinus thrombosis secondary to tonsillectomy. *Auris Nasus Larynx.* 2022;49(4):709–712.
11. Tan AP. Postoperative unilateral internal cerebral vein thrombosis with venous watershed infarcts: case report and review of the literature. *World Neurosurg.* 2020;138:158–162.
12. Moore J, Thomas P, Cousins V, Rosenfeld JV. Diagnosis and management of dural sinus thrombosis following resection of cerebellopontine angle tumors. *J Neurol Surg B Skull Base.* 2014;75:402–408.

CHAPTER

40

What Is the Role of Surgery in Spontaneous Intraparenchymal Hemorrhage?

Mariyam Humayun, MBBS
& J. Ricardo Carhuapoma, MD

Case

A 70-year-old man with a history of hypertension is admitted to the ICU after acute onset headache and hemiplegia, followed rapidly by confusion and lethargy. Blood pressure upon presentation to the emergency department is 190/100. Imaging reveals an intraparenchymal hemorrhage focused on the caudate nucleus on the right side, without associated intraventricular hemorrhage (IVH). Is there a role for surgical intervention?

Key Points

- The role of surgery in spontaneous intraparenchymal hemorrhage is limited.
- All patients need maximal medical therapy with utility of certain procedures restricted to selective patient populations.
- Most existing surgical techniques have not yielded any functional outcome benefits but may be necessary in life-threatening situations.
- Intracerebral hemorrhage has devasting implications, and further advancements in science will help reduce the burden of the disease.

BACKGROUND

Spontaneous intraparenchymal hemorrhage (IPH) accounts for about one-fourth of all stroke cases worldwide.[1] It continues to be associated with a higher mortality and morbidity when compared to ischemic stroke.[2] Treatment options for IPH remain limited in sharp contrast with the progress made in the treatment of ischemic stroke. IPH management focuses primarily on medical therapy including blood-pressure management, reversal of coagulopathy, and cerebral edema management with limited surgical options.[3] Surgical techniques that have been explored in the management of IPH include open craniotomy for clot extraction, minimally invasive techniques for clot aspiration, decompressive craniectomy (DC) for intracranial pressure (ICP) control, and intraventricular catheters for management of IVH.

Blood in the brain not only causes mechanical disruption of structures but also triggers a secondary inflammatory cascade.[4] Necrosis, inflammatory mediators, and blood degradation products in the hemorrhagic bed lead to cytotoxic edema, disruption of blood-brain barrier and neurotoxicity.[3] Presence of pathologic blood in the brain parenchyma also disrupts the volumetric equilibrium, as established by the Monroe-Kellie doctrine, leading to elevated ICP and herniation syndromes. Perihematomal region is also characterized by oligemia and edema. This area has been described as a penumbra that may be potentially salvageable with timely intervention.[4]

EVIDENCE AND REVIEW

Supratentorial ICH

Hematoma evacuation in ICH has been explored since the 1960s. The hope was that clot removal will preserve the penumbra and improve outcomes. The procedure was quite controversial until the Surgical Trial in Intracerebral Haemorrhage (STICH-I) trial in 2005. This randomized clinical trial included patients with spontaneous supratentorial intracerebral hemorrhage who presented with a hematoma diameter >2 cm and Glasgow coma scale (GCS) ≥5.[4] It compared conservative medical management to early surgical intervention within 24 hours of randomization. Most neurosurgeons used an open craniotomy technique to drain the blood. Mortality and functional outcome evaluated by a dichotomized extended Glasgow outcome score (eGOS) did not show any significant differences between the two groups. Subgroup analysis showed a trend toward improved outcomes if the hematoma was ≤1 cm from the cortical surface for which a second series, STITCH-II, was designed.

STITCH-II evaluated the role of early surgical intervention in superficial lobar IPH without IVH; this trial also failed to show any significant improvement in clinical improvement though a marginal nonsignificant trend toward improvement in mortality was seen.[5] There was high crossover rate from the medical to surgical group in both studies which could have confounded the possible benefit in the surgical group. These trials were able to establish the safety of neurosurgical procedures in this patient population, but overall data showed that craniotomies for clot extraction did not help in improving functional outcomes.

In contrast to clot evacuation, DC in supratentorial IPH is not well-studied as an alternative to clot evacuation. The rational to utilize decompressive surgery in this population would be to alleviate severe cerebral edema for risk of imminent herniation. Role of hemicraniectomy has been studied thoroughly in ischemic strokes, with functional and mortality benefit documented in a subset of patients. Some animal models and smaller human studies have shown promising results in IPH.[6] A review study also showed possible clinical benefit for decompressive hemicraniectomy with hematoma evacuation in large hemispheric hemorrhagic strokes though further research is needed to establish their safety and efficacy.[6]

Minimally invasive surgeries (MIS) to drain hematomas have also been explored since. Minimally Invasive Surgery with Thrombolysis in Intracerebral hemorrhage Evacuation (MISTIE-III), a large clinical trial, used a catheter-based clot extraction technique with alteplase administration; 45% of patients in the intervention group versus 41% in the control achieved a favorable modified Rankin score (mRS 0-3) at 1-year follow-up (absolute risk difference 4%, 95% CI: 4-12). Despite a significant reduction in the hematoma size and lower 365-day mortality, no benefit in functional outcome was detected in the intervention group. The study did show a possible correlation between the extent of clot removal and functional outcome.[7]

MIS may be considered over craniotomy to improve mortality in patients with IPH > 20 to 30 cc in volume and GCS of 5 to 12, with uncertain benefit for functional outcomes.[8] Several ongoing trials including the Early Minimally Invasive Removal of Intra Cerebral Hemorrhage (ENRICH), Minimally Invasive Endoscopic Surgical Treatment with Apollo/Artemis in Patients with Brain Hemorrhage (INVEST), and the Dutch Intracerebral Hemorrhage Surgery Trial (DIST) might change clinical practice in the future.

Infratentorial Hemorrhage

Posterior fossa hemorrhages account for 9% to 15% of all intracranial hemorrhages,[9] with cerebellum being the most common location.[10] Given the limited space in the infratentorial region, cerebellar hemorrhage can rapidly lead to brain herniation syndromes. It can also cause mass effect or compression of the fourth ventricle, with consequent development of obstructive hydrocephalus.[9] These patients need to be closely monitored for brain stem compression as surgical intervention can be lifesaving in case of clinical or radiographic deterioration. Existing studies have failed to show improved neurological outcomes with surgical evacuation.[11] Use of external ventricular drain (EVD) in cerebellar hemorrhage is controversial. While it can be helpful in cases of obstructive hydrocephalus, EVD placement without a suboccipital craniotomy is typically not advised and can be injurious in patients with obliterated cisterns.[7] For hemorrhages in the brainstem, evacuation is usually not helpful, given the risk of damage to key tracts and centers in the small space. Further studies are needed to better define the role of surgery in cerebellar hemorrhage, with particular emphasis toward patient selection and type and timing of intervention.

The Role of Invasive Intracranial Pressure Monitoring in IPH

ICP monitoring is not routinely practiced in IPH. An observational study noted that 65% (67/103) of IPH patients had at least one episode of ICP elevation ≥20 mm Hg when intracranial probes were used. Patients with ICP monitors were treated to maintain ICP and cerebral perfusion pressure (CPP) goals and those without ICP monitors were managed based on clinical or radiographic changes. The study showed a trend toward improvement in mortality and functional outcome in the ICP monitoring group after baseline variables were adjusted in both groups,[12] while another retrospective cohort with close to 800 matched patients did not show any improvement in mortality or functional outcomes with ICP monitoring.[13]

Intraventricular Hemorrhage

IVH encountered with IPH is associated with a higher mortality and morbidity.[14] Presence of IVH is one of the five determinants for the ICH score,[15] widely used by neurologists for prognostication of this disease. EVD improves mortality in large IVH and should be placed in patients with depressed mental status.[8] A randomized, double-blinded placebo-controlled trial investigated the use of thrombolytics via an EVD for IVH associated with nontraumatic hemorrhages. They included patients with complete obstruction of the third and fourth ventricles and an intracerebral hemorrhage volume of <30 cc.

Analysis of the 500 enrolled patients showed no difference in functional outcomes measured by a dichotomized mRS score. Intervention group did report a decrease in case fatality and a higher likelihood of achieving mRS < 3 if a larger amount of clot was cleared. Alteplase was not associated with higher number of adverse events and was deemed safe to use.[16] Thus, it is reasonable to use intraventricular thrombolytics for IVH patients with GCS > 3 and small intracerebral hemorrhage.[8] Further research is needed to clarify whether catheter-directed thrombolysis can improve functional outcomes, if effective clot reduction can be achieved.[16] Benefit of neuro-endoscopy to clear IVH in addition to EVD and thrombolytics remains uncertain.[8]

AVAILABLE GUIDELINES

The 2022 American Heart Association/American Stroke Association (AHA/ASA) guidelines serve as a basis for surgical decision making around spontaneous IPH. For supratentorial hemorrhages, they state that the usefulness of surgery is not currently well established. For posterior fossa hemorrhages, they recommend surgical decompression with clot evacuation for cerebellar IPH > 30 cc or at risk for brainstem compression.[8]

In terms of ICP monitoring, given the lack of robust data, AHA/ASA guidelines state that it might be reasonable to monitor ICPs in a subset of patients: poor GCS score (GCS ≤ 8) or presence of hydrocephalus.[8] ICP monitoring can be done with an intraparenchymal monitor versus an EVD. Goal ICP should be <20 mm Hg with CPP targets between 50 and 70 mm Hg. EVDs, though more invasive, can help in draining intraventricular blood or diverting CSF in hydrocephalus, particularly in patients with depressed mental status.[8]

REFERENCES

1. Krishnamurthi RV, Ikeda T, Feigin VL. Global, regional and country-specific burden of ischaemic stroke, intracerebral haemorrhage and subarachnoid haemorrhage: a systematic analysis of the Global Burden of Disease Study 2017. *Neuroepidemiology.* 2020;54(2):171–179. doi: 10.1159/000506396. Epub 2020 Feb 20. PMID: 32079017.
2. Krishnamurthi RV, Feigin VL, Forouzanfar MH, et al. Global and regional burden of first-ever ischaemic and haemorrhagic stroke during 1990-2010: findings from the Global Burden of Disease Study 2010. *Lancet Glob Health.* 2013 Nov;1(5):e259–e281. doi: 10.1016/S2214-109X(13)70089-5. Epub 2013 Oct 24. PMID: 25104492; PMCID: PMC4181351.
3. Qureshi AI, Mendelow AD, Hanley DF. Intracerebral haemorrhage. *Lancet.* 2009 May 9;373(9675):1632–1644. doi: 10.1016/S0140-6736(09)60371-8. PMID: 19427958; PMCID: PMC3138486.
4. Mendelow AD, Gregson BA, Fernandes HM, et al. Early surgery versus initial conservative treatment in patients with spontaneous supratentorial intracerebral haematomas in the International Surgical Trial in Intracerebral Haemorrhage (STICH): a randomised trial. Lancet. 2005 Jan 29-Feb 4;365(9457): 387–397. doi: 10.1016/S0140-6736(05)17826-X. PMID: 15680453.
5. Mendelow AD, Gregson BA, Rowan EN, et al. Early surgery versus initial conservative treatment in patients with spontaneous supratentorial lobar intracerebral haematomas (STICH II): a randomised trial. *Lancet.* 2013 Aug 3;382(9890):397–408. doi: 10.1016/S0140-6736(13)60986-1. Epub 2013 May 29. Erratum in: *Lancet.* 2013 Aug 3;382(9890):396. Erratum in: *Lancet.* 2021 Sep 18;398(10305):1042. PMID: 23726393; PMCID: PMC3906609.
6. Takeuchi S, Wada K, Nagatani K, Otani N, Mori K. Decompressive hemicraniectomy for spontaneous intracerebral hemorrhage. *Neurosurg Focus.* 2013 May;34(5):E5. doi: 10.3171/2013.2.FOCUS12424. PMID: 23634924.
7. Hanley DF, Thompson RE, Rosenblum M, et al. Efficacy and safety of minimally invasive surgery with thrombolysis in intracerebral haemorrhage evacuation (MISTIE III): a randomised, controlled, open-label, blinded endpoint phase 3 trial. *Lancet.* 2019 Mar 9;393(10175):1021–1032. doi: 10.1016/S0140-6736(19)30195-3. Epub 2019 Feb 7. Erratum in: *Lancet.* 2019 Apr 20;393(10181):1596. PMID: 30739747; PMCID: PMC6894906.
8. Greenberg SM, Ziai WC, Cordonnier C, et al. 2022 Guideline for the management of patients with spontaneous intracerebral hemorrhage: a guideline from the American Heart Association/American Stroke Association. *Stroke.* 2022 Jul;53(7):e282–e361. doi: 10.1161/STR.0000000000000407. Epub 2022 May 17. PMID: 35579034.
9. Luney MS, English SW, Longworth A, et al. Acute posterior cranial fossa hemorrhage-is surgical decompression better than expectant medical management? *Neurocrit Care.* 2016 Dec;25(3):365–370. doi: 10.1007/s12028-015-0217-7. PMID: 27071924; PMCID: PMC5138260.
10. Chen R, Wang X, Anderson CS, et al. Infratentorial intracerebral hemorrhage. *Stroke.* 2019 May;50(5):1257–1259. doi: 10.1161/STROKEAHA.118.023766. PMID: 30890109.
11. Kuramatsu JB, Biffi A, Gerner ST, et al. Association of surgical hematoma evacuation vs conservative treatment with functional outcome in patients with cerebellar intracerebral hemorrhage. *JAMA.* 2019 Oct 8; 322(14):1392–1403. doi: 10.1001/jama.2019.13014. PMID: 31593272; PMCID: PMC6784768.
12. Ren J, Wu X, Huang J, et al. Intracranial pressure monitoring-aided management associated with favorable outcomes in patients with hypertension-related spontaneous intracerebral hemorrhage. Transl Stroke Res. 2020 Dec;11(6):1253–1263. doi: 10.1007/s12975-020-00798-w. Epub 2020 Mar 6. PMID: 32144586.
13. Chen CJ, Ding D, Ironside N, et al. Intracranial pressure monitoring in patients with spontaneous intracerebral hemorrhage. *J Neurosurg.* 2019 May 31;132(6):1854–1864. doi: 10.3171/2019.3.JNS19545. PMID: 31151113.
14. Tuhrim S, Horowitz DR, Sacher M, Godbold JH. Volume of ventricular blood is an important determinant of outcome in supratentorial intracerebral hemorrhage. *Crit Care Med.* 1999 Mar;27(3):617–621. doi: 10.1097/00003246-199903000-00045. PMID: 10199544.
15. Hemphill JC 3rd, Bonovich DC, Besmertis L, Manley GT, Johnston SC. The ICH score: a simple, reliable grading scale for intracerebral hemorrhage. *Stroke.* 2001 Apr;32(4):891–897. doi: 10.1161/01.str.32.4.891. PMID: 11283388.
16. Hanley DF, Lane K, McBee N, et al. Thrombolytic removal of intraventricular haemorrhage in treatment of severe stroke: results of the randomised, multicentre, multiregion, placebo-controlled CLEAR III trial. *Lancet.* 2017 Feb 11;389(10069):603–611. doi: 10.1016/S0140-6736(16)32410-2. Epub 2017 Jan 10. PMID: 28081952; PMCID: PMC6108339.

CHAPTER

41

How Can We Limit Postop Complications After Arteriovenous Malformation Resection?

Juan C. Vicenty-Padilla, MD,
Pui Man Rosalind Lai, MD, & Nirav J. Patel, MD

Case

A 22-year-old man was admitted following elective resection of an incidentally discovered left opercular arteriovenous malformation (AVM) measuring 3.5 cm and draining via the superficial venous system (Spetzler-Martin Grade III) (Figure 41–1).

Key Points

- The postoperative care of brain arteriovenous malformations (bAVMs) is a continuation of the treatment that was initiated in the operating room.
- The most disastrous complication after resection of these entities is development of delayed intracerebral hemorrhage due to the phenomenon known as arteriovenous capillary hypertension.
- In the case of low-grade bAVMs, maintenance of normotension probably suffices to avoid this complication.
- However, in the case of high-grade bAVMs, a protocol of strict blood pressure and cerebral perfusion control is mandated for at least 7 days or until the feeding arterial system is remodeled to a normal caliber.
- Sedation and analgesia are powerful aids in blood pressure control but must be limited as possible.

The procedure was uncomplicated, and the patient was left intubated for deliberate postoperative hypotension. Exam revealed no focal deficits. Immediate postoperative computed tomography (CT) angiography demonstrated no residual nidus.

However, on the postoperative day 7, the patient experienced an ictus of generalized tonic-clonic seizures after a brief period of blood pressure parameters relaxation. Nonenhanced CT demonstrated evidence of intracerebral hemorrhage (Figure 41–2). A digital subtraction angiogram revealed no evidence of residual nidus (Figures 41–3 and 41–4). How could this and other postoperative complications from bAVM surgery be avoided?

BACKGROUND

Brain arteriovenous malformations (bAVMs) embody a spectrum of peculiar entities in cerebrovascular pathology. Its treatment represents a challenge for those involved and demands an in-depth knowledge of elements beyond angio-architecture, location, and surgical techniques. In most cases, when performed in expert centers dedicated to its treatment, surgery for bAVMs will result in an overall benefit for the patient.[1] Unlike for other pathologies of the brain, the intensive care unit course of a bAVM patient is not just "postoperative." More accurately, the care provided after surgical resection is a continuity of the treatment effort to successfully cure these patients.

An understanding of the anatomical, developmental, and, most importantly, the hemodynamic characteristics of bAVMs is paramount to predict and avoid potential complications after resection. In this chapter, we aim to describe the fundamentals of managing patients with bAVMs after surgery.

Pathophysiology and Hemodynamics of Brain Arteriovenous Malformations

Intracerebral hematomas, seizures, headaches, and neurologic deficits are among some of the common presentations of cerebral AVMs.[2,3] Although no two bAVMs are equal, all share a unique

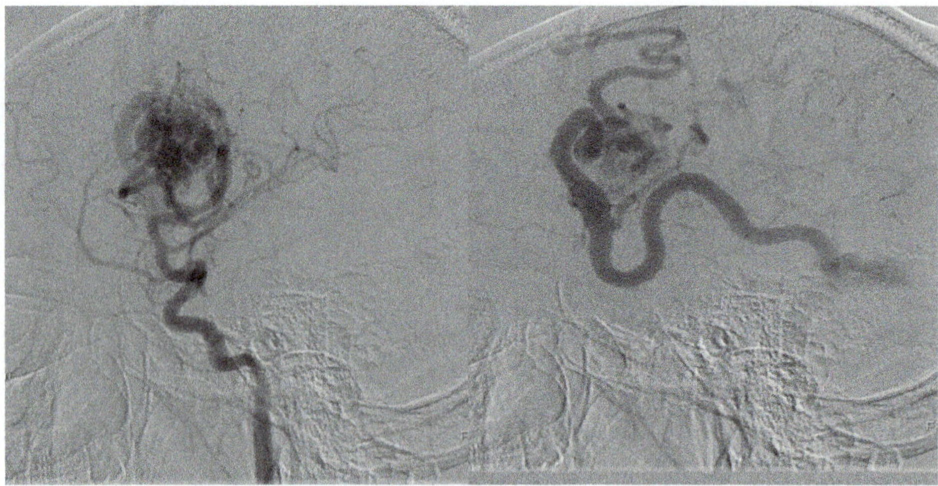

FIGURE 41–1 Left internal carotid injection on lateral projection demonstrating the lesion.

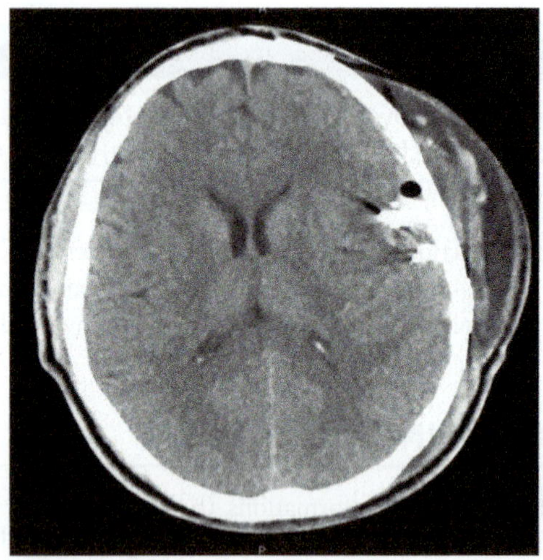

FIGURE 41–2 Postoperative computed tomography (CT) demonstrating clip artifact and no evidence of hemorrhage.

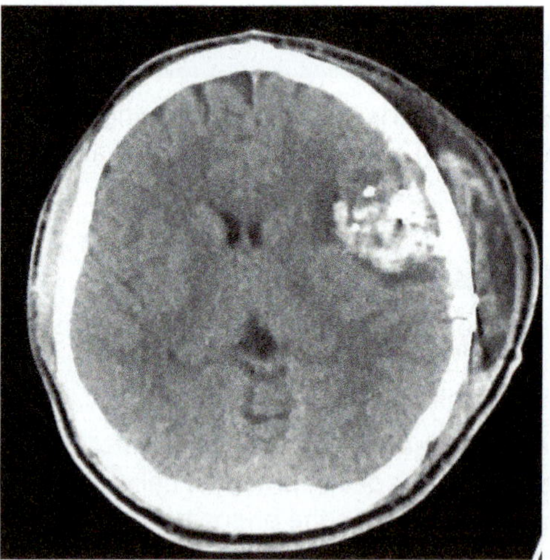

FIGURE 41–3 Nonenhanced computed tomography (CT) demonstrating a delayed intracerebral hemorrhage.

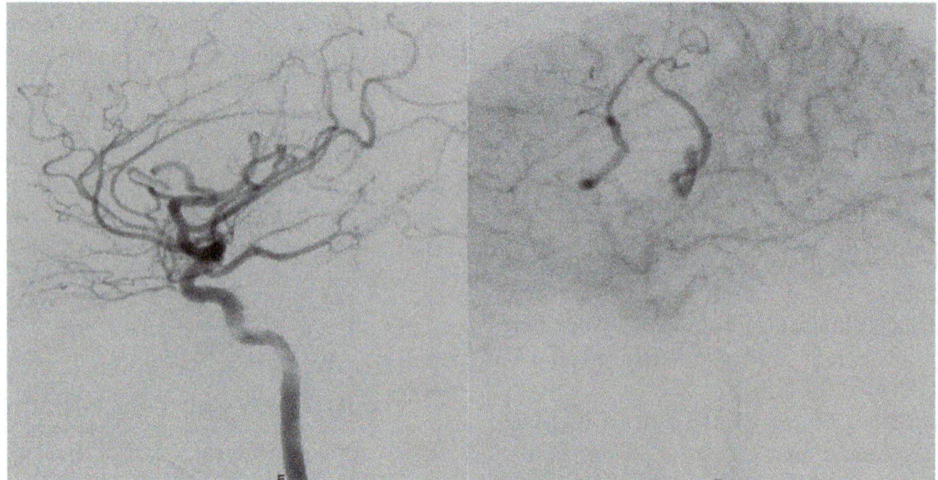

FIGURE 41–4 Postoperative Digital Substraction Angiogram (DSA) with no evidence of residual nidus. Mild venous stagnation observed.

characteristic; their gamut of presentations and symptoms result from alterations of normal cerebral hemodynamics.[4–6]

In its most basic form, AVMs represent a connection between an artery and a vein that has skipped the typical intervening capillaries and its associated small vessel system (ie arterioles and venules).[7,8] The consequence of this misconnection leads to an attempt at homeostasis by the brain that will result in all the aspects of "maturation" of a bAVM (ie, enlargement, aneurysms, and steal).

It is thought that this fistulous connection is established when normal genetic signals fail to produce the normal capillary net during angiogenesis.[9] This small vessel arrangement represents the most important point of resistance to flow in the cerebrovascular system, and therefore, its absence represents a drastic drop of resistance across the fistula. On the arterial side, the result is a lower feeding vessel hemostatic pressure and an increased shear stress which leads to remodeling and enlargement (or formation of aneurysms) that will accommodate greater flow.[10] The variations in the feeding vessels sizes and drop in resistance create alternating intranidal pressures and turbulent flow that serve to buffer normal arterial hemostatic pressures from being transmitted to the venous side.[11] As a consequence, the venous side experiences increased transmural pressures and turbulence that lead to endothelial and morphological remodeling in the form of varicosities and tortuosities.[4–6,12] The product of the lower arterial pressure and venous hypertension is chronic perinidal hypoperfusion that leads to hypoxia and gliosis. Furthermore, it causes the release of neo-angiogenic factors such as vascular endothelial growth factor (VEGF) that will sustain the growth of the malformation, thus creating a vicious cycle.[8,13]

This cascade of events also leads to important hemodynamic models of paramount importance that explain why bAVM patients develop hyperemic syndromes or hemorrhages in the perioperative period. In 1978, Spetzler et al described the phenomenon known as normal perfusion pressure breakthrough, a concept that theorized that the chronic hypotension of the perinidal vessels leads to the loss of their intrinsic autoregulation and therefore exposes the patient to the risk of hyperemia, edema, and hemorrhage once the shunting effect is abolished upon bAVM resection.[14] As of this publication, current evidence has demonstrated that rather than a lack of autoregulation, what happens is that the threshold of normal pressure autoregulation is lowered while still maintaining some degree of vasoreactivity and probably coexisting with the phenomenon of occlusive hyperemia.[15–18] This last theory establishes the possibility that the perinidal hyperemia and edema observed after resection of bAVMs may be related to venous outflow obstruction secondary to thrombosis and/or subsequent arterial stagnation with an ensuing worsening of cerebral hypoperfusion.[19]

The phenomena of normal prefusion pressure breakthrough and occlusive hyperemia are vital in understanding the pathophysiologic development of bAVMs.[14,19] Morgan et al. have described that both phenomena probably coexist in a unifying concept described as "Arterial-capillary-venous hypertensive syndrome."[21] The notion behind this is that whether there is increased arterial pressure, venous stagnation, or both, there is a common pathophysiologic disturbance that results in local, markedly increased perinidal capillary intravascular pressure.[21] This, of course, represents a big threat for the development of intracerebral hemorrhage if not managed appropriately.

Fortunately for both patients and physicians, these changes are reversible and a return of morphological and normal hemodynamic parameters can be slowly observed after successful obliteration of the fistula.[22,23] That is to say, a decrease in the caliber after resection of the fistula is not a sign of vasospasm. Rather is a return to a normal caliber. Knowing these important hemodynamic concepts also enables us to understand how certain bAVMs can present and what complications may be associated. For example, small bAVMs are usually monocompartmental in nature; that is, one single vessel feeding a nidus drained by one or more veins.[13] This usually results in higher feeding artery hemostatic pressures due to higher flow resistance when compared to larger multicompartment lesions (>1 feeding artery and >1 draining vein) and thus higher incidence of hemorrhagic presentation for these small lesions.[24,25] In contrast, larger multicompartment bAVMs may be associated to lower arterial pressures and resistance and therefore more disposed to generate a steal phenomenon. It thus results logical to extrapolate that a presentation of arteriovenous capillary hypertension will be far more common in the postoperative period after resection of larger bAVMs.

EVIDENCE AND REVIEW

Team Building

Fundamentally, the care of bAVM patients in the intensive care unit is a principal part in the treatment. Lack of attention to detail and poor communication of patient-specific goals of care may lead to disastrous results. All team members must be cognizant of this and therefore understand that their participation may alter dramatically the patient's course. Proper team building should aim for open communication, comprehension of all aims, awareness of warning signs, deep understanding of the pathology, and creation of patient- and institution-specific protocols among others. Sharing the responsibility among all team members will result in better outcomes. Given this important observation, in the following text we describe the most important elements in the postintervention care of bAVM patients.

General Monitoring and Precautions

The authors recommend comprehensive monitoring of bAVM patients in the perioperative period. Monitoring of blood pressure, heart rate, oxygen saturation, temperature, glucose, and input/outputs is of paramount importance. Commonly the regular monitoring of hemoglobin, coagulation markers, electrolytes, and arterial blood gases is necessary. Special cases will require placement of a ventriculostomy with an attached external ventriculostomy device, and therefore, monitoring of output as well as regular measurement of intracranial and cerebral perfusion pressures will be required. Additionally, some patients will be followed in the perioperative period with a continuous electroencephalogram and transcranial dopplers.[22,26]

Distinct attention to prophylaxis of gastric ulcers, deep venous thrombosis, infections, and decubitus ulcers will guarantee improved outcomes. Note that head elevation, patient rotation or ambulation, adequate nutrition, and rehab are also vital.

It is the authors preference to avoid the use of heparin as a prophylaxis of deep venous thrombi in order to promote the thrombosis of any residual nidus. Instead, close monitoring with lower extremity non invasive studies and placement of an inferior vena cava filter can be employed.

Blood Pressure Control

The authors would like to stress the importance that complications in dealing with bAVMs may surface from both the intraoperative and postoperative care. Among the various complications, one of the most feared is the development of delayed intracerebral hemorrhage. This risk is estimated to be close to 20%.[21,27–29] As previously described, the concept of arterial-capillary-venous hypertension plays a key role in the development of intracerebral hemorrhage after resection of bAVMs.[21,30] As such, if the surgeon is confident that adequate hemostasis and complete resection have been achieved, one of the most important factors (if not the most important) in controlling hemorrhage in the perioperative period is strict systemic blood pressure control.[21,30–32]

The strictness in blood pressure control will be dictated by the nature of the bAVM in question. In other words, a "high-grade bAVM" with multiple dilated feeding arteries and/or thrombosed variceal draining veins will need a much more rigorous control. Achieving such balance may require central venous access for placement of both titratable vasopressors and antihypertensives.[31] In general, in our institution, we follow the protocol suggested by Morgan et al.[31]

- Low-grade bAVMs (Spetzler-Martin [SM] I, II, and III < 3.5): Systolic blood pressure < 140 mm Hg
- High-grade bAVMs (Spetzler Martin Grades III [>3.5], IV and V): Mean arterial pressure < 70 mm Hg

Also, adequate control may require multiple antihypertensive medications via multiple administration routes and mechanisms of action. That is, for example, a patient may require an intravenous calcium channel blocker as well as an oral beta blocker and/or a diuretic. In our institution, we have readily available intravenous calcium channel blockers such as nicardipine, clevidipine, or diltiazem to be initiated in the operative room. Other agents such as sodium nitroprusside may provide fast and effective control; however, judicious use needs to be contemplated due to the risk of paradoxical brain edema and systemic toxicity.[33] Intravenous coadministration of vasopressors such as norepinephrine or phenylephrine may assist in achieving a goal of cerebral perfusion pressure of at least 60 mm Hg when needed.[31,34]

Of note, in optimal situations, blood pressure control is to be reached with antihypertensive medications only. However, often times, mainly in cases of higher grade bAVMs, further maneuvers such as sedation, analgesia, paralysis, and/or cerebrospinal fluid derivation may be warranted. Liberalization of blood pressure will largely depend on the morphological aspects of the lesion. In an interesting study, Morgan et al demonstrated that bAVMs under 3 cm have a return to normal feeding vessel size within 7 days.[23]

Morgan et al suggested that the control of blood pressure initiates prior to surgery via loading of oral beta blockers or other agents and may extend up to a minimum of 7 days in high-grade bAVMs or as soon as the patient is in a Glasgow coma scale of 15 with concomitant normal intracranial pressures.[31]

A proper protocol of blood pressure control has been shown to decrease delayed intracerebral hemorrhage from 20% to 4%.[40]

Sedation and Analgesia

A patient that is awake and/or in pain can have systematic repercussions that may directly lead to complications in the perioperative period—specifically, spikes in systemic blood pressure. These blood pressure spikes will lead to development of delayed intracerebral hemorrhage in high-grade bAVM patients. Inevitably, after bAVM resection, an awake but disoriented patient may pull out essential monitors, strain, and increase the metabolic stress of the perinidal tissue. Pain leads to increased blood pressure, Valsalva, tachycardia, and restlessness. All these changes will ultimately precipitate worsening of the known arteriovenous hypertension to which bAVM patients are at risk and therefore represent a risk for delayed intraparenchymal hemorrhage.[30,35,36]

The use of analgesia and sedation must be tailored on an individual basis. In the authors' experience, increasing needs for analgesia and sedation positively correlate with the grade of the bAVM in question. Since in the majority of cases that intravenous sedation is needed there is requisite of intubation, we recommend avoiding or limiting it when possible due to the infectious, thrombotic, and deconditioning risks associated to it. In other words, sedation and analgesia must be fitted for those cases where systemic blood pressure control cannot be achieved with antihypertensive medications alone. In the cases where it is used, its recommended to uptitrate the dosage prior to bedside procedures or position changes.

Seizure Prophylaxis

Seizures are estimated to occur in 20% to 29% of the bAVM patients.[3,37] Some of these may be present from the preoperative period as an established epilepsy or "de novo" seizures, whereas others may develop as "de novo" seizures after microsurgical resection. Regardless of its nature, seizures in the postoperative period may precipitate dreaded complications that can result in arteriovenous hypertension and therefore present a high risk for delayed intracerebral hemorrhage as well as other risks.

As with other concepts in the treatment of bAVMs, we must take into consideration its inherent nature. In a study conducted by Piepgras et al, there was a positive association of more seizures among the bAVMs larger than 3 cm.[38] Therefore, an extra level of suspicion and prophylaxis must be maintained for the high-grade bAVMs.

In general, patients with no preoperative seizures can be maintained with an antiepileptic drug medication prophylaxis for the early postoperative period (7-10 days) whereas those with established epilepsy are kept on their regular medication until further considerations.[39] In our institution, we regularly use Levetiracetam 500 to 1,000 mg for early seizure prophylaxis.

Intracranial Pressure Monitoring

There is no doubt that the risk of arteriovenous hypertension increases as the bAVM grade progresses. Along with it, the risk of delayed intracerebral hemorrhage and edema increases. In many cases, high-grade bAVMs will require deep sedation, analgesia, or induced coma to control said risks.[32] Morgan et al specifically described the target goal of cerebral perfusion pressure at >50 mm Hg and <60 mm Hg after resection of high-grade bAVMs.[31]

If needed, the authors prefer using a ventriculostomy with an attached ventriculostomy device for monitoring, mainly because of its cerebrospinal fluid diversion capabilities. The catheter is then slowly weaned off as soon as the patient is successfully extubated.

REFERENCES

1. Morgan MK, Davidson AS, Assaad NNA, Stoodley MA. Critical review of brain AVM surgery, surgical results and natural history in 2017. *Acta Neurochir (Wien)*. 2017;159(8):1457–1478. doi:10.1007/s00701-017-3217-x
2. Karbe A-G, Vajkoczy P. Postoperative management and follow-up after resection of arteriovenous malformations. *J Neurosurg Sci.* 2018;62(4): 484–489. doi:10.23736/S0390-5616.18.04417-X
3. Osbun JW, Reynolds MR, Barrow DL. Arteriovenous malformations: epidemiology, clinical presentation, and diagnostic evaluation. *Handb Clin Neurol.* 2017;143:25–29. doi:10.1016/B978-0-444-63640-9.00003-5
4. Morgan M, Winder M. Haemodynamics of arteriovenous malformations of the brain and consequences of resection: a review. *J Clin Neurosci Off J Neurosurg Soc Australas.* 2001;8(3):216–224. doi:10.1054/jocn.2000.0795
5. Fennell VS, Martirosyan NL, Atwal GS, et al.: Hemodynamics associated with intracerebral arteriovenous malformations: the effects of treatment modalities. *Neurosurgery.* 2018;83(4):611–621. doi:10.1093/neuros/nyx560
6. Kader A, Young WL. The effects of intracranial arteriovenous malformations on cerebral hemodynamics. *Neurosurg Clin N Am.* 1996;7(4):767–781.
7. Laakso A, Hernesniemi J. Arteriovenous malformations: epidemiology and clinical presentation. *Neurosurg Clin N Am.* 2012;23(1):1–6. doi:10.1016/j.nec.2011.09.012
8. Mouchtouris N, Jabbour PM, Starke RM, et al.: Biology of cerebral arteriovenous malformations with a focus on inflammation. *J Cereb Blood Flow Metab.* 2015;35(2):167–175. doi:10.1038/jcbfm.2014.179
9. Lawton MT, Rutledge WC, Kim H, et al.: Brain arteriovenous malformations. *Nat Rev Dis Prim.* 2015;1:15008. doi:10.1038/nrdp.2015.8
10. Shakur SF, Amin-Hanjani S, Mostafa H, Charbel FT, Alaraj A. Hemodynamic characteristics of cerebral arteriovenous malformation feeder vessels with and without aneurysms. *Stroke.* 2015;46(7):1997–1999. doi:10.1161/STROKEAHA.115.009545
11. Young WL, Kader A, Pile-Spellman J, Ornstein E, Stein BM. Arteriovenous malformation draining vein physiology and determinants of transnidal pressure gradients. The Columbia University AVM Study Project. *Neurosurgery.* 1994;35(3):386–389. doi:10.1227/00006123-199409000-00005
12. Shakur SF, Hussein AE, Amin-Hanjani S, Valyi-Nagy T, Charbel FT, Alaraj A. Cerebral arteriovenous malformation flow is associated with venous intimal hyperplasia. *Stroke.* 2017;48(4):1088–1091. doi:10.1161/STROKEAHA.116.015666
13. Moftakhar P, Hauptman JS, Malkasian D, Martin NA. Cerebral arteriovenous malformations. Part 2: physiology. *Neurosurg Focus.* 2009;26(5):E11. doi:10.3171/2009.2.FOCUS09317
14. Spetzler RF, Wilson CB, Weinstein P, Mehdorn M, Townsend J, Telles D. Normal perfusion pressure breakthrough theory. *Clin Neurosurg.* 1978;25: 651–672. doi:10.1093/neurosurgery/25.cn_suppl_1.651
15. Zacharia BE, Bruce S, Appelboom G, Connolly ESJ. Occlusive hyperemia versus normal perfusion pressure breakthrough after treatment of cranial arteriovenous malformations. *Neurosurg Clin N Am.* 2012;23(1):147–151. doi:10.1016/j.nec.2011.09.005
16. Nagasawa S, Kawanishi M, Kondoh S, et al.: Normal perfusion pressure hyperperfusion in cerebral arteriovenous malformation surgery: model study on the hemodynamics and mechanisms. *J Clin Neurosci Off J Neurosurg Soc Australas.* 1998;5 Suppl:30–32. doi:10.1016/s0967-5868(98)90007-8
17. Gutierrez-Gonzalez R, Perez-Zamarron A, Rodriguez-Boto G. Normal perfusion pressure breakthrough phenomenon: experimental models. *Neurosurg Rev.* 2014;37(4):559–567. doi:10.1007/s10143-014-0549-3
18. Rangel-Castilla L, Spetzler RF, Nakaji P. Normal perfusion pressure breakthrough theory: a reappraisal after 35 years. *Neurosurg Rev.* 2015;38(3): 395–399. doi:10.1007/s10143-014-0600-4
19. al-Rodhan NR, Sundt TMJ, Piepgras DG, Nichols DA, Rufenacht D, Stevens LN. Occlusive hyperemia: a theory for the hemodynamic complications following resection of intracerebral arteriovenous malformations. *J Neurosurg.* 1993;78(2):167–175. doi:10.3171/jns.1993.78.2.0167
20. Sekhon LH, Morgan MK, Spence I. Normal perfusion pressure breakthrough: the role of capillaries. *J Neurosurg.* 1997;86(3):519–524. doi:10.3171/jns.1997.86.3.0519
21. Morgan MK, Sekhon LH, Finfer S, Grinnell V. Delayed neurological deterioration following resection of arteriovenous malformations of the brain. *J Neurosurg.* 1999;90(4):695–701. doi:10.3171/jns.1999.90.4.0695
22. Jo K-I, Kim J-S, Hong S-C, Lee J-I. Hemodynamic changes in arteriovenous malformations after radiosurgery: transcranial Doppler evaluation. *World Neurosurg.* 2012;77(2):316–321. doi:10.1016/j.wneu.2011.06.061
23. Morgan MK, Guilfoyle M, Kirollos R, Heller GZ. Remodeling of the feeding arterial system after surgery for resection of brain arteriovenous malformations: an observational study. *Neurosurgery.* 2019;84(1):84–94. doi:10.1093/neuros/nyy007
24. Spetzler RF, Hargraves RW, McCormick PW, Zabramski JM, Flom RA, Zimmerman RS. Relationship of perfusion pressure and size to risk of hemorrhage from arteriovenous malformations. *J Neurosurg.* 1992;76(6): 918–923. doi:10.3171/jns.1992.76.6.0918
25. Duong DH, Young WL, Vang MC, et al.: Feeding artery pressure and venous drainage pattern are primary determinants of hemorrhage from cerebral arteriovenous malformations. *Stroke.* 1998;29(6):1167–1176. doi:10.1161/01.STR.29.6.1167
26. Kaspera W, Majchrzak H. [Evaluation of blood supply dynamics and possibilities of cerebral arteriovenous malformations (AVM) imaging by means of transcranial color-coded duplex sonography (TCCS)]. *Neurol Neurochir Pol.* 2002;36(4):735–748.
27. Pertuiset B, Sichez JP, Philippon J, Fohanno D, Horn Y. [Mortality and morbidity after complete surgical removal of 162 intracranial arteriovenous malformations (author's transl)]. *Rev Neurol (Paris).* 1979;135(4):319–327.
28. Batjer HH, Devous MDS, Seibert GB, et al.: Intracranial arteriovenous malformation: relationships between clinical and radiographic factors and cerebral blood flow. *Neurol Med Chir (Tokyo).* 1989;29(5):395–400. doi:10.2176/nmc.29.395
29. Niini T, Laakso A, Tanskanen P, Niemela M, Luostarinen T. Perioperative treatment of brain arteriovenous malformations between 2006 and 2014: the Helsinki protocol. *Neurocrit Care.* 2019;31(2):346–356. doi:10.1007/s12028-019-00674-y
30. Morgan MK, Winder M, Little NS, Finfer S, Ritson E. Delayed hemorrhage following resection of an arteriovenous malformation in the brain. *J Neurosurg.* 2003;99(6):967–971. doi:10.3171/jns.2003.99.6.0967
31. Morgan MK, Wiedmann MKH, Assaad NNA, Parr MJA, Heller GZ. Deliberate employment of postoperative hypotension for brain arteriovenous malformation surgery and the incidence of delayed postoperative hemorrhage: a prospective cohort study. *J Neurosurg.* 2017;127(5):1025–1040. doi:10.3171/2016.9.JNS161333

32. Day AL, Friedman WA, Sypert GW, Mickle JP. Successful treatment of the normal perfusion pressure breakthrough syndrome. *Neurosurgery.* 1982;11(5):625–630. doi:10.1227/00006123-198211000-00007
33. Rose JC, Mayer SA. Optimizing blood pressure in neurological emergencies. *Neurocrit Care.* 2004;1(3):287–299. doi:10.1385/NCC:1:3:287
34. Delgado T, Wolfe B, Davis G, Ansari S. Safety of peripheral administration of phenylephrine in a neurologic intensive care unit: a pilot study. *J Crit Care.* 2016;34:107–110. doi:10.1016/j.jcrc.2016.04.004
35. Hemphill JC 3rd, Greenberg SM, Anderson CS, et al.: Guidelines for the management of spontaneous intracerebral hemorrhage: a guideline for healthcare professionals from the American Heart Association/American Stroke Association. *Stroke.* 2015;46(7):2032–2060. doi:10.1161/STR.0000000000000069
36. Egawa S, Hifumi T, Kawakita K, et al.: Impact of neurointensivist-managed intensive care unit implementation on patient outcomes after aneurysmal subarachnoid hemorrhage. *J Crit Care.* 2016;32:52–55. doi:10.1016/j.jcrc.2015.11.008
37. Can A, Gross BA, Du R. The natural history of cerebral arteriovenous malformations. *Handb Clin Neurol.* 2017;143:15–24. doi:10.1016/B978-0-444-63640-9.00002-3
38. Piepgras DG, Sundt TMJ, Ragoowansi AT, Stevens L. Seizure outcome in patients with surgically treated cerebral arteriovenous malformations. *J Neurosurg.* 1993;78(1):5–11. doi:10.3171/jns.1993.78.1.0005
39. Schramm J. Seizures associated with cerebral arteriovenous malformations. *Handb Clin Neurol.* 2017;143:31–40. doi:10.1016/B978-0-444-63640-9.00004-7
40. Morgan MK. Surgical management. *Handb Clin Neurol.* 2017;143:41–57. doi:10.1016/B978-0-444-63640-9.00005-9

CHAPTER

42

What Is the Role for Nimodipine in Perimesencephalic Subarachnoid Hemorrhage?

Ofer Sadan, MD, PhD & Feras Akbik, MD, PhD

Case

A 45-year-old man presents after sudden onset severe headache, with computed tomography (CT) scan of the head revealing subarachnoid hemorrhage limited to the basilar cisterns. CT angiogram followed by digital subtraction angiogram did not reveal any underlying aneurysm or other vascular lesions. He is admitted to the ICU for close monitoring. Should he be started in nimodipine to reduce the risk of delayed cerebral ischemia in this case of presumed perimesencephalic subarachnoid hemorrhage?

Key Points

- Perimesencephalic subarachnoid hemorrhage (pSAH) is a distinct subset of angiogram-negative SAH with hemorrhage restricted to the basal cisterns and holds a different natural history than aneurysmal SAH (aSAH) or diffuse angiogram-negative SAH.
- Symptomatic vasospasm and delayed cerebral ischemia (DCI) are uncommon in pSAH.
- Oral nimodipine for a 21-day course reduces the risk of DCI in aSAH by Class 1A evidence but has not been shown to hold similar effect in pSAH.

BACKGROUND

Preventing delayed cerebral ischemia (DCI) is a major treatment goal in subarachnoid hemorrhage (SAH) patients. Strong evidence supports the use of oral nimodipine to prevent DCI in aneurysmal SAH (aSAH). Nevertheless, not all SAH is due to aneurysmal rupture, and it remains unclear how to approach DCI prevention in angiogram-negative patterns of SAH, particularly in patients with a perimesencephalic pattern of SAH (pSAH). Here we explore our current understanding of DCI, natural history of pSAH, and the utility of nimodipine prophylaxis in pSAH patients.

Insights into Delayed Cerebral Ischemia from Aneurysmal Subarachnoid Hemorrhage

Aneurysmal SAH is a life-threatening hemorrhagic stroke with in-hospital mortality rates as high as 20%.[1–3] Of the survivors, ~30% suffer secondary ischemic complications in the weeks that follow the initial insult.[4] DCI has been shown to be associated with worse functional outcomes across multiple cohorts and clinical trials[5–8] and represents a therapeutic target to minimize secondary injury after SAH.

Several mechanisms were suggested to contribute to the development of DCI, with initial interest focusing on cerebral vasospasm.[9] Similar to DCI, this usually occurs in a delayed fashion after aneurysmal rupture, but the onset of vasospasm typically precedes DCI.

The proposed mechanism suggests that arterial vasospasm reduces cerebral blood flow locally, which in turn leads to ischemia and sometimes infarction. This precipitated enormous interest in therapeutically treating cerebral vasospasm to minimize DCI and secondary injury. Unfortunately, multiple interventions have succeeded in treating cerebral vasospasm without modifying DCI rates or patient outcomes.[10–12] This may be due to limited power in resolving differences and/or a set of entirely separate mechanisms that are triggered by SAH to precipitate DCI.

For instance, hemoglobin breakdown in the subarachnoid space leads to oxidative stress and nitric oxide scavenging, and the end result is local vasoconstriction.[13] Indeed, the hemoglobin concertation in the cerebrospinal fluid (CSF) of SAH patients has been correlated to the risk for DCI.[13] Furthermore, the modified Fisher scale, which is based on the blood pattern and burden on imaging, demonstrates a high correlation with the development of DCI.[14]

Another proposed mechanism for DCI is spreading cortical depolarization. Intense neuronal depolarization waves can be observed using invasive electrode strips for electroencephalogram (EEG) monitoring, most commonly in the subdural space. These waves could only be seen by invasive monitoring, while scalp EEG cannot identify them in a robust manner.[15] It remains unclear if spreading depolarization is a manifestation of an ischemic event or a cause for one. Regardless, such an occurrence was found to be correlated with the development of DCI and poor outcome. Interestingly, DCI events in the settings of spreading depolarization occurred independently from cerebral vasospasm.[16] Cilostazol, an emerging intervention to decrease the risk for DCI in aSAH, was found to decrease spreading depolarization events.[17]

EVIDENCE AND REVIEW

From a treatment standpoint, the only Class 1A intervention to reduce DCI is a preventive regimen of oral nimodipine. Nimodipine, a calcium channel blocker and a vasodilator, was shown to reduce rate of DCI and improve long-term functional outcomes in aSAH patients.[18,19] Interestingly, there was no effect on the rates of cerebral vasospasm. In the largest clinical trial, from 1989, DCI decreased from 33% in the control arm to 22% in the intervention one. Poor outcome defined as death, vegetative state, or severe disability in that trial was seen in 33% in the control group and in 20% in the nimodipine group.[19] These results from clinical trials conducted in the 1980s were recently corroborated in meta-analysis.[20] Therefore, clinical guidelines to treat SAH patients recommend treating these patients with a prophylactic 21 days regimen of oral nimodipine.[21] However, these trials, and therefore recommendations, are specifically for SAH resulting from aneurysmal etiology only.

Perimesencephalic Subarachnoid Hemorrhage (pSAH)

A total of 10% to 15% of patients with nontraumatic SAH does not have an underlying aneurysm or macrovascular etiology to explain the hemorrhage pattern. These patients have historically been lumped together as a homogenous pool of angiogram-negative or idiopathic SAH. A more sophisticated approach takes the bleed pattern into account to provide both diagnostic and prognostic implications.[22–24] While diffuse, or aneurysmal, pattern of hemorrhage carries significant risk for DCI and poor outcomes, pSAH is different.

pSAH is a distinct pattern of angiogram-negative SAH in which the hemorrhage is restricted to the basal cisterns. Although rates vary from center to center, pSAH represents 30% to 66% of patients with angiogram-negative SAH.[22,23] These patients have a distinct natural history in contrast with aSAH patients and patients with a diffuse pattern of angiogram-negative SAH (dSAH, Figure 42–1). Critical care complications, neurologic complications, and functional outcomes are far more benign in pSAH patients than dSAH and aSAH patients.[22,23] pSAH patients rarely require cerebrospinal fluid diversion, rarely experience radiographic vasospasm, and have excellent functional outcomes with the overwhelming majority being discharged home.

This distinct natural history suggests a distinct etiology. Given the relatively mild clinical course and lack of correlation with typical vascular risk factors, venous hemorrhage has often been postulated as a cause of pSAH. Consistent with this, atypical deep venous drainage patterns are enriched in patients with pSAH. Rather than the typical Galenic-venous drainage system, patients with pSAH are significantly more likely to have discontinuous, fetal-type veinous drainage directly into dural sinuses rather than the vein of Galen.[25] Moreover, when present, these atypical drainage patterns are typically associated with an eccentric, ipsilateral pSAH.[25] Although only suggestive, these radiographic data support the clinical supposition that the distinct natural history is due to a venous etiology.

The risk of DCI in pSAH is more controversial. Reports vary regarding the incidence, but the rate of convincing DCI is exceedingly low.[26] Given the restriction of blood products in the basal cisterns and low incidence of vasospasm, it is difficult to extrapolate isolated foci of cortical or subcortical diffusion restriction to pSAH-induced DCI. An alternative explanation

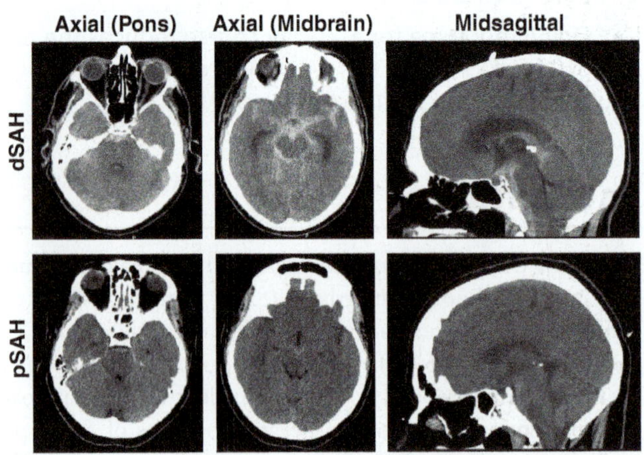

FIGURE 42–1 Illustrative scans demonstrating the difference in bleeding pattern between diffuse angiogram-negative subarachnoid hemorrhage (dSAH) and perimesencephalic subarachnoid hemorrhage (pSAH). Two axial cuts are presented at the level of the pons and at the level of the midbrain, along with a midsagittal cut.

may be that these are catheter-related emboli from the initial diagnostic angiogram. Consistent with this, when MRIs are routinely acquired after diagnostic cerebral angiograms, ~23% of patients will have evidence of a microembolism, complicating the interpretation of these isolated diffusion-weighted imaging (DWI) foci on MRI in the setting of pSAH.[27] When convincingly present, DCI in pSAH patients typically follows a lacunar-type pattern of brainstem infarction, likely due to local vasospasm of small, perforating arteries that are directly affected by the local clot burden.[26] There are currently five convincing reports in the literature, with four others reported but with incomplete clinical information.[23,26]

In this setting, what is the yield of nimodipine in DCI prevention for pSAH? The decision to treat or not to treat pSAH patients is a question of risk and benefit, and no data exists to definitively support treatment with nimodipine in this specific patient population. On the one hand, DCI in pSAH is exceptionally rare and appears to follow a distinct presentation than the typical cases of DCI seen in aSAH (or even from other types of angiogram-negative SAH).[23,26] Patients with pSAH tend to have excellent outcomes regardless of any interventions. Furthermore, nimodipine also incurs risk. In one prospective study following aneurysmal and angio-negative patients, nimodipine regimen was given at full only at 57% of the days. Inability to deliver nimodipine was related to hypotension, a common adverse event related to nimodipine.[28] Similarly, given the changes that have evolved over the past 35 years of supportive neurocritical care for aSAH, there is an ongoing debate regarding the risk of a nimodipine course for patients with low risk for DCI.[29] On the other hand, nimodipine treatment is aimed at reducing the risk for DCI, a complication highly associated with worse outcomes following SAH. Although rare in pSAH patients, it is still described.[23]

AVAILABLE GUIDELINES

For angiographically confirmed pSAH patients, our practice is to empirically start nimodipine, although it is reasonable to defer. We do not complete a 21-day course due to the low likelihood of benefit, risks of hypotension, cumbersome every 4-hour dosing interval as an outpatient, and cost considerations for patients. We perform an initial catheter angiogram upon presentation and an interval noninvasive angiogram at postbleed day 7 to minimize the risk of a missed angiographic source. Similarly, we use daily transcranial doppler ultrasounds or an interval CT angiogram on day 3 to 5 to surveil for vasospasm. At this point, in patients who have no underlying aneurysm and without evidence of radiographic vasospasm, we discharge patients and discontinue nimodipine upon discharge. Since vasospasm is a significant risk factor for DCI, especially if it develops in the first few days,[9] one could decide to continue nimodipine treatment in the rare cases who develop vasospasm. In the absence thereof, the majority of pSAH patients are unlikely to benefit from a 21-day course of nimodipine.

REFERENCES

1. Rincon F, Rossenwasser RH, Dumont A. The epidemiology of admissions of nontraumatic subarachnoid hemorrhage in the United States. *Neurosurgery*. 2013;73:217–222.
2. Udy AA, Vladic C, Saxby ER, et al.: Subarachnoid hemorrhage patients admitted to intensive care in Australia and New Zealand: a multicenter cohort analysis of in-hospital mortality over 15 years. *Crit. Care Med.* 2017;45:e138–e145.
3. Samuels OB, Sadan O, Feng C, et al.: Aneurysmal subarachnoid hemorrhage: trends, outcomes, and predictions from a 15-year perspective of a single neurocritical care unit. *Neurosurgery*. 2021;88:574–583.
4. Weyer GW, Nolan CP, Macdonald RL. Evidence-based cerebral vasospasm management. *Neurosurg. Focus*. 2006;21:E8.
5. Luong CQ, Ngo HM, Hoang HB, et al.: Clinical characteristics and factors relating to poor outcome in patients with aneurysmal subarachnoid hemorrhage in Vietnam: a multicenter prospective cohort study. *PLoS One*. 2021;16:e0256150.
6. Chalard K, Szabo V, Pavillard F, et al.: Long-term outcome in patients with aneurysmal subarachnoid hemorrhage requiring mechanical ventilation. *PLoS One*. 2021;16:e0247942.
7. Raatikainen E, Vahtera A, Kuitunen A, et al.: Prognostic value of the 2010 consensus definition of delayed cerebral ischemia after aneurysmal subarachnoid hemorrhage. *J. Neurol. Sci.* 2021;420:117261.
8. Olsen MH, Orre M, Leisner ACW, et al.: Delayed cerebral ischaemia in patients with aneurysmal subarachnoid haemorrhage: Functional outcome and long-term mortality. *Acta Anaesthesiol. Scand.* 2019;63:1191–1199.
9. Snider SB, Migdady I, LaRose SL, et al.: Transcranial-doppler-measured vasospasm severity is associated with delayed cerebral infarction after subarachnoid hemorrhage. *Neurocrit. Care*. 2022;36:815–821.
10. Macdonald RL, Higashida RT, Keller E, et al.: Randomized trial of clazosentan in patients with aneurysmal subarachnoid hemorrhage undergoing endovascular coiling. *Stroke*. 2012;43:1463–1469.
11. Jang YG, Ilodigwe D, Macdonald RL. Metaanalysis of tirilazad mesylate in patients with aneurysmal subarachnoid hemorrhage. *Neurocrit. Care*. 2009;10:141–147.
12. Carlson AP, Hänggi D, Wong GK, et al.: Single-dose intraventricular nimodipine microparticles versus oral nimodipine for aneurysmal subarachnoid hemorrhage. *Stroke*. 2020;51:1142–1149.
13. Akeret K, Buzzi RM, Schaer CA, et al.: Cerebrospinal fluid hemoglobin drives subarachnoid hemorrhage-related secondary brain injury. *J. Cereb. Blood Flow Metab.* 2021;41:3000–3015.
14. Frontera JA, Claassen J, Schmidt JM,et al.: Prediction of symptomatic vasospasm after subarachnoid hemorrhage: the modified fisher scale. *Neurosurgery*. 2006;59:21–26.
15. Sivakumar S, Tsetsou S, Patel AB, et al.: Cortical spreading depolarizations and clinically measured scalp EEG activity after aneurysmal subarachnoid hemorrhage and traumatic brain injury. *Neurocrit. Care*. 2022;37: 49–59
16. Sugimoto K, Chung DY. Spreading depolarizations and subarachnoid hemorrhage. *Neurotherapeutics*. 2020;17:497–510.
17. Sugimoto K, Nomura S, Shirao S, et al.: Cilostazol decreases duration of spreading depolarization and spreading ischemia after aneurysmal subarachnoid hemorrhage. *Ann. Neurol.* 2018;84:873–885.
18. Allen GS, Ahn HS, Preziosi TJ, et al.: Cerebral arterial spasm–a controlled trial of nimodipine in patients with subarachnoid hemorrhage. *N. Engl. J. Med.* 1983;308:619–624.
19. Pickard JD, Murray GD, Illingworth R, et al.: Effect of oral nimodipine on cerebral infarction and outcome after subarachnoid haemorrhage: British aneurysm nimodipine trial. *BMJ*. 1989;298:636–642.
20. Velat GJ, Kimball MM, Mocco JD, Hoh BL. Vasospasm after aneurysmal subarachnoid hemorrhage: review of randomized controlled trials and meta-analyses in the literature. *World Neurosurg.* 2011;76:446–454.
21. Hoh BL, Ko NU, Amin-Hanjani S, Hsiang-Yi Chou S, Cruz-Flores S, Dangayach NS, Derdeyn CP, Du R, Hänggi D, Hetts SW, et al. 2023 Guideline for the Management of Patients With Aneurysmal Subarachnoid Hemorrhage: A Guideline From the American Heart Association/American Stroke Association. *Stroke*. 2023;54:e314–e370.

22. Nesvick CL, Oushy S, Rinaldo L, Wijdicks EF, Lanzino G, Rabinstein AA. Clinical complications and outcomes of angiographically negative subarachnoid hemorrhage. *Neurology*. 2019;92:E2385–E2394.
23. Akbik F, Pimentel-Farias C, Press DA, et al.: Diffuse angiogram-negative subarachnoid hemorrhage is associated with an intermediate clinical course. *Neurocritical Care*. 2022;36:1002–1010.
24. Rinkel GJ, van Gijn J, Wijdicks EF. Subarachnoid hemorrhage without detectable aneurysm. A review of the causes. *Stroke*. 1993;24: 1403–1409.
25. Van Der Schaaf IC, Velthuis BK, Gouw A, Rinkel GJE. Venous drainage in perimesencephalic hemorrhage. *Stroke*. 2004;35:1614–1618.
26. Mensing LA, Vergouwen MDI, Laban KG, et al.: Perimesencephalic hemorrhage: a review of epidemiology, risk factors, presumed cause, clinical course, and outcome. *Stroke*. 2018;49:1363–1370.
27. Bendszus M, Stoll G. Silent cerebral ischaemia: hidden fingerprints of invasive medical procedures. *Lancet. Neurol.* [Internet]. 2006 [cited 2022 Jun 27];5:364–372. Available from: https://pubmed.ncbi.nlm.nih.gov/16545753/
28. Kieninger M, Gruber M, Knott I, et al.: Incidence of arterial hypotension in patients receiving peroral or continuous intra-arterial nimodipine after aneurysmal or perimesencephalic subarachnoid hemorrhage. *Neurocrit. Care* [Internet]. 2019 [cited 2022 Jun 27];31:32–39. Available from: https://pubmed.ncbi.nlm.nih.gov/30725331/
29. Chen CJ, Turnage C, Sokolowski JD, Kumar JS, Kalani MY, Park MS. Dangers of outpatient nimodipine use after spontaneous subarachnoid hemorrhage in accordance with the Comprehensive Stroke Center guidelines. *J. Clin. Neurosci.* [Internet]. 2018 [cited 2022 Jun 27];52:151–152. Available from: https://pubmed.ncbi.nlm.nih.gov/29656002/

CHAPTER

43

How Should We Manage Vasospasm After Aneurysmal Subarachnoid Hemorrhage

Walid K. Salah, BA, Karol P. Budohoski, MD, PhD, & Ramesh Grandhi, MD

Case

A 52-year-old woman is in the intensive care unit (ICU) 6 days after suffering a subarachnoid hemorrhage from a ruptured posterior communicating artery aneurysm. The aneurysm has since been secured with endovascular coiling. She begins to have worsening contralateral weakness with a fluctuating mental status and is found to have ischemia secondary cerebral vasospasm. How can this best be treated?

Key Points

- Oral nimodipine, maintenance of euvolemia, avoidance of anemia, and hypertension in cases of deterioration secondary to delayed cerebral ischemia (DCI) remain the mainstays of medical treatment for aneurysmal subarachnoid hemorrhage (SAH).
- Future randomized controlled trials are needed to assist in developing better frameworks and standardizations for the way we manage cerebral vasospasm (CVS) today.

Specifically, because intra-arterial and intrathecal modalities have demonstrated promising results in early investigative efforts, our hope is the data from randomized controlled trials will support their use and utility as effective modalities to improve outcomes in this population of patients.

BACKGROUND

Delayed cerebral ischemia (DCI), which is frequently associated with cerebral vasospasm (CVS), remains one of the most common complications following an aneurysmal subarachnoid hemorrhage (SAH).[1] DCI is now recognized as the most significant cause of death and disability after SAH, leading to a 7% to 15% mortality rate[2,3] and severe disability in another 7% of patients.[4] Interestingly, although up to 70% of angiograms at day 7 demonstrate CVS, DCI only occurs in 20% to 30% of patients experiencing aneurysmal SAH.[5–7] DCI and angiographic CVS usually occur between days 7 and 14 but has been reported up to day 21.[7] Despite our increasing understanding of the pathophysiology of CVS and DCI (Figure 43–1), best practices for the diagnosis, prevention, and treatment remained poorly defined. All of these pose significant dilemmas in day-to-day management of patients with aneurysmal SAH.

The diagnosis of CVS and DCI is typically made based on a combination of clinical features supported by imaging. A variety of treatment modalities are commonly used to manage CVS; however, there remains a paucity of evidence behind their use, and to date there is no widely recognized prevention strategy apart from maintaining euvolemia and close-to-normal physiology while the patient is in the ICU. The purpose of this chapter is to outline common treatment modalities for CVS and DCI and the evidence supporting their use.

EVIDENCE AND REVIEW

Hemodynamic Management

For over 50 years, the mainstay of treatment for CVS was induced hypervolemia, hypertension, and hemodilution (commonly referred to as triple-H).[8] The use of such hemodynamic measures was based on the work of Denny-Brown in 1951 demonstrating that patients with severe narrowing of cerebral blood vessels and concomitant hypotension have significantly worse symptoms.[9] Therefore, induced hypertension seemed to be the natural treatment. Further work based on Hagen-Poiseuille's law (Figure 43–2) demonstrated that an increase in blood flow

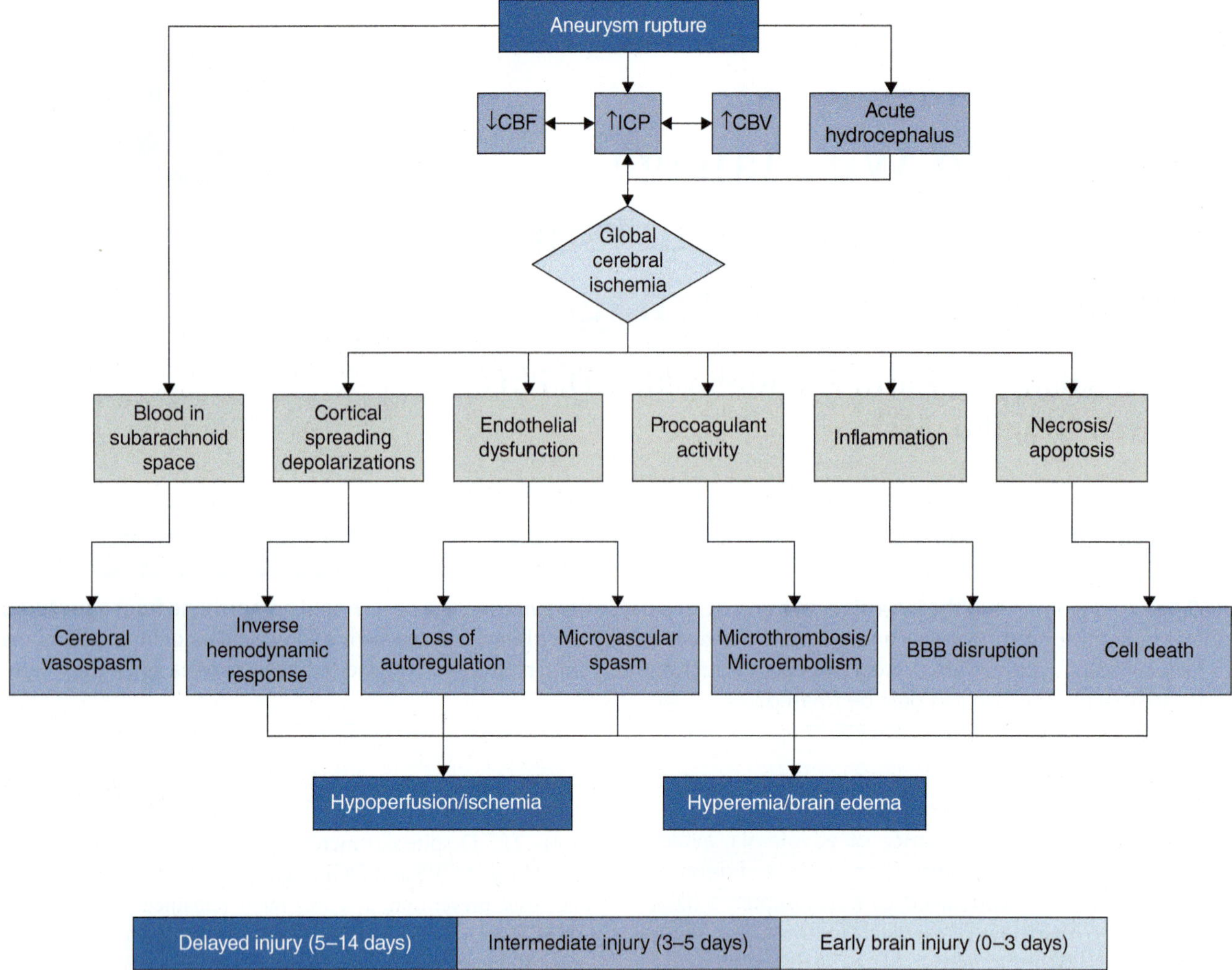

FIGURE 43–1 The multifactorial pathophysiology of delayed cerebral ischemia. CBF, cerebral blood flow; ICP, intracranial pressure; CBV, cerebral blood volume; BBB, blood-brain barrier.

can be achieved with increased pressure as well as hemodilution, establishing triple-H therapy.[8] There are many observational studies as well as anecdotal evidence of remarkable reversal of neurological symptoms with triple-H therapy.[8,10–12] However, one systematic review noted an increase in complications (primarily pulmonary edema) with hypervolemic therapy.[13] Furthermore, hemodilution was found to have no effect on increasing cerebral blood flow and rates of DCI.[13] The component of triple-H therapy that has the most evidence for improving cerebral blood flow and reducing ischemia is induced hypertension.[13–17] Thus, recommendations from the Neurocritical Care Society's

$$\Delta p = \frac{8\mu L Q}{\pi R^4}$$

FIGURE 43–2 Hagen-Poiseuille's law adapted for blood vessels.[8] Δp, blood pressure difference; μ, blood viscosity; L, length of the blood vessel; Q, blood flow rate; R, radius of the vessel.

Multidisciplinary Consensus Conference on management of patients following SAH include the maintenance of euvolemia because many patients are hypovolemic after SAH, avoiding hemodilution, and monitoring hemoglobin concentration to treat anemia.[18] With regard to induced hypertension, it is only recommended if the patient demonstrates signs of deterioration secondary to DCI.[15]

Calcium Channel Blockers

Oral nimodipine remains the mainstay of treatment for SAH and is the only drug approved in the United States for this use.[19] There is convincing evidence that suggests nimodipine does reduce delayed neurological deterioration after SAH and poor outcomes.[2,3,20,21] However, multiple studies have demonstrated that it does not reduce mortality.[3,20,21] Furthermore, the literature remains mixed on whether nimodipine has a significant effect on vasospasm.[2,3,20,21] Some authors suggest that studies did not angiographically confirm vasospasm during the development of DCI, which may have confounded the role nimodipine has on vasospasm.[20] Among other explanations for why nimodipine improves outcomes, independent of vasospasm, is the profibrinolytic effect of nimodipine, which has been found to decrease the levels of plasminogen activator inhibitor 1, thereby potentially reducing microclot burden.[20,22,23] Another school of thought suggests that nimodipine plays a role in the conversion of cortical spreading ischemia to cortical spreading hyperemia.[24] A third possibility is that Ca2+ antagonists in neuronal cells prevent the pathological activation of proteases, endonucleases, and other enzymes that ultimately result in neuronal injury and death.[21] Interestingly, however, a variety of routes to administer Ca2+ antagonists have been investigated, mainly intravenous nicardipine and intraventricular nimodipine, which were both found to be inferior to oral nimodipine.[3,19] Although the literature has demonstrated that oral nimodipine is safe at a dose of 60 mg every 4 hours, it is important to monitor patients for side effects secondary to nimodipine, the most common of which is hypotension (which could very well exacerbate DCI).[21,25,26]

Statins

The use of statins to improve outcomes in patients experiencing SAH has come into question. Earlier studies suggested that statins might play a role in decreasing CVS and DCI and mortality[27]; however, the largest international, multi-institutional randomized controlled trial assessing the role of simvastatin in patients with SAH demonstrated different findings.[28] The study looked at 6-month outcomes, mainly modified Rankin Scale scores (adjusted for age and World Federation of Neurological Surgery grade on admission), in 801 patients randomized to receive a placebo or 40 mg of simvastatin. The study did not detect any benefit in DCI or clinical outcomes from the use of simvastatin.[28] This has been confirmed in other studies, and therefore, statins are currently not routinely used after SAH.[21,28,29]

Endothelin Receptor Antagonists

On the basis of animal models that implicated endothelin-A receptors in having a major role in the pathophysiology of vasospasm,[30] recent efforts have focused on clazosentan, an endothelin-A receptor antagonist, as a potential treatment for vasospasm. In the CONCIOUS-1 trial, intravenous clazosentan was associated with a reduction in angiographic vasospasm and a decrease in morbidity and mortality[31]; however, the CONSCIOUS-2 phase III double-blinded randomized controlled trial demonstrated no significant effects on vasospasm-related outcomes.[32] This finding supports the theory that vasospasm is multifactorial and likely not the only contributor to DCI. Nevertheless, it is important to note that the benefits of clazosentan's reduction of angiographic vasospasm may be masked by the drug's adverse effects (pulmonary edema, anemia, and hypotension, all of which contribute to cerebral ischemia), which were more common in the clazosentan group than the placebo group.[21,32]

Magnesium

Magnesium sulfate has been used widely in the prevention of preeclampsia and eclampsia-induced vasospasm.[33] It is believed that magnesium acts as a noncompetitive antagonist of calcium channels and as an N-methyl-D-aspartate receptor antagonist that leads to vasodilation.[21] In experimental SAH, magnesium sulfate demonstrated promising results in reducing CVS.[34] However, the MASH-2 (Magnesium for Aneurysmal Subarachnoid Hemorrhage) trial, a multicenter randomized controlled trial of 1,204 patients, found that intravenous magnesium sulfate did not improve outcomes after SAH. The authors concluded that routine administration of magnesium could not be supported for this purpose.[35]

Endovascular Balloon Angioplasty

Endovascular balloon angioplasty (EBA) remains one of the mainstay rescue treatments for vasospasm with demonstrated utility.[14,36–41] When used as rescue treatment, EBA decreases DCI, improves outcomes, and decreases morbidity and mortality rates;[14,36–41] however, definitive conclusions cannot be drawn because no randomized controlled trials exist.[36] Additionally, questions regarding the appropriate timing for EBA and patient selection need further investigation. Most studies seem to agree that earlier intervention using balloon angioplasty results in more favorable outcomes;[41–43] however, there is no accepted time frame for the use of medical therapy before transitioning to EBA for CVS refractory to medical treatment. In terms of patient selection, it was widely believed that preprocedural hypodensities/ischemia might preclude patients from EBA; however, one study reported that 15% of preprocedural hypodensities were reversed with balloon angioplasty.[41] Additionally, neurological improvement occurred in 60% of patients with preprocedural hypodensities and 50% had favorable outcomes at discharge. Furthermore, none of the patients with preprocedural hypodensities treated with EBA ended up with hemorrhagic conversion. Conversely, the odds of neurologic recovery and/or good outcomes were five times lower in the patient group with preprocedural hypodensities, indicating that EBA would not be appropriate for some patients.[41] This furthers the dilemma because appropriate selection of patients for EBA becomes even more challenging. Finally, EBA can only be done in patients with focal spasm involving a single vessel that corresponds with clinical symptoms and/or perfusion deficits. This limits the role of EBA in many patients where CVS affects multiple arterial territories including more distal branches.

The prophylactic use of EBA was investigated in a phase II multi-institutional randomized trial.[44] The trial targeted the supraclinoid internal carotid artery, basilar artery, and middle cerebral artery (MCA) M1 segments. Although prophylactic use of transluminal balloon angioplasty within 96 hours of

SAH demonstrated a reduction in vasospasm, outcomes were no different between intervention and control groups.[44,45] In the intervention group of 85 patients, 4 had procedure-related vessel perforation, resulting in the death of 3 patients. Without evidence supporting positive impacts on outcomes, it remains difficult to justify the risks of EBA in a prophylactic setting.

Intra-arterial Pharmacotherapy

Given the role oral calcium channel blockers have in improving outcomes in SAH, intra-arterial verapamil has been explored as a potential preventive treatment modality for vasospasm. Both animal models and small trials have demonstrated promising results with intra-arterial verapamil.[46–49] In one study, intra-arterial verapamil was administered to 86 patients who were found to have symptomatic decline or increased transcranial Doppler (TCD) velocities.[47] Of these, 52% experienced clinical improvement after administration. Although animal models have shown a dose-dependent relationship between intra-arterial verapamil and vertebral vasodilation, the optimum dose in patients has not been settled.[47,50–52] Studies have also shown that administration of low-dose verapamil (2.5-22 mg/procedure) results in neurologic improvement in up to 40% of patients within 24 hours.[47] Support for the efficacy of high-dose verapamil is limited by the small number of clinical series and lack of randomized controlled trials to date. Most studies have indicated that low-dose intra-arterial verapamil is a safe treatment modality following lack of improvement using more traditional treatments (eg, nimodipine).[47] However, when it comes to high-dose intra-arterial verapamil, hemodynamic and intracranial pressure monitoring are crucial for at least 12 hours after treatment.[53] Although no changes to brain tissue oxygenation have been demonstrated, significant increases in intracranial pressure and brain glucose and reductions in cerebral perfusion pressure and mean arterial pressure with high-dose intra-arterial verapamil have been demonstrated.[53] It is also important to note that the literature does cite instances of bradycardia, episodic hypotension, and ictal events with the use of high-dose intra-arterial verapamil.[47,54] One study actually found that intra-arterial nicardipine was just as effective in improving outcomes and reversing hypodensities as balloon angioplasty.[41] Nevertheless, the effects of nicardipine were not as long-lasting and required more frequent administration when compared with balloon angioplasty. However, the lack of large randomized controlled trials limits our knowledge and ability to make conclusions on the effectiveness and utility of intra-arterial verapamil.[41,47]

Intrathecal Management

One of the most promising treatment modalities that has recently been gaining traction is intrathecal vasospasm treatment via lumbar drain or external ventricular drain.[55] The obvious advantage of intrathecal administration of drugs is their ability to reach higher concentrations in the CSF and avoid the blood–brain barrier. A systematic review of nine studies with a total of 377 patients receiving intrathecal nicardipine for vasospasm leading to DCI demonstrated a decrease in angiographic and symptomatic vasospasm and a reduction in mean flow velocities on TCD.[56] The nine studies TCD velocities demonstrated varying rates of decreases in vasospasm in comparison with controls. One specific study demonstrated an absolute risk reduction of 22% in those who received intrathecal nicardipine (7% treatment arm vs. 29% control arm).[57] A separate study of 1,351 patients found that treatment of CVS with intrathecal nicardipine decreased TCDs in 77.3% of patients; the odds ratio for DCI was .61, and the odds ratio to have a favorable functional outcome was 2.17.[58] The most common dosing regimen used in the literature was 4 mg of nicardipine intrathecally every 12 hours.[56] Not only has preliminary data been successful at demonstrating the use of intrathecal nicardipine as a preventive measure, but there is also promising evidence that this treatment plays an important role when used as a rescue agent.[55,59] Agents other than nicardipine are also being analyzed (eg, milrinone, verapamil, nitric oxide, and cilostazol), but at this time, the data on these agents are very limited.[55] Although the available data are promising, the lack of randomized controlled trials to date makes it difficult to draw conclusions on whether intrathecal agents should be used in prevention, rescue therapy, or in combination with other treatment modalities.

REFERENCES

1. Suarez JI, Tarr RW, Selman WR. Aneurysmal subarachnoid hemorrhage. *N Engl J Med*. 2006;354(4):387–396.
2. Pickard JD, Murray GD, Illingworth R, et al. Effect of oral nimodipine on cerebral infarction and outcome after subarachnoid haemorrhage: British Aneurysm Nimodipine Trial. *BMJ*. 1989;298(6674):636–642.
3. Weyer GW, Nolan CP, Macdonald RL. Evidence-based cerebral vasospasm management. *Neurosurg Focus*. 2006;21(3):E8.
4. Kassell NF, Torner JC, Haley EC, Jr., et al. The International Cooperative Study on the Timing of Aneurysm Surgery. Part 1: Overall management results. *J Neurosurg*. 1990;73(1):18–36.
5. Rowland MJ, Hadjipavlou G, Kelly M, et al. Delayed cerebral ischaemia after subarachnoid haemorrhage: looking beyond vasospasm. *Br J Anaesth*. 2012;109(3):315–329.
6. Suarez JI. Diagnosis and Management of Subarachnoid Hemorrhage. *Continuum (Minneap Minn)*. 2015;21(5 Neurocritical Care):1263–1287.
7. Sen J, Afinowi R, Kitchen N, Belli A. Intracranial hemorrhage: aneurysmal, idiopathic, and hypertensive. In: Schapira A, Byrne E, Frackowiak R, et al., eds. *Neurology and Clinical Neuroscience*. Philadelphia: Mosby; 2007: 587–594.
8. Sen J, Belli A, Albon H, et al. Triple-H therapy in the management of aneurysmal subarachnoid haemorrhage. *Lancet Neurol*. 2003;2(10): 614–621.
9. Denny-Brown D. The treatment of recurrent cerebrovascular symptoms and the question of "vasospasm." *Med Clin North Am*. 1951;35(5): 1457–1474.
10. Awad IA, Carter LP, Spetzler RF, et al. Clinical vasospasm after subarachnoid hemorrhage: response to hypervolemic hemodilution and arterial hypertension. *Stroke*. 1987;18(2):365–372.
11. Kassell NF, Peerless SJ, Durward QJ, et al. Treatment of ischemic deficits from vasospasm with intravascular volume expansion and induced arterial hypertension. *Neurosurgery*. 1982;11(3):337–343.
12. Giannotta SL, McGillicuddy JE, Kindt GW. Diagnosis and treatment of postoperative cerebral vasospasm. *Surg Neurol*. 1977;8(4):286–290.

13. Dankbaar JW, Slooter AJ, Rinkel GJ, Schaaf IC. Effect of different components of triple-H therapy on cerebral perfusion in patients with aneurysmal subarachnoid haemorrhage: a systematic review. *Crit Care*. 2010;14(1):R23.
14. Macdonald RL. Delayed neurological deterioration after subarachnoid haemorrhage. *Nat Rev Neurol*. 2014;10(1):44–58.
15. Treggiari MM. Participants in the International Multi-disciplinary Consensus Conference on the Critical Care Management of Subarachnoid Hemorrhage. Hemodynamic management of subarachnoid hemorrhage. *Neurocrit Care*. 2011;15(2):329–335.
16. Muench E, Horn P, Bauhuf C, et al. Effects of hypervolemia and hypertension on regional cerebral blood flow, intracranial pressure, and brain tissue oxygenation after subarachnoid hemorrhage. *Crit Care Med*. 2007;35(8):1844–1851; quiz 1852.
17. Raabe A, Beck J, Keller M, et al. Relative importance of hypertension compared with hypervolemia for increasing cerebral oxygenation in patients with cerebral vasospasm after subarachnoid hemorrhage. *J Neurosurg*. 2005;103(6):974–981.
18. Diringer MN, Bleck TP, Claude Hemphill J, 3rd, et al. Critical care management of patients following aneurysmal subarachnoid hemorrhage: recommendations from the Neurocritical Care Society's Multidisciplinary Consensus Conference. *Neurocrit Care*. 2011;15(2):211–240.
19. Carlson AP, Hanggi D, Wong GK, et al. Single-dose intraventricular nimodipine microparticles versus oral nimodipine for aneurysmal subarachnoid hemorrhage. *Stroke*. 2020;51(4):1142–1149.
20. Etminan N, Vergouwen MD, Ilodigwe D, Macdonald RL. Effect of pharmaceutical treatment on vasospasm, delayed cerebral ischemia, and clinical outcome in patients with aneurysmal subarachnoid hemorrhage: a systematic review and meta-analysis. *J Cereb Blood Flow Metab*. 2011;31(6):1443–1451.
21. Young AM, Karri SK, Helmy A, et al. Pharmacologic management of subarachnoid hemorrhage. *World Neurosurg*. 2015;84(1):28–35.
22. Roos YB, Levi M, Carroll TA, et al. Nimodipine increases fibrinolytic activity in patients with aneurysmal subarachnoid hemorrhage. *Stroke*. 2001;32(8):1860–1862.
23. Vergouwen MD, Vermeulen M, de Haan RJ, et al. Dihydropyridine calcium antagonists increase fibrinolytic activity: a systematic review. *J Cereb Blood Flow Metab*. 2007;27(7):1293–1308.
24. Dreier JP, Korner K, Ebert N, et al. Nitric oxide scavenging by hemoglobin or nitric oxide synthase inhibition by N-nitro-L-arginine induces cortical spreading ischemia when K+ is increased in the subarachnoid space. *J Cereb Blood Flow Metab*. 1998;18(9):978–990.
25. Budohoski KP, Guilfoyle M, Helmy A, et al. The pathophysiology and treatment of delayed cerebral ischaemia following subarachnoid haemorrhage. *J Neurol Neurosurg Psychiatry*. 2014;85(12):1343–1353.
26. Harders A, Kakarieka A, Braakman R, German tSAH Study Group. Traumatic subarachnoid hemorrhage and its treatment with nimodipine. *J Neurosurg*. 1996;85(1):82–89.
27. Sillberg VA, Wells GA, Perry JJ. Do statins improve outcomes and reduce the incidence of vasospasm after aneurysmal subarachnoid hemorrhage: a meta-analysis. *Stroke*. 2008;39(9):2622–2626.
28. Kirkpatrick PJ, Turner CL, Smith C, et al. Simvastatin in aneurysmal subarachnoid haemorrhage (STASH): a multicentre randomised phase 3 trial. *Lancet Neurol*. 2014;13(7):666–675.
29. Vergouwen MD, de Haan RJ, Vermeulen M, Roos YB. Effect of statin treatment on vasospasm, delayed cerebral ischemia, and functional outcome in patients with aneurysmal subarachnoid hemorrhage: a systematic review and meta-analysis update. *Stroke*. 2010;41(1):e47–52.
30. Vatter H, Konczalla J, Seifert V. Endothelin related pathophysiology in cerebral vasospasm: what happens to the cerebral vessels? *Acta Neurochir Suppl*. 2011;110(Pt 1):177–180.
31. Macdonald RL, Kassell NF, Mayer S, et al. Clazosentan to overcome neurological ischemia and infarction occurring after subarachnoid hemorrhage (CONSCIOUS-1): randomized, double-blind, placebo-controlled phase 2 dose-finding trial. *Stroke*. 2008;39(11):3015–3021.
32. Macdonald RL, Higashida RT, Keller E, et al. Clazosentan, an endothelin receptor antagonist, in patients with aneurysmal subarachnoid haemorrhage undergoing surgical clipping: a randomised, double-blind, placebo-controlled phase 3 trial (CONSCIOUS-2). *Lancet Neurol*. 2011;10(7):618–625.
33. Naidu S, Payne AJ, Moodley J, et al. Randomised study assessing the effect of phenytoin and magnesium sulphate on maternal cerebral circulation in eclampsia using transcranial Doppler ultrasound. *Br J Obstet Gynaecol*. 1996;103(2):111–116.
34. van den Bergh WM, Dijkhuizen RM, Rinkel GJ. Potentials of magnesium treatment in subarachnoid haemorrhage. *Magnes Res*. 2004;17(4):301–313.
35. Dorhout Mees SM, Algra A, Vandertop WP, et al. Magnesium for aneurysmal subarachnoid haemorrhage (MASH-2): a randomised placebo-controlled trial. *Lancet*. 2012;380(9836):44–49.
36. Dalai S, Limaye US, Maturu MVS, et al. Role of transluminal balloon angioplasty for the treatment of vasospasm due to aneurysmal subarachnoid haemorrhage: a multicentric Indian experience. *Cureus*. 2022;14(9):e29311.
37. Chaudhry NS, Orning JL, Shakur SF, et al. Safety and efficacy of balloon angioplasty of the anterior cerebral artery for vasospasm treatment after subarachnoid hemorrhage. *Interv Neuroradiol*. 2017;23(4):372–377.
38. Jun P, Ko NU, English JD, et al. Endovascular treatment of medically refractory cerebral vasospasm following aneurysmal subarachnoid hemorrhage. *AJNR Am J Neuroradiol*. 2010;31(10):1911–1916.
39. Hayashi K, Hirao T, Sakai N, et al. Current status of endovascular treatment for vasospasm following subarachnoid hemorrhage: analysis of JR-NET2. *Neurol Med Chir (Tokyo)*. 2014;54(2):107–112.
40. Polin RS, Coenen VA, Hansen CA, et al. Efficacy of transluminal angioplasty for the management of symptomatic cerebral vasospasm following aneurysmal subarachnoid hemorrhage. *J Neurosurg*. 2000;92(2):284–290.
41. Chalouhi N, Tjoumakaris S, Thakkar V, et al. Endovascular management of cerebral vasospasm following aneurysm rupture: outcomes and predictors in 116 patients. *Clin Neurol Neurosurg*. 2014;118:26–31.
42. Jabbarli R, Pierscianek D, Rolz R, et al. Endovascular treatment of cerebral vasospasm after subarachnoid hemorrhage: more is more. *Neurology*. 2019;93(5):e458–e466.
43. Rosenwasser RH, Armonda RA, Thomas JE, et al. Therapeutic modalities for the management of cerebral vasospasm: timing of endovascular options. *Neurosurgery*. 1999;44(5):975–979; discussion 979-980.
44. Zwienenberg-Lee M, Hartman J, Rudisill N, et al. Effect of prophylactic transluminal balloon angioplasty on cerebral vasospasm and outcome in patients with Fisher grade III subarachnoid hemorrhage: results of a phase II multicenter, randomized, clinical trial. *Stroke*. 2008;39(6):1759–1765.
45. Findlay JM, Nisar J, Darsaut T. Cerebral vasospasm: a review. *Can J Neurol Sci*. 2016;43(1):15–32.
46. Maniskas ME, Roberts JM, Aron I, et al. Stroke neuroprotection revisited: intra-arterial verapamil is profoundly neuroprotective in experimental acute ischemic stroke. *J Cereb Blood Flow Metab*. 2016;36(4):721–730.
47. Mao G, Gigliotti MJ, Esplin N, Sexton K. The clinical impact and safety profile of high-dose intra-arterial verapamil treatment for cerebral vasospasm following aneurysmal subarachnoid hemorrhage. *Clin Neurol Neurosurg*. 2021;202:106546.
48. Albanese E, Russo A, Quiroga M, et al. Ultrahigh-dose intraarterial infusion of verapamil through an indwelling microcatheter for medically refractory severe vasospasm: initial experience. Clinical article. *J Neurosurg*. 2010;113(4):913–922.
49. Mikeladze KG, Okishev DN, Belousova OB, et al. Intra-arterial administration of verapamil for the prevention and treatment of cerebral angiospasm. *Acta Neurochir Suppl*. 2020;127:179–183.
50. Abruzzo T, Moran C, Blackham KA, et al. Invasive interventional management of post-hemorrhagic cerebral vasospasm in patients with aneurysmal subarachnoid hemorrhage. *J Neurointerv Surg*. 2012;4(3):169–177.
51. Takayasu M, Bassett JE, Dacey RG, Jr. Effects of calcium antagonists on intracerebral penetrating arterioles in rats. *J Neurosurg*. 1988;69(1):104–109.
52. Takayasu M, Suzuki Y, Shibuya M, et al. The effects of HA compound calcium antagonists on delayed cerebral vasospasm in dogs. *J Neurosurg*. 1986;65(1):80–85.
53. Stuart RM, Helbok R, Kurtz P, et al. High-dose intra-arterial verapamil for the treatment of cerebral vasospasm after subarachnoid hemorrhage: prolonged effects on hemodynamic parameters and brain metabolism. *Neurosurgery*. 2011;68(2):337–345; discussion 345.
54. Rahme R, Abruzzo TA, Zuccarello M, Ringer A. Intra-arterial veramil-induced seizures: drug toxicity or rapid reperfusion? *Can J Neurol Sci*. 2012;39(4):550–552.
55. Grossen AA, Ernst GL, Bauer AM. Update on intrathecal management of cerebral vasospasm: a systematic review and meta-analysis. *Neurosurg Focus*. 2022;52(3):E10.

56. Hafeez S, Grandhi R. Systematic review of intrathecal nicardipine for the treatment of cerebral vasospasm in aneurysmal subarachnoid hemorrhage. *Neurocrit Care.* 2019;31(2):399–405.
57. Toyota A, Nishizawa Y. [Cerebral vasospasm after subarachnoid hemorrhage, and inhibitory effect of nicardipine investigated by means of transcranial Doppler ultrasonography]. *No Shinkei Geka.* 1991;19(12):1143–1150.
58. Sadan O, Waddel H, Moore R, et al. Does intrathecal nicardipine for cerebral vasospasm following subarachnoid hemorrhage correlate with reduced delayed cerebral ischemia? A retrospective propensity score-based analysis. *J Neurosurg.* 2022;136(1):115–124.
59. Grandhi R, Menacho ST, Ravindra VM, et al. Correlation of intraventricular nicardipine for refractory vasospasm in aneurysmal subarachnoid hemorrhage with improved neurophysiology on intracranial multimodality monitoring: illustrative case. *J Neurosurg Case Lessons.* 2022;3(22):CASE22113.

CHAPTER

44

How Can We Optimize Recovery After Ischemic Stroke?

Priya Srikanth, MD, PhD & David J. Lin, MD

Case

Several days after a right-sided middle cerebral artery (MCA) stroke in a 61-year-old woman, the care team is meeting with the patient's family. She is stable and is due to be transferred to a lower acuity floor soon. The family asks, "what can we do to maximize her chances to recover from this?"

Key Points

- Medically appropriate patients without concern for blood-pressure-dependent cerebral perfusion or elevated intracranial pressure may be suitable for early mobilization upon admission. Clinicians should consider the evidence of potential harm from increased out-of-bed mobilization, especially for those with large cerebral injuries, in the very early period after stroke.
- Rehabilitation within the initial weeks of stroke is imperative to capitalize on increased neuroplasticity during this window. Recent studies show promise that similar amounts of therapy delivered in the acute to subacute phase after brain injury have larger positive effects than the same therapy delivered in the chronic phase. Whether increasing rehabilitation intensity in the hyperacute phase (ie, during intensive care unit [ICU] stay) is beneficial remains unknown. Standard practice involves starting with lower intensity rehabilitation within days of admission and increasing intensity as tolerated upon discharge.[1] This remains a ripe area for future study.
- Inpatient serotonin reuptake inhibitor (SSRI) initiation for patients with comorbid mood disorders should continue to be strongly considered especially in patients with motor impairments, given the potential dual effect on neurologic recovery.

BACKGROUND

Stroke is the leading cause of acquired neurologic disability.[2] While remarkable advances have been made in acute stroke care,[3–7] strategies to enhance recovery and rehabilitation after stroke remain limited.[8] Poststroke epochs can be divided into acute (hours-days), subacute (days-weeks), and chronic (months-years) based on tissue responses and biological processes that emerge during these time windows. In contrast to acute stroke treatments in which the goal is to limit neurologic injury by salvaging threatened brain tissue, the goal of stroke recovery treatments is to promote neural repair by targeting surviving neural tissue.

Stroke recovery begins during the acute hospital admission and continues throughout the inpatient rehabilitation and outpatient settings. The rate of recovery of poststroke deficits is generally highest in the first 3 to 6 months after stroke, though patients can continue to improve even years after stroke,[1,9] especially with dedicated therapy.[10] Based on data suggesting that different deficits (ie, motor vs. language vs. cognitive) recover to different degrees with varying time courses, domain-specific outcomes and therapies are best suited for measuring and treating stroke recovery, respectively.[11,12] Multidisciplinary rehabilitation with physical, occupational, and speech therapies is currently the most effective intervention available to maximize poststroke recovery.[8] Despite decades of delivery of acute rehabilitation as the standard of care, the ideal timing, dose, and intensity of rehabilitation therapy after stroke have yet to be elucidated.

While clinical guidelines, based on preclinical literature, have promoted early mobilization after stroke for nearly 20 years,[13] there is a relative paucity of human data demonstrating the specific timing of rehabilitation to optimize neurorecovery. Here we will highlight clinical studies that have examined the impact of early interventions on poststroke recovery, largely in ischemic stroke. We focus on dose and timing. Our goal is to consolidate findings from clinical studies into recommendations for best clinical practice.

EVIDENCE AND REVIEW

Is Early Mobilization Beneficial?

Multiple small, randomized studies have investigated the effect of early mobilization after stroke. The phase II AVERT study found that rehabilitation within 24 hours from stroke was safe and feasible[14] though without a significant difference in favorable outcome. VERITAS similarly demonstrated safety and feasibility of early mobilization within 36 hours of stroke onset.[15] A pooled analysis of AVERT and VERITAS demonstrated increased odds of independence 3 months after stroke.[16] Both trials supported a lower incidence of immobility-related adverse events (ie, venous thromboembolism, pneumonia, and falls) with very early mobilization. Other small studies corroborated safety of very early mobilization, though with variable effects on functional outcome.[17–21] A major limitation of these data is the limited sample size of each study.

Despite early evidence showing a potentially positive impact of very early mobilization, the larger phase III AVERT study did not support these results. In a multicenter trial encompassing 2,104 patients with ischemic or hemorrhagic stroke, intensive mobilization within 24 hours of stroke was associated with *reduced* odds of favorable outcome at 3 months.[22] It is critical to differentiate therapy dose and timing from out-of-bed mobilization, the latter of which was the focus of AVERT. The therapy group spent more time out of bed than the usual care group because the therapy was specifically focused on out-of-bed activities such as sitting, standing, and walking. The underlying pathophysiology leading to worsened outcomes in the early mobilization group is unknown. Early postural shifts after stroke may have a detrimental effect on cerebral perfusion in a subset of patients, especially those with larger strokes and intracerebral hemorrhages. Indeed a subanalysis showed these patients specifically did worse with mobilization.[23] Altogether, AVERT provides a cautionary lesson that early intensive out-of-bed mobilization may worsen outcomes, especially in patients with larger strokes and hemorrhages. Importantly, AVERT was not designed to provide generalizable lessons about dose and timing of *rehabilitation* after stroke.

A recent Cochrane review concluded that evidence does not support a role for early mobilization in improving mortality or functional outcomes after stroke.[24] In the general intensive care unit (ICU) population, one large study found that early active mobilization during mechanical ventilation did not improve mortality or time out of the hospital but did increase mobilization-related adverse events such as arrythmia, altered blood pressure, or hypoxia.[25] Future studies are needed to determine if very early introduction of brief repeated sessions, focusing on increased session number without increasing total mobilization time, might be beneficial for certain patients.[23] Pertinent outcomes of interest would include not only functional outcomes but also modality-specific, impairment-based outcomes (ie, Fugl-Meyer upper extremity score changes[26]) as well as hospitalization duration and mobilization- and immobility-related adverse events.[27]

Rehabilitation Timing: Is Earlier Always Better?

Recovery is typically fastest in the initial several weeks poststroke.[28] Preclinical rodent studies have demonstrated a sensitive period for rehabilitation in the first 2 weeks after stroke, during which rehabilitation has an augmented effect.[29] Whether this holds true in humans remains unknown. Most existing analyses are limited to the subacute to chronic phase of recovery. Within the subacute period, earlier inpatient stroke rehabilitation has been associated with improved functional outcomes.[30,31] Secondary analysis of the EXCITE trial, studying constraint-induced movement therapy (CIMT) 3 to 9 months after stroke, also suggested that patients who received earlier rehabilitation demonstrated improved outcomes.[32]

The Critical Periods After Stroke Study (CPASS) was a phase II study designed to investigate the effects of variable rehabilitation timing on upper extremity motor outcomes.[33] Patients with stroke were randomized to receive an additional 20 hours of upper extremity therapy at three time points: ≤ 30 days (acute), 2 to 3 months (subacute), or ≥ 6 months (chronic) after stroke, compared to controls receiving standard of care motor rehabilitation. Both acute and subacute delivery of upper extremity therapy were associated with better motor recovery at 1 year. In contrast, rehabilitation delivered in the chronic stage did not demonstrate improvement compared to standard of care.[34] CPASS, for the first time, supported the existence of a poststroke sensitive period in human neurorecovery during the acute or subacute period after stroke. It should be noted that the definition of "acute" rehabilitation was up to 30 days from stroke onset, considerably longer than many other studies.

The effect of very early rehabilitation within days of admission (eg, in the ICU) versus rehabilitation after weeks is not yet clear. One study of task-specific upper limb rehabilitation within the 1st week after ischemic stroke demonstrated no significant change in outcomes but showed decreased variability in recovery with early rehabilitation.[35] A recent randomized study comparing standard care with or without rehabilitation within 48 hours of intracerebral hemorrhage found improved mortality and functional outcomes with early rehabilitation.[36] While small studies suggest that early rehabilitation initiation is safe and may augment patient outcomes, further studies will be required to assess the safety and efficacy of very early rehabilitation.

Rehabilitation Intensity: Does Higher Intensity Improve Outcomes?

Independent of therapy timing, the optimal intensity of rehabilitation after stroke poses another question. Animal studies indeed demonstrate a dose-response curve for rehabilitation, plasticity, and recovery.[37–39] Does this relationship exist in humans? Older systematic reviews have supported a potential benefit of increased rehabilitation intensity on poststroke outcomes, though notably limited by heterogeneous patient populations and confounding factors.[40,41]

Recent controlled studies have yet to demonstrate a benefit of increased rehabilitation intensity. One group found that an increased number of task-specific repetitions did not improve motor outcomes in the chronic phase after stroke.[42] The ICARE study evaluated the effect of intensive occupational therapy in the subacute to chronic period after stroke (2-15 weeks). In this analysis, increased occupational therapy intensity was not associated with any significant change in recovery.[43] In the acute phase after stroke, another study compared the efficacy of 2-hour versus 45-minute daily multidisciplinary therapy for hemiplegic patients and showed no difference in outcomes.[44]

CIMT, wherein patients are forced to use the paretic extremity, has emerged as a method of high-intensity poststroke rehabilitation. Prior studies in the subacute to chronic period have demonstrated improved motor recovery with CIMT.[45,46] The VECTORS trial compared traditional therapy to dose-matched or high-intensity CIMT during acute rehabilitation, on average 10 days from stroke onset.[47] While dose-matched CIMT did not change functional outcomes, high-intensity CIMT resulted in worsened motor outcomes at 90 days. Some limitations in the VECTORS patient population should be noted, including substantial differences across groups in gender balance, number of prior strokes, and dominant limb involvement. But taken at face value, the results raise concern for harm with higher intensity rehabilitation—the mechanism of which is unclear. It is possible that increased demand on vulnerable perilesional brain areas exacerbates neurologic injury, as has been shown in animal models.[48,49]

Based on current evidence, the ideal intensity of rehabilitation after stroke is still undetermined. There may be detrimental effects of overly intense rehabilitation in the acute recovery period, so caution should be exercised immediately after stroke. There remains a possibility that intensive rehabilitation may accelerate poststroke recovery, even in the absence of changing the long-term outcome.[50,51] Narrowing patient selection, targeted interventions, and outcomes tailored to neurologic deficits may uncover specific patients who would benefit from early intensive therapies.

Pharmacologic Interventions

Multiple medications have been studied in poststroke neurorecovery, including serotonergic agents, dopaminergic agents, and amphetamines.[52–56] Selective serotonin reuptake inhibitors (SSRIs) have shown the most promise. The FLAME trial found that fluoxetine initiation in hemiparetic patients within 10 days after stroke improved motor recovery.[57] Three larger follow-up studies—FOCUS, AFFINITY, and EFFECTS—showed no difference in functional outcomes after stroke but did demonstrate an increased risk of fractures with fluoxetine treatment.[58–60] All three were pragmatic trials that enrolled far more heterogenous patients than FLAME, with different domains of stroke deficits, varying stroke severities, and less specific outcome measures. For example, FOCUS enrolled stroke patients regardless of deficit domain and evaluated only modified Rankin scale (mRS) at 6 months, compared to FLAME which specifically assessed motor outcomes in patients with poststroke hemiparesis. Clinically meaningful differences in neurorecovery may therefore have been missed in these follow-up studies. Nevertheless, the potential benefit of fluoxetine on motor recovery should be balanced with the increased risk of fractures at 6 months.

Clinicians should carefully consider initiation of SSRIs in stroke patients with comorbid mood disorders, as depressive symptoms can limit engagement in rehabilitation and are associated with worse outcomes.[61,62] Although SSRI initiation is often deferred to the outpatient setting, initiation in the ICU should be considered, given the possible impact on neurorecovery. Further studies investigating the effects of pharmacologic interventions on stroke recovery are ongoing and may yield increased therapeutic options in the future.[53]

Neurotechnological Interventions

Technology-assisted rehabilitation is a burgeoning area of investigation. A wide array of technologies are of interest, including electrical stimulation (vagal nerve stimulation [VNS], transcranial direct current stimulation [tDCS], epidural electrical stimulation, and deep brain stimulation [DBS]), transcranial magnetic stimulation (TMS), brain–computer interface (BCI) technologies, and robot-assisted therapies. These neurotechnologies have been studied largely in the chronic recovery phase. The field is further complicated by the abundance of variables involved in technology deployment, such as detailed stimulation specifications, stimulation location, and concordance with rehabilitation therapies. It is difficult to compare across studies as details of stimulation techniques often vary. Common mechanistic frameworks are needed to optimize neurotechnological approaches.[63]

Despite several smaller studies with variable results, analyses encompassing multiple trials have failed to show a clear benefit for the use of noninvasive brain stimulation (ie, TMS or tDCS) to augment functional outcomes after stroke.[64–69] Similarly, in the phase III Everest study, epidural stimulation did not improve recovery in a primary intent-to-treat analysis, though in posthoc analyses some subsets of patients appeared to benefit.[70] DBS after stroke has been described in case reports most commonly for maladaptive poststroke neurologic disorders such as dystonia, dyskinesia, tremor, and pain, with positive results.[71] Although rarer, there are also reports of DBS use to alleviate motor impairment after stroke,[72] and the EDEN phase I trial of cerebellar dentate nucleus stimulation for stroke motor recovery is ongoing.[72] Data are presently lacking to support the routine use of brain stimulation to promote neurorehabilitation.

BCI employs invasive or noninvasive techniques to decode neural activity and uses this activity to control external devices.[73–75] Though in early stages, BCI-assisted rehabilitation has shown encouraging results in small cohorts.[74–77] Robot-assisted therapy has also gained attention, and patients have access to several devices marketed for recovery after stroke.[78,79] Larger trials evaluating robot-assisted therapy for upper or lower limb motor recovery after stroke have not found any significant benefit.[80,81] However, the selection of patients with moderate-to-severe impairment may have limited the potential for further recovery. The observed benefits of robotics-assisted therapy in published studies are likely related to the higher rehabilitation intensity with robot-assisted therapy. These effects have not been replicated when rehabilitation dose, frequency, and intensity are matched in controls.[82,83]

BCI and robot-assisted therapy trials are challenging to synthesize, given the extensive variety of device types and implementation as well as barriers to properly controlled and properly blinded trial design inherent to the methods studied. There is no evidence that either BCI or robot-assisted therapy is universally beneficial for neurorecovery.[71,84] It remains possible that a subset of patients with a particular range of neurologic deficits and preserved neural substrate may benefit from these technologies.

VNS serves as a promising example of preclinical to clinical technology translation. In rodent models, VNS promotes neuroplasticity and improves recovery after stroke.[85–89] The VNS-REHAB trial evaluated the effect of VNS paired with rehabilitation after chronic ischemic stroke and showed a modest but clinically significant increase in motor recovery.[90] This resulted in Food and Drug Administration (FDA) approval of a VNS system for chronic stroke recovery, though the suitability of VNS in the acute or subacute period remains to be determined. The translation of preclinical findings to well-controlled clinical studies of VNS provides a model for future investigation of other neurotechnologies.

REFERENCES

1. Belagaje, S. R. Stroke Rehabilitation. *Continuum (Minneap Minn)* 23, 238–253 (2017).
2. Virani, S. S. *et al.* Heart Disease and Stroke Statistics—2021 Update: A Report From the American Heart Association. *Circulation* 143, e254–e743 (2021).
3. Menon, B. K. *et al.* Intravenous Tenecteplase Compared With Alteplase for Acute Ischaemic Stroke in Canada (AcT): A Pragmatic, Multicentre, Open-Label, Registry-Linked, Randomised, Controlled, Non-Inferiority Trial. *Lancet* (2022) doi:10.1016/s0140-6736(22)01054-6.
4. Group, N. I. of N. D. and S. rt-P. S. S. Tissue Plasminogen Activator for Acute Ischemic Stroke. *New Engl J Med* 333, 1581–1588 (1995).
5. Berkhemer, O. A. *et al.* A Randomized Trial of Intraarterial Treatment for Acute Ischemic Stroke. *New Engl J Med* 372, 11–20 (2015).
6. Goyal, M. *et al.* Randomized Assessment of Rapid Endovascular Treatment of Ischemic Stroke. *New Engl J Med* 372, 1019–1030 (2015).
7. Lin, J. & Frontera, J. A. Decompressive Hemicraniectomy for Large Hemispheric Strokes. *Stroke* 52, 1500–1510 (2021).
8. Winstein, C. J. *et al.* Guidelines for Adult Stroke Rehabilitation and Recovery. *Stroke* 47, e98–e169 (2016).
9. Duncan, P. W., Goldstein, L. B., Matchar, D., Divine, G. W. & Feussner, J. Measurement of Motor Recovery After Stroke. Outcome Assessment and Sample Size Requirements. *Stroke* 23, 1084–1089 (1992).
10. Ward, N. S., Brander, F. & Kelly, K. Intensive Upper Limb Neurorehabilitation in Chronic Stroke: Outcomes From the Queen Square programme. *J Neurol Neurosurg Psychiatry* 90, 498 (2019).
11. Cramer, S. C., Koroshetz, W. J. & Finklestein, S. P. The Case for Modality-Specific Outcome Measures in Clinical Trials of Stroke Recovery-Promoting Agents. *Stroke* 38, 1393–1395 (2007).
12. Erler, K. S. *et al.* Association of Modified Rankin Scale With Recovery Phenotypes in Patients With Upper Extremity Weakness After Stroke. *Neurology* 98, e1877–e1885 (2022).
13. Diserens, K., Michel, P. & Bogousslavsky, J. Early Mobilisation After Stroke: Review of the Literature. *Cerebrovasc Dis* 22, 183–190 (2006).
14. Bernhardt, J., Dewey, H., Thrift, A., Collier, J. & Donnan, G. A Very Early Rehabilitation Trial for Stroke (AVERT). *Stroke* 39, 390–396 (2008).
15. Langhorne, P. *et al.* Very Early Rehabilitation or Intensive Telemetry After Stroke: A Pilot Randomised Trial. *Cerebrovasc Dis* 29, 352–360 (2010).
16. Craig, L. E., Bernhardt, J., Langhorne, P. & Wu, O. Early Mobilization After Stroke. *Stroke* 41, 2632–2636 (2010).
17. Chippala, P. & Sharma, R. Effect of Very Early Mobilisation on Functional Status in Patients With Acute Stroke: A Single-Blind, Randomized Controlled Trail. *Clin Rehabil* 30, 669–675 (2015).
18. Sundseth, A., Thommessen, B. & Rønning, O. M. Outcome After Mobilization Within 24 Hours of Acute Stroke. *Stroke* 43, 2389–2394 (2012).
19. Poletto, S. R. *et al.* Early Mobilization in Ischemic Stroke: A Pilot Randomized Trial of Safety and Feasibility in a Public Hospital in Brazil. *Cerebrovasc Dis Extra* 5, 31–40 (2015).
20. Morreale, M. *et al.* Early Versus Delayed Rehabilitation Treatment in Hemiplegic Patients with Ischemic Stroke: Proprioceptive or Cognitive Approach? *Eur J Phys Rehab Med* 52, 81–89 (2015).
21. Herisson, F. *et al.* Early Sitting in Ischemic Stroke Patients (SEVEL): A Randomized Controlled Trial. *Plos One* 11, e0149466 (2016).
22. group, T. A. T. C. Efficacy and Safety of Very Early Mobilisation Within 24 h of Stroke Onset (AVERT): A Randomised Controlled Trial. *Lancet* 386, 46–55 (2015).
23. Langhorne, P., Wu, O., Rodgers, H., Ashburn, A. & Bernhardt, J. A Very Early Rehabilitation Trial After stroke (AVERT): A Phase III, Multicentre, Randomised Controlled Trial. *Health Technol Asses* 21, 1–120 (2017).
24. Langhorne, P., Collier, J. M., Bate, P. J., Thuy, M. N. & Bernhardt, J. Very Early Versus Delayed Mobilisation After Stroke. *Cochrane Database Syst Rev* 2018, CD006187 (2018).
25. Group, T. S. I. and the A. C. T. *et al.* Early Active Mobilization During Mechanical Ventilation in the ICU. *New Engl J Med* 387, 1747–1758 (2022).
26. Fugl-Meyer, A. R., Jääskö, L., Leyman, I., Olsson, S. & Steglind, S. The Post-Stroke Hemiplegic Patient. 1. A Method for Evaluation of Physical Performance. *Scand J Rehabil Med* 7, 13–31 (1975).
27. Li, Z., Zhang, X., Wang, K. & Wen, J. Effects of Early Mobilization After Acute Stroke: A Meta-Analysis of Randomized Control Trials. *J Stroke Cerebrovasc Dis* 27, 1326–1337 (2018).
28. Jørgensen, H. S. *et al.* Outcome and Time Course of Recovery in Stroke. Part II: Time Course of Recovery. The Copenhagen Stroke Study. *Arch Phys Med Rehab* 76, 406–412 (1995).
29. Biernaskie, J., Chernenko, G. & Corbett, D. Efficacy of Rehabilitative Experience Declines With Time After Focal Ischemic Brain Injury. *Journal of Neuroscience* 24, 1245–1254 (2004).
30. Paolucci, S. *et al.* Early Versus Delayed Inpatient Stroke Rehabilitation: A Matched Comparison Conducted in Italy. *Arch Phys Med Rehab* 81, 695–700 (2000).
31. Maulden, S. A., Gassaway, J., Horn, S. D., Smout, R. J. & DeJong, G. Timing of Initiation of Rehabilitation After Stroke. *Arch Phys Med Rehab* 86, 34–40 (2005).
32. Wolf, S. L. *et al.* The EXCITE Stroke Trial. *Stroke* 41, 2309–2315 (2010).
33. Dromerick, A. W. *et al.* Critical Periods After Stroke Study: Translating Animal Stroke Recovery Experiments Into a Clinical Trial. *Front Hum Neurosci* 9, 231 (2015).
34. Dromerick, A. W. *et al.* Critical Period After Stroke Study (CPASS): A Phase II Clinical Trial Testing an Optimal Time for Motor

Recovery After Stroke in Humans. *Proc National Acad Sci* 118, e2026676118 (2021).

35. Hubbard, I. J. *et al.* A Randomized Controlled Trial of the Effect of Early Upper-Limb Training on Stroke Recovery and Brain Activation. *Neurorehab Neural Re* 29, 703–713 (2015).
36. Liu, N. *et al.* Randomized Controlled Trial of Early Rehabilitation After Intracerebral Hemorrhage Stroke. *Stroke* 45, 3502–3507 (2018).
37. Bell, J. A., Wolke, M. L., Ortez, R. C., Jones, T. A. & Kerr, A. L. Training Intensity Affects Motor Rehabilitation Efficacy Following Unilateral Ischemic Insult of the Sensorimotor Cortex in C57BL/6 Mice. *Neurorehab Neural Re* 29, 590–598 (2015).
38. Jeffers, M. S. *et al.* Does Stroke Rehabilitation Really Matter? Part B: An Algorithm for Prescribing an Effective Intensity of Rehabilitation. *Neurorehab Neural Re* 32, 73–83 (2018).
39. MacLellan, C. L. *et al.* A Critical Threshold of Rehabilitation Involving Brain-Derived Neurotrophic Factor Is Required for Poststroke Recovery. *Neurorehab Neural Re* 25, 740–748 (2011).
40. Langhorne, P., Wagenaar, R. & Partridge, C. Physiotherapy After Stroke: More Is Better? *Physiotherapy Res Int* 1, 75–88 (1996).
41. Kwakkel, G., Wagenaar, R. C., Koelman, T. W., Lankhorst, G. J. & Koetsier, J. C. Effects of Intensity of Rehabilitation After Stroke: A Research Synthesis. *Stroke* 28, 1550–1556 (1997).
42. Lang, C. E. *et al.* Dose Response of Task-Specific Upper Limb Training in People at least 6 Months Poststroke: A Phase II, Single-Blind, Randomized, Controlled Trial. *Ann Neurol.* 80, 342–354 (2016).
43. Winstein, C. J. *et al.* Effect of a Task-Oriented Rehabilitation Program on Upper Extremity Recovery Following Motor Stroke: The ICARE Randomized Clinical Trial. *Jama* 315, 571–581 (2016).
44. Lauro, A. D. *et al.* A Randomized Trial on the Efficacy of Intensive Rehabilitation in the Acute Phase of Ischemic Stroke. *J Neurol* 250, 1206–1208 (2003).
45. Wolf, S. L. *et al.* Effect of Constraint-Induced Movement Therapy on Upper Extremity Function 3 to 9 Months After Stroke: The EXCITE Randomized Clinical Trial. *Jama* 296, 2095–2104 (2006).
46. Wolf, S. L. *et al.* Retention of Upper Limb Function in Stroke Survivors who Have Received Constraint-Induced Movement Therapy: The EXCITE Randomised Trial. *Lancet Neurology* 7, 33–40 (2008).
47. Dromerick, A. W. *et al.* Very Early Constraint-Induced Movement During Stroke Rehabilitation (VECTORS). *Neurology* 73, 195–201 (2009).
48. Kozlowski, D. A., James, D. C. & Schallert, T. Use-Dependent Exaggeration of Neuronal Injury after Unilateral Sensorimotor Cortex Lesions. *J Neurosci* 16, 4776–4786 (1996).
49. Humm, J. L., Kozlowski, D. A., James, D. C., Gotts, J. E. & Schallert, T. Use-Dependent Exacerbation of Brain Damage Occurs During an Early Post-Lesion Vulnerable Period. *Brain Res* 783, 286–292 (1998).
50. Kwakkel, G., Wagenaar, R. C., Twisk, J. W., Lankhorst, G. J. & Koetsier, J. C. Intensity of Leg and Arm Training After Primary Middle-Cerebral-Artery Stroke: A Randomised Trial. *Lancet* 354, 191–196 (1999).
51. Kwakkel, G. *et al.* Effects of Unilateral Upper Limb Training in Two Distinct Prognostic Groups Early After Stroke. *Neurorehab Neural Re* 30, 804–816 (2016).
52. Cramer, S. C. Recovery After Stroke. *Continuum (Minneap Minn)* 26, 415–434 (2020).
53. Lin, D. J., Finklestein, S. P. & Cramer, S. C. New Directions in Treatments Targeting Stroke Recovery. *Stroke* 49, 3107–3114 (2018).
54. Scheidtmann, K., Fries, W., Müller, F. & Koenig, E. Effect of Levodopa in Combination With Physiotherapy on Functional Motor Recovery After Stroke: A Prospective, Randomised, Double-Blind Study. *The Lancet* 358, 787–790 (2001).
55. Ford, G. A. *et al.* Safety and Efficacy of Co-Careldopa as an Add-On Therapy to Occupational and Physical Therapy in Patients After Stroke (DARS): A Randomised, Double-Blind, Placebo-Controlled Trial. *Lancet Neurol* 18, 530–538 (2019).
56. Gladstone, D. J. *et al.* Physiotherapy Coupled With Dextroamphetamine for Rehabilitation After Hemiparetic Stroke. *Stroke* 37, 179–185 (2006).
57. Chollet, F. *et al.* Fluoxetine for Motor Recovery After Acute Ischaemic Stroke (FLAME): A Randomised Placebo-Controlled Trial. *Lancet Neurol* 10, 123–130 (2011).
58. Collaboration, F. T. Effects of Fluoxetine on Functional Outcomes After Acute Stroke (FOCUS): A Pragmatic, Double-Blind, Randomised, Controlled Trial. *Lancet* 393, 265–274 (2019).
59. Hankey, G. J. *et al.* Safety and Efficacy of Fluoxetine on Functional Outcome After Acute Stroke (AFFINITY): A Randomised, Double-Blind, Placebo-Controlled Trial. *Lancet Neurology* 19, 651–660 (2020).
60. Collaboration, E. T. *et al.* Safety and Efficacy of Fluoxetine on Functional Recovery After Acute Stroke (EFFECTS): A Randomised, Double-Blind, Placebo-Controlled Trial. *Lancet Neurology* 19, 661–669 (2020).
61. Herrmann, N., Black, S. E., Lawrence, J., Szekely, C. & Szalai, J. P. The Sunnybrook Stroke Study. *Stroke* 29, 618–624 (1998).
62. Andersen, G., Vestergaard, K. & Lauritzen, L. Effective Treatment of Post-stroke Depression With the Selective Serotonin Reuptake Inhibitor Citalopram. *Stroke* 25, 1099–1104 (1994).
63. Ganguly, K., Khanna, P., Morecraft, R. J. & Lin, D. J. Modulation of Neural Co-Firing to Enhance Network Transmission and Improve Motor Function After Stroke. *Neuron* 110, 2363–2385 (2022).
64. Dionísio, A., Duarte, I. C., Patrício, M. & Castelo-Branco, M. The Use of Repetitive Transcranial Magnetic Stimulation for Stroke Rehabilitation: A Systematic Review. *J Stroke Cerebrovasc Dis* 27, 1–31 (2018).
65. Ting, W. K.-C., Fadul, F. A.-R., Fecteau, S. & Ethier, C. Neurostimulation for Stroke Rehabilitation. *Front Neurosci-switz* 15, 649459 (2021).
66. Hao, Z., Wang, D., Zeng, Y. & Liu, M. Repetitive Transcranial Magnetic Stimulation for Improving Function After Stroke. *Cochrane Database Syst Rev* CD008862 (2013) doi:10.1002/14651858.cd008862.pub2.
67. Elsner, B., Kugler, J., Pohl, M. & Mehrholz, J. Transcranial Direct Current Stimulation (tDCS) for Improving Activities of Daily Living, and Physical and Cognitive Functioning, in People After Stroke. *Cochrane Database Syst Rev* 2020, CD009645 (2020).
68. Bai, Z., Zhang, J. & Fong, K. N. K. Effects of Transcranial Magnetic Stimulation in Modulating Cortical Excitability in Patients With Stroke: A Systematic Review and Meta-Analysis. *J Neuroeng Rehabil* 19, 24 (2022).
69. Harvey, R. L. *et al.* Randomized Sham-Controlled Trial of Navigated Repetitive Transcranial Magnetic Stimulation for Motor Recovery in Stroke. *Stroke* 49, 2138–2146 (2018).
70. Levy, R. M. *et al.* Epidural Electrical Stimulation for Stroke Rehabilitation. *Neurorehab Neural Re* 30, 107–119 (2016).
71. Elias, G. J. B., Namasivayam, A. A. & Lozano, A. M. Deep Brain Stimulation for Stroke: Current Uses and Future Directions. *Brain Stimul* 11, 3–28 (2018).
72. Wathen, C. A., Frizon, L. A., Maiti, T. K., Baker, K. B. & Machado, A. G. Deep Brain Stimulation of the Cerebellum for Poststroke Motor Rehabilitation: From Laboratory to Clinical Trial. *Neurosurg Focus* 45, E13 (2018).
73. Hochberg, L. R. *et al.* Reach and Grasp by People With Tetraplegia Using a Neurally Controlled Robotic Arm. *Nature* 485, 372–375 (2012).
74. Ramos-Murguialday, A. *et al.* Brain–Machine Interface in Chronic Stroke Rehabilitation: A Controlled Study. *Ann Neurol.* 74, 100–108 (2013).
75. Sebastián-Romagosa, M. *et al.* Brain Computer Interface Treatment for Motor Rehabilitation of Upper Extremity of Stroke Patients—A Feasibility Study. *Front Neurosci-switz* 14, 591435 (2020).
76. Bockbrader, M. A. *et al.* Brain Computer Interfaces in Rehabilitation Medicine. *Pm&r* 10, S233–S243 (2018).
77. Bundy, D. T. *et al.* Contralesional Brain–Computer Interface Control of a Powered Exoskeleton for Motor Recovery in Chronic Stroke Survivors. *Stroke* 48, 1908–1915 (2017).
78. Hobbs, B. & Artemiadis, P. A Review of Robot-Assisted Lower-Limb Stroke Therapy: Unexplored Paths and Future Directions in Gait Rehabilitation. *Front Neurorobotics* 14, 19 (2020).
79. Duret, C., Grosmaire, A.-G. & Krebs, H. I. Robot-Assisted Therapy in Upper Extremity Hemiparesis: Overview of an Evidence-Based Approach. *Front Neurol* 10, 412 (2019).
80. Lo, A. C. *et al.* Robot-Assisted Therapy for Long-Term Upper-Limb Impairment After Stroke. *New Engl J Medicine* 362, 1772–1783 (2010).
81. Duncan, P. W. *et al.* Body-Weight–Supported Treadmill Rehabilitation After Stroke. *New Engl J Medicine* 364, 2026–2036 (2011).
82. Volpe, B. T. *et al.* Intensive Sensorimotor Arm Training Mediated by Therapist or Robot Improves Hemiparesis in Patients With Chronic Stroke. *Neurorehab Neural Re* 22, 305–310 (2008).

83. Klamroth-Marganska, V. *et al.* Three-Dimensional, Task-Specific Robot Therapy of the Arm After Stroke: A Multicentre, Parallel-Group Randomised Trial. *Lancet Neurol* 13, 159–166 (2014).
84. Mehrholz, J., Pohl, M., Platz, T., Kugler, J. & Elsner, B. Electromechanical and Robot-Assisted Arm Training for Improving Activities of Daily Living, Arm Function, and Arm Muscle Strength After Stroke. *Cochrane Database Syst Rev* 2018, CD006876 (2018).
85. Khodaparast, N. *et al.* Vagus Nerve Stimulation Delivered During Motor Rehabilitation Improves Recovery in a Rat Model of Stroke. *Neurorehab Neural Re* 28, 698–706 (2014).
86. Khodaparast, N. *et al.* Vagus Nerve Stimulation During Rehabilitative Training Improves Forelimb Recovery After Chronic Ischemic Stroke in Rats. *Neurorehab Neural Re* 30, 676–684 (2016).
87. Hays, S. A. *et al.* Vagus Nerve Stimulation During Rehabilitative Training Improves Functional Recovery After Intracerebral Hemorrhage. *Stroke* 45, 3097–3100 (2018).
88. Porter, B. A. *et al.* Repeatedly Pairing Vagus Nerve Stimulation With a Movement Reorganizes Primary Motor Cortex. *Cereb Cortex* 22, 2365–2374 (2012).
89. Meyers, E. C. *et al.* Vagus Nerve Stimulation Enhances Stable Plasticity and Generalization of Stroke Recovery. *Stroke* 49, 710–717 (2018).
90. Dawson, J. *et al.* Vagus Nerve Stimulation Paired With Rehabilitation for Upper Limb Motor Function After Ischaemic Stroke (VNS-REHAB): A Randomised, Blinded, Pivotal, Device Trial. *Lancet* 397, 1545–1553 (2021).

CHAPTER

45

How Do We Manage Intracranial Large-Vessel Dissection?

Jody Manners, MD*, Timothy Miller, MD, & Nicholas A. Morris, MD

Case

A 59-year-old man presented for surgical debulking of a planum sphenoidale meningioma. Changes in neuro-monitoring were encountered during surgical resection of the lesion, and intraoperative Doppler suggested poor flow in the right internal carotid artery (ICA). A follow-up computed tomography (CT) angiogram demonstrated an area of poor opacification of the communicating right ICA while CT perfusion showed a corresponding prolonged Tmax throughout the right cerebral hemisphere. Right ICA catheter angiography confirmed a dissection of the vessel resulting in an associated hemodynamically significant stenosis. How do we manage intracranial large vessel dissection?

Key Points

- Current treatment for intracranial dissection is directed by lesion location, stability, and presence of ischemic or hemorrhagic sequelae.
- Data specifically for thrombolysis in isolated intracranial arterial dissection (IAD) are especially lacking.
- Symptomatic IAD is most frequently treated with antithrombotic agents when ischemia is present.
- Antiplatelet and anticoagulant strategies appear to have similar efficacy regarding prevention of recurrent stroke and transient ischemic attack; however, only observational data are available to inform safety profiles.
- Clinical dogma warns against the use of anticoagulants in patients with intracranial extension due to increased risk of subarachnoid hemorrhage.
- Insufficient evidence is available to guide endovascular treatment decisions regarding mechanical thrombectomy ± stenting of acute ischemic strokes due to IAD. Endovascular intervention for recurrent ischemia despite maximal medical management is also reported, though conclusions for efficacy and safety remain unclear.
- Endovascular or open surgical intervention for ruptured dissecting aneurysm is performed to reduce rerupture rates with observational data supporting such interventions, particularly for higher severity hemorrhage. Insufficient evidence is available to guide endovascular treatment decisions regarding mechanical thrombectomy ± stenting of acute ischemic strokes due to IAD.

For author Jody Manners:

*I am a military service member or federal/contracted employee of the United States government. This work was prepared as part of my official duties. Title 17 U.S.C. 105 provides that 'copyright protection under this title is not available for any work of the United States Government.' Title 17 U.S.C. 101 defines a U.S. Government work as work prepared by a military service member or employee of the U.S. Government as part of that person's official duties. The views expressed in this article reflect the results of research conducted by the author and do not necessarily reflect the official policy or position of the Department of the Navy, Department of Defense, nor the United States Government."

BACKGROUND

Intracranial arterial dissection (IAD) is a well-recognized, albeit infrequent and underdiagnosed etiology of ischemic stroke and subarachnoid hemorrhage. IAD accounts for less than 10% of subarachnoid hemorrhage and an even smaller proportion of ischemic stroke (Giroud et al., 1994; Guillon et al., 1998; Kocaeli et al., 2009; Krings & Choi, 2010; Ro et al., 2009; Sasaki et al., 1991). Risk factors are unknown but postulated to include Asian descent, connective tissue diseases and perhaps preceding minor trauma (Hegedüs, 1984; Inoue et al., 2007; B. M. Kim et al., 2011; S. T. Kim et al., 2016; Kwak et al., 2011; Maski et al., 2011; O'Sullivan et al., 1990; Parlapiano et al., 2020; Prabhakaran & Krakauer, 2006; Sherman et al., 1981). Nearly all patients diagnosed with subarachnoid hemorrhage present with severe, sudden onset headache, often preceded by a milder headache of insidious onset (Figures 45–1 to 45–5) (Mizutani, 2011). A similar prodromal headache is found in patients with unruptured IADs presenting with ischemia or simply headache. Owing to its low incidence, randomized controlled trials and comparative outcome data are lacking to guide treatment decisions for IAD as compared to cervical artery dissection and other etiologies of stroke.

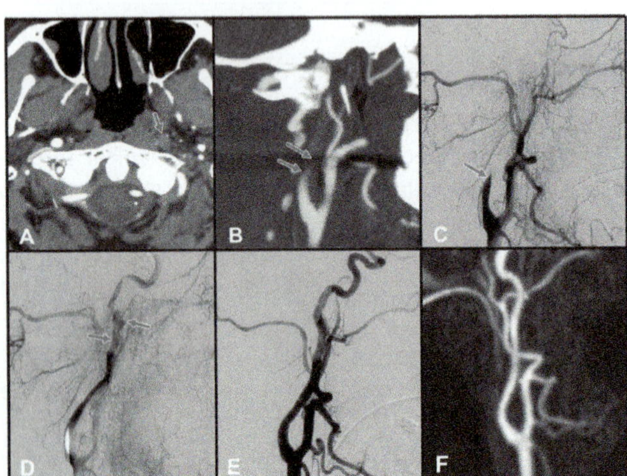

FIGURE 45–1 A 45-year-old man presented with acute ischemic stroke symptoms referable to the left middle cerebral artery territory. There was no history of preceding trauma. Computed tomography (CT) angiography (arrows A and B) demonstrates tapering and apparent occlusion of the cervical left internal carotid artery (ICA). Lateral projection views from a subsequent catheter angiogram performed during injection of contrast into the left common carotid artery redemonstrated marked tapering of the left cervical ICA consistent with spontaneous dissection (arrow C). There was a small amount of stagnant, antegrade flow through the vessel on delayed imaging (D), which showed that the dissection extended into the petrous segment in the skull base (arrow D). The patient subsequently underwent emergent endovascular stenting of the cervical and petrous left ICA segments with restoration of antegrade flow (E). MR angiography (F) performed 3 months later demonstrated excellent remodeling of the left ICA.

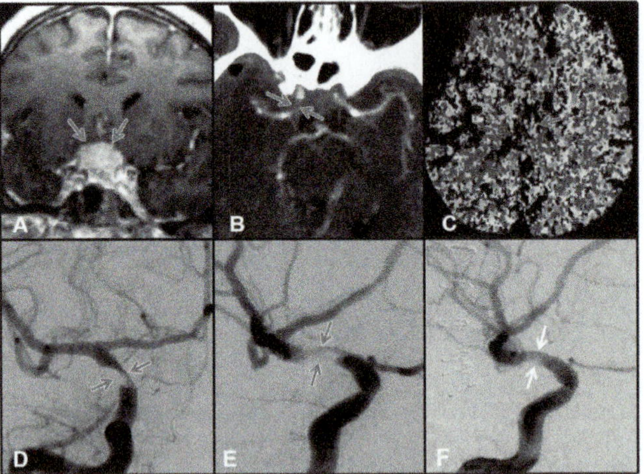

FIGURE 45–2 A 59-year-old man presented for surgical debulking of a planum sphenoidale meningioma as demonstrated on T1-weighted postcontrast MR imaging (black arrows A). Changes in neuromonitoring were encountered during surgical resection of the lesion and intraoperative Doppler suggested poor flow in the right internal carotid artery (ICA). A follow-up computed tomography (CT) angiogram demonstrated an area of poor opacification of the communicating right ICA (black arrows B) while CT perfusion (C) showed a corresponding prolonged Tmax throughout the right cerebral hemisphere. Anterior-Posterior (D) and lateral (E) projections from right ICA catheter angiography confirmed a dissection of the vessel resulting in an associated hemodynamically significant stenosis. The dissection was successfully treated by endovascular stenting in the same session (white arrows F).

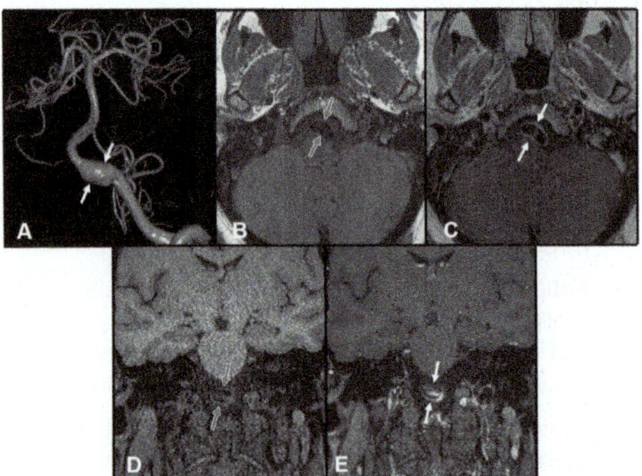

FIGURE 45–3 A 60-year-old woman presented with transient ischemic attacks referable to the posterior, intracranial circulation. 3D rotational angiography performed during injection of contrast into the left vertebral artery demonstrates an area of fusiform dilatation (white arrows A) involving the V4 intracranial segment of the vessel. The differential included simple ectasia versus dissecting aneurysm. Consequently, 3D T1-weighted high-resolution MR vessel wall imaging was performed. Axial pre-(B) and post-(C) contrast imaging demonstrated marked enhancement of the lesion. Coronal pre-(D) and post-(E) contrast imaging from the same study demonstrated a "double lumen," confirming the diagnosis of intracranial dissection. As the patient presented with ischemic symptoms, she was managed conservatively with antiplatelet medication and made an excellent recovery.

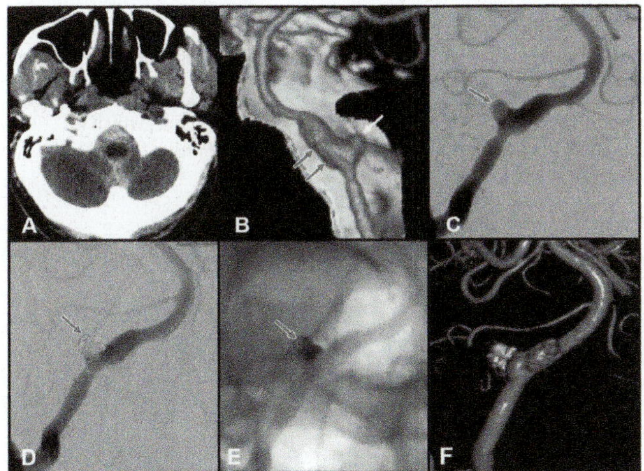

FIGURE 45–4 A 53-year-old man presented with large volume subarachnoid hemorrhage centered in the posterior fossa (A). Posterior view from a shaded surface 3D reconstruction of a computed tomography (CT) angiogram (B) demonstrated a markedly irregular, dissecting aneurysm of the intracranial V4 segment of the right vertebral artery with both fusiform (gray arrows) and saccular (white arrow) component. The dominant saccular component was well demonstrated on right vertebral artery catheter angiography in oblique AP view (gray arrow C). The lesion was subsequently treated with sent-assisted coiling targeting the saccular component (gray arrows D and E). Follow-up AP projection right vertebral artery catheter angiography (F) demonstrated excellent remodeling of the lesion.

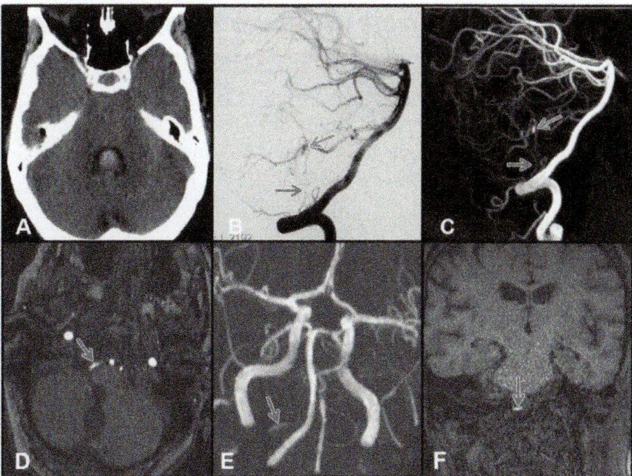

FIGURE 45–5 A 49-year-old woman presented with posterior fossa subarachnoid hemorrhage (A). Lateral (B) and 3D maximum intensity projection (MIP) imaging (C) from a right vertebral artery catheter angiogram demonstrates a small branch arising from the V4 intracranial right vertebral artery (gray arrows) that appeared to supply a dilated vascular structure (gray arrows) suspicious for aneurysm. The latter was in the expected location of the right posterior inferior cerebellar artery (PICA). However, the origin of the right PICA from the vertebral artery was not visualized. Subsequent source 3D time-of-flight (D) and MIP (E) MR angiography imaging demonstrated an area of intrinsic T1-hyperintensity (gray arrows) at the expected location of the anterior medullary segment of the right PICA suspicious for intramural hematoma and dissection. This was confirmed on 3D high-resolution MR vessel wall imaging performed prior to contrast administration (gray arrow F). The patient subsequently underwent surgical exploration where a proximal right PICA dissection was confirmed and treated by surgical trapping.

EVIDENCE AND REVIEW

Diagnosis

Vascular imaging often includes a combination of CT, MRI, and conventional angiography which are required to identify subtle radiographic signs including focal vessel wall irregularities, presence of an intimal flap or false lumen, fusiform dilatation at nonbranching sites (often immediately preceded by luminal narrowing), or intramural hematomas (Kanoto and Hosoya, 2016). Diagnosis can be difficult, and some IADs may mimic atherosclerotic lesions. Magnetic resonance vessel wall imaging holds promise as a technique to improve diagnosis, but no consensus has been reached regarding optimal protocols (Cho et al., 2021).

Prognosis Depends on the Presentation

Patients that develop recurrent symptoms usually follow their initial clinical presentation, that is, those that present with hemorrhage have recurrent hemorrhages and those that present with ischemia have recurrent ischemic events (Ono et al., 2013). The risk for expansion, thrombus formation, or hemorrhage is especially high during the initial phases of the arterial remodeling process but may also occur in a delayed fashion. Patients are also at risk for future dissection in other intracranial arteries. A retrospective study of 190 symptomatic cases found recurrent dissection occurred in 9% of patients after a mean of 3.4 years follow-up, while a review of 143 cases of isolated intracranial dissection found recurrence in 33% of patients when the mean follow-up period extended to 8.2 years (Mizutani, 2011; Ono et al., 2013). Both studies noted a predilection for recurrence early following initial presentation. Ono et al described three stages of recurrence with clinical variability in presentation: the highest incidence occurred within the first month, most frequently manifested by recurrent hemorrhage, whereas late recurrence extended beyond the first year and was marked by mostly nonhemorrhagic symptoms, and a third chronic stage marked by fusiform aneurysm transformation (Ono et al., 2013). Vessel wall healing occurs over several months and can lead to residual stenosis or persistent occlusion, aneurysmal dilation, or full-vessel recanalization.

Treatment

Current treatment for intracranial dissection is directed by lesion location, stability, and presence of ischemic or hemorrhagic sequelae (Table 45-1). Treatment is largely based on observational data without prospective randomized studies and is largely extrapolated from established cervical artery dissection management. Ischemic events are treated with antithrombotic agents to reduce recurrent ischemia which affects 2% to 14% of patients, whereas hemorrhagic complications are treated with surgical or endovascular techniques to reduce the risk of rebleeding, occurring in up to 40% of cases (B. M. Kim et al., 2011; Ono et al., 2013; Takemoto et al., 2010).

TABLE 45–1 Summary of current management strategies of intracranial arterial dissection.

IAD with Ischemia	IAD with Subarachnoid Hemorrhage
• Mechanism: Impaired forward blood flow, occlusion of perforators, emboli of mural hematoma to true lumen, inflammatory mediator release after vessel wall injury • Recurrent ischemia occurs in 2%-14% • Recurrent dissection causing nonhemorrhagic symptoms typically within the first year	• Mechanism: Accumulation of blood in subadventitial space, which is unable to be contained due to reduced elasticity, thinned adventitia of intracranial arteries • Rebleeding in up to 40%; highest risk in first hours/days • Risk of recurrent dissection causing new hemorrhage is highest in first month
Acute Treatment	
Intervention when IAD associated with acute stroke ± large vessel occlusion: Thrombolysis • Overall unknown safety in IAD • No formal recommendation from 2019 AHA Stroke guidelines; thrombolysis considered reasonable in cases of cervical arterial dissection within 4.5-hour window • No formal recommendation from 2021 ESO guidelines; however, expert consensus statement describes that thrombolysis should be considered in IAD by applying standard contraindications of thrombolysis Endovascular intervention • Insufficient evidence to establish routine use of mechanical thrombectomy/stent in IAD • 2021 ESO guideline suggests consideration in cases associated with large vessel occlusion based on location, risk of bleeding *Use of antiplatelet or anticoagulant to reduce thromboembolic sequalae:* • No randomized data to establish preferred agent in isolated IAD; selection varies by provider/institution • 2021 ESO guideline expert consensus statement suggests preference for antiplatelet agents • Antithrombotic agents generally continued 3-6 months; interval imaging may aid in duration (similar to cervical arterial dissection as per 2019 AHA Stroke guidelines)	*Definitive intervention to reduce risk of rebleeding after acute presentation:* Surgical management • Benefit of early intervention per meta-analysis comparing surgical/endovascular intervention vs. medical management reported in 2021 ESO guideline • Utilize deconstructive (parent artery sacrifice) or reconstructive (maintained parent vessel flow) methods • No randomized comparison of outcomes based on technique applied (open vs. endovascular) • Overall increasing favorability of endovascular intervention *Technique based on patient, lesion characteristics, and risks:* Open intervention • Immediate rebleeding risk reduction; may be preferred in complex cases • Various techniques: proximal occlusion/ligation, aneurysm clipping or wrapping, extracranial to intracranial bypass • Requires craniotomy, extensive operative time; may have higher incidence of ischemic complications Endovascular intervention • Expanded availability; avoids pitfalls of craniotomy • Techniques include coil embolization, stenting/flow diversion • Requires skilled center and amenable lesion, long-term use of dual antiplatelet for device patency • May have slightly higher risk of rerupture due to more gradual lesion securement with flow diversion

AHA, American Heart Association; ESO, European Stroke Organization; IAD, intracranial arterial dissection.

Is It Safe to Give Thrombolytics in Patients with Acute Ischemic Stroke Caused by IAD?

The underlying mechanism of IAD-associated occlusion, that is occlusion related to intramural hematoma and dissection flap with or without an intraarterial thrombus, is an important distinction from other thromboembolic etiologies of large vessel occlusion. This difference may be difficult to appreciate on emergent imaging, becoming apparent only after attempts at revascularization or on follow-up imaging. The benefit of thrombolysis or endovascular intervention for revascularization, as well as their associated theoretical harms (expansion of the intramural hematoma after thrombolysis or perforation of the false lumen in the case of endovascular intervention), remains unproven without randomized studies in contrast to other etiologies of large vessel occlusion. Data specifically for thrombolysis in isolated IAD are especially lacking. The American Heart Association 2019 guidelines for the management of acute ischemic stroke consider thrombolysis as reasonably safe in the presence of extracranial cervical artery dissection within the 4.5-hour window but note that the safety of thrombolysis is unknown in the setting of IAD (Powers et al., 2019). The European Stroke Organization, in their 2021 dissection guideline, similarly reports insufficient evidence to provide recommendations but does provide an expert consensus statement that thrombolysis should be considered in patients with acute ischemic stroke caused by IAD after ruling out standard contraindications, including subtle SAH (Debette et al., 2021). A few anecdotal reports demonstrate safety, though reporting bias limits conclusions. The largest series of IAD-associated acute ischemic stroke patients includes only 10 patients. In that series, only five patients received thrombolysis and no patient had SAH or symptomatic ICH, although one patient did have asymptomatic ICH (Bernardo et al., 2019). Observational data in a cervical artery dissection cohort of 55 patients demonstrated worse three-month functional outcomes after intravenous thrombolysis as compared to nondissection patients, though no significant difference in rates of intracranial hemorrhage was found (Engelter et al., 2009). A meta-analysis of 180 patients presenting with stroke due to cervical arterial dissection included 121 (67%) treated with intravenous thrombolysis and 59 (33%) treated with intraarterial thrombolysis and found no significant difference in rates of adverse events or favorable outcome when compared to an unmatched nondissection stroke registry cohort (Zinkstok et al., 2011). While the meta-analysis found only one patient in which intramural hematoma expansion occurred following thrombolysis, it is possible that such events were not fully documented or tracked in the original studies. Caution is warranted in generalizing the experience in cervical artery dissection to IAD, as intradural arteries may be more prone to hemorrhage due to a relative dearth of elastic fibers in the media, little adventitial tissue, and absence of an external elastic lamina (Lee, 1995).

Is There a Role for Endovascular Treatment in Management of Acute Ischemic Strokes due to IAD?

Insufficient evidence is available to guide endovascular treatment decisions regarding mechanical thrombectomy ± stenting of acute ischemic strokes due to IAD. A series of 21 patients with IAD and large vessel occlusion reported seven patients who underwent thrombectomy and another seven who received stent placement without any cases of symptomatic intracranial hemorrhage or delayed ischemia over a median 2-year follow-up period (Labeyrie et al., 2018). Expert consensus from the European Stroke Organization suggests that in acute large vessel occlusions due to IAD, endovascular therapy should be considered after assessing the risk/benefit ratio based on the dissection location and perceived bleeding risk (Debette et al., 2021).

Antiplatelet Versus Anticoagulation for Management of Acute Ischemic Strokes due to IAD

Medical management is favored for secondary prevention of lesions causing ischemia. Antiplatelet or anticoagulant medications are used to reduce thromboembolic sequalae and clot propagation during initial arterial healing. Duration of treatment varies but is generally continued until the risk of ischemia is felt to be significantly reduced or when recanalization is noted on imaging, often at least 3 to 6 months which mirrors extracranial dissection guidelines (Powers et al., 2019). There are no randomized trials to compare antiplatelet versus anticoagulant use in isolated IAD. However, studies of cervical dissection and available retrospective data inclusive of intracranial dissection have shown no significant difference in outcomes with an overall low rate of recurrent ischemia and similar rates of recanalization (Arauz et al., 2013; Daou et al., 2017). Compared to patients with intracranial atherosclerotic disease presenting with stroke, the risk of recurrent stroke is significantly less in those presenting with IAD (Shin et al., 2018). While patients with IAD were excluded, the prospective Cervical Artery Dissection in Stroke Study (CADISS) showed an overall low rate of recurrent stroke when patients were treated with either antiplatelet (2.4%) or anticoagulant (0.8%) which was not significantly different between groups (Markus et al., 2019). In contrast, the Aspirin versus anticoagulation in cervical artery dissection (TREAT-CAD) trial, which did not explicitly exclude IADs but did exclude patients with contraindications to anticoagulation according to the treating physician, did not show that aspirin was noninferior to anticoagulation with vitamin K antagonists in the treatment of cervical artery dissection (Engelter et al., 2021). In that randomized control trial, seven patients in the aspirin group had ischemic strokes as opposed to only one in the anticoagulation group.

Is It Safe to Use Anticoagulants in Acute Stroke Patients due to IAD with Intracranial Extension?

Despite greater potential benefit to reduce clot propagation, clinical dogma warns against the use of anticoagulants in patients with intracranial extension due to increased risk of subarachnoid hemorrhage. It remains unclear if such an increased risk truly exists as there are several retrospective studies in which subarachnoid hemorrhage was not found with anticoagulant use. Metso et al evaluated 76 patients with isolated IAD or cervical artery dissection with intracranial extension who received immediate anticoagulation (bridge intravenous heparin or low-molecular-weight heparin up to 5 days followed by warfarin for 3 months) without any cases of subarachnoid hemorrhage occurring over the follow-up period (Metso et al., 2007). In a nonrandomized retrospective study including 50 patients with isolated IAD or intracranial extension of cervical artery dissection, 26 were treated with anticoagulation and there were no differences in significant adverse events or rates of favorable functional outcome as compared to those treated with antiplatelet agents (Arauz et al., 2013). More recently, in a retrospective study including 74 patients with IAD receiving medical management, rates of hemorrhagic complications were overall rare with only three cases of major intracranial bleeding in patients treated with antiplatelets, anticoagulants, or combined therapy (one event in each treatment group) (Daou et al., 2017). Confounding by indication limits conclusions.

In the absence of standardized management guidelines, treatment remains individualized based on the clinical impression of the potential benefit and risk of medical management. Further, specific choice of antiplatelet (aspirin, clopidogrel, combination) or anticoagulant (heparin, warfarin, direct oral anticoagulants) remains anecdotal, provider, or institution specific. The European Stroke Organization expert consensus statement suggested that for acute symptomatic patients with IAD presenting with ischemia, antiplatelet agents should be preferred to anticoagulants (Debette et al., 2021).

Management of IAD-Associated Subarachnoid Hemorrhage

Patients with IAD-associated subarachnoid hemorrhage at presentation are at high risk of recurrent subarachnoid hemorrhage and experience worse functional outcomes (Mizutani et al., 1995; Ono et al., 2013). Risk of recurrent hemorrhage is greatest in the hours to days following initial injury and associated with significant mortality (Mizutani, 2011; Yamada et al., 2004). Recent meta-analysis of four studies of endovascular or surgical interventions to medical management showed significant benefit to interventional management in terms of subarachnoid hemorrhage recurrence, mortality, and functional outcomes (Debette et al., 2021). Interventional techniques can be summarized as deconstructive (parent artery sacrifice) or reconstructive (maintenance of parent vessel flow, usually with stent placement). Open surgical treatment versus endovascular intervention and their respective outcomes have not been compared in randomized trials, though advancing endovascular procedures have gained favor.

Once the mainstay of surgical treatment, open repair of an intracranial dissection may include proximal occlusion or ligation of the involved artery, clipping or wrapping of the associated aneurysm, or extracranial-intracranial bypass. To reduce potential ischemic complications and guide the repair strategy employed, tolerance for parent artery sacrifice can be tested intraoperatively using transient balloon occlusion (Bond et al., 2021). Data on the use of surgical intervention is less robust for anterior circulation lesions which tend to present more commonly with ischemia (Al-Mufti et al., 2019; Lin et al., 2005; Ohkuma et al., 2003; Pelkonen et al., 2004). Occlusion of a dissecting aneurysm through clipping is difficult and carries a high risk of rupture due to thin adventitia, though bypass surgery may be suited for posterior inferior cerebellar artery involvement or when the contralateral vertebral artery is hypoplastic and the balloon occlusion test is failed (Czabanka et al., 2011). Despite allowing effective treatment, especially for higher complexity cases, the need for craniotomy and extensive operative time during acute presentations reduces the utility of open intervention.

Complications of brain or spinal cord ischemia is the greatest concern for open surgical cases. Debette et al completed an analysis of observational data available from 125 surgical procedures with complication rates reported as follows: ischemia in 18%, rerupture in 0.8%, and cranial nerve palsy in 0.8% (Debette et al., 2015). However, heterogeneity of lesion location and operative procedures for lesion treatment make it difficult to fully assess associated morbidity.

Endovascular management has become a preferred technique for correction at skilled centers due to potential protection from rerupture with reduced need for parent artery sacrifice and absence of associated risks of craniotomy. Strategies include coiling, stent placement or flow diversion to reduce flow through the dissection, followed by dual antiplatelet therapy to maintain device patency (Bond et al., 2021). Parent vessel sacrifice can be performed through coiling embolization if needed. In the analysis by Debette et al of pooled data from 813 endovascular interventions, ischemia was reported in 6.2%, rerupture in 1.8%, and cranial nerve palsy in 0.9% (Debette et al., 2015). Successful management and risk of complications remains dependent on lesion characteristics as well as the endovascular technique employed.

The benefit of surgical intervention, either open or endovascular, seems to be greatest for patients with ruptured dissecting aneurysms at presentation particularly when the severity of hemorrhage is high. In a meta-analysis of endovascular intervention versus conservative treatment (any nonsurgical intervention including antihypertensive management, etc.), Chen et al compared groups of ruptured dissection (149 patients) and unruptured dissection (188 patients) (Chen et al., 2014). Of the patients with rupture, lower mortality (odds ratio [OR] 0.32, confidence interval [CI] 0.15-0.66) and improved rate of good functional recovery (OR 2.22, CI 1.09-4.49) were found in those who received endovascular treatment; however, there was no significant difference in the rate of disability. Patients receiving endovascular intervention for unruptured dissections also showed no difference in death, disability, or functional recovery as compared to those who received only conservative treatment.

Evolving endovascular technique suggests an overall beneficial safety profile when used in patients at high risk of rehemorrhage or in those without hemorrhage but who demonstrate significant mass effect or lesion expansion over time. However, in contrast to the near immediate risk reduction following parent artery sacrifice, risk of rebleeding only gradually decreases following placement of a flow diverter. Residual blood flow through the aneurysm remains after flow diversion, and full occlusion occurs in only 50% at 1 month from the time of intervention (Gory et al., 2019; Kocer et al., 2014).

Surgical intervention, either open or endovascular, remains as a mainstay of treatment particularly for ruptured dissections and is based on favorable outcomes from observational and retrospective data. While evolving endovascular techniques allow for treatment of various dissecting lesion types, careful consideration of patient-specific characteristics should be used to guide therapy. Future comparative studies are needed to clarify benefit and risk of the various interventions that are currently available to patients.

REFERENCES

Al-Mufti, F., Kamal, N., Damodara, N., Nuoman, R., Gupta, R., Alotaibi, N. M., Alkanaq, A., El-Ghanem, M., Keller, I. A., Schonfeld, S., Gupta, G., & Roychowdhury, S. (2019). Updates in the Management of Cerebral Infarctions and Subarachnoid Hemorrhage Secondary to Intracranial Arterial Dissection: A Systematic Review. World Neurosurgery, 121, 51–58. https://doi.org/10.1016/j.wneu.2018.09.153

Arauz, A., Ruiz, A., Pacheco, G., Rojas, P., Rodríguez-Armida, M., Cantú, C., Murillo-Bonilla, L., Ruiz-Sandoval, J. L., & Barinagarrementeria, F. (2013). Aspirin versus anticoagulation in intra- and extracranial vertebral artery dissection. European Journal of Neurology, 20(1), 167–172. https://doi.org/10.1111/j.1468-1331.2012.03825.x

Bernardo, F., Nannoni, S., Strambo, D., Bartolini, B., Michel, P., & Sirimarco, G. (2019). Intravenous thrombolysis in acute ischemic stroke due to intracranial artery dissection: a single-center case series and a review of literature. Journal of Thrombosis and Thrombolysis, 48(4), 679–684. https://doi.org/10.1007/s11239-019-01918-6

Bond, K. M., Krings, T., Lanzino, G., & Brinjikji, W. (2021). Intracranial dissections: A pictorial review of pathophysiology, imaging features, and natural history. Journal of Neuroradiology, 48(3), 176–188. https://doi.org/10.1016/j.neurad.2020.03.007

Chen, Y., Guan, J. J., Liu, A. H., Ding, H., Shao, Y., & Xu, Y. (2014). Outcome of cervicocranial artery dissection with different treatments: A systematic review and meta-analysis. Journal of Stroke and Cerebrovascular Diseases, 23(3). https://doi.org/10.1016/j.jstrokecerebrovasdis.2013.09.026

Cho, S. J., Choi, B. S., Bae, Y. J., Baik, S. H., Sunwoo, L., & Kim, J. H. (2021). Image Findings of Acute to Subacute Craniocervical Arterial Dissection on Magnetic Resonance Vessel Wall Imaging: A Systematic Review and Proportion Meta-Analysis. Frontiers in Neurology, 12, 586735. https://doi.org/10.3389/fneur.2021.586735

Czabanka, M., Ali, M., Schmiedek, P., Vajkoczy, P., & Lawton, M. T. (2011). Vertebral artery-posterior inferior cerebellar artery bypass using a radial artery graft for hemorrhagic dissecting vertebral artery aneurysms: Surgical technique and report of 2 cases. Journal of Neurosurgery, 114(4), 1074–1079. https://doi.org/10.3171/2010.5.JNS091435

Daou, B., Hammer, C., Mouchtouris, N., Starke, R. M., Koduri, S., Yang, S., Jabbour, P., Rosenwasser, R., & Tjoumakaris, S. (2017). Anticoagulation vs antiplatelet treatment in patients with carotid and vertebral artery dissection: A study of 370 patients and literature review. Neurosurgery, 80(3), 368–379. https://doi.org/10.1093/neuros/nyw086

Debette, S., Compter, A., Labeyrie, M.-A., Uyttenboogaart, M., Metso, T. M., Majersik, J. J., Goeggel-Simonetti, B., Engelter, S. T., Pezzini, A., Bijlenga, P., Southerland, A. M., Naggara, O., Béjot, Y., Cole, J. W., Ducros, A., Giacalone, G., Schilling, S., Reiner, P., Sarikaya, H., … Bousser, M.-G. (2015). Epidemiology, pathophysiology, diagnosis, and management of intracranial artery dissection. Lancet Neurology, 14(6), 640–643. https://doi.org/10.1016/S1474-4422(15)00009-5

Debette, S., Mazighi, M., Bijlenga, P., Pezzini, A., Koga, M., Bersano, A., Kõrv, J., Haemmerli, J., Canavero, I., Tekiela, P., Miwa, K., J Seiffge, D., Schilling, S., Lal, A., Arnold, M., Markus, H. S., Engelter, S. T., & Majersik, J. J. (2021). ESO guideline for the management of extracranial and intracranial artery dissection. European Stroke Journal, 6(3), XXXIX. https://doi.org/10.1177/23969873211046475

Engelter, S. T., Rutgers, M. P., Hatz, F., Georgiadis, D., Fluri, F., Sekoranja, L., Schwegler, G., Müller, F., Weder, B., Sarikaya, H., Lüthy, R., Arnold, M., Nedeltchev, K., Reichhart, M., Mattle, H. P., Tettenborn, B., Hungerbühler, H. J., Sztajzel, R., Baumgartner, R. W., … Lyrer, P. A. (2009). Intravenous thrombolysis in stroke attributable to cervical artery dissection. Stroke, 40(12), 3772–3776. https://doi.org/10.1161/STROKEAHA.109.555953

Engelter, S. T., Traenka, C., Gensicke, H., Schaedelin, S. A., Luft, A. R., Simonetti, B. G., Fischer, U., Michel, P., Sirimarco, G., Kägi, G., Vehoff, J., Nedeltchev, K., Kahles, T., Kellert, L., Rosenbaum, S., von Rennenberg, R., Sztajzel, R., Leib, S. L., Jung, S., … Scheitz, J. F. (2021). Aspirin versus anticoagulation in cervical artery dissection (TREAT-CAD): an open-label, randomised, non-inferiority trial. Lancet Neurology, 20(5), 341–350. https://doi.org/10.1016/S1474-4422(21)00044-2

Giroud, M., Fayolle, H., Andre, N., Dumas, R., Becker, F., Martin, D., Baudoin, N., & Krause, D. (1994). Incidence of internal carotid artery dissection in the community of Dijon. Journal of Neurology, Neurosurgery & Psychiatry, 57(11), 1443. https://doi.org/10.1136/JNNP.57.11.1443

Gory, B., Berge, J., Bonafé, A., Pierot, L., Spelle, L., Piotin, M., Biondi, A., Cognard, C., Mounayer, C., Sourour, N., Barbier, C., Desal, H., Herbreteau, D., Chabert, E., Brunel, H., Ricolfi, F., Anxionnat, R., Decullier, E., Huot, L., … Taschner, C. (2019). Flow Diverters for Intracranial Aneurysms. Stroke, 50(12), 3471–3480. https://doi.org/10.1161/STROKEAHA.119.024722

Guillon, B., Levy, C., & Bousser, M.-G. (1998). Internal carotid artery dissection: an update. Journal of Neurological Sciences, Vol. 153.

Hegedüs, K. (1984). Fibromuscular Dysplasia of the Basilar Artery. Archives of Neurology, 41(4), 440–442. https://doi.org/10.1001/archneur.1984.04050160106024

Inoue, T., Nishimura, S., Hayashi, N., Numagami, Y., Takazawa, H., & Nishijima, M. (2007). Postpartum dissecting aneurysm of the posterior cerebral artery. Journal of Clinical Neuroscience, 14(6), 576–581. https://doi.org/10.1016/J.JOCN.2006.04.005

Kanoto, M., & Hosoya, T. (2016). Diagnosis of intracranial artery dissection. Neurologia Medico-Chirurgica, 56(9), 524–533. https://doi.org/10.2176/nmc.ra.2015-0294

Kim, B. M., Kim, S. H., Kim, D. I., Shin, Y. S., Suh, S. H., Kim, D. J., Park, S. I., Park, K. Y., & Ahn, S. S. (2011). Outcomes and prognostic factors of intracranial unruptured vertebrobasilar artery dissection. Neurology, 76(20), 1735–1741. https://doi.org/10.1212/WNL.0b013e31821a7d94

Kim, S. T., Brinjikji, W., Lanzino, G., & Kallmes, D. F. (2016). Neurovascular manifestations of connective-tissue diseases: A review. Interventional Neuroradiology, 22(6), 624–637. https://doi.org/10.1177/1591019916659262

Kocaeli, H., Chaalala, C., Andaluz, N., & Zuccarello, M. (2009). Spontaneous intradural vertebral artery dissection: A single-center experience and review of the literature. Skull Base, 19(3), 209–218. https://doi.org/10.1055/s-0028-1114296

Kocer, N., Islak, C., Kizilkilic, O., Kocak, B., Saglam, M., & Tureci, E. (2014). Flow re-direction endoluminal device in treatment of cerebral aneurysms: Initial experience with short-term follow-up results: Clinical article. Journal of Neurosurgery, 120(5), 1158–1171. https://doi.org/10.3171/2014.1.JNS131442

Krings, T., & Choi, I.-S. (2010). The Many Faces of Intracranial Arterial Dissections. Interventional Neuroradiology, 16, 151–160. www.centauro.it

Kwak, J. H., Choi, J. W., Park, H. J., Chae, E. Y., Park, E. S., Lee, D. H., & Suh, D. C. (2011). Cerebral Artery Dissection: Spectrum of Clinical Presentations Related to Angiographic Findings. Neurointervention, 6(2), 78–83. https://doi.org/10.5469/NEUROINT.2011.6.2.78

Labeyrie, M. A., Civelli, V., Reiner, P., Aymard, A., Saint-Maurice, J. P., Zetchi, A., & Houdart, E. (2018). Prevalence and treatment of spontaneous intracranial artery dissections in patients with acute stroke due to intracranial large vessel occlusion. Journal of NeuroInterventional Surgery, 10(8), 761–764. https://doi.org/10.1136/neurintsurg-2018-013763

Lee, R. M. K. W. (1995). Morphology of cerebral arteries. Pharmacol Ther, 66(1), 149–173. https://doi.org/10.1016/0163-7258(94)00071-a

Lin, C. H., Jeng, J. S., & Yip, P. K. (2005). Middle cerebral artery dissections: Differences between isolated and extended dissections of internal carotid artery. Journal of the Neurological Sciences, 235(1–2), 37–44. https://doi.org/10.1016/j.jns.2005.03.047

Markus, H. S., Levi, C., King, A., Madigan, J., & Norris, J. (2019). Antiplatelet therapy vs anticoagulation therapy in cervical artery dissection: The cervical artery dissection in stroke study (cadiss) randomized clinical trial final results. JAMA Neurology, 76(6), 657–664. https://doi.org/10.1001/jamaneurol.2019.0072

Maski, K. P., Sengupta, S., Silvera, M., & Rivkin, M. J. (2011). Intracranial Artery Dissection in an Adolescent With Marfan Syndrome. Pediatric Neurology, 45(1), 39–41. https://doi.org/10.1016/J.PEDIATRNEUROL.2010.12.011

Metso, T. M., Metso, A. J., Helenius, J., Haapaniemi, E., Salonen, O., Porras, M., Hernesniemi, J., Kaste, M., & Tatlisumak, T. (2007). Prognosis and safety of anticoagulation in intracranial artery dissections in adults. Stroke, 38(6), 1837–1842. https://doi.org/10.1161/STROKEAHA.106.479501

Mizutani, T. (2011). Natural course of intracranial arterial dissections. Journal of Neurosurgery, 114(4), 1037–1044. https://doi.org/10.3171/2010.9.JNS10668

Mizutani, T., Aruga, T., Kirino, T., Miki, Y., Saito, I., & Tsuchida, T. (1995). Recurrent Subarachnoid Hemorrhage from Untreated Ruptured Vertebrobasilar Dissecting Aneurysms. Neurosurgery, 36(5), 905–913. https://doi.org/10.1227/00006123-199505000-00003

Ohkuma, H., Suzuki, S., Shimamura, N., & Nakano, T. (2003). Dissecting aneurysms of the middle cerebral artery: Neuroradiological and clinical features. Neuroradiology, 45(3), 143–148. https://doi.org/10.1007/S00234-002-0919-3/TABLES/3

Ono, H., Nakatomi, H., Tsutsumi, K., Inoue, T., Teraoka, A., Yoshimoto, Y., Ide, T., Kitanaka, C., Ueki, K., Imai, H., & Saito, N. (2013). Symptomatic recurrence of intracranial arterial dissections: Follow-up study of 143 consecutive cases and pathological investigation. Stroke, 44(1), 126–131. https://doi.org/10.1161/STROKEAHA.112.670745/FORMAT/EPUB

O'Sullivan, R. M., Robertson, W. D., Nugent, R. A., Berry, K., & Turnbull, I. M. (1990). Supraclinoid carotid artery dissection following unusual trauma. AJNR. American Journal of Neuroradiology, 11(6), 1150–1152. http://www.ncbi.nlm.nih.gov/pubmed/2124042

Parlapiano, G., di Lorenzo, F., Salehi, L. B., Ruvolo, G., Novelli, G., & Sangiuolo, F. (2020). Neurovascular manifestations in connective tissue diseases: The case of Marfan Syndrome. Mechanisms of Ageing and Development, 191, 111346. https://doi.org/10.1016/J.MAD.2020.111346

Pelkonen, O., Tikkakoski, T., Pyhtinen, J., & Sotaniemi, K. (2004). Cerebral CT and MRI findings in cervicocephalic artery dissection. Acta Radiologica, 45(3), 259–265. https://doi.org/10.1080/02841850410004184

Powers, W. J., Rabinstein, A. A., Ackerson, T., Adeoye, O. M., Bambakidis, N. C., Becker, K., Biller, J., Brown, M., Demaerschalk, B. M., Hoh, B., Jauch, E. C., Kidwell, C. S., Leslie-Mazwi, T. M., Ovbiagele, B., Scott, P. A., Sheth, K. N., Southerland, A. M., Summers, D. V., & Tirschwell, D. L. (2019). Guidelines for the early management of patients with acute ischemic stroke: 2019 update to the 2018 guidelines for the early management of acute ischemic stroke a guideline for healthcare professionals from the American Heart Association/American Stroke Association. Stroke, 50(12), E344–E418. https://doi.org/10.1161/STR.0000000000000211

Prabhakaran, S., & Krakauer, J. W. (2006). Multiple Reversible Episodes of Subcortical Ischemia Following Postcoital Middle Cerebral Artery Dissection. Archives of Neurology, 63(6), 891–893. https://doi.org/10.1001/ARCHNEUR.63.6.891

Ro, A., Kageyama, N., Abe, N., Takatsu, A., & Fukunaga, T. (2009). Intracranial vertebral artery dissection resulting in fatal subarachnoid hemorrhage: Clinical and histopathological investigations from a medicolegal perspective: Clinical article. Journal of Neurosurgery, 110(5), 948–954. https://doi.org/10.3171/2008.11.JNS08951

Sasaki, O., Ogawa, H., Koike, T., Koizumi, T., & Tanaka, R. (1991). A clinicopathological study of dissecting aneurysms of the intracranial vertebral artery. Journal of Neurosurgery, 75(6), 874–882. https://doi.org/10.3171/JNS.1991.75.6.0874

Sherman, D. G., Hart, R. G., & Easton, J. D. (1981). Abrupt change in head position and cerebral infarction. Stroke, 12(1), 2–6. https://doi.org/10.1161/01.STR.12.1.2

Shin, J., Chung, J.-W., Park, M. S., Lee, H., Cha, J., Seo, W.-K., Kim, G.-M., & Bang, O. Y. (2018). Outcomes after ischemic stroke caused by intracranial atherosclerosis vs dissection. Neurology, 91(19), e1751–e1759. https://doi.org/10.1212/WNL.0000000000006459

Takemoto, K., Abe, H., Uda, K., & Inoue, T. (2010). Surgical treatment of intracranial VA dissecting aneurysm. Acta Neurochirurgica, Supplementum, 107, 51–56. https://doi.org/10.1007/978-3-211-99373-6_8

Yamada, M., Kitahara, T., Kurata, A., Fujii, K., & Miyasaka, Y. (2004). Intracranial vertebral artery dissection with subarachnoid hemorrhage: clinical characteristics and outcomes in conservatively treated patients. Journal of Neurosurgery, 101(1), 25–30. https://doi.org/10.3171/JNS.2004.101.1.0025

Zinkstok, S. M., Vergouwen, M. D. I., Engelter, S. T., Lyrer, P. A., Bonati, L. H., Arnold, M., Mattle, H. P., Fischer, U., Sarikaya, H., Baumgartner, R. W., Georgiadis, D., Odier, C., Michel, P., Putaala, J., Griebe, M., Wahlgren, N., Ahmed, N., van Geloven, N., … Nederkoorn, P. J. (2011). Safety and Functional Outcome of Thrombolysis in Dissection-Related Ischemic Stroke: A Meta-Analysis of Individual Patient. Stroke, 42(9), 2515–2520. https://doi.org/10.1161/STROKEAHA.111.617282

SECTION V SEIZURES AND EPILEPSY

CHAPTER

46

How Should We Best Manage Seizures in the NeuroICU?

Alvin S. Das, MD, Jong Woo Lee, MD, PhD,
& Henrikas Vaitkevicius, MD

Case

A 53-year-old woman presents to the emergency department after a motor vehicle accident. On initial exam, her Glasgow coma scale was noted to be 6 and she was not following commands. Noncontrast head computed tomography (CT) revealed the presence of bilateral temporal and inferior frontal contusions. She is admitted to the neurological intensive care unit (NeuroICU) where an intracranial pressure monitor and electroencephalogram (EEG) leads are placed. How should we best manage seizures in the NeuroICU?

Key Points

- Once a seizure is recognized, the focus should be to abolish both the clinical and electrographic components of seizures.
- In conjunction with seizure treatment, a thorough workup to determine the underlying cause or precipitant should be performed.
- The staple of expediated seizure detection and confirmation is continuous electroencephalogram (cEEG).
- In critically ill patients, maintain a high suspicion for nonconvulsive status epilepticus (NCSE) and have a low threshold to obtain cEEG monitoring
- After cardiac arrest, post-anoxic SE is common and can include NCSE, generalized convulsive status epilepticus (GCSE), or myoclonic SE. Patients with traumatic brain injury (TBI) are at an increased risk for developing NCSE.
- Postoperative seizures may be found in as many as 17% of patients, and their incidence varies based on the location and type of procedure.
- Seizures have been reported in up to 31% of patients with intracerebral hemorrhage, half of which are subclinical.
- In patients with status epilepticus, the lowest dose of anesthetics sufficient to control seizures should be used because of the toxicities associated with anesthetic medications.

BACKGROUND

Pathologic electroencephalogram (EEG) patterns including seizures are highly prevalent in neurological intensive care unit (NeuroICU). While considered toxic, these abnormal EEG patterns are frequently a symptom of underlying neuronal dysfunction—metabolic, toxic, or structural etiologies. Regardless of their etiology, however, seizures in the ICU are associated with worse functional outcomes including increased mortality and higher disability at discharge.[1,2] Therefore, rapid identification and early treatment of seizures are crucial and are a core competency for neurointensivists.

EVIDENCE AND REVIEW

Definitions

A seizure refers to the abnormal, hypersynchronous discharge from a population of cortical neurons.[3] Electrographically, this manifests as at least 10 seconds of repetitive generalized or focal spikes, sharp waves, or spike/sharp-wave and slow-wave complexes that evolve in morphology and location and are usually at a frequency > 2.5 Hz.[4,5] Seizures can be classified as either focal, due to their localized origin, or generalized, due to their onset in both cerebral hemispheres.[6] In many cases, focal onset seizures may rapidly evolve to become generalized seizures. Generalized seizures may be classified as convulsive, manifested by prominent tonic-clonic movements, or nonconvulsive, in which seizures are occurring, but the only apparent clinical manifestation is an alteration in consciousness with subtle motor movements of the limbs or eyes.

When clinical or electrographic seizures persist longer than 5 minutes, it is termed **status epilepticus (SE)**. Electroclinical status epilepticus (ECSE) is defined as an electroclinical seizure ≥ 10 continuous minutes or for a total duration of 20% of any 60-minute period of a recording. For practical reasons, recurrent seizure activity without returning to baseline between the seizures is also defined as SE.[7] Generalized convulsive SE is SE that results from ongoing convulsive seizures as manifested by tonic-clonic movements of the extremities and concomitant mental status impairment. If such bilateral tonic-clonic activity lasts for ≥ 5 continuous minutes, it qualifies as ECSE. Nonconvulsive SE (NCSE) is SE that is defined as changes from baseline mental status associated with continuous epileptiform discharges lasting at least 5 minutes. While subtle movements of the limbs or eyes may be observed, there are no obvious apparent clinical manifestations of these seizures. NCSE may arise independently or may be a late stage of convulsive SE. Because NCSE does not present with reliable clinical features, EEG findings remain the hallmark of diagnosis. Due to the wide variability in the presentation of NCSE, several different diagnostic criteria have been proposed, although no standardized definition has emerged. Highlighting every proposed classification scheme for NCSE is beyond the scope of this textbook; however, the most widely adopted criterion is perhaps the Salzburg criteria.[8,9] These criteria state that epileptiform discharges at a frequency > 2.5 Hz are diagnostic of NCSE. However, if the frequency of epileptiform discharges is <2.5 Hz, but there is spatiotemporal evolution, subtle ictal phenomenon, or clinical improvement after the administration of antiseizure medications (ASMs), the diagnosis of NCSE can also be made.[8] Focal SE is defined as SE caused by seizures that involve only one area of the cortex and do not generalize. Based on the area of the cortex that is involved, these may exhibit unilateral motor activity or weakness corresponding to cortical ictal activity. **Refractory status epilepticus** (RSE) includes patients who fail to respond to adequate doses of a benzodiazepine followed by a second-line antiepileptic agent.[7] **Super refractory status epilepticus (SRSE)** is defined as SE that continues or recurs 24 hours after initiating anesthetic agents and includes SE that recurs after weaning anesthetics agents intended for seizure control.[10] These definitions are summarized in Table 46–1.

Workup

The workup for SE should be initiated as soon as the SE is recognized. In the acute setting, basic laboratory workup should be

TABLE 46–1 Classification and definitions of seizures.

Seizure	Transient occurrence of signs and/or symptoms due to abnormal excessive or hypersynchronous neuronal activity in the brain
Focal	Localized origin of seizures
Generalized	Onset of seizures in both cerebral hemispheres
Status epilepticus	Clinical or electrographic seizures > 5 min or seizure activity without a return to baseline
Generalized Convulsive	Tonic-clonic movements of the extremities and concomitant mental status impairment lasting for at least 5 continuous min
Nonconvulsive	Changes from baseline mental status associated with generalized continuous epileptiform discharges lasting at least 5 min and no obvious apparent clinical manifestations of these seizures
Focal	Status epilepticus caused by seizures that involve only one area of the cortex and do not generalize
Refractory status epilepticus	Status epilepticus that persists despite adequate doses of a benzodiazepine followed by a second-line antiepileptic agent
Super refractory status epilepticus	Status epilepticus that continues or recurs 24 h after initiating anesthetic agents and includes seizures that recur after weaning anesthetics agents intended for seizure control

obtained including checking finger stick blood glucose, complete metabolic panel, complete blood count, magnesium, calcium (total and ionized), antiepileptic drug levels (if indicated), and a urine toxicology screen (if suspected). Creatine kinase (CK) and lactate are often increased after generalized seizures, so these levels should also be checked. Once the SE is controlled and the hemodynamics parameters are stable, additional diagnostic studies can be performed to identify common precipitants. In most patients, a noncontract head CT should be obtained to exonerate any acute pathology. If a diagnosis is not achieved by head CT alone, a contrast-enhanced brain magnetic resonance imaging should be performed. In cases of suspected infection, especially in elderly patients, a lumbar puncture is warranted to exonerate meningitis or encephalitis. Moreover, in previously nonepileptic patients who develop SE without any identifiable cause, a lumbar puncture should be strongly considered.

Additional workup based on the clinical presentation may include extended toxicology screening and serum paraneoplastic panels. In situations in which ongoing seizures are suspected but the surface EEG is unremarkable, a brain positron emission tomography (PET) may identify ongoing seizures as manifested by a hypermetabolic focus. In certain instances, such as traumatic brain injury (TBI), depth electrodes can aid in the identification of ongoing seizures that may otherwise be missed by surface electrodes.

Principles of Management

Directed seizure management should include both a focus on the treatment of an underlying precipitant (if one is identified) and treatment of the seizures themselves. If seizures are transient and are the direct result of an underlying cause such as hyponatremia or alcohol withdrawal, antiepileptic medications may not be necessary (beyond abortive benzodiazepines). The primary focus should be on correcting the underlying insulting pathophysiology. However, if a metabolic condition such as diabetic ketoacidosis results in NCSE, treatment should be targeted at both correction of the hyperglycemia and treatment of the NCSE. While the patient will likely not require chronic treatment with ASMs, acute treatment of the NCSE is necessary with ASMs.

In patients without clear clinical signs of seizures, but a high suspicion for seizures, continuous EEG (cEEG) can be employed. Findings on the EEG range from patterns that are clearly ictal and should be treated aggressively to patterns that are benign and may be followed over time. However, there are a host of patterns that are neither clearly ictal or benign, termed the ictal-interictal continuum, in which the management is less clear.[11] Key features that should be evaluated and monitored when the pattern falls within the ictal-interictal continuum are the frequency of the discharges as well as the evolution of the pattern. These discharges have been standardized by the American Clinical Neurophysiology Society and classified based on the appearance of the waveform as well as their localization (Table 46–2).[12] All terms consist of main term 1 followed by 2 as well as any relevant modifiers. The first term (main term 1) in the classification is based on location and includes generalized, lateralized,

TABLE 46–2 American Clinical Neurophysiology Society's critical care EEG terminology.

Rhythmic or periodic patterns	
Main term 1 (Location)	Generalized (G), lateralized (L), bilateral independent (BI), unilateral independent (UI), multifocal (Mf)
Main term 2 (Waveform)	Periodic discharges (PD), rhythmic delta activity (RDA), spike-and-wave or sharp-and-wave (SW)
Modifiers	Prevalence, duration, frequency, number of phases, sharpness, amplitude (voltage), polarity, stimulus-induced (SI) or stimulus-terminated (ST), evolution, plus (+)
Minor modifiers	Sudden onset or gradual onset, "triphasic" morphology, anterior-posterior lag or posterior-anterior lag, polarity

bilateral independent, unilateral independent, or multifocal. The second term (main term 2) is based on the waveform morphology and includes periodic discharges, rhythmic delta activity, or spike wave (includes sharp wave and polyspike wave). Several modifications can be added to these terms to further specify the patterns based on the frequency, amplitude, sharpness, prevalence, or polarity of these discharges. These discharges are mainly descriptors and do not provide information on management. However, some types of discharges are more associated with ictal activity than others (Figure 46–1). If discharges are evolving, especially ones that are more ictal in nature, such as lateralized period discharges, their response to an ASM should be observed even if their frequency is <2.5 Hz. In these instances, a short-acting benzodiazepine or ASM is usually administered to determine whether these patterns warrant aggressive treatment. Sufficient doses of these medications should be given such that the discharges abate. If a clinical change occurs as a result of the ASM therapy, it is reasonable to continue seizure treatment as this meets the criteria for NCSE.

In addition to an ASM challenge, brain PET may help determine whether ictal-interictal continuum patterns should be treated. In one study, approximately 60% of patients with ictal-interictal continuum patterns were found to have fludeoxyglucose (^{18}F)-PET (FDG-PET) hypermetabolism, which predicted electrographic or ECSE with 100% specificity.[13] Furthermore, as the frequency of lateralized periodic discharges increases, FDG uptake increases in parallel.[14] In these circumstances, it is reasonable to consider treatment of lateralized periodic discharges with associated hypermetabolism even if their frequency is <2.5 Hz.

Initial Therapies

Once seizures are recognized, the primary focus should be to abolish both the clinical and electrographic components of seizures. Seizures are a medical emergency and should be treated aggressively in the acute setting with a rapid escalation of therapies. In the outpatient setting, these therapies can

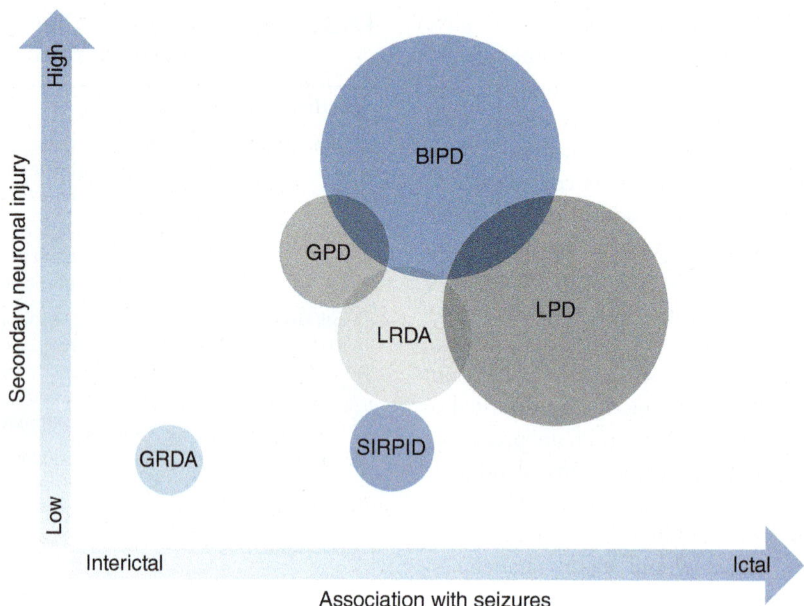

FIGURE 46–1 Ictal-interictal continuum. This figure shows the various discharges (in accordance with ACNS terminology) along the ictal-interictal continuum. The x-axis delineates an increasing association with seizures, and the y-axis denotes an increasing association with neuronal injury as well as mortality. BIPD, bilateral independent periodic discharge; GPDs, generalized periodic discharge; GRDA, generalized rhythmic delta activity; LPD, lateralized periodic discharge; LRDA, lateralized rhythmic delta activity; SIRPID, stimulus-induced rhythmic, periodic, or ictal discharges. Adapted from: Johnson EL, Kaplan PW. *Clin Neurophysiol Pract*. 2017 May 26; 2:107–118.

be tapered conservatively. Because of the heightened aspiration risk during seizures as well as the respiratory depression attributed to ASMs, management of hemodynamics, obtaining intravenous access, and securing the airway should be performed in parallel to seizure control. The first-line ASM therapy for seizures is benzodiazepines. Intravenous lorazepam (at 0.1 mg/kg) is the preferred agent if intravenous access is established and midazolam is the preferred therapy for intramuscular administration.[7] In most circumstances, a long-acting antiepileptic drug such as levetiracetam, fosphenytoin, or valproate should be concomitantly administered to prevent seizures within the next 24 hours. In order to obtain therapeutic levels rapidly, these drugs should be intravenously administered. If patients were taking a certain ASM prior to admission, it is reasonable to administer additional doses of this ASM to target higher than normal therapeutic levels.

If seizures persist despite optimal doses of benzodiazepines and a second-line agent (Table 46–3), additional agents including intravenous anesthetics should be initiated. However, in situations in which patients are hemodynamically stable and are in NCSE or focal status epilepticus, it is also reasonable to add additional second-line intravenous agents or re-bolus previously administered ASMs to avoid intubation. Once patients are deemed to be in RSE, they should be monitored in a critical care setting with cEEG capability. Many of the intravenous anesthetics used to treat refractory seizures can cause hypotension, which may necessitate the use of concomitant vasopressor agents. Furthermore, patients should be monitored on telemetry, given that these agents may cause cardiopulmonary side effects. For the treatment of RSE, the two most widely used anesthetic agents are midazolam and propofol. Other intravenous anesthetics such as pentobarbital should be reserved for later use, given their increased side-effect profile.

Refractory Status Epilepticus Management

Because of the toxicities associated with anesthetic medications, the lowest dose of anesthetics that is sufficient to control seizures should be used. Although practice styles vary, it is reasonable to initially target seizure suppression with intravenous anesthetics. Specifically, this involves titrating the anesthetic medications to a dose that abolishes epileptiform activity on the EEG. Once this dose is established, seizure suppression should be continued for 24 to 48 hours followed by a gradual tapering of the medications. If seizures recur during the weaning process, anesthetic agents should be escalated to either target seizure suppression again or further escalated to target burst suppression. Although neither strategy has demonstrated clear efficacy over the other,[15] a reasonable approach is to target burst suppression after seizure suppression has failed.

Burst suppression is characterized by a discontinuous EEG pattern with bursts of high amplitude activity interspersed between intervals of background suppression.[16] In addition to targeting seizure control, burst suppression interrupts synaptic transmission and can serve as an electrical "reset switch," similar to the effect sedation has on fatal ventricular tachycardia electrical storms.[17] Burst suppression enables temporary electrographic control allowing additional time for the underlying etiologies to be diagnosed and treated. For example, if SE is incited by bacterial meningitis, burst suppression inhibits seizures while

TABLE 46–3 Antiepileptic drugs.

Drug	Loading Dose
First-line agents	
Lorazepam	0.1 mg/kg IV (up to 4 mg/dose); repeat once in 5-10 min as needed (max total dose is 8 mg)
Diazepam	0.15 mg/kg IV (up to 10 mg/dose); repeat every 3-5 min
Midazolam	0.2 mg/kg IM (up to 10 mg/dose)
Second-line agents	
Levetiracetam	40-50 mg/kg IV (max dose 4,000 mg)
Fosphenytoin	15-20 mg PE/kg IV (may give an additional 5 mg/kg)
Phenytoin	15-20 mg/kg IV (may give an additional 5 mg/kg)
Valproic acid	20-40 mg/kg IV (may give an additional 20 mg/kg)
Third-line agents	
Midazolam	0.05-2 mg/kg IV
Propofol	20-83 mcg/kg/min
Ketamine	1.5-4.5 mg/kg IV
Pentobarbital	5-15 mg/kg IV (may give an additional 5-10 mg/kg)
Lidocaine	100 mg IV; may repeat in 30 min
Other frequently used agents	
Lacosamide	300-400 mg IV
Topiramate	200-400 mg PO
Clobazam	5-10 mg PO
Perampanel	2-32 mg PO
Phenobarbital	15-20 mg/kg IV (may give an additional 5-10 mg/kg)

IV = intravenous, PO = by mouth, PE = phenytoin sodium equivalents

antibiotics are reaching therapeutic levels, thereby increasing the chances of successful anesthetic weaning. Also, during this time, "fine tuning" of other parameters can occur, such as electrolyte optimization. In addition, burst suppression allows for seizure control while ASMs and other antiseizure treatments are becoming therapeutic. While the patient is burst suppressed, maintenance ASMs should be optimized so that seizures do not recur after anesthetic weaning. Lastly, burst suppression "buys time" for further diagnostic studies to occur (Figure 46–2).

During burst suppression, it is reasonable to target 8- to 20-second interburst intervals as well as a burst suppression ratio of 80% or greater.[7] If a single agent fails to produce adequate burst suppression, a second intravenous anesthetic agent may be added. Although a common practice is to continue burst suppression for 24 to 48 hours, the optimal duration of burst suppression has not been established. In fact, much shorter periods of burst suppression (<2 hours) have been successfully employed, effectively minimizing the exposure to anesthetic agent toxicities.[18] If seizures recur after a gradual tapering of anesthetics, longer durations of burst suppression can be considered. Furthermore, after multiple failed weaning attempts using a single agent, it is reasonable to consider adding additional intravenous anesthetics. However, this should be done cautiously, as prolonged use of these anesthetic agents exponentially increases the potential for side effects. Sustained use of intravenous anesthetics often results in tolerance and tachyphylaxis such that increasing doses may be required to achieve the same level of burst suppression. Higher doses of medications can concomitantly increase the potential for adverse reactions, especially when multiple ASMs are being administered. Therefore, it is important to frequently assess for medication toxicities and use as minimal doses of anesthetic agents as possible to achieve adequate burst suppression. In many instances, ictal-interictal patterns are encountered during the weaning of anesthetic agents. During these periods, if the EEG background shows reassuring features such as an organizing rhythm without a reversed anterior–posterior gradient, it is reasonable to continue tapering therapy rather than reescalating to continued burst suppression.[19]

A subset of patients will continue to experience seizures despite multiple rounds of burst suppression such that they in are in SRSE. On a molecular level, as seizures progress, evidence suggests that there may be impairment of gamma-aminobutyric acid (GABA) inhibition.[20,21] With sustained excitability, GABA receptors internalize resulting in reduced efficacy of GABAergic agents.[22] Furthermore, there may be increased numbers of α-amino-3-hydroxy-5-methyl-4-isoxazolepropionic acid (AMPA) and N-methyl-D-aspartate receptor (NMDA) receptors at the synaptic membrane.[20] In this setting, agents that target NMDA, such as ketamine, may be effective adjunctive agents.[23] At the current time, there are no drugs capable of blocking internalization of GABA receptors or externalization of excitatory receptors. Beyond ketamine, several experimental therapies have been proposed for SRSE (Table 46–4), although large randomized controlled trials on these therapies are lacking (due to the logistical issues of creating such trials).

EXPERT SUMMARY/GUIDELINES

Continuous Electroencephalogram Monitoring

The staple of expediated seizure detection and confirmation is cEEG. This powerful, noninvasive technique is a dynamic study, unlike commonly used imaging modalities such as magnetic resonance imaging. Recognition of seizures in the critical care setting is challenging, given that a high proportion of abnormal movements are seizure mimics.[24] These include nonepileptic seizures, rigors, tremors, myoclonic jerks, or semipurposeful movements of the extremities. Incorporation of digital video recordings to cEEG can facilitate differentiation between seizures and other nonepileptic spells. Without cEEG monitoring, these seizure mimics are often treated unnecessarily as epileptic seizures, leading to increased sedation and delirium. However, cEEG is complementary to the clinical exam and should never be interpreted in isolation as this may also lead to overtreatment.

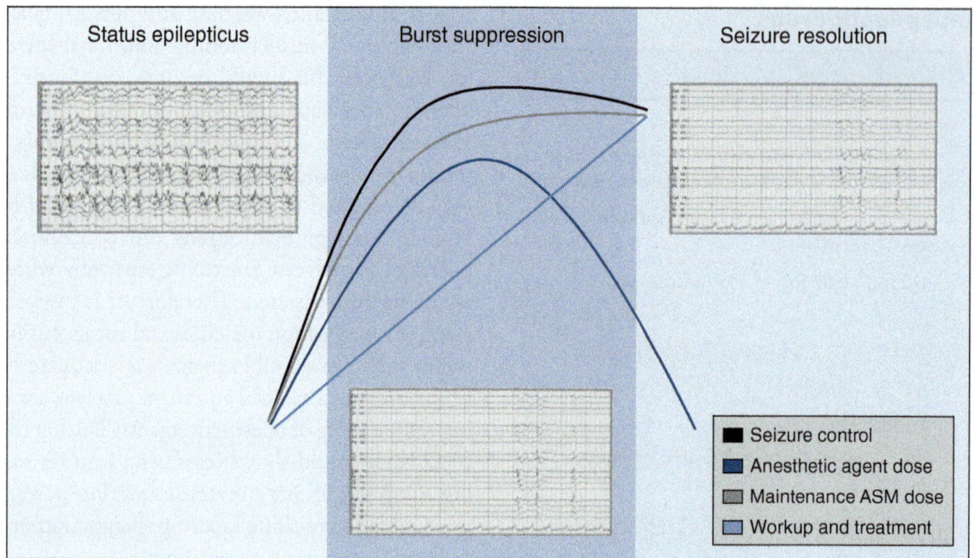

FIGURE 46–2 Burst suppression. The left pane of this figure is the phase of status epilepticus during which time the levels of maintenance ASMs are low, workup is only preliminary, and anesthetics have not yet been initiated. Once anesthetic agents are initiated to a sufficient level, seizure control is gained, and the EEG is in a burst suppression pattern (middle pane). During this time of seizure control, doses of maintenance ASMs and other antiseizure therapeutics are increased to therapeutic concentrations. Treatments have had time to take effect and fine tuning of other clinical parameters (such as electrolyte optimization) can be performed. During this time, additional workup to determine the cause of status epilepticus can be considered. Once these are completed, anesthetic agents are gradually tapered to achieve seizure resolution and awakefulness (right pane).

In addition to excluding nonepileptic events, cEEG is particularly useful for detecting nonconvulsive seizures. In one study, cEEG identified seizures in about 12% to 19% of patients with an unexplained depressed level of consciousness in the ICU.[25,26] The majority (>90%) of these seizures were nonconvulsive, making their diagnosis near impossible without the use of cEEG. Therefore, there should be a high suspicion for nonconvulsive seizures and a low threshold for the routine monitoring of patients in the neuroICU, especially since cEEG is a noninvasive and low-cost tool. In addition to characterizing encephalopathy, cEEG can also identify structural lesions (eg, focal slowing may be indicative of stroke) and can be used to trend arousal. Lastly, cEEG results are affected by changes in blood flow and cerebral metabolism. In this regard, cEEG can detect increased intracranial pressure as manifested by focal slowing, global EEG suppression, or an isoelectric EEG.[27]

TABLE 46–4 Trialed but unproven therapies for super refractory status epilepticus.

Pharmacological	*Nonpharmacological*
Inhaled Anesthetics (isoflurane or desflurane)	Ketogenic diet
Corticosteroids	Acupuncture
Neuroactive steroids	Vagus nerve stimulation
Coenzyme Q-10	Responsive neurostimulation
Bromide	Electroconvulsive therapy
Pyridoxine	Transcranial magnetic stimulation
Magnesium	Plasma exchange
Tocilizumab	Deep brain stimulation
Anakinra	CSF drainage
Intravenous immunoglobulin	Resective neurosurgery
Plasmapheresis	

Duration of cEEG Monitoring

With regard to the duration of monitoring to exonerate seizures, the same study demonstrated that comatose patients required >24 hours of monitoring for the first seizure to be detected.[25] Accordingly, the **Neurocritical Care Society guidelines suggest that at least 48 hours of cEEG monitoring should occur in critically ill patients in a comatose state.**[7] When seizures are detected, cEEG can also be used to monitor treatment response including anesthesia efficacy during burst suppression. It is recommended that **cEEG monitoring occurs 24 hours after the cessation of electrographic seizures or after ASMs are weaned.**[7]

Despite its utility for seizure detection in the ICU, cEEG remains an underutilized tool. Reasons that have prevented its widespread adoption include the costs associated with having an EEG technician available full-time for electrode placement as well as an epileptologist to interpret the data round-the-clock. However, the development of quantitative EEG metrics including compressed spectral array (CSA), amplitude-integrated EEG (aEEG), and density spectral array (DSA) has increased the ability of nurses, residents, and fellows to easily detect seizures

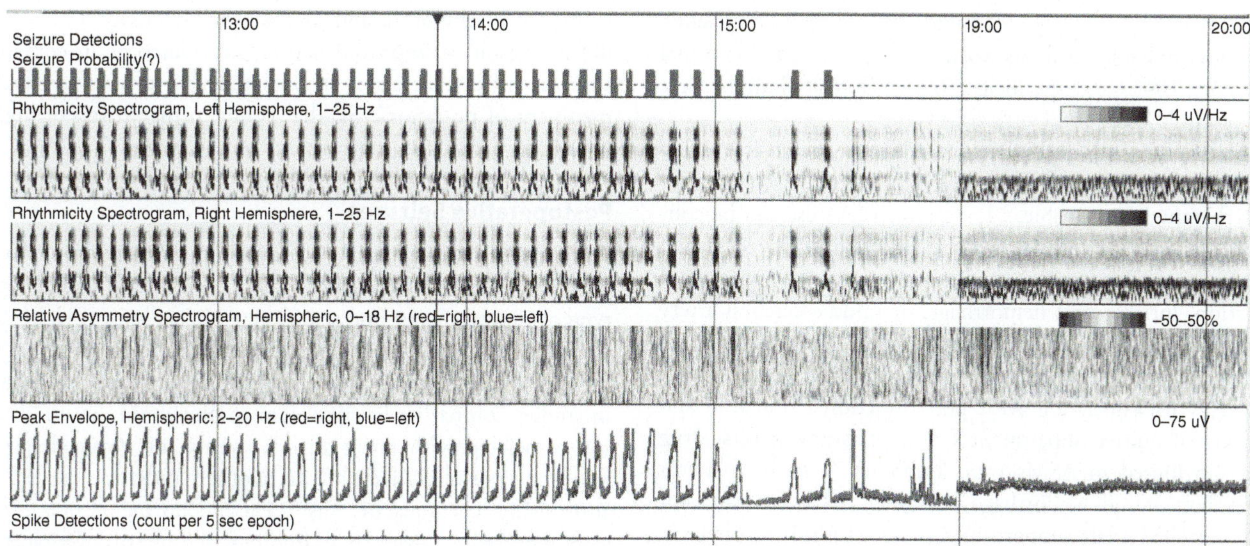

FIGURE 46–3 Electroencephalogram (EEG) spectrogram. This figure illustrates a typical EEG spectrogram which includes information regarding rhythmicity, asymmetry, and seizure probability. Asymmetry trends (third row) are color coded such that red represents activity in which the spectral power of the right hemisphere is greater than that of the left hemisphere, and blue represents regions in which the spectral power is greater in the left hemisphere than the right hemisphere. In this patient, there is a relative abundance of activity in the right hemisphere correlating as seizures on the probability map (top row). As evidenced on the spectrogram, this patient experienced 19 seizures/hour, which resolved after initiation of anesthetic agents.

(Figure 46–3).[28–30] While these tools do not obviate the need for formal EEG review by an experienced electrophysiologist, they provide a rapid means of seizure identification by bedside clinicians, potentially offloading the burden of continuous interpretation. Similarly, the use of commercially available bedside EEG monitors that allow for rapid setup by nurses and residents have also been shown to be efficacious and can mitigate the need for overnight EEG technologists, thereby reducing costs.[31,32]

Special Considerations

Traumatic Brain Injury

Patients with TBI are at an increased risk for developing NCSE. In one study, one-third of adults with TBI who underwent routine cEEG monitoring developed seizures that were detected, on average, 3 days after the trauma.[33] In a pediatric cohort, seizures were found in 42.5% of TBI patients and NCSE was found in 13.8% of patients.[34] In another study of pediatric patients with TBI, seizures were found in 30%, of which 40% experienced only subclinical seizures.[35] In both of these trials, younger age and abusive head trauma were risk factors for seizures. Furthermore, the presence of seizures correlated with longer ICU and hospital stays. Therefore, in patients with TBI, a high level of suspicion for nonconvulsive should be maintained, and routine cEEG of TBI patients should be adopted as a standard practice. Given that the majority of patients in one study developed seizures 3 days after initial presentation,[33] a minimum of 24 hours of cEEG monitoring should be performed. In TBI patients who require an intracranial pressure monitor,[36] it is reasonable to utilize a multimodal monitors that include a depth electrode for the purpose of seizure detection.

Seizures in TBI can elevate intracranial pressure and increase metabolic demand.[37] Current guidelines from the Brain Trauma Foundation recommend using ASM prophylaxis for 7 days.[36] The two agents that have been adopted for this purpose include levetiracetam and phenytoin.[38–40] Early post-traumatic seizures (PTS) are relatively common[41]; however, ASM therapy reduces only early (within 7 days) not late seizures.[42] Moreover, a short course of ASM therapy minimizes the risk for potential side effects. Given that long-term ASM prophylaxis does not reduce the risk of developing post-traumatic epilepsy, and can lead to side effects including cognitive dysfunction,[43] the use of ASMs should be limited to a maximum of 7 days for the sole purpose of preventing early seizures.

Subarachnoid Hemorrhage

Seizures following subarachnoid hemorrhage are common and can be detected in up to 26% of patients using cEEG.[44] In one study, NCSE was found in 8% of patients with subarachnoid hemorrhage who underwent cEEG monitoring despite being on a prophylactic ASM.[45] In these patients, the seizures were highly refractory to therapy and were associated with a poor prognosis. Other EEG findings that have been associated with a poor prognosis include the presence of periodic epileptiform discharges as well as the absence of sleep architecture.[46] In at least two studies, age and higher hemorrhage grade were found to be associated with NCSE.[45,47]

Not only is cEEG useful for seizure identification in subarachnoid hemorrhage but it may also be helpful for detection of cerebral vasospasm. Examining the decreased relative alpha variability have been indicative of vasospasm and can precede vasospasm by several days.[48–51] In one study, the alpha/delta ratio was decreased by 24% in patients with delayed cerebral ischemia compared to 3% for patients without delayed cerebral ischemia (sensitivity 100% and specificity 76%).[52] Similar findings have been reported using intracortical EEG.[53]

ASM prophylaxis for subarachnoid hemorrhage is controversial, but current guidelines suggest that a short course of ASM therapy is reasonable.[54] Long-term ASM use can be considered for patients with known risk factors for delayed seizure disorder including prior seizures, intractable hypertension, infarction, intracerebral hemorrhage, or middle cerebral artery aneurysm.[54,55] Phenytoin should be avoided, given its potential interactions with nimodipine (decreases drug concentration)[56] as well as its association with poor functional outcome and long-term cognitive impairment.[57,58] In one study, adverse drug events attributed to ASMs were found in 23.4% of patients with subarachnoid hemorrhage.[59] Despite a lack of randomized controlled trials supporting the use of ASM prophylaxis, the use of prophylactic ASMs for subarachnoid hemorrhage is still widespread.[60] This may be due to the fact that seizures in patients with subarachnoid hemorrhage could potentially lead to increased rebleeding from an unsecured aneurysm. However, the use of prophylactic ASMs may not necessary lead to reduced seizure frequency.[61]

Intracerebral Hemorrhage

Seizures have been reported in up to 31% of patients with intracerebral hemorrhage, half of which are subclinical.[62] The majority of these seizures usually occur within the first 24 hours of presentation.[58] Therefore, a relatively high suspicion for subclinical seizures should be performed in patients with intracerebral hemorrhage, especially lobar or expanding hemorrhages.[63] Prophylactic ASMs in intracerebral hemorrhage have been associated with poor outcome, and so, the routine use of prophylactic ASMs is not recommended.[64,65]

Anoxia

In hypoxic-ischemic injury, cEEG is useful for both prognostication and seizure monitoring. After cardiac arrest, postanoxic SE is common and can include NCSE, GCSE, or myoclonic SE.[66] Up to one-third of patients who undergo therapeutic hypothermia experience seizures which can occur during hypothermia or rewarming.[67] Myoclonus is also a common occurrence after arrest, and cEEG can distinguish between epileptic myoclonus (a cortical process) and nonepileptic myoclonus (a subcortical process) which are two distinct entities.[66] Since therapeutic hypothermia usually involves the use of paralytics and sedation, which may mask seizures, cEEG is often incorporated into hypothermia protocols. It can also help distinguish seizures from common, nonepileptic movements such as shivering. In addition to seizure detection, cEEG can aid in prognostication such that malignant EEG features are associated with poor outcomes.[68] Findings such as low electrical voltages, burst suppression, and absence of EEG reactivity are all associated with a poor prognosis after cardiac arrest.[69,70] While findings within the ictal-interictal continuum are common after cardiac arrest, treatment of rhythmic and periodic EEG activity with ASMs did not result in improved neurological outcome in comatose survivors of cardiac arrest in one study.[71] However, aggressive treatment of postanoxic SE that is not in the setting of highly malignant EEGs may improve outcome.

Postoperative Seizures

Postoperative seizures may be found in as many as 17% of patients,[72] and their incidence varies based on the location and type of procedure. In one semisystematic analysis of eight randomized trials, the majority of trials reported no benefit for ASM prophylaxis, and adverse event reporting was scarce.[73] However, in studies comparing levetiracetam to phenytoin, levetiracetam was associated with fewer adverse events and reduced seizure frequency postoperatively.[74,75] In another study, the rate of seizures using levetiracetam was 7.3% and no major side effects were reported.[76] Given these findings, the use of levetiracetam in the immediate postoperative period may be safe, although its efficacy warrants further investigation in a clinical trial.

REFERENCES

1. Carrera E, Claassen J, Oddo M, Emerson RG, Mayer SA, Hirsch LJ. Continuous electroencephalographic monitoring in critically ill patients with central nervous system infections. *Archives of Neurology.* 2008;65(12):1612–1618.
2. Jehi L. Consequences of status epilepticus in the intensive care unit: What we know and what we need to know. *Epilepsy Currents.* 2014;14(6):337–338.
3. Bromfield EB, Cavazos JE, Sirven JI, editors. An Introduction to Epilepsy [Internet]. West Hartford (CT): American Epilepsy Society; 2006. Chapter 1, Basic Mechanisms Underlying Seizures and Epilepsy.
4. Jette N, Claassen J, Emerson RG, Hirsch LJ. Frequency and predictors of nonconvulsive seizures during continuous electroencephalographic monitoring in critically ill children. *Archives of Neurology.* 2006;63(12):1750–1755.
5. Chong DJ, Hirsch LJ. Which EEG patterns warrant treatment in the critically ill? Reviewing the evidence for treatment of periodic epileptiform discharges and related patterns. *Journal of Clinical Neurophysiology: Official Publication of the American Electroencephalographic Society.* 2005;22(2):79–91.
6. Fisher RS, Cross JH, French JA, et al.: Operational classification of seizure types by the International League Against Epilepsy: position paper of the ILAE Commission for Classification and Terminology. *Epilepsia.* 2017;58(4):522–530.
7. Brophy GM, Bell R, Claassen J, et al; Neurocritical Care Society Status Epilepticus Guideline Writing Committee. Guidelines for the evaluation and management of status epilepticus. *Neurocritical Care.* 2012;17(1):3–23.
8. Leitinger M, Beniczky S, Rohracher A, et al. Salzburg consensus criteria for non-convulsive status epilepticus—approach to clinical application. *Epilepsy & Behavior: E&B.* 2015;49:158–163.
9. Leitinger M, Trinka E, Gardella E, et al. Diagnostic accuracy of the Salzburg EEG criteria for non-convulsive status epilepticus: a retrospective study. *The Lancet Neurology.* 2016;15(10):1054–1062.
10. Shorvon S, Trinka E. The London-Innsbruck Status Epilepticus Colloquia 2007–2011, and the main advances in the topic of status epilepticus over this period. *Epilepsia.* 2013;54:11–13.
11. Chong DJ, Hirsch LJ. Which EEG patterns warrant treatment in the critically ill? Reviewing the evidence for treatment of periodic epileptiform discharges and related patterns. *Journal of Clinical Neurophysiology: Official Publication of the American Electroencephalographic Society.* 2005; 22(2):79–91.
12. Hirsch LJ, LaRoche SM, Gaspard N, et al. American Clinical Neurophysiology Society's Standardized Critical Care EEG Terminology: 2012 version. *Journal of Clinical Neurophysiology: Official Publication of the American Electroencephalographic Society.* 2013;30(1):1–27.

13. Struck AF, Westover MB, Hall LT, Deck GM, Cole AJ, Rosenthal ES. Metabolic correlates of the ictal-interictal continuum: FDG-PET during continuous EEG. *Neurocritical Care.* 2016;24(3):324–331.
14. Subramaniam T, Jain A, Hall LT, et al. Lateralized periodic discharges frequency correlates with glucose metabolism. *Neurology.* 2019;92(7): e670–e674.
15. Krishnamurthy KB, Drislane FW. Depth of EEG suppression and outcome in barbiturate anesthetic treatment for refractory status epilepticus. *Epilepsia.* 1999;40(6):759–762.
16. Niedermeyer E. The burst-suppression electroencephalogram. *American Journal of Electroneurodiagnostic Technology.* 2009;49(4):333–341.
17. Muser D, Santangeli P, Liang JJ. Management of ventricular tachycardia storm in patients with structural heart disease. *World Journal of Cardiology.* 2017;9(6):521.
18. Das AS, Lee JW, Izzy S, Vaitkevicius H. Ultra-short burst suppression as a "reset switch" for refractory status epilepticus. *Seizure.* 2019;64:41–44.
19. Das AS, Lee JW, Rosenthal ES, Vaitkevicius H. Successful wean despite emergence of ictal-interictal EEG patterns during the weaning of prolonged burst-suppression therapy for super-refractory status epilepticus. *Neurocritical Care.* 2018;29(3):452–462.
20. Naylor DE, Liu H, Wasterlain CG. Trafficking of GABAA receptors, loss of inhibition, and a mechanism for pharmacoresistance in status epilepticus. *Journal of Neuroscience.* 2005;25(34):7724–7733.
21. Goodkin HP, Yeh J-L, Kapur J. Status epilepticus increases the intracellular accumulation of GABAA receptors. *The Journal of Neuroscience: The Official Journal of the Society for Neuroscience.* 2005;25(23):5511–5520.
22. Goodkin HR, Joshi S, Kozhemyakin M, Kapur J. Impact of receptor changes on treatment of status epilepticus. *Epilepsia.* 2007;48 Suppl 8:14–15.
23. Höfler J, Trinka E. Intravenous ketamine in status epilepticus. *Epilepsia.* 2018;59 Suppl 2:198–206.
24. Benbadis SR, Chen S, Melo M. What's shaking in the ICU? The differential diagnosis of seizures in the intensive care setting. *Epilepsia.* 2010;51(11):2338–2340.
25. Claassen J, Mayer SA, Kowalski RG, Emerson RG, Hirsch LJ. Detection of electrographic seizures with continuous EEG monitoring in critically ill patients. *Neurology.* 2004;62(10):1743–1748.
26. Alvarez V, Rodriguez Ruiz AA, LaRoche S, et al. The use and yield of continuous EEG in critically ill patients: a comparative study of three centers. *Clinical Neurophysiology: Official Journal of the International Federation of Clinical Neurophysiology.* 2017;128(4):570–578.
27. Newey CR, Sarwal A, Hantus S. Continuous electroencephalography (cEEG) changes precede clinical changes in a case of progressive cerebral edema. *Neurocritical Care.* 2013;18(2):261–265.
28. Stewart CP, Otsubo H, Ochi A, Sharma R, Hutchison JS, Hahn CD. Seizure identification in the ICU using quantitative EEG displays. *Neurology.* 2010;75(17):1501–1508.
29. Dericioglu N, Yetim E, Bas DF, et al. Non-expert use of quantitative EEG displays for seizure identification in the adult neuro-intensive care unit. *Epilepsy Research.* 2015;109:48–56.
30. Topjian AA, Fry M, Jawad AF, et al. Detection of electrographic seizures by critical care providers using color density spectral array after cardiac arrest is feasible. *Pediatric Critical Care Medicine.* 2015;16(5):461–467.
31. Young GB, Sharpe MD, Savard M, Al Thenayan E, Norton L, Davies-Schinkel C. Seizure detection with a commercially available bedside EEG monitor and the subhairline montage. *Neurocritical Care.* 2009;11(3): 411–416.
32. Hobbs K, Krishnamohan P, Legault C, et al. Rapid bedside evaluation of seizures in the ICU by listening to the sound of brainwaves: a prospective observational clinical trial of Ceribell's brain stethoscope function. *Neurocritical Care.* 2018;29(2):302–312.
33. Ronne-Engstrom E, Winkler T. Continuous EEG monitoring in patients with traumatic brain injury reveals a high incidence of epileptiform activity. *Acta Neurologica Scandinavica.* 2006;114(1):47–53.
34. Arndt DH, Lerner JT, Matsumoto JH, et al. Subclinical early posttraumatic seizures detected by continuous EEG monitoring in a consecutive pediatric cohort. *Epilepsia.* 2013;54(10):1780–1788.
35. O'Neill BR, Handler MH, Tong S, Chapman KE. Incidence of seizures on continuous EEG monitoring following traumatic brain injury in children. *Journal of Neurosurgery: Pediatrics.* 2015;16(2):167–176.
36. Carney N, Totten AM, O'Reilly C, Ullman JS, Hawryluk GW, Bell MJ, Bratton SL, Chesnut R, Harris OA, Kissoon N, Rubiano AM, Shutter L, Tasker RC, Vavilala MS, Wilberger J, Wright DW, Ghajar J. Guidelines for the Management of Severe Traumatic Brain Injury, Fourth Edition. Neurosurgery. 2017 Jan 1;80(1):6-15.
37. Hirsch LJ. Nonconvulsive seizures in traumatic brain injury: what you don't see can hurt you. *Epilepsy Currents.* 2008;8(4):97–99.
38. Torbic H, Forni AA, Anger KE, Degrado JR, Greenwood BC. Use of antiepileptics for seizure prophylaxis after traumatic brain injury. *American Journal of Health-System Pharmacy: AJHP: Official Journal of the American Society of Health-System Pharmacists.* 2013;70(9):759–766.
39. Inaba K, Menaker J, Branco BC, et al. A prospective multicenter comparison of levetiracetam versus phenytoin for early posttraumatic seizure prophylaxis. *The Journal of Trauma and Acute Care Surgery.* 2013;74(3):766–771; discussion 771–773.
40. Szaflarski JP, Sangha KS, Lindsell CJ, et al. Prospective, randomized, single-blinded comparative trial of intravenous levetiracetam. *Neurocritical Care.* 2010;12(2):165–172.
41. Frey LC. Epidemiology of posttraumatic epilepsy: a critical review. *Epilepsia.* 2003;44(s10):11–17.
42. Temkin NR, Dikmen SS, Wilensky AJ, Keihm J, Chabal S, Winn HR. A randomized, double-blind study of phenytoin for the prevention of post-traumatic seizures. *The New England Journal of Medicine.* 1990;323(8):497–502.
43. Dikmen SS, Temkin NR, Miller B, Machamer J, Winn HR. Neurobehavioral effects of phenytoin prophylaxis of posttraumatic seizures. *JAMA.* 1991;265(10):1271–1277.
44. Hart RG, Byer JA, Slaughter JR, Hewett JE, Easton JD. Occurrence and implications of seizures in subarachnoid hemorrhage due to ruptured intracranial aneurysms. *Neurosurgery.* 1981;8(4):417–421.
45. Dennis LJ, Claassen J, Hirsch LJ, et al. Nonconvulsive status epilepticus after subarachnoid hemorrhage. *Neurosurgery.* 2002;51(5):1136–1144.
46. Claassen J, Hirsch LJ, Frontera JA, et al. Prognostic significance of continuous EEG monitoring in patients with poor-grade subarachnoid hemorrhage. *Neurocritical Care.* 2006;4(2):103–112.
47. Little AS, Kerrigan JF, McDougall CG, et al. Nonconvulsive status epilepticus in patients suffering spontaneous subarachnoid hemorrhage. *Journal of Neurosurgery.* 2007;106(5):805–811.
48. Labar DR, Fisch BJ, Pedley TA, Fink ME, Solomon RA. Quantitative EEG monitoring for patients with subarachnoid hemorrhage. *Electroencephalography and Clinical Neurophysiology.* 1991;78(5):325–332.
49. Vespa PM, Nuwer MR, Juhász C, et al. Early detection of vasospasm after acute subarachnoid hemorrhage using continuous EEG ICU monitoring. *Electroencephalography and Clinical Neurophysiology.* 1997;103(6):607–615.
50. Rots ML, van Putten MJAM, Hoedemaekers CWE, Horn J. Continuous EEG monitoring for early detection of delayed cerebral ischemia in subarachnoid hemorrhage: a pilot study. *Neurocritical Care.* 2016;24(2):207–216.
51. Gollwitzer S, Groemer T, Rampp S, et al. Early prediction of delayed cerebral ischemia in subarachnoid hemorrhage based on quantitative EEG: a prospective study in adults. *Clinical neurophysiology: Official Journal of the International Federation of Clinical Neurophysiology.* 2015;126(8): 1514–1523.
52. Claassen J, Hirsch LJ, Kreiter KT, et al. Quantitative continuous EEG for detecting delayed cerebral ischemia in patients with poor-grade subarachnoid hemorrhage. *Clinical Neurophysiology: Official Journal of the International Federation of Clinical Neurophysiology.* 2004;115(12):2699–2710.
53. Stuart RM, Waziri A, Weintraub D, et al. Intracortical EEG for the detection of vasospasm in patients with poor-grade subarachnoid hemorrhage. *Neurocritical Care.* 2010;13(3):355–358.
54. Diringer MN, Bleck TP, Claude Hemphill J, et al. Critical care management following aneurysmal SAH. *Neurocritical Care.* 2011;15:211–240.
55. Connolly ES, Rabinstein AA, Carhuapoma JR, et al. Guidelines for the management of aneurysmal subarachnoid hemorrhage: A guideline for healthcare professionals from the American Heart Association/American Stroke Association. *Stroke.* 2012;43(6):1711–1737.
56. Tartara A, Galimberti CA, Manni R,et al. Differential effects of valproic acid and enzyme-inducing anticonvulsants on nimodipine pharmacokinetics in epileptic patients. *British Journal of Clinical Pharmacology.* 1991;32(3):335–340.

57. Naidech AM, Kreiter KT, Janjua N, et al. Phenytoin exposure is associated with functional and cognitive disability after subarachnoid hemorrhage. *Stroke*. 2005;36(3):583–587.
58. Yerram S, Katyal N, Premkumar K, Nattanmai P, Newey CR. Seizure prophylaxis in the neuroscience intensive care unit. *Journal of Intensive Care*. 2018;6(1):17.
59. Choi KS, Chun HJ, Yi HJ, Ko Y, Kim YS, Kim JM. Seizures and epilepsy following aneurysmal subarachnoid hemorrhage: incidence and risk factors. *Journal of Korean Neurosurgical Society*. 2009;46(2):93–98.
60. Dewan MC, Mocco J. Current practice regarding seizure prophylaxis in aneurysmal subarachnoid hemorrhage across academic centers. *Journal of Neurointerventional Surgery*. 2015;7(2):146–149.
61. Panczykowski D, Pease M, Zhao Y, et al. Prophylactic antiepileptics and seizure incidence following subarachnoid hemorrhage: a propensity score-matched analysis. *Stroke*. 2016;47(7):1754–1760.
62. Claassen J, Jetté N, Chum F, et al. Electrographic seizures and periodic discharges after intracerebral hemorrhage. *Neurology*. 2007;69(13): 1356–1365.
63. Passero S, Rocchi R, Rossi S, Ulivelli M, Vatti G. Seizures after spontaneous supratentorial intracerebral hemorrhage. *Epilepsia*. 2002;43(10):1175–1180.
64. Messé SR, Sansing LH, Cucchiara BL, et al. Prophylactic antiepileptic drug use is associated with poor outcome following ICH. *Neurocritical Care*. 2009;11(1):38–44.
65. Naidech AM, Garg RK, Liebling S, et al. Anticonvulsant use and outcomes after intracerebral hemorrhage. *Stroke*. 2009;40(12):3810–3815.
66. Reynolds AS, Claassen J. Treatment of seizures and postanoxic status epilepticus. *Seminars in Neurology*. 2017;37(1):33–39.
67. Knight WA, Hart KW, Adeoye OM, et al. The incidence of seizures in patients undergoing therapeutic hypothermia after resuscitation from cardiac arrest. *Epilepsy Research*. 2013;106(3):396–402.
68. Westhall E, Rossetti AO, Van Rootselaar AF, et al. Standardized EEG interpretation accurately predicts prognosis after cardiac arrest. *Neurology*. 2016;86(16):1482–1490.
69. Rossetti AO, Urbano LA, Delodder F, Kaplan PW, Oddo M. Prognostic value of continuous EEG monitoring during therapeutic hypothermia after cardiac arrest. *Critical Care*. 2010;14(5):R173.
70. Hofmeijer J, van Putten MJAM. EEG in postanoxic coma: prognostic and diagnostic value. *Clinical Neurophysiology: Official Journal of the International Federation of Clinical Neurophysiology*. 2016;127(4):2047–2055.
71. Ruijter BJ, Keijzer HM, Tjepkema-Cloostermans MC, et al. Treating rhythmic and periodic EEG patterns in comatose survivors of cardiac arrest. *New England Journal of Medicine*. 2022;386(8):724–734.
72. Foy PM, Copeland GP, Shaw MD. The incidence of postoperative seizures. *Acta Neurochirurgica*. 1981;55(3–4):253–264.
73. Greenhalgh J, Weston J, Dundar Y, Nevitt SJ, Marson AG. Antiepileptic drugs as prophylaxis for postcraniotomy seizures. *The Cochrane Database of Systematic Reviews*. 2018;5:CD007286.
74. Milligan TA, Hurwitz S, Bromfield EB. Efficacy and tolerability of levetiracetam versus phenytoin after supratentorial neurosurgery. *Neurology*. 2008;71(9):665–669.
75. Iuchi T, Kuwabara K, Matsumoto M, Kawasaki K, Hasegawa Y, Sakaida T. Levetiracetam versus phenytoin for seizure prophylaxis during and early after craniotomy for brain tumours: a phase II prospective, randomised study. *Journal of Neurology, Neurosurgery, and Psychiatry*. 2015;86(10):1158–1162.
76. Gokhale S, Khan S, McDonagh D, Agrawal A, Friedman A. Levetiracetam seizure prophylaxis in craniotomy patients at high risk for postoperative seizures. *Asian Journal of Neurosurgery*. 2013;8(4):169.

CHAPTER

47

What Is the Utility of Spot EEGs and Other Imaging Tools in the Detection of Seizures?

Jafar Hashem, MD & Jong Woo Lee, MD, PhD

Case

A 45-year-old woman with a history of hypertension was admitted to the intensive care unit (ICU) after surgical resection of the right posterior frontal mass resection. The patient's mental status worsened a few hours after the surgery. Computed tomography (CT) head was done and showed stable postoperative changes. Metabolic workup is unrevealing. Neurosurgery and ICU team suspected a possible nonconvulsive seizure; what's the optimal electroencephalogram (EEG) monitoring duration?

Key Points

- Full montage continuous electroencephalogram (cEEG) remains the gold standard in detecting seizures in neurocritical illness.
- Due to limitations in both technical and labor resource limitations, several different strategies have been employed, including reduced montage/rapid application EEGs, and optimizing both the duration and frequency of EEG monitoring.
- The Continuous EEG Randomized Trial in Adults (CERTA) prospective randomized trial demonstrated that cEEG was associated with a fourfold increase in detection rates of seizures, SE, and more frequent identification of ictal-interictal continuum (IIC) features compared to two 20-minute spot EEGs performed on consecutive days.
- It is suggested that patients be monitored for at least 48 hours if they are comatose and 24 hours if they are not.
- Imaging tools are utilized with increasing frequency in the characterization of seizures and status epilepticus (SE), although its utility is less clear as compared to EEG studies.
- Positron emission tomography (PET) scans may be clinically useful in instances where it is unclear whether refractory focal SE or periodic discharges are the primary pathology or whether these patterns are driven by an underlying structural abnormality, such as neoplasms or autoimmune lesions.

BACKGROUND

Critically ill adults have a high incidence of seizures. Electrographic seizures occur in approximately 10% to 25% of critically ill adults, most of which are nonconvulsive and without overt clinical signs.[1,2] There are significant associations between time spent with seizures or status epilepticus (SE) and worse clinical outcome.[3–5] Nonconvulsive seizures can lead to detrimental hemodynamic and metabolic crises on the brain and potentially contribute to increased intracranial pressure if allowed to continue undetected.[3,6–10] Therefore, timely seizure detection and treatment is critical to prevent further brain injury.

EVIDENCE AND REVIEW

There are several electroencephalogram (EEG) configurations as detailed in Table 47–1. U.S. Food and Drug Administration (FDA) approved several reduced montage EEG (RM-EEG) systems. The use of one such system (Ceribell, 5-electrode pairs configured into eight channels) in the critical care setting demonstrated comparable sensitivity and specificity of seizure detection with a remarkably short time-to-encephalography (5 min) compared to conventional EEG in a clinical trial (Figure 47–1).[11] Discrete low seizure-burden and SE can be detected with a 88% and 100% sensitivity and specificity, respectively.[12]

Status Epilepticus, Seizures, Suppression, Rhythmic Periodic Patterns (RPP) and the Ictal-Interictal Continuum (IIC): What Questions Can Be Answered?

Rapid-replacement EEG system may provide a recording quality that is comparable to conventional EEG in the critical care setting, where the seizures detected on both systems had concordant electrographic morphology and laterality.[18] Comparative observations demonstrate robust performance of RM EEG with sensitivity and specificity exceeding 90% for detection of electrographic seizures and RPP when compared to conventional EEG as well as in cohorts that included postcardiac arrest survivors,[19] with no compromise in interobserver variability.[20]

Earlier studies of RM EEGs have shown similar performance characteristics[21] though other studies have resulted in more modest performance.[22–25] Background features have less robust concordance with FM EEG ranging between 70% and 88% and need to be interpreted with caution. Improvement in concordance and intrarater agreement was seen upon optimization of several methodological factors.[16] RM EEG can often be associated with excessive artifact that may often preclude accurate interpretation. A significant false-positive detection rate of epileptiform discharges up to 31% due to eye movement artifact was noted in one observation. Of note, the sensitivity for seizure detection in non-intensive care unit (ICU) pediatric patients may be reduced and remains to be further elucidated.[26]

There is still limited data regarding the clinical utility of rapid EEG placement in critically ill patients. In critically ill neonates and children, there is a small but statistically significant increase in mortality independently associated with time to continuous EEG (cEEG) initiation.[27] As time to treatment of SE is strongly associated with outcome, it is likely that rapid detection of seizures, particularly SE, will also result in improved outcome.

What's the Optimal EEG Monitoring Duration?

An association has been established between the duration of monitoring and the rate of seizure detection; however, the minimum duration necessary to reliably exclude delayed seizure occurrence is unclear and may vary substantially due to heterogeneity of specific illnesses. Practices have largely followed recommendations based on clinical factors such as coma or prior history of seizures. It is suggested that patients be monitored for at least 48 hours if they are comatose and 24 hours if they are not.[28,29] While such approaches provide general guidance, prolonged EEG monitoring may not be clinically feasible in certain patients such as those who require urgent procedures or critical diagnostic imaging. This led to validated, risk-stratification models that consider individual patient characteristics to predict the risk of subsequently developing seizures. This may shorten unnecessary EEG time and improve the cost-effectiveness of monitoring. The 2HELPS2B score is an easy-to-use, validated, EEG-based seizure risk-stratification tool, where the probability of developing seizures can be accurately predicted based on a 1-hour screening EEG.[30,31] The TERSE algorithm is a promising tool that combines both clinical and EEG approaches to promote

TABLE 47–1 Overview of available systems.

Conventional full-montage (FM) EEG	It is recognized as the gold standard for scalp detection of seizures, but it is not always feasible in emergent or limited-resource settings where specialized technologist support or expert interpretation by neurologists or neurophysiologists is not readily available.
Rapid application FM and reduced montage (RM) EEG	These configurations have emerged for expediting point-of-care testing in the critical care setting. These are easily applied by nonexperts allowing for expeditious treatment initiation. Integrated user-friendly interfaces allow for prompt real-time viewing of the tracing both at the bedside as well as wireless transmission to online servers in real-time for remote evaluation by experts.
Reduced-montage EEG (RM-EEG) and Prefabricated RM EEG	These configurations typically cover the lateral circumference of the scalp. This can be particularly advantageous when structural barriers hinder the placement of an FM EEG (eg, postoperative neurosurgical or trauma patients).
Full-montage EEG (FM EEG)	Full-montage rapid application EEGs with acceptable recording qualities for a few hours have been developed[13–15], but it is unclear whether there is substantial benefit over a rapid application reduced-montage EEG. While FM EEG may be superior for seizure localization owing to widespread coverage with a greater number of EEG channels, RM EEG preserves key features of the traditional EEG system that is necessary for seizure detection.[16] For instance, systems that offer no coverage of the midline and parasagittal regions do not appear to have compromised performance as seizures arising exclusively from these regions in adults are shown to be rare.[17] In addition, delayed seizures detected by conventional EEG were uniformly visible in the temporal chains.[16]

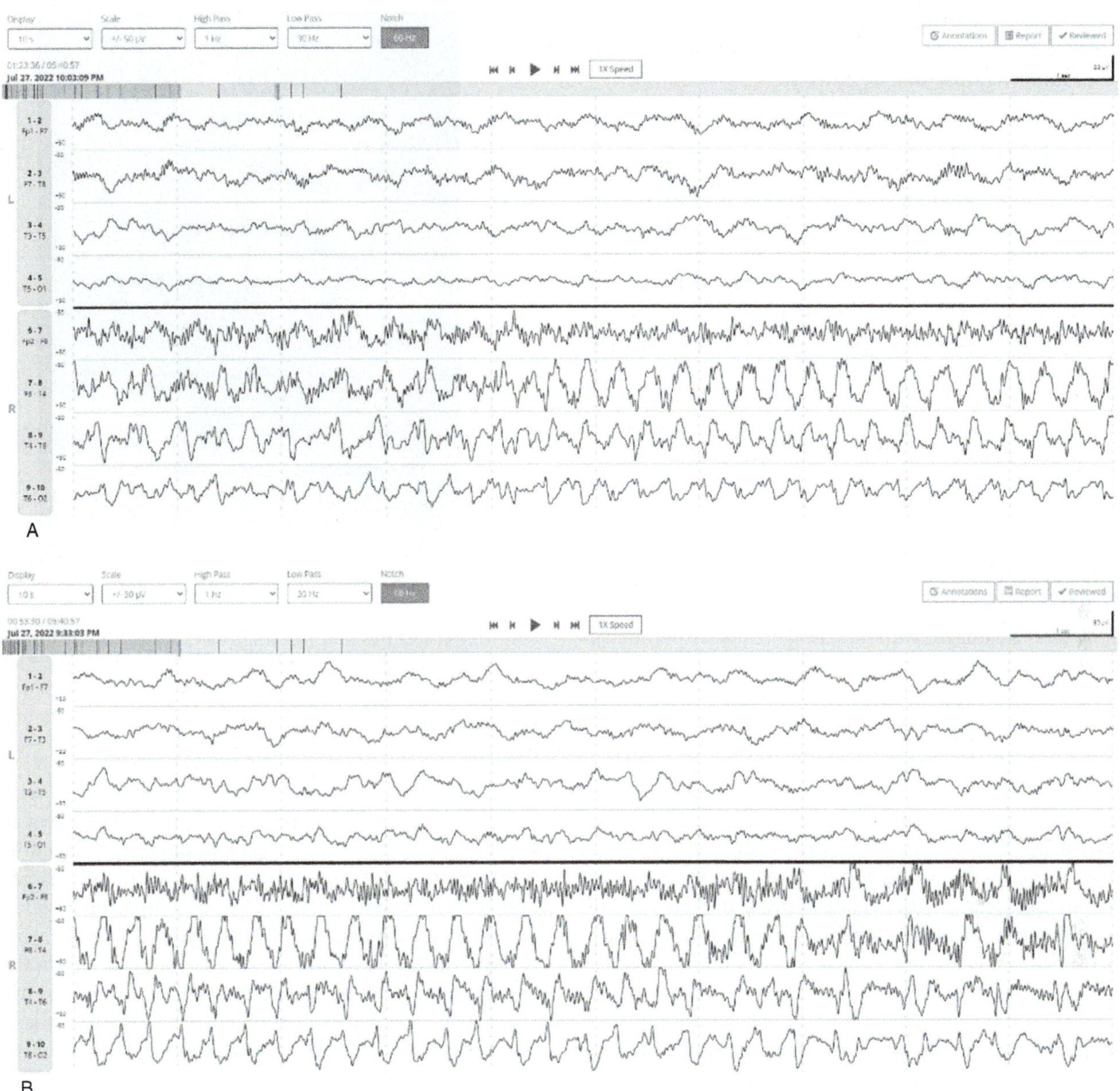

FIGURE 47–1 Ceribell recording consistent with electrographic status epilepticus in a patient presenting with altered mental status (AMS).

predictive accuracy. The model combines pre-EEG clinical features (coma and history of seizures) with EEG risk patterns to accurately determine the shortest duration of EEG necessary to achieve a high detection rate (>95%) of electrographic seizures. However, further validation in independent cohorts is needed.[32]

Regardless of which method is used, the limitations of such algorithms must be recognized. While some have shown excellent performance, no single algorithm achieves perfect sensitivity and specificity. Since the time-to-seizure detection can be markedly delayed by several hours up to several days in certain disease states, clinical judgement and individual patient factors remain critical in determining the optimal monitoring time. It is also important to note that current models are not intended for patients with hypoxic-ischemic brain injury.

Continuous Versus Intermittent EEG Which One Is Recommended?

Both the ACNS and European Society of Intensive Care Medicine suggest cEEG for critically ill patients with altered consciousness as it improves detection of nonconvulsive SE and delayed seizure activity.[30,33,34] Until recently, benefit in clinical outcomes had been only supported by retrospective observational studies.[35,36] The Continuous EEG Randomized Trial in Adults (CERTA) prospective randomized trial demonstrated that cEEG was associated with a fourfold increase in detection rates of seizures, SE, and more frequent identification of IIC features compared to two 20-minute spot EEGs performed on consecutive days.[37] Despite leading to improved diagnostics and increased modification in antiseizure therapy, the use of cEEG did not translate into reduced mortality or improved functional outcomes. The effect of cEEG monitoring on long-term functional outcome remains to be determined.

Conventional Versus Intracranial EEG

The sensitivity of scalp EEG is not always adequate for the detection of occult seizures. Whether certain scalp EEG features can predict their occurrence is uncertain and a high index of suspicion is required. Recent data demonstrates the diagnostic utility of intracranial EEG monitoring in the ICU leading to significantly enhanced sensitivity of depth seizure detection, particularly in the traumatic brain injury (TBI) and SAH patient populations.[7] Risk has been shown to be highest ipsilateral to the side of predominant injury in TBI.[7] Approaches include depth electrode (orthogonally or diagonally inserted) and subdural strip or grid electrode placement.

Is There a Role for Neuroimaging in Seizure Detection?

Imaging tools are utilized with increasing frequency in the characterization of seizures and SE, although its utility is less clear as compared to EEG studies.

A. MRI

MRI changes are most notable for changes in diffusion-weighted imaging changes, at times accompanied by T2/FLAIR changes, and occur in ~11% to 12% of patients with SE.[38,39] Location of lesions may localize with EEG findings, including the hippocampus ipsilateral to the seizure focus and gyral patterns, or may be present in more distal areas involved in the epileptic network including crossed cerebellar diaschisis, subcortical white matter, thalamus, and the splenium of the corpus callosum (Figure 47–2).[38–41] Long duration of SE and presence of lateralized periodic discharges were associated with MRI changes. These changes are transient in most, but not all, patients, and resolution may take several weeks.[39,42]

MRI of abnormal perfusion may play a key in the management of SE, particularly in determining the region of focus in focal seizures.[40,43–45] In certain situations, computed tomography (CT) perfusion in fact may be preferred due to its greater availability and more rapid acquisition time.[46] The colocalization of diffusion and perfusion changes over areas of prolonged ictal activity suggests that hyperperfusion serves as a compensatory mechanism to the high metabolic state, yet insufficient to prevent compromise caused by the hypermetabolic state, leading to a decoupling of blood flow and metabolism. This results in anerobic metabolism, failure of the Na/K ATPase pump, loss of cellular gradient, and cellular edema. These cellular changes are reflected in abnormalities in diffusion imaging.[40,47]

Importantly, MRI is often critical in quickly determining the underlying etiology of SE. The treatment/reversal of the causative etiology is most often the most effective method of both controlling seizures and limiting brain injury to optimize long-term outcome.

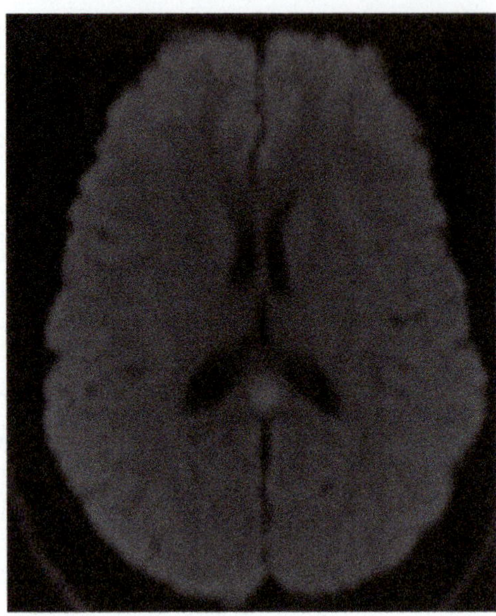

FIGURE 47–2 Transient lesion in the splenium of the corpus callosum in a patient with acute frequent seizures.

B. Nuclear Imaging

The most employed functional imaging modality in this population is the use of fluorodeoxyglucose positron emission tomography (FDG-PET). PET scans have demonstrated increased uptake in patients with rhythmic and periodic discharges[8] (Figure 47–3). Furthermore, the higher the frequency of the discharges, the higher the uptake,[48] demonstrating a hypermetabolic state created by these discharges that may lead to relative ischemia.

Hypermetabolic states have also been demonstrated in patients with frank SE. Furthermore, PET scans have demonstrated that hypermetabolism extends past the focus of the seizure but to areas that are functionally connected. The demonstration of crossed cerebellar diaschisis dramatically presents that the risk for a hypermetabolic state in the contralateral cerebellum.

PET scans may be of particular clinical utility as an ancillary test in patients with medication refractory suspected SE. In a case series of eight patients, Siciari et al demonstrated the utility of the FDG-PET scan in establishing the diagnosis of focal SE, defining the ictal zone for surgical evaluation, or clarifying incongruent clinical, MRI, or EEG features.[49] Rarely, PET scans may demonstrate a focus in patients with clinical epileptic manifestations but without corroborating EEG and MRI scans.[50] The identification of a seizure focus in patients with medically refractory and super refractory SE may be amenable to surgical resection. Multiple case series have demonstrated the utility of FDG-PET in that capacity. However, overall, the results of such surgical interventions have not been as regularly favorable as anticipated for reasons that are still unclear. One possibility is that SE may activate a broader network, which may counteract the ability to identify the offending lesion or, if identified, be impervious to surgical resection.

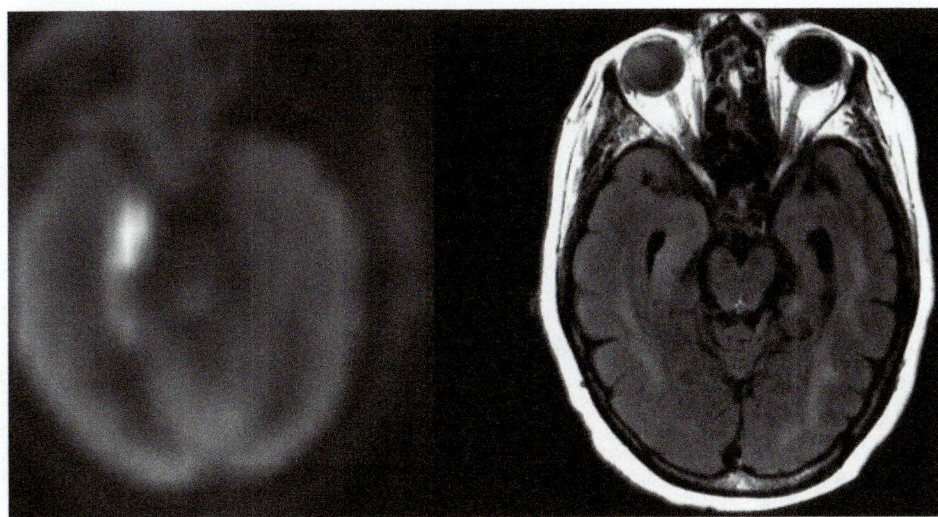

FIGURE 47–3 FDG-PET and MRI FLAIR lesion in a patient with right temporal status epilepticus.

PET scans may also be clinically useful in instances where it is unclear whether refractory focal SE or periodic discharges are the primary pathology or whether these patterns are driven by an underlying structural abnormality, such as neoplasms or autoimmune lesions. In instances where a hypermetabolic focus on a PET scan is present, the patient may undergo a repeat scan after burst suppression of the electrographic events is achieved. A resolution of the hypermetabolic focus likely indicates that the epileptic event is the primary driver of these discharges, whereas persistence of the hypermetabolic focus would imply that the structural lesion may be the primary pathology. Treatment therefore can be directed either toward escalating the antiseizure medication regimen or toward the structural lesion.[51]

C. Other Modalities

Other nuclear imaging techniques have been less frequently utilized. Single photon emission computed tomography (SPECT) tracers are utilized to assess blood flow and, similar to perfusion MRI, have been utilized to determine focal regions of hyperemia in patients in SE.[52] Although SPECT scans obviate the need for on-site cyclotrons, as compared to PET scans, both their spatial resolution and signal to noise ratio are lower and are thus less frequently utilized.

REFERENCES

1. Rodriguez Ruiz AA, Vlachy J, Lee JW, et al. Association of periodic and rhythmic electroencephalographic patterns with seizures in critically ill patients. *JAMA Neurol.* 2017;74:181–188. doi: 10.1001/jamaneurol.2016.4990.
2. Westover MB, Shafi MM, Bianchi MT, et al. The probability of seizures during EEG monitoring in critically ill adults. *Clin Neurophysiol.* 2015;126(3):463–471. Epub 2014/08/02. doi: 10.1016/j.clinph.2014.05.037. PubMed PMID: 25082090; PMCID: PMC4289643.
3. Vespa PM, Nuwer MR, Nenov V, et al. Increased incidence and impact of nonconvulsive and convulsive seizures after traumatic brain injury as detected by continuous electroencephalographic monitoring. *J Neurosurg.* 1999;91(5):750–760. Epub 1999/11/30. doi: 10.3171/jns.1999.91.5.0750. PubMed PMID: 10541231; PMCID: PMC4347935.
4. Claassen J, Hirsch LJ, Frontera JA, et al. Prognostic significance of continuous EEG monitoring in patients with poor-grade subarachnoid hemorrhage. *Neurocrit Care.* 2006;4(2):103–112. Epub 2006/04/22. doi: 10.1385/NCC:4:2:103. PubMed PMID: 16627897.
5. Vespa PM, McArthur DL, Xu Y, et al. Nonconvulsive seizures after traumatic brain injury are associated with hippocampal atrophy. *Neurology.* 2010;75(9):792–798. Epub 2010/09/02. doi: 10.1212/WNL.0b013e3181f07334. PubMed PMID: 20805525; PMCID: PMC2938965.
6. Ferlini L, Su F, Creteur J, Taccone FS, Gaspard N. Cerebral and systemic hemodynamic effect of recurring seizures. *Sci Rep.* 2021;11(1):22209. Epub 2021/11/17. doi: 10.1038/s41598-021-01704-6. PubMed PMID: 34782705; PMCID: PMC8593180.
7. Vespa P, Tubi M, Claassen J, et al. Metabolic crisis occurs with seizures and periodic discharges after brain trauma. *Ann Neurol.* 2016;79:579–590. doi: 10.1002/ana.24606. PubMed PMID: 26814699.
8. Struck AF, Westover MB, Hall LT, Deck GM, Cole AJ, Rosenthal ES. Metabolic correlates of the ictal-interictal continuum: FDG-PET during continuous EEG. *Neurocrit Care.* 2016;24:324–331. doi: 10.1007/s12028-016-0245-y. PubMed PMID: 27169855.
9. Payne ET, Zhao XY, Frndova H, et al. Seizure burden is independently associated with short term outcome in critically ill children. *Brain.* 2014;137:1429–1438. doi: 10.1093/brain/awu042. PubMed PMID: 24595203.
10. De Marchis GM, Pugin D, Meyers E, et al. Seizure burden in subarachnoid hemorrhage associated with functional and cognitive outcome. *Neurology.* 2016;86:253–260. doi: 10.1212/WNL.0000000000002281. PubMed PMID: 26701381.
11. Vespa PM, Olson DM, John S, et al. Evaluating the clinical impact of rapid response electroencephalography: The DECIDE multicenter prospective observational clinical study. *Crit Care Med.* 2020;48(9):1249–1257. Epub 2020/07/04. doi: 10.1097/CCM.0000000000004428. PubMed PMID: 32618687; PMCID: PMC7735649.
12. Kamousi B, Karunakaran S, Gururangan K, et al. Monitoring the burden of seizures and highly epileptiform patterns in critical care with a novel machine learning method. *Neurocrit Care.* 2021;34(3):908–917. Epub 2020/10/08. doi: 10.1007/s12028-020-01120-0. PubMed PMID: 33025543; PMCID: PMC8021593.
13. Ladino LD, Voll A, Dash D, et al. StatNet electroencephalogram: a fast and reliable option to diagnose nonconvulsive status epilepticus in emergency setting. *Can J Neurol Sci.* 2016;43(2):254–260. Epub 2016/02/13. doi: 10.1017/cjn.2015.391. PubMed PMID: 26864547.
14. Slater JD, Kalamangalam GP, Hope O. Quality assessment of electroencephalography obtained from a "dry electrode" system. *J Neurosci Methods.* 2012;208(2):134–137. Epub 2012/05/29. doi: 10.1016/j.jneumeth.2012.05.011. PubMed PMID: 22633894.
15. McKay JH, Feyissa AM, Sener U, et al. Time is brain: the use of EEG electrode caps to rapidly diagnose nonconvulsive status epilepticus. *J Clin Neurophysiol.* 2019;36(6):460–466. Epub 2019/07/25. doi: 10.1097/WNP.0000000000000603. PubMed PMID: 31335565.

16. Westover MB, Gururangan K, Markert MS, et al. Diagnostic value of electroencephalography with ten electrodes in critically ill patients. *Neurocrit Care*. 2020;33(2):479–490. Epub 2020/02/09. doi: 10.1007/s12028-019-00911-4. PubMed PMID: 32034656; PMCID: PMC7416437.
17. Gururangan K, Parvizi J. Midline and parasagittal seizures are rare in adult patients. *Neurocrit Care*. 2020;32(1):193–197. Epub 2019/08/16. doi: 10.1007/s12028-019-00804-6. PubMed PMID: 31414373; PMCID: PMC7012956.
18. Kamousi B, Grant AM, Bachelder B, Yi J, Hajinoroozi M, Woo R. Comparing the quality of signals recorded with a rapid response EEG and conventional clinical EEG systems. *Clin Neurophysiol Pract*. 2019;4:69–75. Epub 2019/04/13. doi: 10.1016/j.cnp.2019.02.002. PubMed PMID: 30976727; PMCID: PMC6444024.
19. Rittenberger JC, Weissman A, Baldwin M, et al. Preliminary experience with point-of-care EEG in post-cardiac arrest patients. *Resuscitation*. 2019;135:98–102. Epub 2019/01/04. doi: 10.1016/j.resuscitation.2018.12.022. PubMed PMID: 30605711.
20. Backman S, Cronberg T, Rosen I, Westhall E. Reduced EEG montage has a high accuracy in the post cardiac arrest setting. *Clin Neurophysiol*. 2020;131(9):2216–2223. Epub 2020/07/28. doi: 10.1016/j.clinph.2020.06.021. PubMed PMID: 32711346.
21. Karakis I, Montouris GD, Otis JA, et al. A quick and reliable EEG montage for the detection of seizures in the critical care setting. *J Clin Neurophysiol*. 2010;27:100–105. doi: 10.1097/WNP.0b013e3181d649e4. PubMed PMID: 20234318.
22. Kolls BJ, Husain AM. Assessment of hairline EEG as a screening tool for nonconvulsive status epilepticus. *Epilepsia*. 2007;48:959–965. Epub 2007/04/17. doi: 10.1111/j.1528-1167.2007.01078.x. PubMed PMID: 17433054.
23. Bubrick EJ, Bromfield EB, Dworetzky BA. Utilization of below-the-hairline EEG in detecting subclinical seizures. *Clin EEG Neurosci*. 2010;41:15–18. PubMed PMID: 20307011.
24. Ma BB, Johnson EL, Ritzl EK. Sensitivity of a reduced EEG montage for seizure detection in the neurocritical care setting. *J Clin Neurophysiol*. 2018;35(3):256–262. Epub 2018/02/23. doi: 10.1097/WNP.0000000000000463. PubMed PMID: 29470192.
25. Herta J, Koren J, Furbass F, Hartmann M, Gruber A, Baumgartner C. Reduced electrode arrays for the automated detection of rhythmic and periodic patterns in the intensive care unit: Frequently tried, frequently failed? *Clin Neurophysiol*. 2017;128(8):1524–1531. Epub 2017/05/16. doi: 10.1016/j.clinph.2017.04.012. PubMed PMID: 28501415.
26. Tacke M, Janson K, Vill K, et al. Effects of a reduction of the number of electrodes in the EEG montage on the number of identified seizure patterns. *Sci Rep*. 2022;12(1):4621. Epub 2022/03/19. doi: 10.1038/s41598-022-08628-9. PubMed PMID: 35301386; PMCID: PMC8930978.
27. Sanchez Fernandez I, Sansevere AJ, Guerriero RM, et al. Time to electroencephalography is independently associated with outcome in critically ill neonates and children. *Epilepsia*. 2017;58(3):420–428. Epub 2017/01/29. doi: 10.1111/epi.13653. PubMed PMID: 28130784; PMCID: PMC6736634.
28. Abend NS, Gutierrez-Colina AM, Topjian AA, et al. Nonconvulsive seizures are common in critically ill children. *Neurology*. 2011;76(12):1071–1077. Epub 2011/02/11. doi: 10.1212/WNL.0b013e318211c19e. PubMed PMID: 21307352; PMCID: PMC3068008.
29. Claassen J, Mayer SA, Kowalski RG, Emerson RG, Hirsch LJ. Detection of electrographic seizures with continuous EEG monitoring in critically ill patients. *Neurology*. 2004;62:1743–1748. Epub 2004/05/26. PubMed PMID: 15159471.
30. Struck AF, Tabaeizadeh M, Schmitt SE, et al. Assessment of the validity of the 2HELPS2B score for inpatient seizure risk prediction. *JAMA Neurol*. 2020;77(4):500–507. Epub 2020/01/14. doi: 10.1001/jamaneurol.2019.4656. PubMed PMID: 31930362; PMCID: PMC6990873.
31. Struck AF, Ustun B, Ruiz AR, et al. Association of an electroencephalography-based risk score with seizure probability in hospitalized patients. *JAMA Neurol*. 2017;53705:1–6. Epub 2017/10/21. doi: 10.1001/jamaneurol.2017.2459. PubMed PMID: 29052706.
32. Cisse FA, Osman GM, Legros B, et al. Validation of an algorithm of time-dependent electro-clinical risk stratification for electrographic seizures (TERSE) in critically ill patients. *Clin Neurophysiol*. 2020;131(8):1956–1961. Epub 2020/07/06. doi: 10.1016/j.clinph.2020.05.031. PubMed PMID: 32622337.
33. Herman ST, Abend NS, Bleck TP, et al. Consensus statement on continuous EEG in critically ill adults and children, part II: personnel, technical specifications, and clinical practice. *J Clin Neurophysiol*. 2015;32:96–108.
34. Herman ST, Abend NS, Bleck TP, et al. Consensus statement on continuous EEG in critically Ill adults and children, part I: Indications. *J Clin Neurophysiol*. 2015;32:87–95. doi: 10.1097/WNP.0000000000000166. PubMed PMID: 25626777.
35. Hill CE, Blank LJ, Thibault D, et al. Continuous EEG is associated with favorable hospitalization outcomes for critically ill patients. *Neurology*. 2018. Epub 2018/12/07. doi: 10.1212/WNL.0000000000006689. PubMed PMID: 30504428.
36. Ney JP, van der Goes DN, Nuwer MR, Nelson L, Eccher MA. Continuous and routine EEG in intensive care: utilization and outcomes, United States 2005-2009. *Neurology*. 2013;81:2002–2008. doi: 10.1212/01.wnl.0000436948.93399.2a. PubMed PMID: 24186910.
37. Rossetti AO, Schindler K, Sutter R, et al. Continuous vs routine electroencephalogram in critically ill adults with altered consciousness and no recent seizure. *JAMA Neurology*. 2020. doi: 10.1001/jamaneurol.2020.2264.
38. Milligan TA, Zamani A, Bromfield E. Frequency and patterns of MRI abnormalities due to status epilepticus. *Seizure*. 2009;18:104–108. doi: 10.1016/j.seizure.2008.07.004. PubMed PMID: 18723376.
39. Giovannini G, Kuchukhidze G, McCoy MR, Meletti S, Trinka E. Neuroimaging alterations related to status epilepticus in an adult population: definition of MRI findings and clinical-EEG correlation. *Epilepsia*. 2018;59 Suppl 2:120–127. Epub 2018/08/22. doi: 10.1111/epi.14493. PubMed PMID: 30129213.
40. Szabo K, Poepel A, Pohlmann-Eden B, et al. Diffusion-weighted and perfusion MRI demonstrates parenchymal changes in complex partial status epilepticus. *Brain*. 2005;128(Pt 6):1369–1376. Epub 2005/03/04. doi: 10.1093/brain/awh454. PubMed PMID: 15743871.
41. Mariajoseph FP, Sagar P, Muthusamy S, Amukotuwa S, Seneviratne U. Seizure-induced reversible MRI abnormalities in status epilepticus: a systematic review. *Seizure*. 2021;92:166–173. Epub 2021/09/16. doi: 10.1016/j.seizure.2021.09.002. PubMed PMID: 34525432.
42. Cianfoni A, Caulo M, Cerase A, et al. Seizure-induced brain lesions: a wide spectrum of variably reversible MRI abnormalities. *Eur J Radiol*. 2013;82(11):1964–72. Epub 2013/06/22. doi: 10.1016/j.ejrad.2013.05.020. PubMed PMID: 23787273.
43. El-Koussy M, Mathis J, Lovblad KO, Stepper F, Kiefer C, Schroth G. Focal status epilepticus: follow-up by perfusion- and diffusion MRI. *Eur Radiol*. 2002;12(3):568–574. Epub 2002/03/01. doi: 10.1007/s003300100999. PubMed PMID: 11870471.
44. Kanazawa Y, Morioka T, Arakawa S, Furuta Y, Nakanishi A, Kitazono T. Nonconvulsive partial status epilepticus mimicking recurrent infarction revealed by diffusion-weighted and arterial spin labeling perfusion magnetic resonance images. *J Stroke Cerebrovasc Dis*. 2015;24(4):731–738. Epub 2015/03/01. doi: 10.1016/j.jstrokecerebrovasdis.2014.09.026. PubMed PMID: 25724245.
45. Shimogawa T, Morioka T, Sayama T, et al. The initial use of arterial spin labeling perfusion and diffusion-weighted magnetic resonance images in the diagnosis of nonconvulsive partial status epileptics. *Epilepsy Res*. 2017;129:162–173. Epub 2017/01/17. doi: 10.1016/j.eplepsyres.2016.12.008. PubMed PMID: 28092848.
46. Payabvash S, Oswood MC, Truwit CL, McKinney AM. Acute CT perfusion changes in seizure patients presenting to the emergency department with stroke-like symptoms: correlation with clinical and electroencephalography findings. *Clin Radiol*. 2015;70(10):1136–1143. Epub 2015/07/15. doi: 10.1016/j.crad.2015.06.078. PubMed PMID: 26155937.
47. Meletti S, Monti G, Mirandola L, Vaudano AE, Giovannini G. Neuroimaging of status epilepticus. *Epilepsia*. 2018;59 Suppl 2:113–119. Epub 2018/08/31. doi: 10.1111/epi.14499. PubMed PMID: 30160066.
48. Subramaniam T, Jain A, Hall LT, Cole AJ, Westover MB, Rosenthal ES, Struck AF. Lateralized periodic discharges frequency correlates with glucose metabolism. *Neurology*. 2019;92(7):e670–e674. Epub 2019/01/13. doi: 10.1212/WNL.0000000000006903. PubMed PMID: 30635488; PMCID: PMC6382363.

49. Siclari F, Prior JO, Rossetti AO. Ictal cerebral positron emission tomography (PET) in focal status epilepticus. *Epilepsy Res.* 2013; 105:356–361. doi: 10.1016/j.eplepsyres.2013.03.006. PubMed PMID: 23582605.
50. Dong C, Sriram S, Delbeke D, et al. Aphasic or amnesic status epilepticus detected on PET but not EEG. *Epilepsia.* 2009;50(2):251–255. Epub 2008/09/20. doi: 10.1111/j.1528-1167.2008.01782.x. PubMed PMID: 18801038.
51. Akbik F, Robertson M, Das AS, Singhal T, Lee JW, Vaitkevicius H. The PET sandwich: using serial FDG-PET scans with interval burst suppression to assess ictal components of disease. *Neurocrit Care.* 2020. Epub 2020/04/08. doi: 10.1007/s12028-020-00956-w. PubMed PMID: 32253731.
52. Jaraba S, Reynes-Llompart G, Sala-Padro J, et al. Usefulness of HMPAO-SPECT in the diagnosis of nonconvulsive status epilepticus. *Epilepsy Behav.* 2019;101(Pt B):106544. Epub 2019/11/23. doi: 10.1016/j.yebeh.2019.106544. PubMed PMID: 31753769.

CHAPTER

48

What Is the Role of Antiseizure Medication in Seizure Prophylaxis After Routine Craniotomy?

Alexander G. Yearley, BA, Steven Tobochnik, MD, & Michael A. Mooney, MD

Case

A 44-year-old woman with no prior history of epilepsy presented to the emergency department after a bilateral tonic-clonic seizure. Brain imaging revealed an enhancing mass at the anterior skull base with surrounding vasogenic edema, consistent with an olfactory groove meningioma (Figure 48–1). The patient was started on levetiracetam and dexamethasone. She was taken to the operating room and gross total resection was achieved. Pathology confirmed a World Health Organization grade 1 meningioma with a high proliferative index. She was discharged home on postoperative day 4 on levetiracetam with no further seizure activity. At her postoperative follow-up visit, she reported mildly increased emotional lability and inquired how long she will require antiseizure medication.

Key Points

- Antiseizure prophylaxis is not recommended in patients with brain tumors who have not had prior seizures.
- Antiseizure prophylaxis in the initial 7 days after traumatic brain injury decreases early risk of seizures but not delayed risk.
- Patients with epilepsy should be continued on their maintenance antiseizure medications (ASMs).
- Trials on the use of prophylactic ASMs after craniotomy differ in the timing and dosage of ASM administration, availability of therapeutic drug monitoring, follow-up length, randomization, and outcome reporting.[1]

BACKGROUND

Seizures are associated with significant morbidity and mortality. A single seizure not only adversely impacts a patient's health but can also contribute to a decreased quality of life due to restricted driving privileges among other activities.[2–5] While most patients fully recover, postoperative seizures have been linked to decreased cognitive function, re-intubation, prolonged hospitalization, readmission, brain injury, and death.[6–8] Craniotomies make up the vast majority of the estimated 665,000 nonelective neurosurgical cases that occur in the United States and Canada every year.[9] Postcraniotomy seizures are defined as any seizure occurring following a craniotomy; these are often subdivided into immediate seizures that occur within 24 hours, early seizures that occur within 1 week, and late seizures that occur >1 week after surgery.

There has been significant interest in identifying patients at risk for postcraniotomy seizures and in developing strategies for management and prevention. These strategies typically involve the use of antiseizure medications (ASMs); however, there exist many unresolved questions surrounding the specific indications for use, choice of drug, dosing, and duration of treatment. As such, this remains a controversial topic with variable approaches to management. This chapter aims to summarize the current body of evidence and highlight areas of general consensus in order to assist clinicians with patient management.

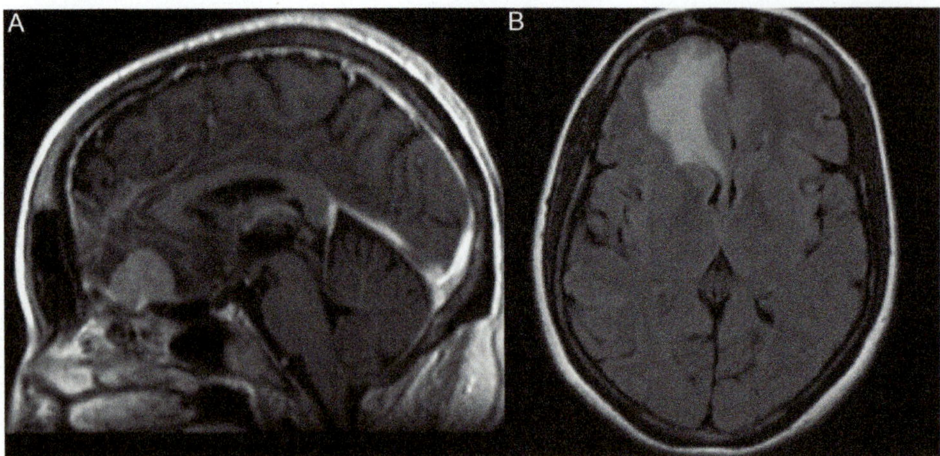

FIGURE 48–1 Preoperative sagittal postcontrast T1-weighted **(A)** and axial T2-FLAIR **(B)** MR sequences depicting a 2-cm olfactory groove meningioma with surrounding vasogenic edema.

EVIDENCE AND REVIEW

Epidemiology

Rates of postcraniotomy seizures vary by type of craniotomy, pathology, and preexisting risk factors. One study of 1,103 patients undergoing a supratentorial nontraumatic craniotomy reported a postoperative seizure incidence as high as 15% to 20%.[4] More recent work has shown that postcraniotomy seizure incidence ranges from 5% to 50% based on the surgical pathology.[5,10–20]

Seizures are frequently associated with brain tumors, with rates ranging from approximately 10% in primary central nervous system (CNS) lymphoma to nearly 100% in dysembryoplastic neuroepithelial tumors.[21] Incidence of seizures following craniotomy for primary brain tumors similarly varies by tumor histology. In patients with meningioma, 1% to 12% experience new-onset seizures following surgery, compared to 24% to 39% in grade 4 gliomas and 33% to 62% in grade 2 to 3 gliomas.[15,16,22–26]

Rates of postcraniotomy seizures are also widely variable for nontumor intracranial pathologies. In surgically treated chronic subdural hematomas, postoperative seizures have been reported in 4% to 19% of cases.[17,18] The incidence of postoperative seizure in intracranial aneurysm or arteriovenous malformation repair has been reported as 3% to 42% and 6% to 50%, respectively.[19,20,27,28]

Risk Factors

A history of preoperative seizure is a well-established and durable risk factor for postoperative seizures.[29,30] However, given that most of these patients are already maintained on ASMs, the role of additional antiseizure prophylaxis is uncertain. While the identification of additional risk factors is an area of active investigation, some work has been done to guide risk stratification, particularly in patients with brain tumors. Studies of patients undergoing supratentorial meningioma resection identified poor preoperative seizure control, presence of epilepsy for >1 year, a history of previous radiation, and presence of residual tumor as risk factors for postcraniotomy seizures.[22,31] There is some disagreement on the impact of tumor size, with certain studies associating larger tumors with an increased risk of seizure while others found the opposite trend.[16,30,32] More work is needed in this space to identify additional risk factors, particularly with respect to tumor genetic and molecular features that may predict postcraniotomy seizures.

Evidence for Prophylaxis

The use of ASMs for postcraniotomy seizure prophylaxis in the absence of prior seizures remains controversial. To date, there is no definitive evidence supporting this practice. A Cochrane Database systematic review of 10 randomized controlled trials (RCTs) investigating the effect of prophylactic ASMs in patients undergoing craniotomies for different indications found limited evidence that ASMs are either effective or not effective in preventing seizures.[1] In fact, when examining both incidence of death and late seizures following craniotomy, no trials have found significant differences between ASM prophylaxis and control groups.[2,13,33–36] While two RCTs did identify a reduced incidence of early seizures after craniotomy with phenytoin prophylaxis, seven other trials found no significant reduction with ASM prophylaxis.[2,13,33–39] The uncertainty surrounding use of these medications is further augmented by the development of newer ASMs with improved tolerability and fewer drug interactions compared to those used in the majority of RCTs. While most trials have found no significant difference in tolerability between ASMs, some studies have suggested that phenytoin is associated with increased adverse effects compared to other ASMs.[2,13,33,35–39]

Postoperative ASM prophylaxis has been more extensively studied in brain tumor patients relative to other pathologies. Three separate systematic reviews covering a total of 69 studies of postcraniotomy ASM prophylaxis in meningioma patients failed to find a significant difference in postoperative seizure incidence.[22,40,41] A meta-analysis of ASM prophylaxis trials in primary glial tumors, cerebral metastases, and meningiomas also concluded that ASMs had no effect on seizure prevention up to 6 months after surgery.[42] However, a meta-analysis of four RCTs by Joiner et al[43] evaluating ASM prophylaxis after cranial tumor resection found that while isolated RCTs did not demonstrate a benefit of chemoprophylaxis, when pooled, perioperative ASMs yielded a significant reduction in risk of early seizures compared with placebo. This discrepancy between studies may be explained by exclusion of nonoperative patients and separation of early and late seizures in the analysis by Joiner et al.[43]

These conflicting data highlight the need for further investigation into the role of ASM prophylaxis. As detailed below, controversy in clinical decision-making exists due to a lack of agreement between evidence-based guidelines and current practices.

In Clinical Practice

Surveys of practicing neurosurgeons reveal a strong bias toward the use of ASM prophylaxis after craniotomy. Multiple studies seeking to evaluate the practice patterns of neurosurgeons in the United States found that 63% to 80% of neurosurgeons report prescribing ASM prophylaxis after surgery for a supratentorial brain tumor.[44–46] While data only exist in the field of neuro-oncology, it is conceivable that similar trends exist in other areas of neurosurgery. Levetiracetam is the most commonly used ASM by 78% to 85% of respondents, with phenytoin used less commonly by 20% of respondents.[45,47] Number of years in practice was the strongest predictor for the use of ASM prophylaxis.[44] Patients with primary malignancies, secondary metastases, and those being discharged with home services were more likely to receive prophylaxis while those undergoing biopsy procedures or transsphenoidal surgery were less likely.[44,47] This apparent lack of clinical equipoise must be considered in the design of future controlled studies.

Table 48–1 provides seizure prophylaxis recommendations stratified by pathology based on the current body of literature.

TABLE 48–1 Evidence-based recommendations for postcraniotomy seizure prophylaxis by indication.

Indication	Recommendation
Primary and metastatic brain tumors	No ASM prophylaxis is indicated in patients without history of seizures[22,35,40–42,48–50]
Traumatic brain injury	ASM prophylaxis for the first 7 days after injury[51–62]
History of epilepsy	Adhere to preoperative ASM regimen[63–65]
Unruptured intracranial aneurysm	No consensus recommendation[66,67]
Subdural hematoma evacuation	No consensus recommendation[17,68,69]

ASM, Anti-Seizure Medication

Anti-Seizure Medication Choice

With many ASMs available, drug choice varies by indication and patient-specific contraindications. The choice also partially reflects physician preference, with recent work showing that, over time, the field has moved away from carbamazepine and phenytoin toward levetiracetam and lamotrigine.[70]

General principles that should always be considered when choosing an ASM are as follows:

1. Strong cytochrome P450 inducers (eg, carbamazepine, phenytoin, phenobarbital, primidone) should be avoided in patients with malignancy due to potential interaction with chemotherapy.
2. Less sedating medications are preferred to decrease postoperative delirium.
3. ASMs with intravenous formulations may be preferred in the perioperative period.
4. Adverse effect profiles and patient-specific contraindications to individual medications should be considered (Table 48–2).

ASM choice is also influenced by the patient's underlying pathology. In patients with brain tumors, levetiracetam and lamotrigine are recommended by the European Association of Neuro-Oncology for their efficacy, favorable adverse effect profiles, and minimal interactions with oncologic treatments.[49,84] Levetiracetam is most commonly used in clinical practice with 78% to 90% of physicians who treat brain-tumor related epilepsy citing it as their first choice.[47,85] Lacosamide, lamotrigine, valproic acid, and clobazam are also common well-tolerated alternatives.[47,48,85,86] However, valproic acid must be used with added caution, given its CYP inhibitor properties. Several retrospective studies have shown a survival benefit of ASMs, especially levetiracetam, in high-grade glioma patients independent of their antiseizure effects.[87–90] However, this is an active area of investigation and other work contradicts these findings.[91–93]

While few other pathologies have been as heavily investigated as brain tumors, some recommendations exist for seizure prophylaxis in traumatic brain injury. The American Academy of Neurology recommends prophylaxis with phenytoin.[62] However, multiple studies have shown no treatment benefit with phenytoin use over other ASMs such as levetiracetam or valproic acid.[55,57]

Duration of Treatment

Little consensus exists as to the optimal duration for postcraniotomy seizure prophylaxis. Surveys of practicing neurosurgeons have found wide variation in the duration of ASM prescription with 18% to 25% of respondents administering ASMs for <7 days, 35% to 37% for 2 to 6 weeks, and 13% to 36% for >6 weeks.[44,45] Studies suggest that 67% of postoperative seizures occur within a month of surgery and 75% of patients who develop seizures do so within a year of surgery.[11] While it is estimated that only 8% of patients have a first seizure >2 years after surgery, for some conditions, such as cerebral abscesses or arteriovenous malformations, there remains a high risk of epilepsy even after 5 years.[11,94]

The duration of ASM treatment is driven by the presence and timing of seizures (Figure 48–2). If the patient has no history of seizures and no seizures have occurred at 1 week after

TABLE 48–2 Summary of contraindications and adverse effects of commonly prescribed antiseizure medications. SJS, Stevens-Johnson syndrome.

Medication	Contraindications	Common Adverse Effects
Phenytoin/fosphenytoin (PO, IV)	Pregnancy[71]	Neurotoxicity, teratogenicity, gingival hypertrophy, hirsutism, rash, folic acid depletion, decreased bone density, SJS syndrome[72]
Valproic acid (PO, IV)	Liver failure, pregnancy[73]	Hepatotoxicity, teratogenicity, metabolic syndrome, thrombocytopenia, bleeding, alopecia, tremor[74,75]
Levetiracetam/brivaracetam (PO, IV)	Psychiatric illness (minor contraindication)[76]	Hallucinations, apathy, emotional lability, agitation, irritability, hostility, fatigue, somnolence, dizziness, infection[77]
Lacosamide (PO, IV)	PR interval > 200 ms[78]	Dizziness, ataxia, cardiac arrhythmia, syncope, hypersensitivity reactions[79]
Lamotrigine (PO)	—	Drowsiness, insomnia, headache, diplopia, SJS syndrome[80]
Perampanel (PO)	Psychiatric illness (minor contraindication)[81]	Dizziness, somnolence, fatigue, irritability, falls, nausea, weight gain, vertigo, ataxia, gait disturbances[81]
Clobazam (PO)	Myasthenia gravis, narrow-angle glaucoma, severe hepatic or respiratory disease, sleep apnea, history of substance abuse[82]	Sedation, somnolence, drowsiness, headache, nausea, pyrexia, lethargy, aggression, drooling, irritability, ataxia, constipation, dry mouth, blurred vision, depression, insomnia, amnesia[82,83]

surgery, it is recommended to discontinue seizure prophylaxis at this time. The principal indication for prolonged ASM prophylaxis is if the patient meets the diagnostic criteria for epilepsy.[95] Many cases of unprovoked late postoperative seizures with a brain lesion qualify as epilepsy based on one seizure and a 60% risk of recurrence. Additionally, limited data extrapolated from outcomes of acute symptomatic seizures suggest that if seizures occur preoperatively and the lesion is completely removed or if exclusively early postoperative seizures occur, an intermediate course of ASMs, typically 3 to 6 months, may be adequate.[96]

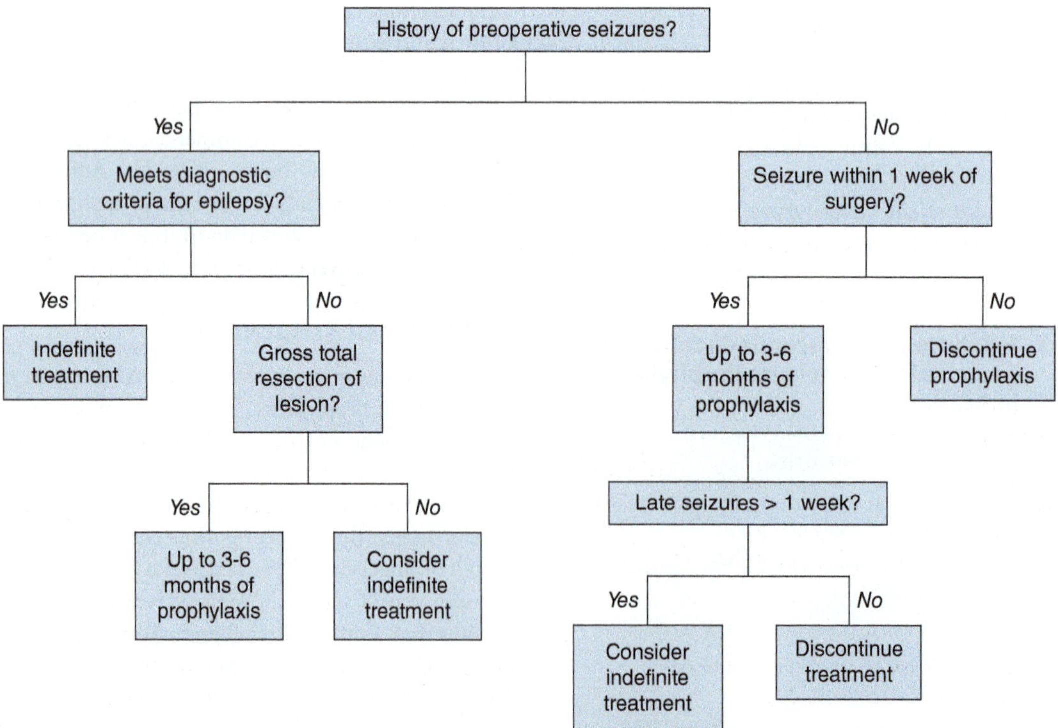

FIGURE 48–2 Algorithm for duration of postcraniotomy antiseizure medication treatment. Limited data exist to determine the optimal durations of treatment in patients with seizures without a definite epilepsy diagnosis.

TABLE 48–3 Summary of professional society guidelines concerning the use of antiseizure medications for postcraniotomy seizure prophylaxis.

Society	Scope	Guideline
European Association of Neuro-Oncology	Diffuse gliomas of adulthood	1. Patients who have suffered epileptic seizures should receive anticonvulsant drugs preoperatively. 2. Primary prophylaxis does not reduce the risk of a first seizure in patients with low- or high-grade glioma without a history of seizures and is not recommended.[48,49]
Society for Neuro-Oncology, European Association of Neuro-Oncology, American Academy of Neurology	Brain tumors	1. In patients with brain tumors undergoing surgery, there is insufficient evidence to recommend prescribing ASMs to reduce the risk of seizures in the peri- or postoperative period. 2. In patients with brain tumors who have not had seizures, there is insufficient evidence to support using tumor location, histology (primary vs. metastatic), grade, molecular features, or imaging characteristics when deciding whether or not to prescribe prophylactic ASMs.[50]
American Society of Clinical Oncology, Society for Neuro-Oncology	Metastatic brain tumors	1. Routine postcraniotomy antiseizure medication use for seizure-free patients with brain metastases is not recommended.[111]
Institut national d'excellence en santé et en services sociaux Quebec, Ontario Neurotrauma Foundation	Traumatic brain injury	1. Anticonvulsants are indicated to reduce the incidence of post-traumatic seizures in the first 7 days post-injury.[112]

ASM, Antiseizure medication

Future Directions

Recent advances have led to new treatments and the opportunity for targeted therapies. Novel ASMs such as perampanel, brivaracetam, eslicarbazepine, and cenobamate have been recently introduced and generally offer equivalent or improved efficacy with fewer adverse effects than many older ASMs.[97] For example, brivaracetam has a higher target affinity for synaptic vesicle glycoprotein 2A (SV2A) than levetiracetam, with a similar pharmacological profile.[98]

In brain-tumor-related epilepsy, a bidirectional relationship between glioma growth and glutamatergic peritumoral neuronal activity has been demonstrated in animal models.[99–102] In preclinical studies, treatment with perampanel, an AMPA receptor antagonist, decreased tumor growth.[99,103] In several recent clinical studies, perampanel has also led to improved seizure control in patients with uncontrolled tumor-related seizures.[104,105]

Other efforts include work to develop machine learning algorithms and identify biomarkers that can predict the development of seizures and response to treatment.[106–108] For instance, in preliminary studies, SV2A expression was positively correlated with seizure response to levetiracetam and inversely correlated with the development of neuropsychiatric adverse effects to levetiracetam.[109,110] These early findings support the potential for future targeted therapies, such that clinicians will be better able to tailor medication timing, dose, and duration to individual patients.

AVAILABLE GUIDELINES

Table 48–3 provides a summary of society evidence–based guidelines.

REFERENCES

1. Greenhalgh, J., Weston, J., Dundar, Y., Nevitt, S. J. & Marson, A. G. Antiepileptic drugs as prophylaxis for postcraniotomy seizures. *Cochrane Database Syst Rev* **4**, Cd007286 (2020). https://doi.org:10.1002/14651858.CD007286.pub5
2. Beenen, L. F., Lindeboom, J., Kasteleijn-Nolst Trenité, D. G., *et al.* Comparative double blind clinical trial of phenytoin and sodium valproate as anticonvulsant prophylaxis after craniotomy: efficacy, tolerability, and cognitive effects. *J Neurol Neurosurg Psychiatry* **67**, 474–480 (1999). https://doi.org:10.1136/jnnp.67.4.474
3. Drazkowski, J. An overview of epilepsy and driving. *Epilepsia* **48**, 10–12 (2007). https://doi.org:10.1111/j.1528-1167.2007.01392.x
4. Foy, P. M., Copeland, G. P. & Shaw, M. D. M. The incidence of postoperative seizures. *Acta Neurochirurgica* **55**, 253–264 (1981). https://doi.org:10.1007/BF01808441
5. Glantz, M. J., Cole, B. F., Forsyth, P. A., *et al.* Practice parameter: anticonvulsant prophylaxis in patients with newly diagnosed brain tumors. Report of the Quality Standards Subcommittee of the American Academy of Neurology. *Neurology* **54**, 1886–1893 (2000). https://doi.org:10.1212/wnl.54.10.1886
6. Dube, S. K., Rath, G. P., Bharti, S. J., *et al.* Causes of tracheal re-intubation after craniotomy: a prospective study. *Saudi J Anaesth* **7**, 410–414 (2013). https://doi.org:10.4103/1658-354x.121056
7. Agbi, C. B. & Bernstein, M. Seizure prophylaxis for brain tumour patients. Brief review and guide for family physicians. *Can Fam Physician* **39**, 1153–1156, 1159-1160, 1163-1154 (1993).
8. Dasenbrock, H. H., Yan, S. C., Smith, T. R., *et al.* Readmission after craniotomy for tumor: a national surgical quality improvement program analysis. *Neurosurgery* **80**, 551–562 (2017). https://doi.org:10.1093/neuros/nyw062
9. Dewan, M. C., Rattani, A., Fieggen, G., *et al.* Global neurosurgery: the current capacity and deficit in the provision of essential neurosurgical care. Executive summary of the Global Neurosurgery Initiative at the Program in Global Surgery and Social Change. *J Neurosurg* **130**, 1055–1064 (2018). https://doi.org:10.3171/2017.11.Jns171500
10. Cabral, R., King, T. T. & Scott, D. F. Incidence of postoperative epilepsy after a transtentorial approach to acoustic nerve tumours. *J Neurol Neurosurg Psychiatry* **39**, 663–665 (1976). https://doi.org:10.1136/jnnp.39.7.663

11. Cabral, R. J., King, T. T. & Scott, D. F. Epilepsy after two different neurosurgical approaches to the treatment of ruptured intracranial aneurysm. *J Neurol Neurosurg Psychiatry* **39**, 1052–1056 (1976). https://doi.org:10.1136/jnnp.39.11.1052
12. Cohen, N., Strauss, G., Lew, R., Silver, D. & Recht, L. Should prophylactic anticonvulsants be administered to patients with newly-diagnosed cerebral metastases? A retrospective analysis. *J Clin Oncol* **6**, 1621–1624 (1988). https://doi.org:10.1200/jco.1988.6.10.1621
13. North, J. B., Penhall, R. K., Hanieh, A., Frewin, D. B. & Taylor, W. B. Phenytoin and postoperative epilepsy. A double-blind study. *J Neurosurg* **58**, 672–677 (1983). https://doi.org:10.3171/jns.1983.58.5.0672
14. North, J. B., Hanieh, A., Challen, R. G., Penhall, R. K., Hann, C. S. & Frewin, D. B. Postoperative epilepsy: a double-blind trial of phenytoin after craniotomy. *Lancet* **1**, 384–386 (1980). https://doi.org:10.1016/s0140-6736(80)90941-1
15. Boarini, D. J., Beck, D. W. & VanGilder, J. C. Postoperative prophylactic anticonvulsant therapy in cerebral gliomas. *Neurosurgery* **16**, 290–292 (1985). https://doi.org:10.1227/00006123-198503000-00002
16. Telfeian, A. E., Philips, M. F., Crino, P. B. & Judy, K. D. Postoperative epilepsy in patients undergoing craniotomy for glioblastoma multiforme. *J Exp Clin Cancer Res* **20**, 5–10 (2001).
17. Ohno, K., Maehara, T., Ichimura, K., Suzuki, R., Hirakawa, K. & Monma, S. Low incidence of seizures in patients with chronic subdural haematoma. *J Neurol Neurosurg Psychiatry* **56**, 1231–1233 (1993). https://doi.org:10.1136/jnnp.56.11.1231
18. Sabo, R. A., Hanigan, W. C. & Aldag, J. C. Chronic subdural hematomas and seizures: the role of prophylactic anticonvulsive medication. *Surg Neurol* **43**, 579–582 (1995). https://doi.org:10.1016/0090-3019(95)00155-7
19. Korosue, K., Hara, Y., Tamaki, N. & Heros, R. C. Long-term prognosis of seizures after complete surgical resection of AVMs of the brain. *Japanese J Neurosurg* **3**, 10–17 (1994).
20. Foy, P. M., Copeland, G. P. & Shaw, M. D. The natural history of postoperative seizures. *Acta Neurochir (Wien)* **57**, 15–22 (1981). https://doi.org:10.1007/bf01665108
21. van Breemen, M. S., Wilms, E. B. & Vecht, C. J. Epilepsy in patients with brain tumours: epidemiology, mechanisms, and management. *Lancet Neurol* **6**, 421–430 (2007). https://doi.org:10.1016/s1474-4422(07)70103-5
22. Englot, D. J., Magill, S. T., Han, S. J., Chang, E. F., Berger, M. S. & McDermott, M. W. Seizures in supratentorial meningioma: a systematic review and meta-analysis. *J Neurosurg* **124**, 1552–1561 (2016). https://doi.org:10.3171/2015.4.Jns142742
23. Sughrue, M. E., Rutkowski, M. J., Chang, E. F., *et al.* Postoperative seizures following the resection of convexity meningiomas: are prophylactic anticonvulsants indicated? Clinical article. *J Neurosurg* **114**, 705–709 (2011). https://doi.org:10.3171/2010.5.Jns091972
24. Neal, A., Morokoff, A., O'Brien, T. J. & Kwan, P. Postoperative seizure control in patients with tumor-associated epilepsy. *Epilepsia* **57**, 1779–1788 (2016). https://doi.org:10.1111/epi.13562
25. Chang, E. F., Potts, M. B., Keles, G. E., *et al.* Seizure characteristics and control following resection in 332 patients with low-grade gliomas. *J Neurosurg* **108**, 227–235 (2008). https://doi.org:10.3171/jns/2008/108/2/0227
26. You, G., Sha, Z.-Y., Yan, W., *et al.* Seizure characteristics and outcomes in 508 Chinese adult patients undergoing primary resection of low-grade gliomas: a clinicopathological study. *Neuro Oncol* **14**, 230–241 (2012). https://doi.org:10.1093/neuonc/nor205
27. Parkinson, D. & Bachers, G. Arteriovenous malformations. Summary of 100 consecutive supratentorial cases. *J Neurosurg* **53**, 285–299 (1980). https://doi.org:10.3171/jns.1980.53.3.0285
28. Rhoney, D. H., Tipps, L. B., Murry, K. R., Basham, M. C., Michael, D. B. & Coplin, W. M. Anticonvulsant prophylaxis and timing of seizures after aneurysmal subarachnoid hemorrhage. *Neurology* **55**, 258–265 (2000). https://doi.org:10.1212/wnl.55.2.258
29. Wirsching, H. G., Morel, C., Gmür, C., *et al.* Predicting outcome of epilepsy after meningioma resection. *Neuro Oncol* **18**, 1002–1010 (2016). https://doi.org:10.1093/neuonc/nov303
30. Al-Dorzi, H. M., Alruwaita, A. A., Marae, B. O., *et al.* Incidence, risk factors and outcomes of seizures occurring after craniotomy for primary brain tumor resection. *Neurosciences (Riyadh)* **22**, 107–113 (2017). https://doi.org:10.17712/nsj.2017.2.20160570
31. Englot, D. J., Berger, M. S., Barbaro, N. M. & Chang, E. F. Predictors of seizure freedom after resection of supratentorial low-grade gliomas. A review. *J Neurosurg* **115**, 240–244 (2011). https://doi.org:10.3171/2011.3.Jns1153
32. Lee, J. W., Wen, P. Y., Hurwitz, S., *et al.* Morphological characteristics of brain tumors causing seizures. *Arch Neurol* **67**, 336–342 (2010). https://doi.org:10.1001/archneurol.2010.2
33. Franceschetti, S., Binelli, S., Casazza, M., *et al.* Influence of surgery and antiepileptic drugs on seizures symptomatic of cerebral tumours. *Acta Neurochir (Wien)* **103**, 47–51 (1990). https://doi.org:10.1007/bf01420191
34. Nakamura, N. A randomized controlled trial of zonisamide in postoperative epilepsy: a report of the Cooperative Group Study. *Japanese J Neurosurg* **8**, 647–656 (1999).
35. Wu, A. S., Trinh, V. T., Suki, D., *et al.* A prospective randomized trial of perioperative seizure prophylaxis in patients with intraparenchymal brain tumors. *J Neurosurg* **118**, 873–883 (2013). https://doi.org:10.3171/2012.12.Jns111970
36. Fuller, K. L., Wang, Y. Y., Cook, M. J., Murphy, M. A. & D'Souza, W. J. Tolerability, safety, and side effects of levetiracetam versus phenytoin in intravenous and total prophylactic regimen among craniotomy patients: a prospective randomized study. *Epilepsia* **54**, 45–57 (2013). https://doi.org:10.1111/j.1528-1167.2012.03563.x
37. Iuchi, T., Kuwabara, K., Matsumoto, M., Kawasaki, K., Hasegawa, Y. & Sakaida, T. Levetiracetam versus phenytoin for seizure prophylaxis during and early after craniotomy for brain tumours: a phase II prospective, randomised study. *J Neurol Neurosurg Psychiatry* **86**, 1158–1162 (2015). https://doi.org:10.1136/jnnp-2014-308584
38. Zhang, Y., Zhou, L. F., Du, G.L., *et al.* Phenytoin or sodium valproate for prophylaxis of postoperative epilepsy: a randomized comparison. *Chin J Nerv Ment Dis* **26**, 33 (2000).
39. Lee, S. T., Lui, T.-N., Chang, C.-N., *et al.* Prophylactic anticonvulsants for prevention of immediate and early postcraniotomy seizures. *Surg Neurol* **31**, 361–364 (1989). https://doi.org:10.1016/0090-3019(89)90067-0
40. Komotar, R. J., Raper, D. M., Starke, R. M., Iorgulescu, J. B. & Gutin, P. H. Prophylactic antiepileptic drug therapy in patients undergoing supratentorial meningioma resection: a systematic analysis of efficacy. *J Neurosurg* **115**, 483–490 (2011). https://doi.org:10.3171/2011.4.Jns101585
41. Islim, A. I., McKeever, S., Kusu-Orkar, T. E. & Jenkinson, M. D. The role of prophylactic antiepileptic drugs for seizure prophylaxis in meningioma surgery: a systematic review. *J Clin Neurosci* **43**, 47–53 (2017). https://doi.org:10.1016/j.jocn.2017.05.020
42. Sirven, J. I., Wingerchuk, D. M., Drazkowski, J. F., Lyons, M. K. & Zimmerman, R. S. Seizure prophylaxis in patients with brain tumors: a meta-analysis. *Mayo Clin Proc* **79**, 1489–1494 (2004). https://doi.org:10.4065/79.12.1489
43. Joiner, E. F., Youngerman, B. E., Hudson, T. S., *et al.* Effectiveness of perioperative antiepileptic drug prophylaxis for early and late seizures following oncologic neurosurgery: a meta-analysis. *J Neurosurg* **130**, 1274–1282 (2018). https://doi.org:10.3171/2017.10.Jns172236
44. Siomin, V., Angelov, L., Li, L. & Vogelbaum, M. A. Results of a survey of neurosurgical practice patterns regarding the prophylactic use of antiepilepsy drugs in patients with brain tumors. *J Neurooncol* **74**, 211–215 (2005). https://doi.org:10.1007/s11060-004-6912-4
45. Dewan, M. C., Thompson, R. C., Kalkanis, S. N., Barker, F. G., 2nd & Hadjipanayis, C. G. Prophylactic antiepileptic drug administration following brain tumor resection: results of a recent AANS/CNS Section on Tumors survey. *J Neurosurg* **126**, 1772–1778 (2017). https://doi.org:10.3171/2016.4.Jns16245
46. Glantz, M. J., Cole, B. F., Friedberg, M. H., *et al.* A randomized, blinded, placebo-controlled trial of divalproex sodium prophylaxis in adults with newly diagnosed brain tumors. *Neurology* **46**, 985–991 (1996). https://doi.org:10.1212/wnl.46.4.985
47. Youngerman, B. E., Joiner, E. F., Wang, X., *et al.* Patterns of seizure prophylaxis after oncologic neurosurgery. *J Neurooncol* **146**, 171–180 (2020). https://doi.org:10.1007/s11060-019-03362-1
48. Weller, M., van den Bent, M., Preusser, M., *et al.* EANO guidelines on the diagnosis and treatment of diffuse gliomas of adulthood. *Nat Rev Clin Oncol* **18**, 170–186 (2021). https://doi.org:10.1038/s41571-020-00447-z

49. Roth, P., Pace, A., Le Rhun, E., *et al.* Neurological and vascular complications of primary and secondary brain tumours: EANO-ESMO Clinical Practice Guidelines for prophylaxis, diagnosis, treatment and follow-up. *Ann Oncol* **32**, 171–182 (2021). https://doi.org:10.1016/j.annonc.2020.11.003
50. Walbert, T., Harrison, R. A., Schiff, D., *et al.* SNO and EANO practice guideline update: Anticonvulsant prophylaxis in patients with newly diagnosed brain tumors. *Neuro-Oncology* **23**, 1835–1844 (2021). https://doi.org:10.1093/neuonc/noab152
51. Thompson, K., Pohlmann-Eden, B., Campbell, L. A. & Abel, H. Pharmacological treatments for preventing epilepsy following traumatic head injury. *Cochrane Database of Systematic Reviews* **2015** (2015). https://doi.org:10.1002/14651858.CD009900.pub2
52. Manaka, S. Cooperative prospective study on posttraumatic epilepsy: risk factors and the effect of prophylactic anticonvulsant. *Jpn J Psychiatry Neurol* **46**, 311–315 (1992). https://doi.org:10.1111/j.1440-1819.1992.tb00865.x
53. McQueen, J. K., Blackwood, D. H., Harris, P., Kalbag, R. M. & Johnson, A. L. Low risk of late post-traumatic seizures following severe head injury: implications for clinical trials of prophylaxis. *J Neurol Neurosurg Psychiatry* **46**, 899–904 (1983). https://doi.org:10.1136/jnnp.46.10.899
54. Pechadre, J. C., Lauxerois, M., Colnet, G., *et al.* [Prevention of late post-traumatic epilepsy by phenytoin in severe brain injuries. 2 years' follow-up]. *Presse Med* **20**, 841–845 (1991).
55. Szaflarski, J. P., Sangha, K. S., Lindsell, C. J. & Shutter, L. A. Prospective, randomized, single-blinded comparative trial of intravenous levetiracetam versus phenytoin for seizure prophylaxis. *Neurocrit Care* **12**, 165–172 (2010). https://doi.org:10.1007/s12028-009-9304-y
56. Temkin, N. R., Dikmen, S. S., Wilensky, A. J., Keihm, J., Chabal, S. & Richard Winn, H. A randomized, double-blind study of phenytoin for the prevention of post-traumatic seizures. *N Engl J Med* **323**, 497–502 (1990). https://doi.org:10.1056/nejm199008233230801
57. Temkin, N. R., Dikmen, S. S., Anderson, G. D., *et al.* Valproate therapy for prevention of posttraumatic seizures: a randomized trial. *J Neurosurg* **91**, 593–600 (1999). https://doi.org:10.3171/jns.1999.91.4.0593
58. Temkin, N. R., Anderson, G. D., Richard Winn, H., *et al.* Magnesium sulfate for neuroprotection after traumatic brain injury: a randomised controlled trial. *Lancet Neurol* **6**, 29–38 (2007). https://doi.org:10.1016/s1474-4422(06)70630-5
59. Young, B., Rapp, R. P., Norton, J. A., Haack, D., Tibbs, P. A. & Bean, J. R. Failure of prophylactically administered phenytoin to prevent early posttraumatic seizures. *J Neurosurg* **58**, 231–235 (1983). https://doi.org:10.3171/jns.1983.58.2.0231
60. Young, B., Rapp, R. P., Norton, J. A., Haack, D., Tibbs, P. A. & Bean, J. R. Failure of prophylactically administered phenytoin to prevent late posttraumatic seizures. *J Neurosurg* **58**, 236–241 (1983). https://doi.org:10.3171/jns.1983.58.2.0236
61. Young, K. D., Okada, P. J. & Sokolove, P. E. A randomized, double-blinded, placebo-controlled trial of phenytoin for the prevention of early posttraumatic seizures in children with moderate to severe blunt head injury. *Ann Emerg Med* **43**, 435–446 (2004). https://doi.org:10.1016/j.annemergmed.2003.09.016
62. Chang, B. S. & Lowenstein, D. H. Practice parameter: antiepileptic drug prophylaxis in severe traumatic brain injury. *Neurology* **60**, 10 (2003). https://doi.org:10.1212/01.WNL.0000031432.05543.14
63. Mirian, C., Møller Pedersen, M., Sabers, A. & Mathiesen, T. Antiepileptic drugs as prophylaxis for de novo brain tumour-related epilepsy after craniotomy: a systematic review and meta-analysis of harm and benefits. *J Neurol, Neurosurg Psychiatry* **90**, 599 (2019). https://doi.org:10.1136/jnnp-2018-319609
64. Niesen, A. D., Jacob, A. K., Aho, L. E., *et al.* Perioperative seizures in patients with a history of a seizure disorder. *Anesth Analg* **111**, 729–735 (2010). https://doi.org:10.1213/ANE.0b013e3181e534a4
65. Perks, A., Cheema, S. & Mohanraj, R. Anaesthesia and epilepsy. *Br J Anaesth* **108**, 562–571 (2012). https://doi.org:10.1093/bja/aes027
66. Daou, B. J., Maher, C. O., Holste, K., *et al.* Seizure prophylaxis in unruptured aneurysm repair: a randomized controlled trial. *J Stroke Cerebrovasc Dis* **29**, 105171 (2020). https://doi.org:10.1016/j.jstrokecerebrovasdis.2020.105171
67. Baker, C. J., Prestigiacomo, C. J. & Solomon, R. A. Short-term perioperative anticonvulsant prophylaxis for the surgical treatment of low-risk patients with intracranial aneurysms. *Neurosurgery* **37**, 863–870; discussion 870-861 (1995). https://doi.org:10.1227/00006123-199511000-00003
68. Ducruet, A. F., Grobelny, B. T., Zacharia, B. E., *et al.* The surgical management of chronic subdural hematoma. *Neurosurg Rev* **35**, 155–169; discussion 169 (2012). https://doi.org:10.1007/s10143-011-0349-y
69. Rubin, G. & Rappaport, Z. H. Epilepsy in chronic subdural haematoma. *Acta Neurochirurgica* **123**, 39–42 (1993). https://doi.org:10.1007/BF01476283
70. Chen, Z., Brodie, M. J., Liew, D. & Kwan, P. Treatment outcomes in patients with newly diagnosed epilepsy treated with established and new antiepileptic drugs: a 30-year longitudinal cohort study. *JAMA neurology* **75**, 279–286 (2018). https://doi.org:10.1001/jamaneurol.2017.3949
71. Hanson, J. W. & Smith, D. W. Fetal hydantoin syndrome. *Lancet* **1**, 692 (1976). https://doi.org:10.1016/s0140-6736(76)92805-1
72. Rzany, B., Correia, O., Kelly, J. P., Naldi, L., Auquier, A. & Stern, R.,. Risk of Stevens-Johnson syndrome and toxic epidermal necrolysis during first weeks of antiepileptic therapy: a case-control study. Study Group of the International Case Control Study on Severe Cutaneous Adverse Reactions. *Lancet* **353**, 2190–2194 (1999). https://doi.org:10.1016/s0140-6736(98)05418-x
73. Subbarao, B. S., Silverman, A., & Eapen, B. C. Seizure Medications. StatPearls. *StatPearls* Publishing (2022).
74. Biton, V., Mirza, W., Montouris, G., Vuong, A., Hammer, A. E., Barrett, P. S. Weight change associated with valproate and lamotrigine monotherapy in patients with epilepsy. *Neurology* **56**, 172–177 (2001). https://doi.org:10.1212/wnl.56.2.172
75. Kim, J. Y. & Lee, H. W. Metabolic and hormonal disturbances in women with epilepsy on antiepileptic drug monotherapy. *Epilepsia* **48**, 1366–1370 (2007). https://doi.org:10.1111/j.1528-1167.2007.01052.x
76. van der Meer, P. B., Dirven, L., Fiocco, M., *et al.* First-line antiepileptic drug treatment in glioma patients with epilepsy: Levetiracetam vs valproic acid. *Epilepsia* **62**, 1119–1129 (2021). https://doi.org:10.1111/epi.16880
77. Delanty, N., Jones, J. & Tonner, F. Adjunctive levetiracetam in children, adolescents, and adults with primary generalized seizures: open-label, noncomparative, multicenter, long-term follow-up study. *Epilepsia* **53**, 111–119 (2012). https://doi.org:10.1111/j.1528-1167.2011.03300.x
78. Rudd, G. D., Haverkamp, W., Mason, J. W., *et al.* Lacosamide cardiac safety: clinical trials in patients with partial-onset seizures. *Acta Neurol Scand* **132**, 355–363 (2015). https://doi.org:10.1111/ane.12414
79. Luk, M. E., Tatum, W. O., Patel, A. V., Nau, K. M. & Freeman, W. D. The safety of lacosamide for treatment of seizures and seizure prophylaxis in adult hospitalized patients. *Neurohospitalist* **2**, 77–81 (2012). https://doi.org:10.1177/1941874412446200
80. Smith, P. E. M. Initial management of seizure in adults. *N Engl J Med* **385**, 251–263 (2021). https://doi.org:10.1056/NEJMcp2024526
81. Cada, D. J., Levien, T. L. & Baker, D. E. Perampanel. *Hosp Pharm* **48**, 321–331 (2013). https://doi.org:10.1310/hpj4804-321.test
82. Humayun, M. J., Samanta, D. & Carson, R. P. Clobazam. *StatPearls*. StatPearls Publishing (2022).
83. Ng, Y. T., Conry, J. A., Drummond, R., Stolle, J. & Weinberg, M. A. Randomized, phase III study results of clobazam in Lennox-Gastaut syndrome. *Neurology* **77**, 1473–1481 (2011). https://doi.org:10.1212/WNL.0b013e318232de76
84. de Bruin, M. E., van der Meer, P. B., Dirven, L., Taphoorn, M. J. B. & Koekkoek, J. A. F. Efficacy of antiepileptic drugs in glioma patients with epilepsy: a systematic review. *Neurooncol Pract* **8**, 501–517 (2021). https://doi.org:10.1093/nop/npab030
85. van der Meer, P. B., Dirven, L., van den Bent, M. J., *et al.* Prescription preferences of antiepileptic drugs in brain tumor patients: an international survey among EANO members. *Neuro-Oncology Practice* **9**, 105–113 (2022). https://doi.org:10.1093/nop/npab059
86. Rudà, R., Pellerino, A., Franchino, F., *et al.* Lacosamide in patients with gliomas and uncontrolled seizures: results from an observational study. *J Neurooncol* **136**, 105–114 (2018). https://doi.org:10.1007/s11060-017-2628-0
87. Weller, M., Gorlia, T., Cairncross, J. G., *et al.* Prolonged survival with valproic acid use in the EORTC/NCIC temozolomide trial for glioblastoma. *Neurology* **77**, 1156–1164 (2011). https://doi.org:10.1212/WNL.0b013e31822f02e1

88. Kim, Y. H., Kim, T., Joo, J.-D., *et al.* Survival benefit of levetiracetam in patients treated with concomitant chemoradiotherapy and adjuvant chemotherapy with temozolomide for glioblastoma multiforme. *Cancer* **121**, 2926–2932 (2015). https://doi.org:10.1002/cncr.29439
89. Jabbarli, R., Ahmadipour, Y., Rauschenbach, L., *et al.* How about levetiracetam in glioblastoma? An institutional experience and meta-analysis. *Cancers (Basel)* **13** (2021). https://doi.org:10.3390/cancers13153770
90. Pallud, J., Huberfeld, G., Dezamis, E., *et al.* Effect of levetiracetam use duration on overall survival of isocitrate dehydrogenase wild-type glioblastoma in adults: an observational study. *Neurology* **98**, e125–e140 (2022). https://doi.org:10.1212/wnl.0000000000013005
91. Happold, C., Gorlia, T., Chinot, O., *et al.* Does valproic acid or levetiracetam improve survival in glioblastoma? A pooled analysis of prospective clinical trials in newly diagnosed glioblastoma. *J Clin Oncol* **34**, 731–739 (2016). https://doi.org:10.1200/jco.2015.63.6563
92. Knudsen-Baas, K. M., Engeland, A., Gilhus, N. E., Storstein, A. M. & Owe, J. F. Does the choice of antiepileptic drug affect survival in glioblastoma patients? *J Neurooncol* **129**, 461–469 (2016). https://doi.org:10.1007/s11060-016-2191-0
93. Iwamoto, F. M., Kreisl, T. N., Kim, L., *et al.* Phase 2 trial of talampanel, a glutamate receptor inhibitor, for adults with recurrent malignant gliomas. *Cancer* **116**, 1776–1782 (2010). https://doi.org:10.1002/cncr.24957
94. Shaw, M. D. & Foy, P. M. Epilepsy after craniotomy and the place of prophylactic anticonvulsant drugs: discussion paper. *J R Soc Med* **84**, 221–223 (1991).
95. Fisher, R. S., Acevedo, C., Arzimanoglou, A., *et al.* ILAE official report: a practical clinical definition of epilepsy. *Epilepsia* **55**, 475–482 (2014). https://doi.org:10.1111/epi.12550
96. Gunawardane, N. & Fields, M. Acute Symptomatic seizures and provoked seizures: to treat or not to treat? *Curr Treat Options Neurol* **20**, 41 (2018). https://doi.org:10.1007/s11940-018-0525-2
97. Perucca, E. The pharmacological treatment of epilepsy: recent advances and future perspectives. *Acta Epileptologica* **3**, 22 (2021). https://doi.org:10.1186/s42494-021-00055-z
98. Steinhoff, B. J. & Staack, A. M. Levetiracetam and brivaracetam: a review of evidence from clinical trials and clinical experience. *Ther Adv Neurol Disord* **12**, 1756286419873518 (2019). https://doi.org:10.1177/1756286419873518
99. Venkatesh, H. S., Morishita, W., Geraghty, A. C., *et al.* Electrical and synaptic integration of glioma into neural circuits. *Nature* **573**, 539–545 (2019). https://doi.org:10.1038/s41586-019-1563-y
100. Venkatesh, H. S., Johung, T. B., Caretti, V., *et al.* Neuronal activity promotes glioma growth through neuroligin-3 secretion. *Cell* **161**, 803–816 (2015). https://doi.org:10.1016/j.cell.2015.04.012
101. Venkatesh, H. S., Tam, L. T., Woo, P. J., *et al.* Targeting neuronal activity-regulated neuroligin-3 dependency in high-grade glioma. *Nature* **549**, 533–537 (2017). https://doi.org:10.1038/nature24014
102. Venkataramani, V., Tanev, D. I., Strahle, C., *et al.* Glutamatergic synaptic input to glioma cells drives brain tumour progression. *Nature* **573**, 532–538 (2019). https://doi.org:10.1038/s41586-019-1564-x
103. Lange, F., Weßlau, K., Porath, K., *et al.* AMPA receptor antagonist perampanel affects glioblastoma cell growth and glutamate release in vitro. *PLoS One* **14**, e0211644 (2019). https://doi.org:10.1371/journal.pone.0211644
104. Coppola, A., Zarabla, A., Maialetti, A., *et al.* Perampanel confirms to be effective and well-tolerated as an add-on treatment in patients with brain tumor-related epilepsy (PERADET Study). *Front Neurol* **11**, 592 (2020). https://doi.org:10.3389/fneur.2020.00592
105. Vecht, C., Duran-Peña, A., Houillier, C., Durand, T., Capelle, L. & Huberfeld, G. Seizure response to perampanel in drug-resistant epilepsy with gliomas: early observations. *J Neurooncol* **133**, 603–607 (2017). https://doi.org:10.1007/s11060-017-2473-1
106. Delen, D., Davazdahemami, B., Eryarsoy, E., Tomak, L. & Valluru, A. Using predictive analytics to identify drug-resistant epilepsy patients. *Health Informatics J* **26**, 449–460 (2020). https://doi.org:10.1177/1460458219833120
107. Devinsky, O., Dilley, C., Ozery-Flato, M., *et al.* Changing the approach to treatment choice in epilepsy using big data. *Epilepsy Behav* **56**, 32–37 (2016). https://doi.org:10.1016/j.yebeh.2015.12.039
108. Chen, Z., Rollo, B., Antonic-Baker, A., *et al.* New era of personalised epilepsy management. *BMJ* **371**, m3658 (2020). https://doi.org:10.1136/bmj.m3658
109. Contreras-García, I. J., Gómez-Lira, G., Phillips-Farfán, B. V., *et al.* Synaptic vesicle protein 2A expression in glutamatergic terminals is associated with the response to levetiracetam treatment. *Brain Sci* **11** (2021). https://doi.org:10.3390/brainsci11050531
110. Romoli, M., Mandarano, M., Romozzi, M., *et al.* Synaptic vesicle protein 2A tumoral expression predicts levetiracetam adverse events. *J Neurol* **266**, 2273–2276 (2019). https://doi.org:10.1007/s00415-019-09410-0
111. Olson, J. J., Kalkanis, S. N. & Ryken, T. C. Congress of neurological surgeons systematic review and evidence-based guidelines for the treatment of adults with metastatic brain tumors: executive summary. *Neurosurgery* **84**, 550–552 (2019). https://doi.org:10.1093/neuros/nyy540
112. Bayley M, S. B., Lamontagne M.E, Marshall S, et al. INESSS-ONF clinical practice guideline for the rehabilitation of adults with moderate to severe traumatic brain injury. Ontario Neurotrauma Foundation, Toronto, ON (2016).

CHAPTER

49

How Do We Manage Focal Status Epilepticus?

Anthony N. Mefford, MD, Neel S. Singhal, MD, PhD, & Elan L. Guterman, MD, MAS

Case

A 45-year-old man with history of herpes simplex virus encephalitis and migraine headache presented to emergency room with left face, arm, and leg ongoing myoclonic twitching. Computed tomography (CT) head showed no acute changes. He was treated with Ativan and loaded with Keppra which resulted in improvement of his twitching. Maintenance Keppra was continued, and further workup was done including MRI brain showed gliosis and atrophy of the right temporal lobe. On the floor, the patient's symptoms reoccurred as he became more altered with worsened dysarthria, twitching of left eyelid, lips, and contractions of the left arm and leg. The patient was loaded with Depakote with no significant improvement in his jerks. Electroencephalograph (EEG) was done 1 hour after his symptoms worsened and showed semirhythmic, irregular, high-amplitude delta activity, predominantly lateralized over the right centro-temporal regions. How should we manage patients with focal status epilepticus?

Key Points

- Focal status epilepticus (FSE) is a neurological emergency, with early treatment leading to more rapid cessation of seizures and lower likelihood of progressing to refractory SE.
- Presentations of FSE are heterogenous and can be difficult to diagnose; therefore, clinicians need to have a high index of suspicion in patients at risk for FSE.
- Overall, there is no single best second-line intravenous (IV) antiepileptic drug (AED) for FSE. The first- and second-line treatments for FSE are the same to those used in generalized convulsive status epilepticus (GCSE); however, the management of refractory FSE needs to be tailored depending on patient-specific variables.
- When combining multiple AEDs, it is important to keep in mind which AEDs can be synergistic or antagonistic with one another, depending on their drug-drug interactions and pharmacokinetics.
- In GCSE, there is established risk of irreversible neurological injury related to ongoing seizure activity. However, data and expert opinion suggest FSE has a lower risk of irreversible neurological injury than GCSE. Therefore, the risks of sedating anesthetic medications and intubation in FSE may outweigh the risk of continued focal seizure activity.
- As additional clinical data emerge, the optimal approach for FSE will become more clearly defined.

BACKGROUND

While the management of generalized convulsive status epilepticus (GCSE) has been well defined, the approach to focal status epilepticus (FSE) is less established and some aspects of management remain controversial.[1–6] Most basic science and clinical studies of status epilepticus (SE) have focused on GCSE, with a relative paucity of high-quality studies examining other forms of SE including nonconvulsive status epilepticus (NCSE) and FSE. Therefore, findings and management strategies for GCSE must be extrapolated to FSE to guide clinical management where specific data are lacking.

FSE is a state of prolonged or repetitive focal-onset seizures.[7–10] The generally accepted definition of FSE is ongoing or repeated

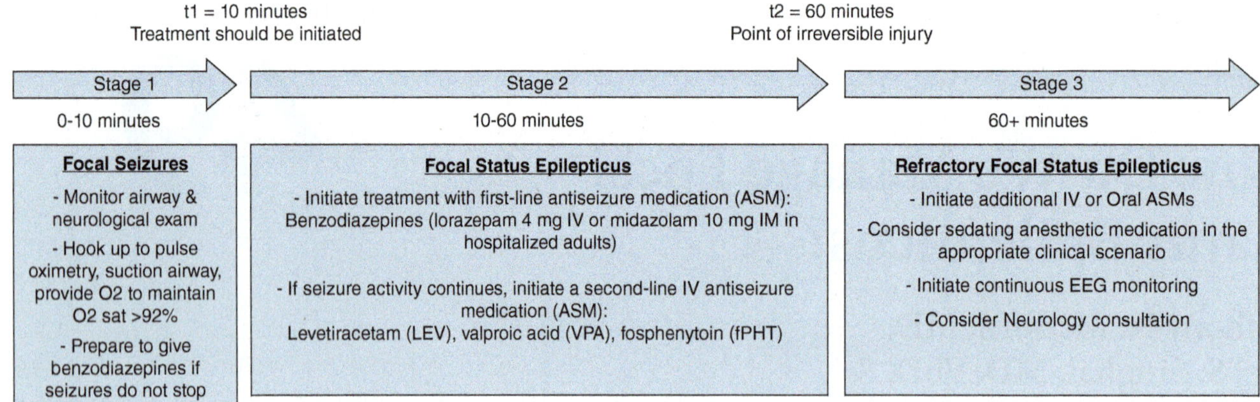

FIGURE 49–1 Time course and treatment algorithm of focal status epilepticus (FSE).

seizure activity for 10 minutes or greater without an intervening return to clinical baseline. Expert consensus is that long-term neurologic consequences develop when focal seizure activity has persisted for 60 minutes or longer (Figure 49–1) and treatment should be initiated well before this time point (Box 49-1).[11–17]

EVIDENCE AND REVIEW

When to Be Concerned?

Clinical symptoms of FSE often vary across patients but are stereotyped within a patient. Patients may report episodic twitching or weakness. They may also report continuous symptoms as is the case with aura continua.[7] Clinical signs of FSE are similarly varied and can include a change in mental status, sensory symptoms, or repetitive movements such as unilateral jerking, twitching, or sustained contraction.[7–10] A focused neurological exam assessing mental status including level of arousal, orientation, language, and motor function is important.[18–21] Cranial nerve findings include gaze preference or deviation, eye movement abnormalities such as nystagmus or oculoclonic movements, mydriasis, head deviation, and facial motor movements or asymmetry.[22,23] Motor findings include rhythmic clonus, tonic posturing, or myoclonus in the extremities, typically in a unilateral distribution.[24,25] Additionally, there can be vital sign abnormalities including hypertension, tachycardia/bradycardia, or tachypnea. The presence of these clinical neurological findings without an alternative explanation, especially in the setting of a known intracranial abnormality, should raise concern for FSE.

BOX 49–1 High-yield diagnostics for evaluation of FSE.

- ☐ Serum labs for seizure triggers: complete blood counts, metabolic panel, liver function tests, glucose, urinalysis, urine toxicology, ethanol level
- ☐ Antiseizure medication serum levels:
  - ☐ Rapid AED levels: valproic acid, phenytoin (total level), phenobarbital
  - ☐ Others (longer return time): oxcarbazepine, carbamazepine, levetiracetam, lamotrigine
- ☐ Neuroimaging: MRI brain with and without contrast; consider CT brain without contrast if MRI delayed
- ☐ CSF studies:
  - ☐ Basic: cell count + differential, protein, glucose, IgG index, oligoclonal bands
  - ☐ Consider additional evaluation for autoimmune or infectious causes of encephalitis as indicated
- ☐ EEG: Continuous video-EEG preferred

One particular form of FSE that can be difficult to diagnose is a subtype of focal motor SE known as Epilepsia Partialis Continua (EPC).[26] EPC typically manifests as waxing-waning twitching localized to single muscles or muscle groups on one hemibody. These seizures can last minutes or longer and can even continue for days. They are frequently associated with structural brain lesions. They can also be especially refractory to treatment with typical antiseizure medications (ASM). EPC is difficult to diagnose because the movements are subtle, and the electrical field is small; thus, these seizures can be missed by electroencephalograph (EEG) monitoring. This often raises the possibility that the movements are nonepileptic; thus, it is important for the neurocritical care physician to be able to distinguish EPC from other abnormal movements. Common abnormal movements observed in the neurologic intensive care unit (NeuroICU) that are nonepileptic include tremor, noncortical myoclonus, shivering, and asterixis.

Another form of FSE that can be difficult to diagnose is focal NCSE. Focal convulsive SE (CSE) can progress to focal nonconvulsive SE which can have subtle clinical findings that are easily missed while examining a patient.[27] At times, the only clinical finding is persistent altered mental status (AMS); therefore, persistent AMS after multiple focal seizures should raise concern for ongoing subtle or subclinical FSE.

In settings where a patient has unexplained abnormal movements or persistent AMS, EEG monitoring is important to further evaluate for FSE and guide clinical management.[28] EEG can accurately distinguish seizure and nonseizure-related activity, except in some cases of EPC; thus, EEG studies demonstrating underlying seizure activity provide further support for initiating ASM, while studies revealing an absence of seizure activity help avoid unnecessary treatment.

What Are the Common Etiologies?

An important initial branch point in determining the underlying cause of FSE is whether the patient has established epilepsy or de novo seizures, given the most common etiologies of seizure and FSE differ considerably in these two patient populations. The most common causes of FSE in patients with established epilepsy are medication nonadherence, infections, breakthrough seizures in the setting of medically refractory epilepsy, or worsening of an underlying pathology—for instance, an enlarging glioma.[29–35]

In patients with FSE with no prior history of epilepsy, FSE is further subdivided into cryptogenic FSE (without a clear etiology) and symptomatic FSE (due to an acute, often structural process). The most common cause of cryptogenic FSE is new onset epilepsy. The most common causes of symptomatic FSE are hypoxic-anoxic brain injury, traumatic brain injury, stroke, intracranial hemorrhage, malignancy, and encephalitis (infectious or autoimmune).[29–35] Of note, seizures due to metabolic abnormalities typically lead to generalized, as opposed to focal seizures. However, certain metabolic disturbances, in particular hypoglycemia and hyperglycemia, are important causes of focal seizures that can present as FSE.

How Aggressively to Treat?

The treatment of FSE depends on (1) the suspected underlying cause of FSE and (2) the patient's clinical status. Whether the patient is intubated at onset of FSE, and the availability of EEG monitoring are two of many important factors guiding treatment. Consultation with neurology is typically recommended to assist in determining the appropriate approach to treatment on a case-by-case basis. We provide a general framework below.

Shorter time to treatment of SE leads to more rapid cessation of seizure activity and decreased risk of progression to refractory SE.[36] Thus, rapid treatment is a priority for all forms of SE, including FSE. However, treatments for SE have significant risks including decreased mental status, respiratory depression, hypotension, cardiac arrhythmias, metabolic disturbances, and liver injury. Further there are varying degrees of risk associated with first-line, second-line, and third-line agents. Benzodiazepines and ASMs generally have a lower risk profile, while third-line therapy with sedating anesthetic medications is associated with higher risk. It is important to balance the risk of these different treatment options against the risks of untreated seizures during clinical care.

In GCSE, there is established risk of irreversible neurological injury related to ongoing seizure activity, with experimental models and pathologic studies showing neuronal damage resulting from severe metabolic dysfunction during generalized convulsive seizure activity.[14,15] In FSE, the risk is less well established. Data and expert opinion suggest FSE has a lower risk of irreversible neurological injury than GCSE.[11–13,16] Thus, patients with FSE should still receive urgent treatment with first-line benzodiazepines and second-line ASM. However, balancing the risks and benefits of starting third-line anesthetic therapy when SE is refractory to first- and second-line treatments is different for patients with GCSE and FSE. FSE requires a more measured approach balancing the risks of ongoing seizure activity with the risks of more aggressive treatments.

In GCSE, providers are expected to take an aggressive approach to treatment. This includes escalating to interventions with higher risks, including starting intravenous (IV) anesthetic medications within 60 minutes and performing endotracheal intubation and ventilatory support. In FSE, the risks of sedating anesthetic medications and intubation may outweigh the risk of continued focal seizure activity.[36,37] The field lacks high-quality data to guide management, but the authors recommend taking the current clinical status of the patient into consideration. If a patient is already intubated and receiving anesthetic medications for an alternate indication, then the risk of adjusting the anesthetic infusion to achieve better seizure control is low and this should be done. In contrast, if a patient has preserved consciousness and is breathing without ventilatory support, then providers should aim to avoid starting IV anesthetic medications and intubating the patient to achieve seizure control. Instead, providers can administer additional ASM until seizure control is achieved. These different options are further discussed below.

Of note, some studies suggest adjusting treatment based upon the underlying etiology of SE, favoring nonaggressive treatment for SE due to conditions with lower morbidity such as absence epilepsy or medication discontinuation and more aggressive treatment for SE due to conditions with significant risk of seizure-induced neurological damage such as intracerebral hemorrhage.[36]

What Medications to Use Initially?

There is agreement among most experts that first- and second-line treatments of FSE should mirror those used in GCSE. First-line treatment includes early administration of IV or intramuscular (IM) benzodiazepines in the first 5 to 10 minutes of persistent focal seizure activity.[38–41] If seizures continue, second-line treatment involves administration of IV ASM, such as fosphenytoin, valproate, or levetiracetam.[38,42,43] Additionally, there is growing evidence for the use of IV lacosamide for SE.[44–49] Overall, there is no single best second-line IV ASM for FSE.[43] A medication may be chosen based on the treating provider's clinical experience, the patient's preexisting medications for chronic epilepsy, or to avoid interactions with other medications.

What If Seizures Continue?

There is limited data to guide the management of FSE beyond first-line and second-line treatments. For a patient who is not intubated, providers should consider starting additional ASMs before escalating to more aggressive treatment with an IV

TABLE 49–1 Interactions between combinations of common antiseizure medications used for FSE.

	VPA	PHT	LEV	LCM	TPM	OXC	CBZ	ESL	CLB	PER	BRV
VPA											
PHT											
LEV											
LCM											
TPM											
OXC											
CBZ											
ESL											
CLB											
PER											
BRV											

	Significant interaction, avoid combination
	Consider therapy modification
	Monitor therapy
	No interaction or no action needed

The combination of multiple antiseizure medications (ASMs) can lead to CNS depression.

anesthetic medication.[37,50] Subsequent ASMs can be administered intravenously or orally. The most common IV ASMs are those used for initial second-line therapy and discussed above: fosphenytoin, valproate, levetiracetam, and lacosamide. Fosphenytoin and valproate interact with one another; thus, they should not be combined. Other combinations of IV ASMs are generally well-tolerated. Providers can also use regularly scheduled benzodiazepines as an alternative IV ASM option.

Historically, the most common oral ASMs used for FSE were topiramate, carbamazepine, and oxcarbazepine because their dose can all be increased rapidly.[51–54] Other oral ASMs including eslicarbazepine, clobazam, perampanel, and brivaracetam are used increasingly often and have growing evidence of efficacy in SE.[55,56] Lamotrigine is commonly used for focal epilepsy, but the dose needs to be increased slowly; thus, it is not an ideal medication for treatment of FSE where patients need to achieve therapeutic serum levels as quickly as possible.

When combining multiple ASMs, it is important to keep in mind which ASMs can be synergistic or antagonistic with one another, depending on their drug-drug interactions and pharmacokinetics (see Table 49–1).[57,58] Close attention should be paid to hepatic enzyme inducers (phenytoin, carbamazepine, and phenobarbital) and inhibitors (valproate), which can lead to alterations in levels of other ASMs as well as other medications. Because of the frequency of drug interactions and altered drug metabolism among patients in the ICU, it is important to monitor serum levels of ASMs when available. This ensures appropriate therapeutic dosing and allows providers to adjust the dose more precisely if the patient's seizures remain uncontrolled. The ASM levels that are most commonly available for monitoring are valproate, phenytoin, phenobarbital, and carbamazepine.

If FSE continues despite multiple ASMs, providers must balance risks and benefits of starting an anesthetic medication and intubating the patient in the ICU.[36,37,59] There are limited data comparing the efficacy of different anesthetics in treating FSE. The most common medications are propofol, midazolam, and ketamine.[60]

For super refractory FSE, there are small trials that have examined several adjunctive treatments including electroconvulsive therapy (ECT),[61] therapeutic hypothermia,[62] ketogenic diet,[63] surgical resection,[64] multiple subpial transections (MST),[65,66] vagal nerve stimulation (VNS), deep brain stimulation (DBS), neurosteroids such as allopregnanolone,[67] and transmagnetic stimulation (TMS).[35] Finally, it is important to consider that for causes of symptomatic FSE such as secondary to intracranial hemorrhage, autoimmune encephalitis, metabolic derangements, or vitamin deficiencies, treatment should be focused on the specific underlying etiology to remove the provoking factor for seizures.

REFERENCES

1. Cherian, A., & Thomas, S. V. (2009). Status epilepticus. *Annals of Indian Academy of Neurology, 12*(3), 140.
2. Meierkord, H., Boon, P., Engelsen, B., Göcke, K., Shorvon, S., Tinuper, P., & Holtkamp, M. (2010). EFNS guideline on the management of status epilepticus in adults. *European Journal of Neurology, 17*(3), 348–355.
3. Trinka E., Cock H., Hesdorffer D., Rossetti A. O., Scheffer I. E., Shinnar S., Shorvon S., & Lowenstein D. H. (2015). A definition and classification of status epilepticus. - Report of the ILAE Task Force on Classification of Status Epilepticus. *Epilepsia, 56,* 1515–1523.
4. Brophy, G. M., Bell, R., Claassen, J., Alldredge, B., Bleck, T. P., Glauser, T., Laroche, S. M., Riviello, J. J. Jr, Shutter, L., Sperling, M. R., Treiman, D. M., Vespa, P. M., & Neurocritical Care Society Status Epilepticus

Guideline Writing Committee. (2012). Guidelines for the evaluation and management of status epilepticus. *Neurocrit Care, 17*, 3–23.

5. Betjemann, J. P., & Lowenstein, D. H. (2015). Status epilepticus in adults. *The Lancet Neurology, 14*(6), 615–624.
6. González, N. H., González, A. B., Requejo, V. H., & Díaz, J. D. (2021). Focal status epilepticus: a review of pharmacological treatment. *Neurología (English Edition)*.
7. Scholtes, F. B., Renier, W. O., & Meinardi, H. (1996). Simple partial status epilepticus: causes, treatment, and outcome in 47 patients. *Journal of Neurology, Neurosurgery & Psychiatry, 61*(1), 90–92.
8. Drislane, F. W., Blum, A. S., & Schomer, D. L. (1999). Focal status epilepticus: clinical features and significance of different EEG patterns. *Epilepsia, 40*(9), 1254–1260.
9. Meierkord, H., & Holtkamp, M. (2007). Non-convulsive status epilepticus in adults: clinical forms and treatment. *The Lancet Neurology, 6*(4), 329–339.
10. Rossetti, A. O., Trinka, E., Stähli, C., & Novy, J. (2016). New ILAE versus previous clinical status epilepticus semiologic classification: Analysis of a hospital-based cohort. *Epilepsia, 57*(7), 1036–1041.
11. Aminoff, M. J. (1998). Do nonconvulsive seizures damage the brain?—No. *Archives of Neurology, 55*(1), 119–120.
12. de Curtis, M., Rossetti, A. O., Verde, D. V., van Vliet, E. A., & Ekdahl, C. T. (2021). Brain pathology in focal status epilepticus: evidence from experimental models. *Neuroscience & Biobehavioral Reviews, 131*, 834–846.
13. Kaplan, P. W. (2000). No, some types of nonconvulsive status epilepticus cause little permanent neurologic sequelae (or: "the cure may be worse than the disease"). *Neurophysiologie Clinique/Clinical Neurophysiology, 30*(6), 377–382.
14. Wasterlain, C. G., Fujikawa, D. G., Penix, L., & Sankar, R. (1993). Pathophysiological mechanisms of brain damage from status epilepticus. *Epilepsia, 34*, S37–S53.
15. Walker, M. C. (2018). Pathophysiology of status epilepticus. *Neuroscience Letters, 667*, 84–91.
16. Young, G. B., & Jordan, K. G. (1998). Do nonconvulsive seizures damage the brain?—Yes. *Archives of Neurology, 55*(1), 117–119.
17. Lowenstein, D. H., Bleck, T., & Macdonald, R. L. (1999). It's time to revise the definition of status epilepticus. *Epilepsia, 40* (1), 120–122.
18. Kirshner, H. S., Hughes, T., Fakhoury, T., & Abou-Khalil, B. (1995). Aphasia secondary to partial status epilepticus of the basal temporal language area. *Neurology, 45*(8), 1616–1618.
19. Chung, P. W., Seo, D. W., Kwon, J. C., Kim, H., & Na, D. L. (2002). Nonconvulsive status epilepticus presenting as a subacute progressive aphasia. *Seizure, 11*(7), 449–454.
20. Kaplan, P. W., & Stagg, R. (2011). Frontal lobe nonconvulsive status epilepticus: a case of epileptic stuttering, aphemia, and aphasia—not a sign of psychogenic nonepileptic seizures. *Epilepsy & Behavior, 21*(2), 191–195.
21. Tombini, M., Koch, G., Placidi, F., Sancesario, G., Marciani, M. G., & Bernardi, G. (2005). Temporal lobe epileptic activity mimicking dementia: a case report. *European Journal of Neurology, 12*(10), 805–806.
22. Espay, A. J., Schmithorst, V. J., & Szaflarski, J. P. (2008). Chronic isolated hemifacial spasm as a manifestation of epilepsia partialis continua. *Epilepsy & Behavior, 12*(2), 332–336.
23. Towfigh, A., Mostofi, N., & Motamedi, G. K. (2007). Poststroke partial seizures presenting as hemifacial spasm. *Movement Disorders: Official Journal of the Movement Disorder Society, 22*(13), 1981–1982.
24. Hilkens, P. H. E., & De Weerd, A. W. (1995). Non-convulsive status epilepticus as cause for focal neurological deficit. *Acta Neurologica Scandinavica, 92*(3), 193–197.
25. Zyss, J., Xie-Brustolin, J., Ryvlin, P., Peysson, S., Beschet, A., Sappey-Marinier, D., ... & Thobois, S. (2007). Epilepsia partialis continua with dystonic hand movement in a patient with a malformation of cortical development. *Movement Disorders: Official Journal of the Movement Disorder Society, 22*(12), 1793–1796.
26. Schomer, D. L. (1993). Focal status epilepticus and epilepsia partialis continua in adults and children. *Epilepsia, 34*, S29–S36.
27. DeLorenzo, R. J., Waterhouse, E. J., Towne, A. R., Boggs, J. G., Ko, D., DeLorenzo, G. A., Brown, A, & Garnett, L. (1998). Persistent nonconvulsive status epilepticus after the control of convulsive status epilepticus. *Epilepsia, 39*(8), 833–840.
28. Privitera, M., Hoffman, M., Moore, J. L., & Jester, D. (1994). EEG detection of nontonic-clonic status epilepticus in patients with altered consciousness. *Epilepsy Research, 18*(2), 155–166.
29. Lowenstein, D. H., & Alldredge, B. K. (1993). Status epilepticus at an urban public hospital in the 1980s. *Neurology, 43*(3 Part 1), 483–483.
30. DeLorenzo, R. J., Pellock, J. M., Towne, A. R., & Boggs, J. G. (1995). Epidemiology of status epilepticus. *Journal of Clinical Neurophysiology: Official Publication of the American Electroencephalographic Society, 12*(4), 316–325.
31. Krumholz, A., Sung, G. Y., Fisher, R. S., Barry, E., Bergey, G. K., & Grattan, L. M. (1995). Complex partial status epilepticus accompanied by serious morbidity and mortality. *Neurology, 45*(8), 1499–1504.
32. DeLorenzo, R. J., Hauser, W. A., Towne, A. R., Boggs, J. G., Pellock, J. M., Penberthy, L., Garnett, L., Fortner, C. A., & Ko, D. (1996). A prospective, population-based epidemiologic study of status epilepticus in Richmond, Virginia. *Neurology, 46*(4), 1029–1035.
33. Vespa, P. M., Nuwer, M. R., Nenov, V., Ronne-Engstrom, E., Hovda, D. A., Bergsneider, M., Kelly, D. F., Martin, N. A., & Becker, D. P. (1999). Increased incidence and impact of nonconvulsive and convulsive seizures after traumatic brain injury as detected by continuous electroencephalographic monitoring. *Journal of Neurosurgery, 91*(5), 750–760.
34. Leitinger, M., Trinka, E., Giovannini, G., Zimmermann, G., Florea, C., Rohracher, A., ... & Siebert, U. (2019). Epidemiology of status epilepticus in adults: a population-based study on incidence, causes, and outcomes. *Epilepsia, 60*(1), 53–62.
35. Rai, S., & Drislane, F. W. (2018). Treatment of refractory and super-refractory status epilepticus. *Neurotherapeutics, 15*(3), 697–712.
36. Ferguson, M., Bianchi, M. T., Sutter, R., Rosenthal, E. S., Cash, S. S., Kaplan, P. W., & Westover, M. B. (2013). Calculating the risk benefit equation for aggressive treatment of non-convulsive status epilepticus. *Neurocritical Care, 18*(2), 216–227.
37. Sutter, R., Marsch, S., Fuhr, P., Kaplan, P. W., & Rüegg, S. (2014). Anesthetic drugs in status epilepticus: risk or rescue?: a 6-year cohort study. *Neurology, 82*(8), 656–664.
38. Treiman, D. M., Meyers, P. D., Walton, N. Y., Collins, J. F., Colling, C., Rowan, A. J., ... & Mamdani, M. B. (1998). A comparison of four treatments for generalized convulsive status epilepticus. *New England Journal of Medicine, 339*(12), 792–798.
39. Silbergleit, R., Durkalski, V., Lowenstein, D., Conwit, R., Pancioli, A., Palesch, Y., & Barsan, W. (2012). Intramuscular versus intravenous therapy for prehospital status epilepticus. *New England Journal of Medicine, 366*(7), 591–600.
40. Rantsch, K., Walter, U., Wittstock, M., Benecke, R., & Rösche, J. (2013). Treatment and course of different subtypes of status epilepticus. *Epilepsy Research, 107*(1-2), 156–162.
41. Kellinghaus, C., Rossetti, A. O., Trinka, E., Lang, N., May, T. W., Unterberger, I., ... & Rosenow, F. (2019). Factors predicting cessation of status epilepticus in clinical practice: data from a prospective observational registry (SENSE). *Annals of Neurology, 85*(3), 421–432.
42. Kapur, J., Elm, J., Chamberlain, J. M., Barsan, W., Cloyd, J., Lowenstein, D., ... & Silbergleit, R; NETT and PECARN. Investigators. (2019). Randomized trial of three anticonvulsant medications for status epilepticus. *New England Journal of Medicine, 381*(22), 2103–2113.
43. Chamberlain, J. M., Kapur, J., Shinnar, S., Elm, J., Holsti, M., Babcock, L., ... & Su, C. M.; Pediatric Emergency Care Applied Research Network investigators (2020). Efficacy of levetiracetam, fosphenytoin, and valproate for established status epilepticus by age group (ESETT): a double-blind, responsive-adaptive, randomised controlled trial. *The Lancet, 395*(10231), 1217–1224.
44. Kellinghaus, C., Berning, S., Immisch, I., Larch, J., Rosenow, F., Rossetti, A. O., Tilz, C..., & Trinka, E. (2011). Intravenous lacosamide for treatment of status epilepticus. *Acta Neurologica Scandinavica, 123*(2), 137–141.
45. Hawkes, M. A., Suárez, M. F., Ugarnes, G., & D'Giano, C. (2013). Single-dose oral lacosamide in refractory simple partial status epilepticus: case report and review. *Clinical Neuropharmacology, 36*(4), 138–140.
46. Spalletti, M., Comanducci, A., Vagaggini, A., Bucciardini, L., Grippo, A., & Amantini, A. (2013). Efficacy of lacosamide on seizures and myoclonus in a patient with epilepsia partialis continua. *Epileptic Disorders, 15*(2), 193–196.

47. Höfler, J., & Trinka, E. (2013). Lacosamide as a new treatment option in status epilepticus. *Epilepsia, 54*(3), 393–404.
48. Kellinghaus, C., Berning, S., & Stögbauer, F. (2014). Intravenous lacosamide or phenytoin for treatment of refractory status epilepticus. *Acta Neurologica Scandinavica, 129*(5), 294–299.
49. Strzelczyk, A., Zöllner, J. P., Willems, L. M., Jost, J., Paule, E., Schubert-Bast, S., Rosenow, F., & Bauer, S. (2017). Lacosamide in status epilepticus: systematic review of current evidence. *Epilepsia, 58*(6), 933–950.
50. Holtkamp, M. (2018). Pharmacotherapy for refractory and super-refractory status epilepticus in adults. *Drugs, 78*(3), 307–326.
51. Towne, A. R., Garnett, L. K., Waterhouse, E. J., Morton, L. D., & DeLorenzo, R. J. (2003). The use of topiramate in refractory status epilepticus. *Neurology, 60*(2), 332–334.
52. Kellinghaus, C., Berning, S., & Stögbauer, F. (2014). Use of oxcarbazepine for treatment of refractory status epilepticus. *Seizure, 23*(2), 151–154.
53. Patel, V., Cordato, D. J., Malkan, A., & Beran, R. G. (2014). Rectal carbamazepine as effective long-acting treatment after cluster seizures and status epilepticus. *Epilepsy & Behavior, 31*, 31–33.
54. Fechner, A., Hubert, K., Jahnke, K., Knake, S., Konczalla, J., Menzler, K., Ronellenfitsch, M. W., Rosenow, F., & Strzelczyk, A. (2019). Treatment of refractory and superrefractory status epilepticus with topiramate: a cohort study of 106 patients and a review of the literature. *Epilepsia, 60*(12), 2448–2458.
55. Redecker, J., Wittstock, M., Benecke, R., & Rösche, J. (2015). Efficacy of perampanel in refractory nonconvulsive status epilepticus and simple partial status epilepticus. *Epilepsy & Behavior, 45*, 176–179.
56. Farrokh, S., Bon, J., Erdman, M., & Tesoro, E. (2019). Use of newer anticonvulsants for the treatment of status epilepticus. *Pharmacotherapy: The Journal of Human Pharmacology and Drug Therapy, 39*(3), 297–316.
57. Perucca, E. (2006). Clinically relevant drug interactions with antiepileptic drugs. *British Journal of Clinical Pharmacology, 61*(3), 246–255.
58. I Johannessen, S., & Johannessen Landmark, C. (2010). Antiepileptic drug interactions-principles and clinical implications. *Current Neuropharmacology, 8*(3), 254–267.
59. Kowalski, R. G., Ziai, W. C., Rees, R. N., Werner Jr, J. K., Kim, G., Goodwin, H., & Geocadin, R. G. (2012). Third-line antiepileptic therapy and outcome in status epilepticus: the impact of vasopressor use and prolonged mechanical ventilation. *Critical Care Medicine, 40*(9), 2677–2684.
60. Claassen, J., Hirsch, L. J., Emerson, R. G., & Mayer, S. A. (2002). Treatment of refractory status epilepticus with pentobarbital, propofol, or midazolam: a systematic review. *Epilepsia, 43*(2), 146–153.
61. Zeiler, F. A., Matuszczak, M., Teitelbaum, J., Gillman, L. M., & Kazina, C. J. (2016). Electroconvulsive therapy for refractory status epilepticus: a systematic review. *Seizure, 35*, 23–32.
62. Corry, J. J., Dhar, R., Murphy, T., & Diringer, M. N. (2008). Hypothermia for refractory status epilepticus. *Neurocritical Care, 9*(2), 189–197.
63. Cervenka, M. C., Hocker, S., Koenig, M., Bar, B., Henry-Barron, B., Kossoff, E. H., ... & Geocadin, R. G. (2017). Phase I/II multicenter ketogenic diet study for adult superrefractory status epilepticus. *Neurology, 88*(10), 938–943.
64. Basha, M. M., Suchdev, K., Dhakar, M., Kupsky, W. J., Mittal, S., & Shah, A. K. (2017). Acute resective surgery for the treatment of refractory status epilepticus. *Neurocritical Care, 27*(3), 370–380.
65. Desbiens, R., Berkovic, S. F., Dubeau, F., Andermann, F., Laxer, K. D., Harvey, S., ... & Barbaro, N. M. (1993). Life-threatening focal status epilepticus due to occult cortical dysplasia. *Archives of Neurology, 50*(7), 695–700.
66. Molyneux, P., Barker, R., Thom, M., Van Paesschen, W., Harkness, W., & Duncan, J. (1998). Successful treatment of intractable epilepsia partialis continua with multiple subpial transections. *Journal of Neurology, Neurosurgery, and Psychiatry, 65*(1), 137.
67. Rosenthal, E. S., Claassen, J., Wainwright, M. S., Husain, A. M., Vaitkevicius, H., Raines, S., ... & Kanes, S. J. (2017). Brexanolone as adjunctive therapy in super-refractory status epilepticus. *Annals of Neurology, 82*(3), 342–352.

CHAPTER

50

How Should We Think About Management of Electrographic Status Epilepticus and Rhythmic and Periodic Patterns On The Ictal Interictal Continuum?

Manuel Melo Bicchi, MD,
Emily J. Gilmore, MD, FNCS, FACNS,
& Ayham Alkhachroum, MD

Case

Four days after resection of a right temporal high-grade glioma, a patient develops altered mental status over a period of 48 hours. This is characterized by fluctuating but worsening confusion and level of consciousness, with inconsistent contralateral weakness. Electroencephalogram readings show global diffuse slowing, with lateralized periodic discharges that localize to the right temporal region. How are we to think about the management of such a patient?

Key Points

- Patients with altered level of awareness should be screened with electroencephalogram (EEG) to rule out electrographic seizures (ESz) and electrographic status epilepticus (ESE). Continuous EEG should be used when available. However, in centers with limited resources, routine EEG is a valid alternative.
- Treatment should be based on the EEG findings, etiology, and clinical status of the patient, typically reserving the use of anesthetic agents for those with impaired awareness and acute brain injury, and convulsive SE.
- Challenging electrographic patterns such as the interictal continuum (IIC) and/or generalized periodic discharge (GPDs) with triphasic wave (TW) morphology should be identified to avoid under- or overtreatment.

BACKGROUND

The definition of status epilepticus (SE) has evolved since the early 1960s with progressively shortened timelines for earlier diagnosis and treatment.[1] Treatment should be initiated promptly to reduce the risk of developing refractory and super refractory SE as well as to minimize the risk of irreversible injury. Refractory status epilepticus (RSE) and super refractory status epilepticus (SRSE) are established clinical terms used in clinical practice.[2] RSE is characterized by continuous ictal activity not controlled after first- (often benzodiazepines) and second-line antiseizure medications (ASMs).[3] SRSE is characterized by persistent ictal activity lasting 24 hours after the initiation or withdrawal of anesthetic agents.[4]

Electrographic seizures (ESz) correspond to epileptiform discharges averaging >2.5 Hz for ≥10 seconds or any pattern with unequivocal evolution lasting ≥10 seconds.[5] The Salzburg Consensus Criteria was developed by a group of experts proposing a

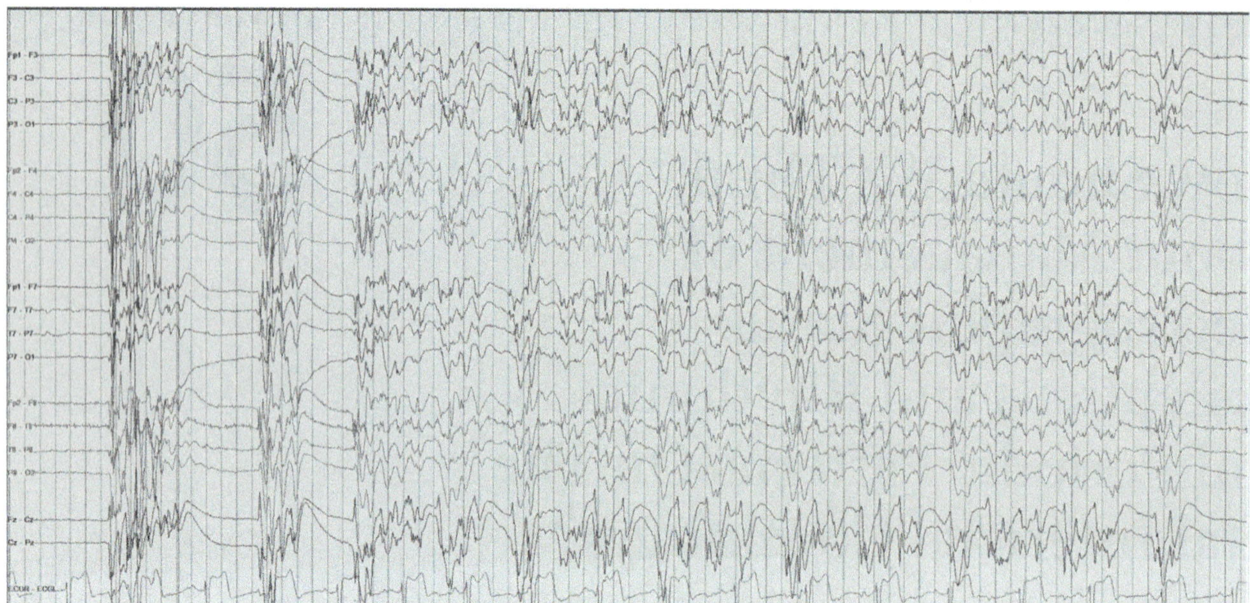

FIGURE 50–1 A 66-year-old woman who presented after hypoxic brain injury. Bipolar montage EEG (sensitivity low frequency filter [LFF] 1 Hz, high frequency filter [HFF] 70 Hz, notch 60 Hz, sensitivity 7 uV/mm, timebase 30 mm/s) shows 2.5 to 3 Hz generalized polyspike-wave (GSW) consistent with electrographic status epilepticus.

systematic diagnostic criteria for electrographic status epilepticus (ESE) which includes epileptiform discharges > 2.5 Hz or epileptiform discharges ≤ 2.5 Hz or rhythmic delta/theta activity (>0.5 Hz) associated with any of the following: subtle clinical phenomena, spatiotemporal evolution on electroencephalogram (EEG), or clinical and EEG improvement after ASM or benzodiazepine trial.[6–8] This consensus criteria were validated in several studies[9–11] and incorporated into the American Clinical Neurophysiology Society (ACNS) critical care terminology.[5] Figure 50–1 shows an example of ESE.

Critically ill patients are at increased risk of seizures which occur in 20% to 50% of patients admitted to the intensive care unit (ICU).[12–15] Clinicians should have an increased level of suspicion for the diagnosis of ESz and ESE in comatose patients. Subtle clinical signs such as hippus (pupillary oscillations regardless of light intensity), gaze deviation, nystagmoid eye movements, and muscle twitching (especially facial) should prompt further EEG monitoring.[16,17] ESz can occur in subarachnoid hemorrhage (SAH) (11%-15%), hemorrhagic and ischemic strokes (28%-30% and 6%-10%, respectively), traumatic brain injury (TBI) (22%), intracranial tumors (13%-51%), hyperglycemia (6%-25%), amongst others.[18–23]

EVIDENCE AND REVIEW

How Do I Treat Patients with Ictal Events?

Once seizures are confirmed on EEG, treatment should be initiated promptly. Unlike convulsive SE, with well-defined treatment guidelines and randomized controlled trial (RCT),[24–32] the treatment of ESz and ESE still remains obscured by the limited number of clinical trials. The European Guidelines recommend treating ESE like convulsive SE.[27] Different landmark trials primarily included convulsive SE. Nonetheless, ESE was included in the analysis as a result from convulsive seizures (progression from convulsive to nonconvulsive SE), providing information on the efficacy of ASMs for the treatment of ESE. For example, the SE Veterans Affairs study randomized 384 patients with convulsive SE and 134 with ESE to diazepam followed by phenytoin, lorazepam, phenobarbital, and phenytoin. Successful treatment was seen with lorazepam (65%), phenobarbital (58%), diazepam and phenytoin (56%), and phenytoin (43%). There were no statistically significant differences among the treatment in patients with ESE (P = .91). Additionally, the ESE treatment success rate was lower when compared to convulsive SE (7.7%-24.2% vs. 43.6%-64.9%).[29] The TRENdS study was a multicenter RCT of 74 patients with ESz (excluded patients with SE) showing noninferiority of lacosamide to fosphenytoin with similar adverse event profile.[33] Another RCT (ESETT trial) evaluating the efficacy of levetiracetam, phenytoin, and valproate included convulsive SE and those with nystagmoid or rhythmic eye movements in patients who were refractory to benzodiazepines. There was no statistically significant difference in success rates (phenytoin 45%, valproate 46%, and levetiracetam 47%).[30] The RAMPART trial was an RCT comparing the efficacy of intramuscular (IM) midazolam with that of intravenous (IV) lorazepam in patients with convulsive SE. Seizures were controlled in 73% of patients with IM midazolam and in 63% in the IV lorazepam group (P < .001) showing IM midazolam noninferiority.[34] While this study only included convulsive SE, it is imperative to treat seizures early on to prevent progression to ESz and ESE.[35] Figure 50–2 and Table 50–1 provide a treatment algorithm[29–33,36] and other ASMs[37–42] used for the management of SE, respectively.

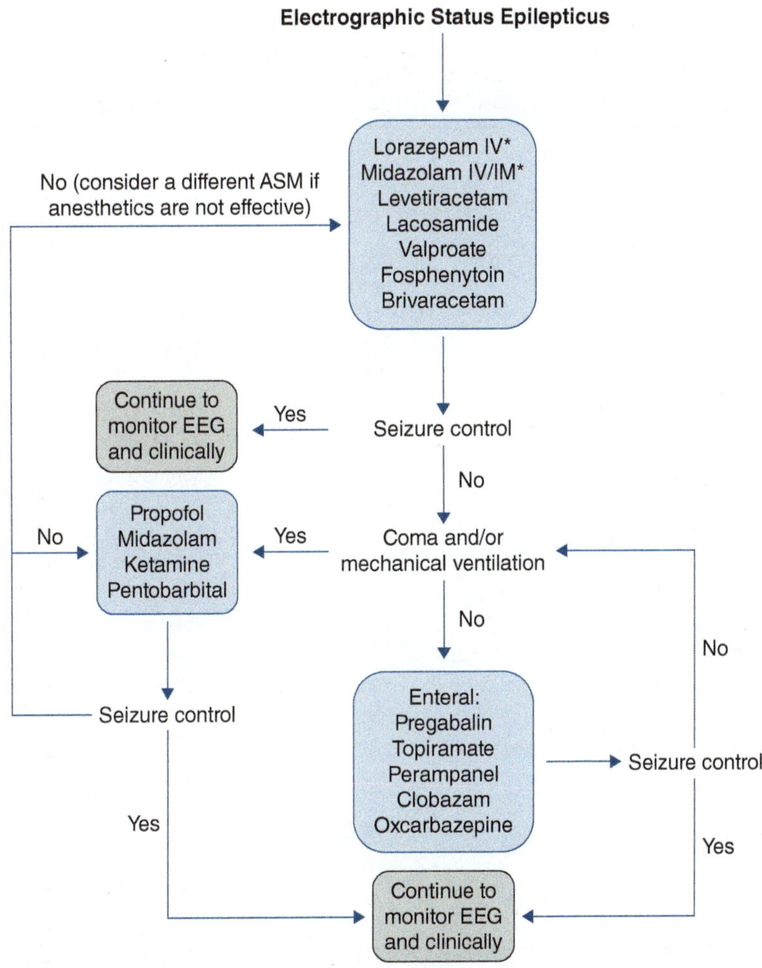

FIGURE 50–2 Treatment algorithm for electrographic status epilepticus and electrographic seizures in adults.

It remains debatable whether ESE (especially when focal) should be treated as aggressively as convulsive SE (ie, with anesthetic agents).[43,44] The authors of this manuscript typically reserve the aggressive use of anesthetic agents for patients with convulsive SE or impaired awareness ESE (focal or generalized) with concomitant acute brain injury. In contrast to convulsive SE, the management of ESE is heterogeneous and will vary based on the EEG findings, etiology, clinical status of the patient, and the overall prognosis. A balanced decision between the risk and benefit of treatments should be decided on as a case-by-case basis to avoid under- and overtreatment as seizures can be associated with increased morbidity as can their treatment. In a prospective study of 109 patients (42% ischemic and 57% hemorrhagic stroke) who underwent continuous EEG (cEEG), ESz occurred in 28% of patients with hemorrhagic stroke with increased risk of midline shift and worse outcomes.[19] In a retrospective study of 402 patients with SAH, seizures were seen in 12% of patients and associated with worse functional and cognitive outcomes at 3 months.[45] Moreover, ESz are associated with elevated neuron-specific enolase (marker of neuronal injury), brain hypoxia, and increased intracranial pressure.[46,47] Aggressive treatment decision should be based on the likelihood that the neurological deficit or encephalopathy is a direct result of the EEG findings, which can be challenging in comatose and critically ill patients. The use of prolonged anesthesia and mechanical ventilation is not without risks. In a prospective study of 25 episodes of ESE in critically ill patients undergoing aggressive treatment versus conservative approach, the use of benzodiazepines was associated with prolonged hospital stay without improved outcome.[48] Other studies have identified that increased mortality is associated with the acute medical condition, mental status impairment, and not the EEG findings.[49,50]

The management of RSE and SRSE not only includes seizure control but also preventing complications from prolonged sedation and immobilization (pulmonary embolism, sepsis, ileus, pressure ulcers, etc.).[51] A retrospective analysis of 63 consecutive episodes of nonanoxic RSE established that seizure suppression when compared to EEG suppression (burst suppression or isoelectric background) was associated with better functional outcome.[52] The Neurocritical Care Society guidelines

TABLE 50–1 Antiseizure medications for patients with NCS and NCSE.

	Antiseizure Medication	Mechanism of Action	Loading Dose	Maintenance Dose	Adverse Effects	Comments
Enteral ASM	Topiramate	Sodium channel blockade. Some effect on GABA potentiation	400-800 mg	200-800 mg/d in divided doses	Somnolence, metabolic acidosis, hyperammonemia	Requires dose adjustment in renal and/or hepatic dysfunction
	Oxcarbazepine	Sodium channel blockade	600-1,200 mg	600-1,200 mg in divided doses	Dose-dependent hyponatremia, dizziness	
	Pregabalin	P/Q-type calcium channel blockade	360 mg	360 mg/d in divided doses	Somnolence, dizziness	
	Perampanel	AMPA glutamate receptor antagonist	8-12 mg	4-10 mg/d in divided doses	Dizziness, somnolence, transaminitis	
	Clobazam	GABA potentiation	20-40 mg	20-40 mg/d in divided doses	Somnolence	
Parenteral ASM	Phenobarbital	Facilitation of chloride influx. GABA potentiation	20 mg/kg IV	1-3 mg/kg/d divided q12h	Sedation, hypotension, respiratory depression	Long half-life may mask neurological exam in comatose patients
	Fosphenytoin	Sodium channel blockade	20 mg/kg IV PE	200-600 mg/d in divided doses	Cardiac arrhythmias, hypotension	Requires dose adjustment in hepatic dysfunction
	Lacosamide	Sodium channel blockade	200-600 mg	300-600 mg/d in divided doses	Cardiac conduction block	Administer under telemetry
	Valproic acid	Sodium channel blockade. GABA potentiation	20-40 mg/kg IV	2,000-4,000 mg/d in divided doses	Hepatotoxicity, platelet dysfunction	Requires dose adjustment in hepatic dysfunction
	Brivaracetam	Binding to SV2a protein	200-400 mg	200-600 mg/d in divided doses	Somnolence	Available in IV formulation
	Lorazepam	Enhances GABAergic neurons	0.1 mg/kg IV up to 4 mg per dose, may repeat in 5 min	n/a	Sedation, hypotension, respiratory depression	Use early in the treatment course
	Midazolam	Enhances GABAergic neurons	0.2 mg/kg IV may repeat in 5 min. Maximum 10 mg	0.05-3 mg/kg/h	Sedation, hypotension, respiratory depression	Use early in the treatment course. May be used IM if no IV access. Will need dose adjustment in patients with kidney injury
	Propofol	GABA potentiation	1-2 mg/kg IV	1.8-12 mg/kg/h	Propofol infusion syndrome (bradycardia, metabolic acidosis, hyperlipidemia, renal failure, hepatomegaly)	Avoid high doses for >48 h.
	Ketamine	NMDA receptor antagonist that blocks glutamate	1-3 mg/kg IV load	1-10 mg/kg/h	Cardiac arrhythmias, metabolic acidosis	No effect on intracranial pressure

ASM, antiseizure medication; IV, intravenous; IM, intramuscular; GABA (γ-aminobutyric acid), AMPA (α-amino-3-hydroxy-5-methyl-4-isoxazolepropionic acid), SV2a (Synaptic vesicle a), NMDA (N-methyl-D-aspartate).

recommend maintaining electrographic suppression or seizure control for 24 to 48 hours, followed by gradual withdrawal of anesthetics.[24] A retrospective study of 182 patients with RSE that analyzed the relationship between duration of therapeutic coma and outcome concluded that longer duration of therapeutic coma (>35 hours) was independently associated with seizure recurrence when attempting to wean off anesthetics but not with functional neurologic outcome, in-hospital complications, or mortality. Additionally, higher doses of anesthetics (deeper sedation) were independently associated with fewer in-hospital complications and shorter duration of mechanical ventilation, suggesting that shorter (<35 hours) and deeper sedation from therapeutic coma may be more effective than the currently recommended guidelines of 24 to 48 hours.[53]

What Are the Most Seen and Challenging Electrographic Patterns in the ICU?

Common electrographic patterns seen in the ICU include rhythmic and periodic discharges. Periodic discharges are separated by an interdischarge interval and can be classified as generalized and lateralized. If associated with "plus" features (ie, superimposed fast, rhythmic delta, and/or both) and/or higher frequency, they are associated with increased risk of seizures.[54] LPDs are commonly seen in structural brain lesions such as ischemic/hemorrhagic stroke, infection, trauma, and mass lesions, typically being ipsilateral to the lesion.[55] When compared to LPDs, GPDs can be seen in toxic-metabolic syndromes, hypoxic ischemic encephalopathy, and sepsis.[56] Less so than LPDs, GPDs >1.5 Hz with "plus" modifiers have also been associated with the development of seizures.[54] BIPDs (bilateral independent periodic discharge) are less common than LPDs, characterized by repetitive asynchronous PDs occurring simultaneously in bilateral hemispheres. They are commonly seen in CNS infections, stroke, and anoxic encephalopathy. Seizures can be identified in 45% to 78% of patients, with 36% mortality.[57,58] mfPDs (multifocal periodic discharges) are characterized by three independent lateralized patterns with at least one in each hemisphere. Unilateral independent patterns are characterized by two independent and simultaneous rhythmic and periodic patterns (RPP) in the same hemisphere. These were recently included in the 2021 ACNS Standardized Critical Care EEG terminology[5] (see Figure 50–3).

Compared to PDs, RDA (rhythmic delta activity) is characterized by a uniform waveform without an interdischarge interval, which can be lateralized or generalized. LRDA (lateralized rhythmic delta activity) can be seen in SAH and intracranial hemorrhage.[59] Seizures can be seen in approximately 63% of patients with LRDA, having a similar clinical significance as LPDs.[59] GRDA (generalized rhythmic delta activity) is less likely to be associated with increased risk of seizures regardless of plus modifier.[54]

GPDs with triphasic wave (TW) morphology are characterized by an initial low-amplitude negative phase, followed by a high-amplitude positive phase, and third positive phase have been typically associated with toxic metabolic derangements (sepsis and hepatic encephalopathy), drug-toxicity (cefepime and baclofen), stroke, amongst others.[60] However, studies have reported an association between TWs and ESz in up to 28% of patients with GPDs with TW morphology (higher risk identified in patients with focality on EEG, interburst suppression, history of epilepsy, and abnormal neuroimaging).[61] Another study identified seizures in 25% of patients with GPDs with TWs compared with 26% in those without TWs.[62]

Rhythmic (LRDA and GRDA) and periodic (LPDs, GPDs, BIPDs, mfPDs, and UIPDs) patterns not meeting criteria for ESz can create management dilemmas. Some of these patterns fall under the umbrella of ictal interictal continuum (IIC), an electrographic pattern that does not qualify as ESE but may be contributing to the encephalopathic process and results in a subsequent neuronal injury (possible ESE). IIC is characterized by at least 10 seconds of (1) any PD or spike/sharp-wave (SW) occurring at 1 to 2.5 Hz without spatial evolution or clinical correlate, (2) any PD or SW at 0.5 to 1 Hz and a plus modifier, and (3) any LRDA occurring at >1 Hz with a plus modifier. Note that GRDA is not included in the IIC description.[5] There is cumulative evidence that these patterns may cause worse functional outcomes secondary to cerebral hypermetabolism and hypoxia, particularly those >2 Hz.[63–65]

The "electro paraclinical gap" concept may aid in the decision-making process.[66] This gap occurs when the imaging and/or laboratory results do not sufficiently explain the EEG findings (ie, high suspicion for ESE requiring treatment). In addition, when diagnostic uncertainty exists as is often the case with patterns are on the IIC, an ASM or benzodiazepine trial is often warranted. Less sedating IV agents such as valproate, fosphenytoin, levetiracetam, brivaracetam, and lacosamide may also be used. The trial is considered diagnostic of ESz if there is concomitant electrographic and clinical improvement, although the latter, required for the definitive diagnosis, is rarely seen in clinical practice.[67,68] More often than not, patients fall into the possible ESE category where there is an EEG improvement but no

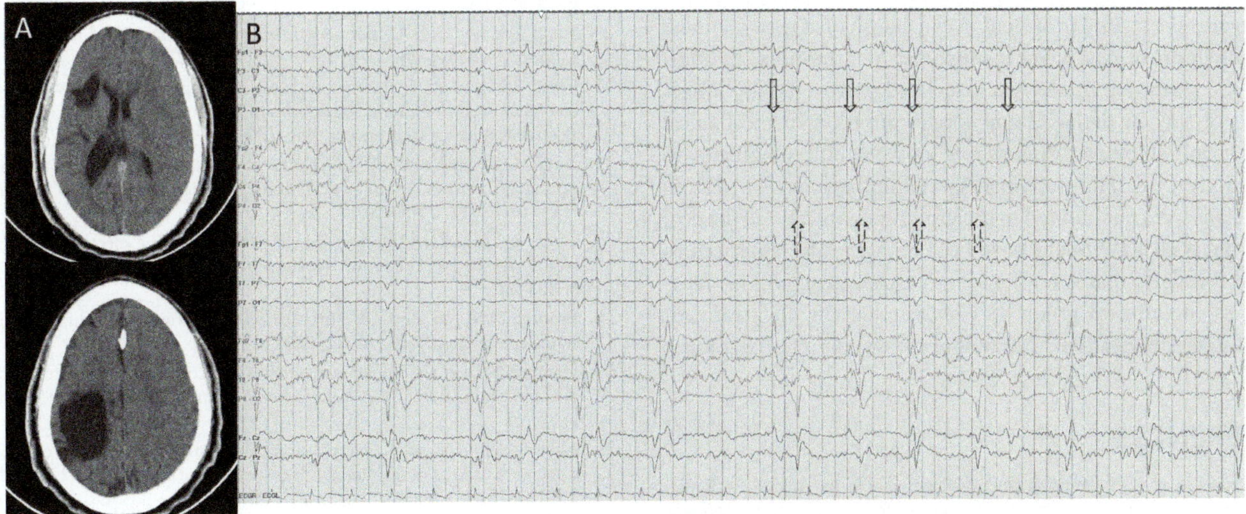

FIGURE 50–3 A 44-year-old man with history of remote severe traumatic brain injury presented with left hemibody twitching after missing his antiseizure medications. (A) Axial CT brain shows chronic right frontal and frontoparietal large encephalomalacia. (B) Bipolar EEG montage (sensitivity LFF 1 Hz, HFF 70 Hz, Notch 60 Hz, sensitivity 7 uV/mm, timebase 30 mm/sec) showing right hemispheric unilateral independent periodic discharges in frontal (solid arrow) and posterior quadrant region (dashed arrow).

clinical improvement. These patients should be monitored with cEEG to ensure the potentially harmful pattern does not return. Importantly, clinicians should keep in mind when interpreting the trial that the lack of improvement, or slow improvement, can be encountered in both metabolic processes and ESz or ESE and that both conditions may exist concomitantly.[69]

Future Directions

Efforts to address later stages of SE have been undergoing to avoid the use of anesthetic agents, when they are not indicated, as these are associated to prolonged mechanical ventilation, infections, increased mortality, etc.[70] The use of neurosteroids acting on $GABA_A$ (γ-aminobutyric acid-a) receptors has shown promising results. For example, in an open-label, phase 2 trial, 17 patients with convulsive or ESE who failed to respond to ≥1 second-line intravenous ASM (ie, RSE) were treated with ganaxolone. Sixteen (94%) patients achieved and maintained seizure cessation for 24 hours following ganaxolone administration.[71] Similarly, in an open-label study, 25 patients with ESE who failed to respond to third-line agents (ie, SRSE) after 24 hours were treated with brexanolone. Twenty-two patients were included in the analysis, 17 (77%) patients were able to successfully wean off anesthetics after brexanolone infusion. Sixteen (73%) successfully weaned off anesthetics within 5 days of initiating brexanolone infusion without anesthetic reinstatement in the following 24 hours.[72] An ongoing phase 3 RCT (RAndomized Therapy In Status Epilepticus Trial—NCT04391569) is enrolling patients with SE. The primary outcome measures are SE cessation within 30 minutes following ganaxolone initiation and proportion of patients with no progression to anesthetics within 36 hours following drug infusion.

In a large multicenter open-label trial, investigators randomized 172 patients who suffered cardiac arrest and EEG with rhythmic and periodic patterns to antiseizure-treatment group plus standard of care or standard of care alone. Results showed that aggressive seizure treatment over a period of at least 48 hours did not improve neurological outcomes at 3 months. In addition, the treatment group was associated with a slightly longer length of stay in the ICU and longer duration of mechanical ventilation.[73] However, this should not preclude physicians to actively treat SE. The study had several limitations: (1) treating physicians were not blinded to the group assignment, (2) the goal to suppress all RPP might have been an aggressive approach to suppress activity that is not known to cause harm, and (3) mortality in the control group was higher than in the treatment group suggesting early withdrawal of life-sustaining therapies.

REFERENCES

1. Trinka, E., et al., *A* definition and classification of status epilepticus–Report of the ILAE Task Force on Classification of Status Epilepticus. *Epilepsia*, 2015. **56**(10): p. 1515–1523.
2. Hirsch, L.J., et al., Proposed consensus definitions for new-onset refractory status epilepticus (NORSE), febrile infection-related epilepsy syndrome (FIRES), and related conditions. *Epilepsia*, 2018. **59**(4): p. 739–744.
3. Bleck, T.P., Refractory status epilepticus. *Curr Opin Crit Care*, 2005. **11**(2): p. 117–120.
4. Shorvon, S. and M. Ferlisi, The treatment of super-refractory status epilepticus: a critical review of available therapies and a clinical treatment protocol. *Bra*, 2011. **134**(Pt 10): p. 2802–2818.
5. Hirsch, L.J., et al., American Clinical Neurophysiology Society's standardized critical care EEG terminology: 2021 Version. *J Clin Neurophysiol*, 2021. **38**(1): p. 1–29.
6. Shorvon, S. and E. Trinka, The 5th London-Innsbruck Colloquium on status epilepticus and acute seizures. *Epilepsy Behav*, 2015. **49**: p. 1–3.
7. Beniczky, S., et al., Unified EEG terminology and criteria for nonconvulsive status epilepticus. *Epilepsia*, 2013. **54 Suppl 6**: p. 28–29.
8. Leitinger, M., et al., Diagnostic accuracy of the Salzburg EEG criteria for non-convulsive status epilepticus: a retrospective study. *The Lancet Neurology*, 2016. **15**(10): p. 1054–1062.
9. Krogstad, M.H., et al., Nonconvulsive status epilepticus: validating the Salzburg criteria against an expert EEG examiner. *J Clin Neurophysiol*, 2019. **36**(2): p. 141–145.
10. Leitinger, M., et al., Salzburg criteria for nonconvulsive status epilepticus: Details matter. *Epilepsia*, 2019. **60**(11): p. 2334–2336.
11. Othman, A.S., S. Meletti, and G. Giovannini, The EEG diagnosis of NCSE: concordance between clinical practice and Salzburg criteria for NCSE. *Seizure*, 2020. **79**: p. 1–7.
12. Jordan, K.G., Nonconvulsive status epilepticus in acute brain injury. *J Clin Neurophysiol*, 1999. **16**(4): p. 332–340; discussion 353.
13. Privitera, M., et al., EEG detection of nontonic-clonic status epilepticus in patients with altered consciousness. *Epilepsy Res*, 1994. **18**(2): p. 155–166.
14. Sutter, R., Are we prepared to detect subtle and nonconvulsive status epilepticus in critically ill patients? *J Clin Neurophysiol*, 2016. **33**(1): p. 25–31.
15. Appavu, B. and J.J. Riviello, Electroencephalographic patterns in neurocritical care: pathologic contributors or epiphenomena? *Neurocrit Care*, 2018. **29**(1): p. 9–19.
16. Jirsch, J. and L.J. Hirsch, Nonconvulsive seizures: developing a rational approach to the diagnosis and management in the critically ill population. *Clin Neurophysiol*, 2007. **118**(8): p. 1660–1670.
17. Schmitt, S.E., Utility of clinical features for the diagnosis of seizures in the intensive care unit. *J Clin Neurophysiol*, 2017. **34**(2): p. 158–161.
18. Claassen, J., et al., Prognostic significance of continuous EEG monitoring in patients with poor-grade subarachnoid hemorrhage. *Neurocrit Care*, 2006. **4**(2): p. 103–112.
19. Vespa, P.M., et al., Acute seizures after intracerebral hemorrhage: a factor in progressive midline shift and outcome. *Neurology*, 2003. **60**(9): p. 1441–1446.
20. Sung, C.Y. and N.S. Chu, Epileptic seizures in intracerebral haemorrhage. *J Neurol Neurosurg Psychiatry*, 1989. **52**(11): p. 1273–1276.
21. Vespa, P.M., et al., Increased incidence and impact of nonconvulsive and convulsive seizures after traumatic brain injury as detected by continuous electroencephalographic monitoring. *J Neurosurg*, 1999. **91**(5): p. 750–760.
22. Singh, G., J.H. Rees, and J.W. Sander, Seizures and epilepsy in oncological practice: causes, course, mechanisms and treatment. *J Neurol Neurosurg Psychiatry*, 2007. **78**(4): p. 342–349.
23. Clouston, P.D., L.M. DeAngelis, and J.B. Posner, The spectrum of neurological disease in patients with systemic cancer. *Ann Neurol*, 1992. **31**(3): p. 268–273.
24. Brophy, G.M., et al., Guidelines for the evaluation and management of status epilepticus. *Neurocrit Care*, 2012. **17**(1): p. 3–23.
25. Herman, S.T., et al., Consensus statement on continuous EEG in critically ill adults and children, part I: indications. *J Clin Neurophysiol*, 2015. **32**(2): p. 87–95.
26. Alkhachroum, A., et al., Electroencephalogram in the intensive care unit: a focused look at acute brain injury. *Intensive Care Med*, 2022. **48**(10): p. 1443–1462.
27. Meierkord, H., et al., EFNS guideline on the management of status epilepticus in adults. *Eur J Neurol*, 2010. **17**(3): p. 348–355.
28. Glauser, T., et al., Evidence-based guideline: treatment of convulsive status epilepticus in children and adults: report of the Guideline Committee of the American Epilepsy Society. *Epilepsy Curr*, 2016. **16**(1): p. 48–61.

29. Treiman, D.M., et al., A comparison of four treatments for generalized convulsive status epilepticus. Veterans Affairs Status Epilepticus Cooperative Study Group. *N Engl J Med*, 1998. **339**(12): p. 792–798.
30. Kapur, J., et al., Randomized trial of three anticonvulsant medications for status epilepticus. *N Engl J Med*, 2019. **381**(22): p. 2103–2113.
31. Dalziel, S.R., et al., Levetiracetam versus phenytoin for second-line treatment of convulsive status epilepticus in children (ConSEPT): an open-label, multicentre, randomised controlled trial. *Lancet*, 2019. **393**(10186): p. 2135–2145.
32. Lyttle, M.D., et al., Levetiracetam versus phenytoin for second-line treatment of paediatric convulsive status epilepticus (EcLiPSE): a multicentre, open-label, randomised trial. *Lancet*, 2019. **393**(10186): p. 2125–2134.
33. Husain, A.M., et al., Randomized trial of lacosamide versus fosphenytoin for nonconvulsive seizures. *Ann Neurol*, 2018. **83**(6): p. 1174–1185.
34. Silbergleit, R., et al., Intramuscular versus intravenous therapy for prehospital status epilepticus. *N Engl J Med*, 2012. **366**(7): p. 591–600.
35. DeLorenzo, R.J., et al., Persistent nonconvulsive status epilepticus after the control of convulsive status epilepticus. *Epilepsia*, 1998. **39**(8): p. 833–840.
36. Alkhachroum, A., et al., Ketamine to treat super-refractory status epilepticus. *Neurology*, 2020. **95**(16): p. e2286–e2294.
37. Fechner, A., et al., Treatment of refractory and superrefractory status epilepticus with topiramate: a cohort study of 106 patients and a review of the literature. *Epilepsia*, 2019. **60**(12): p. 2448–2458.
38. Swisher, C.B., M. Doreswamy, and A.M. Husain, Use of pregabalin for nonconvulsive seizures and nonconvulsive status epilepticus. *Seizure*, 2013. **22**(2): p. 116–118.
39. Strzelczyk, A., et al., Perampanel for treatment of status epilepticus in Austria, Finland, Germany, and Spain. *Acta Neurol Scand*, 2019. **139**(4): p. 369–376.
40. Madžar, D., et al., Effects of clobazam for treatment of refractory status epilepticus. *BMC Neurol*, 2016. **16**(1): p. 202.
41. Santamarina, E., et al., Use of intravenous brivaracetam in status epilepticus: A multicenter registry. *Epilepsia*, 2019. **60**(8): p. 1593–1601.
42. Busl, K.M., et al., Pregabalin for recurrent seizures in critical illness: a promising adjunctive therapy, especially for cyclic seizures. *Neurocrit Care*, 2022. **37**(1): p. 140–148.
43. Chong, D.J. and L.J. Hirsch, Which EEG patterns warrant treatment in the critically ill? Reviewing the evidence for treatment of periodic epileptiform discharges and related patterns. *J Clin Neurophysiol*, 2005. **22**(2): p. 79–91.
44. Rossetti, A.O., L.J. Hirsch, and F.W. Drislane, Nonconvulsive seizures and nonconvulsive status epilepticus in the neuro ICU should or should not be treated aggressively: A debate. *Clin Neurophysiol Pract*, 2019. **4**: p. 170–177.
45. De Marchis, G.M., et al., Seizure burden in subarachnoid hemorrhage associated with functional and cognitive outcome. *Neurology*, 2016. **86**(3): p. 253–260.
46. Claassen, J., et al., Nonconvulsive seizures after subarachnoid hemorrhage: multimodal detection and outcomes. *Ann Neurol*, 2013. **74**(1): p. 53–64.
47. DeGiorgio, C.M., et al., Serum neuron-specific enolase in the major subtypes of status epilepticus. *Neurology*, 1999. **52**(4): p. 746–749.
48. Litt, B., et al., Nonconvulsive status epilepticus in the critically ill elderly. *Epilepsia*, 1998. **39**(11): p. 1194–202.
49. Shneker, B.F. and N.B. Fountain, Assessment of acute morbidity and mortality in nonconvulsive status epilepticus. *Neurology*, 2003. **61**(8): p. 1066–1073.
50. Rossetti, A.O., G. Logroscino, and E.B. Bromfield, Refractory status epilepticus: effect of treatment aggressiveness on prognosis. *Arch Neurol*, 2005. **62**(11): p. 1698–1702.
51. Hocker, S., E.F. Wijdicks, and A.A. Rabinstein, Refractory status epilepticus: new insights in presentation, treatment, and outcome. *Neurol Res*, 2013. **35**(2): p. 163–168.
52. Hocker, S.E., et al., Predictors of outcome in refractory status epilepticus. *JAMA Neurol*, 2013. **70**(1): p. 72–77.
53. Muhlhofer, W.G., et al., Duration of therapeutic coma and outcome of refractory status epilepticus. *Epilepsia*, 2019. **60**(5): p. 921–934.
54. Rodriguez Ruiz, A., et al., Association of periodic and rhythmic electroencephalographic patterns with seizures in critically ill patients. *JAMA Neurol*, 2017. **74**(2): p. 181–188.
55. Hartings, J.A., A.J. Williams, and F.C. Tortella, Occurrence of nonconvulsive seizures, periodic epileptiform discharges, and intermittent rhythmic delta activity in rat focal ischemia. *Exp Neurol*, 2003. **179**(2): p. 139–149.
56. Foreman, B., et al., Generalized periodic discharges in the critically ill: a case-control study of 200 patients. *Neurology*, 2012. **79**(19): p. 1951–1960.
57. Osman, G., et al., Bilateral independent periodic discharges are associated with electrographic seizures and poor outcome: a case-control study. *Clin Neurophysiol*, 2018. **129**(11): p. 2284–2289.
58. de la Paz, D. and R.P. Brenner, Bilateral independent periodic lateralized epileptiform discharges: clinical significance. *Arch Neurol*, 1981. **38**(11): p. 713–715.
59. Gaspard, N., et al., Similarity of lateralized rhythmic delta activity to periodic lateralized epileptiform discharges in critically ill patients. *JAMA Neurol*, 2013. **70**(10): p. 1288–1295.
60. Bicchi, M.M., A. Alkhachroum, and A.M. Kanner, Status triphasicus versus status epilepticus? *J Clin Neurophysiol*, 2021. **38**(5): p. 376–383.
61. Alkhachroum, A.M., et al., Generalized periodic discharges with and without triphasic morphology. *J Clin Neurophysiol*, 2018. **35**(2): p. 144–150.
62. Foreman, B., et al., Generalized periodic discharges and 'triphasic waves': a blinded evaluation of inter-rater agreement and clinical significance. *Clin Neurophysiol*, 2016. **127**(2): p. 1073–1080.
63. Witsch, J., et al., Electroencephalographic periodic discharges and frequency-dependent brain tissue hypoxia in acute brain injury. *JAMA Neurol*, 2017. **74**(3): p. 301–309.
64. Vespa, P., et al., Metabolic crisis occurs with seizures and periodic discharges after brain trauma. *Ann Neurol*, 2016. **79**(4): p. 579–590.
65. Struck, A.F., et al., Metabolic correlates of the ictal-interictal continuum: FDG-PET during continuous EEG. *Neurocrit Care*, 2016. **24**(3): p. 324–331.
66. Trinka, E. and M. Leitinger, Management of status epilepticus, refractory status epilepticus, and super-refractory status epilepticus. *Continuum (Minneap Minn)*, 2022. **28**(2): p. 559–602.
67. Rossetti, A.O. and E.B. Bromfield, Levetiracetam in the treatment of status epilepticus in adults: a study of 13 episodes. *Eur Neurol*, 2005. **54**(1): p. 34–38.
68. Towne, A.R., et al., The use of topiramate in refractory status epilepticus. Neurology, 2003. **60**(2): p. 332–334.
69. O'Rourke, D., et al., Response rates to anticonvulsant trials in patients with triphasic-wave EEG patterns of uncertain significance. *Neurocrit Care*, 2016. **24**(2): p. 233–239.
70. Sutter, R., et al., Anesthetic drugs in status epilepticus: risk or rescue? A 6-year cohort study. *Neurology*, 2014. **82**(8): p. 656–664.
71. Vaitkevicius, H., et al., Intravenous ganaxolone for the treatment of refractory status epilepticus: Results from an open-label, dose-finding, phase 2 trial. *Epilepsia*, 2022. **63**(9): p. 2381–2391.
72. Rosenthal, E.S., et al., Brexanolone as adjunctive therapy in super-refractory status epilepticus. *Ann Neurol*, 2017. **82**(3): p. 342–352.
73. Ruijter, B.J., et al., Treating rhythmic and periodic EEG patterns in comatose survivors of cardiac arrest. *N Engl J Med*, 2022. **386**(8): p. 724–734.

CHAPTER

51

When Should We Attempt Surgical Management in Patients with Status Epilepticus from a Focal Lesion?

Justine Cormier, MD & Jennifer A. Kim, MD, PhD

Case

A previously healthy 42-year-old man presented to the hospital with a 6-week history of episodes of left arm tonic flexion, left hemifacial jerking, and slow head turn to the left followed by 20 to 30 minutes of confusion. These episodes had increased in frequency and duration, occurring 3 to 4 times daily, with seizures lasting up to 15 minutes and postictal confusion lasting up to an hour. Electroencephalography (EEG) showed abundant interictal right frontotemporal sharp waves. He was initially treated with levetiracetam with no improvement in EEG or seizure burden. A number of other antiseizure medications (ASMs) were also trialed and similarly ineffective, including valproic acid, phenytoin, lacosamide, clobazam, and phenobarbital. Over his admission, the motor component of his seizures became less prominent; however, he had frequent periods of disorientation and disinhibition and worsening encephalopathy. His EEG showed frequent right frontotemporal seizures and later, focal nonconvulsive status epilepticus (NCSE). He required intubation for airway protection, at which point he was also trialed on propofol, midazolam, and ketamine infusions, ultimately achieving a burst-suppression pattern. Each attempt to wean anesthetics resulted in recurrence of NCSE. Magnetic resonance imaging (MRI) on day 5 showed subtle right frontal lobe hyperintensity on T2-weighted images without diffusion restriction or contrast enhancement. These findings correlated with the location of seizure onset on EEG and were felt to be ictal-related. Lumbar puncture demonstrated unremarkable cerebrospinal fluid (CSF) except for slightly elevated protein to 62 mg/dL. Should we attempt focal resection of the presumed seizure focus?

Key Points

- While resective surgery has been shown to be an effective treatment option for some patients with refractory focal epilepsy, data on its efficacy in super refractory SE (SRSE) are heterogenous and limited to case reports and small case series.
- The American Epilepsy Society (AES) Super Refractory Status Epilepticus Taskforce has made the following statement, "... focal surgical resection is recommended for patients with a well-localized ictal zone in non-eloquent cortex and persistence of convulsive or non-convulsive SRSE and failure of proper pharmacological therapy (level U, class IV studies)."[1]
- The optimal timing of surgical intervention is unclear. The best approach is one that exhausts medical therapies first.
- Most patients in the literature who benefited from a surgical approach had surgery between 1 and 3 weeks from SE onset, although more robust, prospective studies are needed to further elucidate which patients may benefit most and to clarify optimal timing.

BACKGROUND

Status epilepticus (SE) is a neurological emergency with potential for significant morbidity and mortality if not recognized and treated early. Although reports in the literature vary, it is estimated that rates of SE in the United States range from 18 to 41 per 100,000 patients per year in a bimodal distribution, most affecting those in the first year of life and over 60 years old.[2] One 2020 review of the epidemiology of SE[2] reported an overall 30-day mortality rate of approximately 21% across all age groups; however, it was noted that in-hospital mortality in pediatric cases (1.3%-3.5%) was lower than in adult cases (6.5%-29.6%). A major prognostic factor in SE is the response to treatment. When SE is refractory to two intravenous (IV) antiseizure medications (ASMs), including a benzodiazepine, it is referred to as refractory status epilepticus (RSE), and when it persists despite 24 hours of anesthetic treatment, or when it recurs with withdrawal of anesthetics, it is termed super refractory SE (SRSE). Reports suggest that 23% to 48% of SE cases progress to RSE, and 15% to 22% of RSE progresses to SRSE.[1,3] SRSE is associated with substantial risk of poor outcome, with mortality rates up to 35% and risk of neurologic deficit up to 26%.[1,4,5] Over the last several years, alternative treatment strategies for patients with SRSE have begun to be explored.

While resective surgery has been shown to be an effective treatment option for some patients with refractory focal epilepsy, data on its efficacy in SRSE are heterogenous and limited to case reports and small case series. Although limited, some of this data suggest that surgery may be a promising treatment option for patients with either an established or highly suspected focal lesion. Multiple surgical approaches have been utilized including focal resection, uni- or multilobar lobectomy, multiple subpial transections (MST), corpus callostomy, anatomical or functional hemispherectomy, and neurostimulation in patients with a broad range of ages, etiologies, duration of RSE or SRSE, and outcomes. Despite the heterogeneity of the literature and lack of randomized control trials (RCTs), the American Epilepsy Society (AES) Super Refractory Status Epilepticus Taskforce has made the following statement, "... focal surgical resection is recommended for patients with a well-localized ictal zone in non-eloquent cortex and persistence of convulsive or nonconvulsive SRSE and failure of proper pharmacological therapy (level U, class IV studies)."[1]

The aim of this chapter is to summarize the available data on surgical approaches to treatment of SRSE that is presumed to be from a focal lesion or onset zone and to propose a suggested approach to patient selection.

EVIDENCE AND REVIEW

Patient Population and Surgical Approaches

There have been many case reports and case series over the last 30 years describing various surgical approaches to SRSE, including 68 patients in which there was a proven or highly suspected focal seizure onset. These patients spanned the pediatric and adult literature (aged 1 mo-68 y) and included predominantly patients with known epilepsy (n = 51),[3,6-25] although 17 of these were patients with de novo seizures.[3,7,15,25-33] Most (n = 32) underwent focal resection,[3,6-8,11,13-16,18,23,25,26,30] although 12 underwent lobectomy,[6-8,10,15,21,27,32] 3 had MST only,[8,22,24] and 10 had either a combination of the above or one of these procedures combined with functional hemispherectomy or anterior corpus callosotomy.[6,8,11,15,17,23,29,31,33] Nine patients required a second procedure for ongoing SE, including repeat resection,[9,18,20,28] resection following MST,[19,20] or lobectomy[8] or hemispherectomy[8,15] following an initial resection. One patient underwent placement of a responsive neurostimulator (RNS) into a focal lesion.[12]

Focal MRI Lesion

Of the 68 patients in the literature who underwent neurosurgical intervention for suspected focal etiology of SRSE, 57 had abnormal findings on magnetic resonance imaging (MRI). Of these, 51 had focal abnormalities, including focal cortical dysplasia (FCD) and other malformations of cortical development (MCD), focal atrophy, intracerebral hemorrhage (ICH), cavernous malformations, calcifications (Sturge Weber Syndrome), or other nonspecific focal contrast enhancement, diffusion restriction, or increased T2 signal.[3,6-9,12-18,20,21,23,25-31] Forty patients with focal MRI lesions also had corresponding focal onset seizures on electroencephalography (EEG), whereas 10 had generalized, multifocal, or holohemispheric seizure onset on EEG, and 1 had no ictal EEG correlate. Many of these patients had additional imaging (Table 51–1) including positron emission tomography (PET, n = 9, 6 were localizing, 3 were not), ictal single-photon emission computed tomography (SPECT, n = 14, 12 were localizing and concordant with other data, 2 were not), and magnetoencephalography (MEG, n = 6, 4 with localized spike clusters and 2 without). Thirty-seven patients had intraoperative electrocorticography recordings (IOER) or extraoperative electrocorticography recordings (EOER) in the form of intracranial grids, strips, or depth electrodes to confirm suspected seizure onset zone and/or to delineate areas of eloquent cortex. While nine patients had surgery based solely on MRI and EEG findings, the majority (n = 42) had at least one additional study to confirm localization of seizure onset.

The majority of patients (n = 45) had resolution of SE after surgery. Two patients had ongoing status that resolved with a second surgery[8,15]—both had initial focal resection, one followed by lobectomy and one by hemispherectomy. Two patients had no benefit from surgery but ultimately had resolution of status with medical intervention 1 to 2 months postoperatively—one was seizure free at follow up, and the other had ongoing seizures (3-4 per mo).[7] Five patients died while inpatient—two did not have resolution of SE with surgery and died from medical complications,[7,26] two had initial resolution of SE with surgery but experienced SE recurrence after 4 to 6 weeks and ultimately

TABLE 51–1 Number of patients with various confirmatory imaging studies broken down by MRI findings (a focal, solitary lesion suspected to be seizure source; multifocal but discrete abnormalities (e.g. tuberous sclerosis tubers), diffuse abnormalities, or a normal MRI). A '+' is a positive, confirmatory focal finding. A '–' is a non-localizing or contradictory finding. The right side displays how many patients had 0, 1, 2, or 3 additional confirmatory studies prior to surgery. PET-positron emission tomography. SPECT–single-photon emission computed tomography. MEG–magnetoencephalography. IOER–intraoperative electrocorticography recordings. EOER–intraoperative electrocorticography recordings (combination of intracranial grid, strip, and/ or depth electrodes).

					# Studies in Additional to EEG and MRI			
MRI Findings	**PET**	**SPECT**	**MEG**	**IOER/EOER**	**0**	**1**	**2**	**3**
Focal solitary lesion	9 (6+, 3–)	14 (12+, 2–)	6 (4+, 2–)	37	9	18	22	2
Multifocal	0	1 (+)	0	2	1	1	1	0
Diffuse	1 (+)	2 (1+, 1–)	0	3	0	1	1	1
Normal	1 (+)	7 (4+, 3–)	1 (+)	11	0	4	5	2

died,[7] and one had resolution of seizures but persistent comatose state due to anti-Hu encephalitis from small cell lung cancer and died on hospital day 54 while on hospice care.[16]

Follow-up data were available for 62/63 patients who survived to discharge, including 45 patients with focal MRI findings, with time to follow-up ranging from 1 month to 7 years. Of these 45 patients, 31 remained seizure free at follow-up,[3,6–9,12–15,17,18,21,27,29–31] four had reduction of baseline seizure frequency,[8,18,23] and 10 had ongoing occasional or frequent seizures with unclear relation to baseline seizure frequency or were patients with de novo seizures.[7,8,15,20,23,25,28,32] All patients had trials of multiple ASMs and anesthetic infusions, ranging from 3 to 14 (median = 6), including steroids and allopregnanolone in some patients and electroconvulsive therapy (ECT) in one. Time from onset of SE to surgery (TTS) ranged from 7 to 54 days (median 21 days). One outlier had surgery after 180 days of SE, but despite this and frequent partial seizures at follow-up, the person was performing well in school and participating in sports and orchestra. The complication rates of SRSE and its treatments were not reliably reported; however, there were 12 patients with reported complications including hypotension (most common, n = 9), infections, deep vein thrombosis, gastrointestinal bleeding/ ulcers, and prolonged intubation requiring tracheostomy and percutaneous gastrostomy tubes.[3,6,12,16,17,20,26,29,31]

While RNS is not typically considered in patients with a single seizure focus, there was one reported patient with FCD in eloquent cortex on MRI and corresponding focal seizures on EEG, ictal SPECT, and EOER who declined resection. He later presented with SRSE, and given previously expressed wishes, resection was deferred. RNS was placed into the FCD with resolution of SE and seizure freedom on follow-up.[12]

There were three patients who had multifocal findings (eg, tuberous sclerosis) but in whom it was felt that one of the lesions was the culprit lesion, given seizure semiology, EEG (all 3), IOER (n = 2), or ictal SPECT (n = 1). All three patients had successful resolution of SE with surgery, and at follow-up, two were seizure free and one had rare, brief seizures without alteration of consciousness.[6,22,26]

Diffuse MRI abnormalities

Of 57 patients with abnormal MRI findings, three had diffuse or holohemispheric abnormalities. Two of them also had nonfocal EEGs[8]—one of whom had a nonlocalizing SPECT, but focal semiology and IOER and underwent resection of the temporo-parietal-occipital junction 112 days after SE onset. SE persisted initially, and the patient required subsequent hemispherectomy with resolution of SE and occasional bilateral tonic-clinic (BTC) seizures at follow-up. The second patient had localizing PET, ictal SPECT, and concordant IOER findings suggesting temporo-parietal-occipital junction onset. Resection was performed on day 28 with resolution of SE and over 50% seizure reduction at follow-up, although no data were available on functional status. The third patient had focal seizures on EEG and EOER (depth electrodes) and underwent anterior temporal lobectomy on day 25 with resolution of status and one focal seizure a month (improved from baseline) at 4-year follow-up.[10]

Normal MRI

There was a small subset of 11 patients with RSE or SRSE who underwent surgery for suspected focal lesion despite a normal MRI.[7,8,11,19,20,24,33] Ten of these patients had focal seizures on EEG, all of whom had at least one other imaging modality to confirm localization. All patients had resolution of SE, with nine achieving seizure freedom at follow-up and one with reduced seizure severity. Two patients had initial MST only, given concern for postoperative neurologic deficits with resection. Both had ongoing SE requiring subsequent focal resection with resolution of SE at that point. The one patient with a nonfocal EEG had both focal semiology and two additional studies to support this suspicion—SPECT and IOER. Given that the seizure focus appeared to overlap with eloquent cortex,

MST over motor area was performed, which resulted in immediate resolution of SE and over 50% reduction in baseline seizure frequency at follow-up. Interestingly, of seven patients who underwent resective surgery despite normal MRI and for whom histopathology data were available, six had findings consistent with FCD. Time to surgery, number of ASMs, and time to follow-up were similar to that reported above for patients with abnormal MRI.

RECOMMENDATIONS

Treatment of SRSE is a challenge in neurocritical care. Patients with super refractory seizures often develop acute complications from the seizures and treatments (infections, hypotension, etc.) and are at risk of long-term neurologic sequelae. Although there are no RCTs to evaluate the efficacy of resective surgery for SRSE, there are data suggesting that a surgical approach can be helpful for some patients when a focal seizure source is suspected. The exact patient population(s) that could most benefit and the optimal timing of a surgical approach are not clear, however. It seems logical that patients who would benefit most would be those with a focal lesion on MRI corresponding to focal seizures on EEG, and available case reports seem to confirm this, as most patients who were seizure free at follow-up had these findings. It must be considered, however, that the data are highly skewed toward this patient population with 42/68 patients meeting these criteria. Finding the optimal surgical target in a patient with a normal MRI or one who has multifocal or diffuse abnormalities is challenging, and not all centers have the capability to perform additional advanced confirmatory imaging such as PET, SPECT, IOER/EOER, or MEG. As such, the number of patients with multifocal, diffuse, or normal findings on MRI who underwent focal resective surgery was markedly lower. Despite this, it should be noted that most patients with a normal or multifocal MRI who had a focal resection given other data suggesting focal onset also had resolution of SE and either seizure freedom or seizure reduction at follow-up (Table 51–2).

Ideally, management of SRSE should be targeted to the underlying source or trigger for the seizures; however, this can be challenging to determine. We recommend a stepwise approach (Figure 51–1). All patients should have a preliminary workup to screen for treatable medical conditions that could trigger seizures. This should include basic serum studies to assess for infectious or autoimmune/inflammatory processes that could be treated with anti-infectives or immune therapy (eg, steroids or IV immunoglobulin) and serum levels of ASMs in all epilepsy patients. Lumbar puncture should be considered when another trigger is not quickly identified, particularly in patients with de novo seizures. All patients should have continuous EEG—or repeated shorter duration EEG in centers without this capability—to attempt to localize the seizure onset area and to assess treatment response as well as MRI brain with and without contrast to evaluate for any abnormality that could provoke seizures. Focal resection should be considered in patients who have EEG and MRI findings suggesting a single focal seizure source outside of eloquent cortex and who have persistent SRSE despite maximal ASM and anesthetic therapy. In patients with only one data point suggesting a focal seizure source (eg, focal seizures on EEG but normal or diffusely abnormal MRI), we recommend consideration of IOER-guided focal resection only if at least one other confirmatory imaging modality—PET, SPECT, MEG, or EOER—supports the suspicion of a focal seizure source. If neither the EEG nor the MRI is suggestive of a single seizure source, but there is strong suspicion based on history or seizure semiology, we recommend consideration of IOER-guided resection **only** if at least two other imaging modalities are strongly supportive of a focal source.

The optimal timing of surgical intervention is unclear. The best approach is one that exhausts medical therapies first, while not waiting so long that patients develop iatrogenic complications or significant neurologic sequelae. However, determination of what is "too long" remains a challenge. Most patients in the literature who benefited from a surgical approach had surgery between 1 and 3 weeks from SE onset, although more robust, prospective studies are needed to further elucidate which patients may benefit most and to clarify optimal timing.

TABLE 51–2 Number of patients with various MRI and EEG findings broken down by seizure outcome. Focal MRI = focal, solitary lesion felt to be seizure source. Multifocal or diffuse = multiple discrete abnormalities (e.g. tuberous sclerosis tubers) or diffuse abnormalities. Focal EEG = EEG findings suggesting of focal seizure onset area. The right side shows how many patients had 0, 1, 2, or 3 additional confirmatory studies prior to surgery. 'Occ'- occasional. 'Freq'- frequent.

Seizure Outcome at Follow-up	Focal MRI	Multifocal or Diffuse MRI	Normal MRI	Focal EEG	# Studies in Additional to EEG and MRI			
					0	1	2	3
Seizure free ($n = 42$)	31	2	9	36	8	21	18	3
Seizure reduction ($n = 8$)	4	4	1	4	1	4	2	1
Ongoing occ./freq. seizures ($n = 12$)	10	1	1	11	0	5	6	1
Death ($n = 5$)	5	0	0	3	1	2	2	0

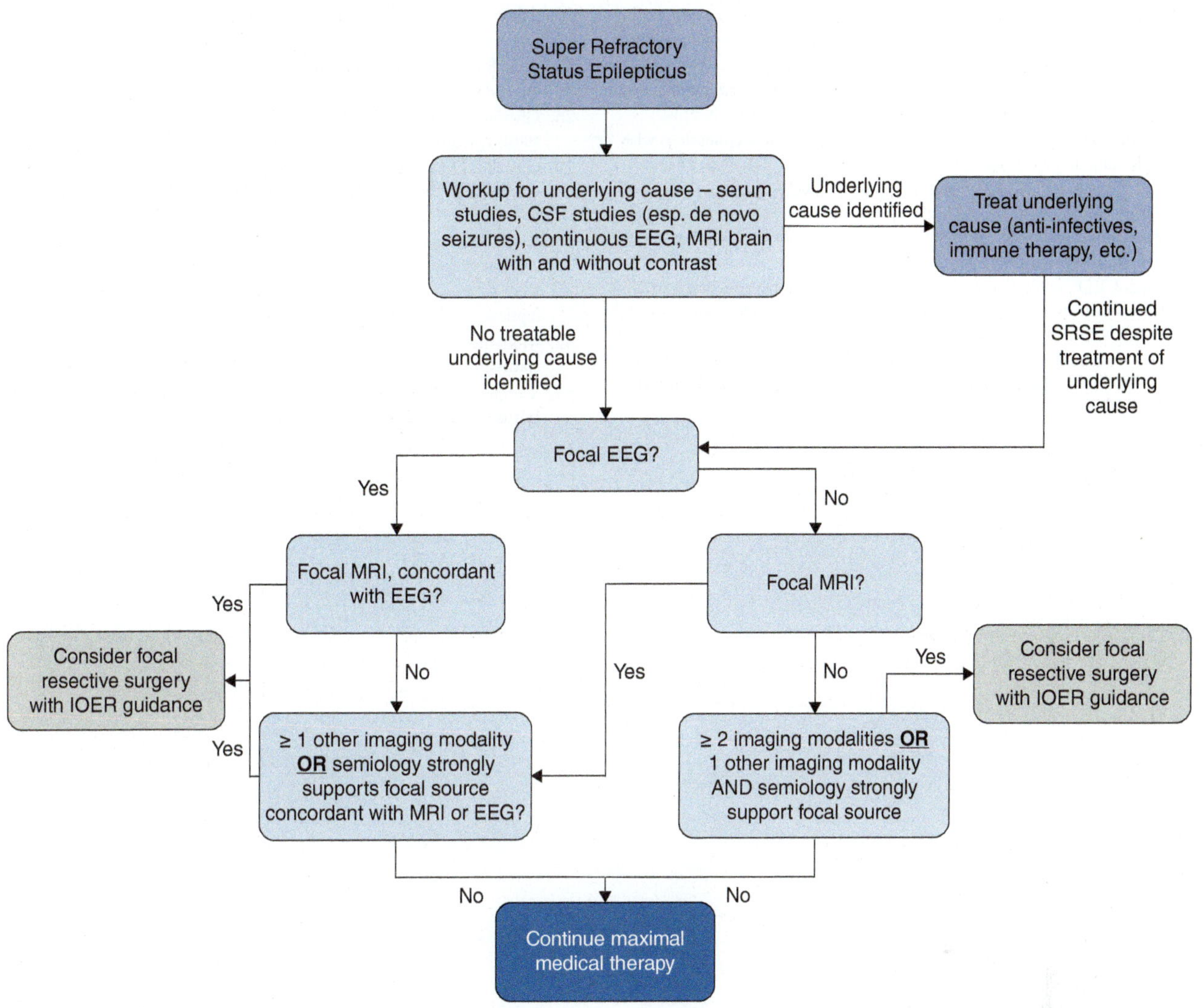

FIGURE 51–1 Suggested approach to determination of possible surgical candidates for SRSE.

REFERENCES

1. Ochoa, J.G., et al., Treatment of super-refractory status epilepticus: a review. *Epilepsy Curr*, 2021. **21**(6): p. 1535759721999670.
2. Lu, M., et al., Epidemiology of status epilepticus in the United States: a systematic review. *Epilepsy Behav*, 2020. **112**: p. 107459.
3. Yonamoto, A., et al., Good seizure outcome after focal resection surgery for super-refractory status epilepticus: report of two cases. *Surg Neurol Int*, 2022. **13**: p. 164.
4. Ferlisi, M. and S. Shorvon, The outcome of therapies in refractory and super-refractory convulsive status epilepticus and recommendations for therapy. *Brain*, 2012. **135**(Pt 8): p. 2314–28.
5. Rai, S. and F.W. Drislane, Treatment of refractory and super-refractory status epilepticus. *Neurotherapeutics*, 2018. **15**(3): p. 697–712.
6. Alexopoulos, A., et al., Resective surgery to treat refractory status epilepticus in children with focal epileptogenesis. *Neurology*, 2005. **64**(3): p. 567–70.
7. Basha, M.M., et al., Acute resective surgery for the treatment of refractory status epilepticus. *Neurocrit Care*, 2017. **27**(3): p. 370–80.
8. Bhatia, S., et al., Surgical treatment of refractory status epilepticus in children: clinical article. *J Neurosurg Pediatr*, 2013. **12**(4): p. 360–6.
9. Chandra, P.S., et al., Fourth ventricular hamartoma presenting with status epilepticus treated with emergency surgery in an infant. *Pediatr Neurosurg*, 2011. **47**(3): p. 217–22.
10. Cuello-Oderiz, C., et al., Surgical treatment of focal symptomatic refractory status epilepticus with and without invasive EEG. *Epilepsy Behav Case Rep*, 2015. **4**: p. 96–8.
11. Desbiens, R., et al., Life-threatening focal status epilepticus due to occult cortical dysplasia. *Arch Neurol*, 1993. **50**(7): p. 695–700.
12. Ernst, L.D., et al., Novel use of responsive neurostimulation (RNS System) in the treatment of super refractory status epilepticus. *J Clin Neurophysiol*, 2019. **36**(3): p. 242–5.
13. Gorman, D.G., et al., Neurosurgical treatment of refractory status epilepticus. *Epilepsia*, 1992. **33**(3): p. 546–9.
14. Jagtap, S.A., et al., Role of epilepsy surgery in refractory status epilepticus in children. *Epilepsy Res*, 2021. **176**: p. 106744.
15. Mohamed, I.S., et al., Magnetoencephalography for surgical treatment of refractory status epilepticus. *Acta Neurol Scand Suppl*, 2007. **186**: p. 29–36.
16. Nahab, F., A. Heller, and S.M. Laroche, Focal cortical resection for complex partial status epilepticus due to a paraneoplastic encephalitis. *Neurologist*, 2008. **14**(1): p. 56–9.
17. Ng, Y.T., et al., The role of neurosurgery in status epilepticus. *Neurocrit Care*, 2007. **7**(1): p. 86–91.
18. Ng, Y.T., J.F. Kerrigan, and H.L. Rekate, Neurosurgical treatment of status epilepticus. *J Neurosurg*, 2006. **105**(5 Suppl): p. 378–81.
19. Ng, Y.T., H.L. Kim, and J.W. Wheless, Successful neurosurgical treatment of childhood complex partial status epilepticus with focal resection. *Epilepsia*, 2003. **44**(3): p. 468–71.

20. Schrader, D.V., P. Steinbok, and M. Connolly, Urgent, resective surgery for medically refractory, convulsive status epilepticus. *Eur J Paediatr Neurol*, 2009. **13**(1): p. 10–7.
21. Weimer, T., et al., Temporal lobectomy for refractory status epilepticus in a case of limbic encephalitis. *J Neurosurg*, 2008. **109**(4): p. 742–5.
22. D'Giano, C.H., et al., Treatment of refractory partial status epilepticus with multiple subpial transection: case report. *Seizure*, 2001. **10**(5): p. 382–5.
23. Lega, B.C., et al., Cortical resection tailored to awake, intraoperative ictal recordings and motor mapping in the treatment of intractable epilepsia partialis continua: technical case report. *Neurosurgery*, 2009. **64**(3 Suppl): p. ons195–6; discussion ons196.
24. Molyneux, P.D., et al., Successful treatment of intractable epilepsia partialis continua with multiple subpial transections. *J Neurol Neurosurg Psychiatry*, 1998. **65**(1): p. 137–8.
25. Zumsteg, D., et al., H2(15)O or 13NH3 PET and electromagnetic tomography (LORETA) during partial status epilepticus. *Neurology*, 2005. **65**(10): p. 1657–60.
26. Atkinson, M., et al., Refractory status epilepticus secondary to CNS vasculitis, a role for epilepsy surgery. *J Neurol Sci*, 2012. **315**(1-2): p. 156–9.
27. Bick, S.K., et al., Anterior temporal lobectomy for refractory status epilepticus in herpes simplex encephalitis. *Neurocrit Care*, 2016. **25**(3): p. 458–63.
28. Cherian, K.A., et al., Extensive apoptosis in a case of intractable infantile status epilepticus. *Epilepsy Res*, 2009. **85**(2-3): p. 305–10.
29. Costello, D.J., et al., Efficacy of surgical treatment of de novo, adult-onset, cryptogenic, refractory focal status epilepticus. *Arch Neurol*, 2006. **63**(6): p. 895–901.
30. Krsek, P., et al., Life-saving epilepsy surgery for status epilepticus caused by cortical dysplasia. *Epileptic Disord*, 2002. **4**(3): p. 203–8.
31. Ma, X., et al., Neurosurgical treatment of medically intractable status epilepticus. *Epilepsy Res*, 2001. **46**(1): p. 33–8.
32. Mohamed, I.S., et al., Surgical treatment for acute symptomatic refractory status epilepticus: a case report. *J Child Neurol*, 2007. **22**(4): p. 435–9.
33. Weimer, T., W. Boling, and A. Palade, Neurosurgical therapy for central area status epilepticus. *W V Med J*, 2012. **108**(5): p. 20–3.

SECTION VI TUMOR

CHAPTER 52

What Are the Optimal Perioperative Blood Pressure Parameters for Patients Undergoing Craniotomy for Tumors?

Sherwin A. Tavakol, MD, MPH &
Ian F. Dunn, MD, FACS, FAANS

Case

A 42-year-old woman with history of hypertension (treated with metoprolol, hydrochlorothiazide-losartan, and clonidine patch), generalized anxiety disorder, and recurrent primary intracranial sarcoma (status post surgical resection and focused radiation) underwent a repeat craniotomy for resection (Figure 52–1A, 1B). In the operating theater, anesthetic induction is employed with intravenous ketamine and remifentanil, and inhaled nitrous oxide is used for maintenance. She underwent a near total resection, with encountering of significant scarring during elevation of the skin flap and dissection of the underlying adherent dura. During closure and emergence, spikes in the systolic blood pressure (SBP) were noted, prompting initiation of a nicardipine infusion. After significant coughing and one episode of emesis during extubation, a scopolamine patch is placed. She continued to be hypertensive and agitated in the postanesthesia care unit and removed her arterial line. Haloperidol is administered for agitation. On transfer to the ICU several hours later, the patient is noted to be snoring, difficult to arouse, weakly withdrawing in all extremities, with anisocoric pupils. Cuff pressure reads 216/114. The patient is taken for an urgent noncontrast CT brain, which reveals a large surgical bed hematoma with cytotoxic edema, subarachnoid hemorrhage, and dilated ventricles (Figure 52–1C, 1D).

Key Points

- Patients undergoing intracranial tumor resection have many reasons to experience volatility in their hemodynamic status.
- Preoperative chronic comorbidities, local physiologic tumor effects, anesthesia, and postcraniotomy emergence, along with a host of postoperative factors, impact patient's blood pressure and therefore cerebral blood flow (CBF).
- Coordination between the neurosurgeon and neurointensivist to determine a patient-specific postoperative blood pressure parameter is paramount to ensure sufficient tissue perfusion and prevent disastrous complications when possible.

INTRODUCTION

The perioperative period of neurosurgical patients undergoing craniotomy for tumor resection is frequently complicated by fluctuations in systemic blood pressure.[1–7] Preoperatively, patients with metabolically active tumors, such as glomus tumors or some functioning pituitary adenomas, those with tumors causing mass effect and significant vasogenic edema leading to dysfunction in cerebral autoregulation, or patients with posterior fossa lesions with resultant brainstem compression can all experience elevated blood pressure prior to surgery. In the operating room, acute hypertensive episodes can be brought on during head-pin application and administration of local anesthetic with epinephrine, brain manipulation, and cortical retraction as well as during emergence. However, the roles of the neurosurgeon and neurointensivist are most likely to converge postoperatively, where the conundrum of the ideal blood pressure parameter can be simplified to toggle between two distinct goals: preventing a hypotension-induced ischemic event and avoiding potential catastrophic postoperative hematoma. This chapter seeks to elucidate causes of perioperative blood pressure fluctuations in patients undergoing craniotomy for tumor resection with normal indices of clotting and to provide conceptual and practical parameters for managing blood pressure, with a particular emphasis on the postoperative period.

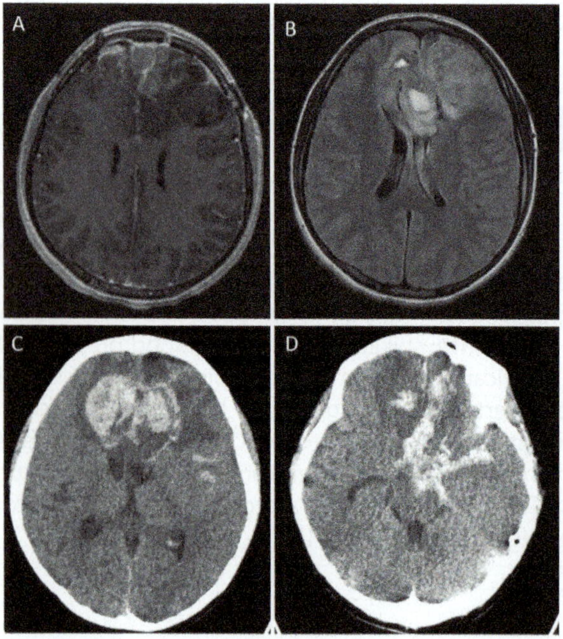

FIGURE 52–1 Pre- and postoperative imaging. (**A**) Axial T1-weighted postcontrast MRI, (**B**) axial T2 FLAIR MRI, (**C and D**) axial noncontrast CT brain showing a large bifrontal tumor bed hematoma with cytotoxic edema and resultant mass effect on the frontal horns of the lateral ventricles and subarachnoid hemorrhage in the left sylvian fissure and basal cisterns.

EVIDENCE AND REVIEW

The Preoperative Setting

Causes of systemic hypertension in the preoperative setting are plentiful. The most common cause is chronic essential hypertension, unrelated to the patient's brain tumor.[7,8] However, in a small subset of patients, tumoral factors can induce elevated blood pressure as well. Glomus tumors, also known as paragangliomas, are typically benign slow-growing tumors that have secretory granules leading to elevated norepinephrine, serotonin, and/or kallikrein. Moreover, functioning pituitary adenomas, including adrenocorticotropic hormone (ACTH)- or thyroid-stimulating hormone (TSH)-secreting adenomas, can cause hypertension through elevation of cortisol and thyroid hormone, respectively. Furthermore, local mass effect, for example as seen in posterior fossa tumors that cause compression of the rostral medulla, can also lead to arterial hypertension.[9–11] Irrespective of the cause of systemic hypertension, however, its effect on cerebral blood flow (CBF) can be heightened by an intracranial tumor's interaction with the cortical microenvironment.[12,13]

In nondiseased brain, blood vessel vasodilation and vasoconstriction occur in response to fluctuations of cerebral perfusion pressure (CPP) to maintain adequate CBF.[14,15] This process is termed cerebrovascular blood pressure autoregulation and is largely driven by the reactivity to the partial pressure of carbon dioxide (CO_2). When systemic blood pressure oscillates on the plateau between the lower and upper margins of autoregulation, CBF is steady. When blood pressure decreases or increases beyond these limits, cerebral vasculature cannot dilate or constrict sufficiently enough to maintain CBF (Figure 52–2). The effect of an intracranial tumor is to further narrow this window of autoregulation, leading to "impaired autoregulation." This has been associated with worse clinical outcomes and likely affects the therapeutic efficacy of treating intracranial hypertension.

The literature is conflicting about the effect of preoperative hypertension on hematoma formation after craniotomy. For example, a total of 69 patients with clinically significant intracerebral hemorrhage (ICH) after intracranial operations out of the

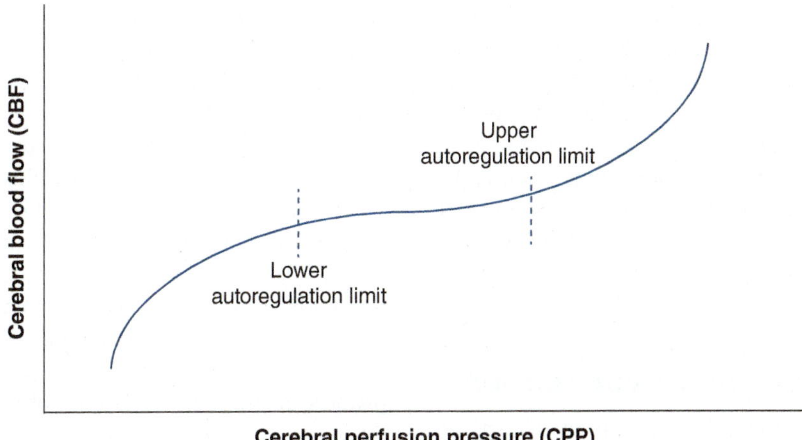

FIGURE 52–2 The cerebrovascular autoregulation curve consists of a plateau across which shifts in cerebral perfusion pressure (CPP) do not lead to significant fluctuations in cerebral blood flow (CBF) by means of tightly modulated vasoreactivity. In practice, cerebral autoregulation is optimized when blood pressure is maintained between dashed lines, a conceptual target that is affected by patient age, clinical status, intracranial pressure, local tumoral factors, etc. When perfusion goes beyond the upper limit of autoregulation, cerebral blood vessels are unable to constrict sufficiently enough to reduce CBF. Conversely, when perfusion dips below the lower autoregulation boundary, cerebral vasculature cannot sufficiently vasodilate to increase blood flow.

Cleveland Clinic Foundation were compared using a 2:1 ratio of matched controls to cases.[1] This study found that a history of hypertension documented in the medical record was similar among cases and controls. However, in a different study out of Beijing Tiantan Hospital in China, 184 patients with clinically significant postcraniotomy ICH were compared 1:1 with matched controls revealing a higher incidence of preoperative hypertension in the ICH group.[16]

The Intraoperative Setting

Fluctuations in blood pressure in the operating room can occur frequently and rapidly, necessitating close dialogue between neurosurgeon and neuroanesthetist at all stages of the case to maintain adequate CBF. Cases requiring preoperative diuresis for cerebral edema can be complicated by volume depletion and resultant hypotension. Particularly stimulating portions of the surgery, including head pinning, skin incision, and periosteal dissection, can lead to sudden and significant episodes of hypertension, especially if the craniotomy is performed on an awake patient.[17] Manipulation of the trigeminal nerve can elicit the trigeminocardiac reflex (TCR), which is a phenomenon that consists of bradycardia (or even asystole) and significant hypotension. A variant of the TCR is the oculocardiac reflex (OCR), or Aschner reflex, which represents bradycardia during surgical stimulation of the ophthalmic branch of the trigeminal nerve via manipulation of ocular/periocular structures or simply during periods of significant globe pressure.[18] Irritation of the vagus nerve during surgical retraction or tumor resection can have similar cardiovascular consequences.[9] Emergence hypertension is another well-documented occurrence after general anesthesia for craniotomy and is thought to be related to sympathetic overdrive with acute and transient increase in blood catecholamine levels and consequent peripheral vasoconstriction.[19,20]

Intraoperative elevations of blood pressure can impede effective hemostasis and lead to elevated intracranial pressure (ICP) resulting in a narrowed operative corridor, an increased need for mechanical retraction, and the cascade of detrimental effects of malignant vasogenic edema.[10,21] Further, intraoperative blood pressure spikes have been shown to be associated with postoperative complications such as ICH. In multiple studies, an intraoperative maximum systolic blood pressure (SBP) >160 mm Hg was associated with an increased odds of clinically significant postoperative ICH.[1,3,4] As opposed to using an absolute blood pressure threshold, assessing elevations in blood pressure in comparison to the patient's preoperative baseline (ie, preventing an increase of >20% from baseline) was also assessed but with mixed results.[16] Assuming an "absolute mechanical vulnerability of intracranial blood vessels" as described by Basali et al using a universal threshold blood pressure parameter may be biologically sound and practically efficacious, given that a lack of preoperative blood pressure measurements may hinder the determination of an accurate baseline for elective craniotomy patients.[1] It is also critical that the surgeon and anesthetist adopt the same lexicon as while surgeons often consider systolic goals, other subspecialists may use mean arterial pressure (MAP) more commonly.

The Postoperative Setting

The early postoperative period after craniotomy for brain tumor resection is a critical time requiring close patient monitoring, strict attention to hemodynamic status, and a high level of suspicion for acute changes in neurological function. Disruption of cerebral autoregulation by intracranial tumor is intensified by surgical breach of the blood-brain barrier (BBB), leading to a passive increase in blood flow with an increase in blood pressure. This can subsequently lead to an increase in ICP or hyperemia-induced escape of intravascular fluid across an already disrupted

BBB. Delicate foci of hemostasis can be affected, leading to potentially serious hematoma formation. Even after postcraniotomy emergence, the postoperative period is replete with potential causes of hypertension, including coughing during endotracheal extubation, incisional pain, and agitation or anxiety. These factors all necessitate close coordination between and attention by the neurosurgeon and the neurointensivist to ensure prevention of a hemodynamic-induced postoperative complication when able, and swift recognition and urgent management of a problem should it occur.[22,23]

Incidence of Postoperative Hypertension

The incidence of postoperative hypertension in neurosurgical patients varies widely in the literature, in large part due to varying blood pressure parameters and the proportion of particular demographic characteristics, such as age, gender, and preoperative hypertension. When a postoperative SBP goal of 90 to 130 was sought, 60% to 90% of neurosurgical patients required some form of antihypertensive therapy in one study.[20] In other reports, less restrictive SBP parameters (ie, SBP < 140 or SBP < 160) naturally necessitated hypertensive treatment more infrequently (21%-57% of patients).[19]

Incidence of Postoperative Hematoma

The incidence of clinically significant hematoma requiring surgical evacuation after craniotomy ranges from 0.48% to 3.9%.[1–4,16,22,23] In multiple studies, intrinsic tumor resection has been found to be the most frequent indication for craniotomy after which a clinically significant ICH occurs (up to 6.5%).[1,22] When hemorrhage does occur, it can be located at the operative site or in remote areas.[4] Regardless of location, however, outcomes after ICH are poor. In one report, only 13% of patients with postoperative ICH were found to have a good outcome and 55% were dead or severely disabled by 6 months.[4] A complicating feature in the temporal analysis of the relationship between postoperative hematoma formation and hypertension is that an elevated blood pressure can herald or be a consequence of an ICH.

Postoperative hematomas can be arterial or venous in origin as well as a combination of the two.[4,16] Whereas an arterial bleed or the disruption of a vessel's hemostatic plug can lead to brisk hematoma development, slow venous oozing can contribute to both clinically insignificant surgical bed hematomas and delayed intracranial hemorrhages. For tumors near or invading venous structures including cerebral sinuses, it is of paramount importance that adequate intraoperative hemostasis be confirmed to prevent the development of a postoperative hematoma and that critical veins are not sacrificed that may lead to venous hypertension and subsequent hemorrhage.

Timing of Postoperative Blood Pressure Control

The majority of hypertensive episodes that occur in the 12-hour period prior to ICH occurred within 6 hours of the bleed.[1] Additionally, incidence of elevated blood pressure in the 4 hours prior to ICH was higher than the 4 hours after ICH, arguing against ICH being the cause of hypertension (HTN) in these patients. Most interventions for postoperative hypertension occur within the first 24-hour period, with some literature showing that elevated blood pressure begins most commonly between 10 and 20 minutes from the end of surgery.[1,3] However, patients with preexisting HTN may require postoperative treatment of elevated blood pressure up to 72 hours after surgery.[6,7] In fact, in one study assessing the need for intensive care unit (ICU)-level admission after elective craniotomy, the most common postoperative critical care need was the use of an intravenous blood pressure medication drip (76.4% of ICU admissions).[3]

Incidence of Postoperative Ischemia

While much attention is given to the concern for an intracranial bleed, postoperative ischemic lesions are also commonly identified on routine postoperative MRIs and can be the source of new neurological deficits after surgery. In one study, 31% of patients experienced postoperative ischemic lesions after resection of a newly diagnosed glioma, and 80% of patients experienced the same after surgery for a recurrent glioma. Despite these high rates of diffusion restriction on imaging, far fewer patients experienced permanent new or worsening of neurological deficits after tumor resection. In highly select patients where there was a clinical concern for arterial vasospasm as judged by the need for significant intraoperative manipulation of arteries, MAP therapy for 48 hours after surgery has even been considered to reduce the chance of cerebral ischemia. Further, in the setting of craniotomy for ICH, brain tissue oxygen tension was prospectively monitored and lower SBP and CPP were significantly associated with higher risk for brain tissue hypoxia. While not feasible in all patients, prevention of hypotension or hypovolemia after tumor resection, particularly in patients where risk of ischemia is high, should be prioritized.[24–27]

AVAILABLE GUIDELINES

No national guidelines exist for blood pressure control after a craniotomy for tumor resection. Instead, institution- and surgeon-dependent preference predominate. Basic considerations include balancing the risk of hemorrhage with that of a hypotensive ischemic event, while weighing patients' chronic comorbid conditions (eg, coronary artery disease, congestive heart failure, and chronic kidney disease) and the competing effect these may have on a patient's hemodynamic requirements. A broad goal of maintaining SBP between 90 and 140 is likely a safe and reasonable parameter for at least the first 24 hours after craniotomy for tumor resection. However, as is always the case, patient-specific features should be taken into consideration when determining blood pressure parameters. For patients with preoperative uncontrolled hypertension, those where there was intraoperative concern for vessel manipulation, or in situations of increased ICP, it may be prudent to allow for a higher upper limit. For those with coagulopathy, intraoperative concern for insufficient hemostasis, or known remote hemorrhagic lesions, a narrower blood pressure goal maintained past the first 24 hours could be considered.

REFERENCES

1. Basali, A., Mascha, E. J., Kalfas, I., & Schubert, A. (2000). Relation between perioperative hypertension and intracranial hemorrhage after craniotomy. *Anesthesiology*, 93(1), 48–54. https://doi.org/10.1097/00000542-200007000-00012
2. Perez, C. A., Stutzman, S., Jansen, T., Perera, A., Jannusch, S., Atem, F., & Aiyagari, V. (2020). Elevated blood pressure after craniotomy: a prospective observational study. *J Crit Care*, 60, 235–240. https://doi.org/10.1016/j.jcrc.2020.08.013
3. Hanak, B. W., Walcott, B. P., Nahed, B. V., Muzikansky, A., Mian, M. K., Kimberly, W. T., & Curry, W. T. (2014). Postoperative intensive care unit requirements after elective craniotomy. *World Neurosurg*, 81(1), 165–172. https://doi.org/10.1016/j.wneu.2012.11.068
4. Kalfas, I. H., & Little, J. R. (1988). Postoperative hemorrhage: a survey of 4992 intracranial procedures. *Neurosurgery*, 23(3), 343–347. https://doi.org/10.1227/00006123-198809000-00010
5. Bilotta, F., Lam, A. M., Doronzio, A., Cuzzone, V., Delfini, R., & Rosa, G. (2008). Esmolol blunts postoperative hemodynamic changes after propofol-remifentanil total intravenous fast-track neuroanesthesia for intracranial surgery. *J Clin Anesth*, 20(6), 426–430. https://doi.org/10.1016/j.jclinane.2008.04.006
6. Bebawy, J. F., Houston, C. C., Kosky, J. L., Badri, A. M., Hemmer, L. B., Moreland, N. C., ... Gupta, D. K. (2015). Nicardipine is superior to esmolol for the management of postcraniotomy emergence hypertension: a randomized open-label study. *Anesth Analg*, 120(1), 186–192. https://doi.org/10.1213/ANE.0000000000000473
7. Gal, T. J., & Cooperman, L. H. (1975). Hypertension in the immediate postoperative period. *Br J Anaesth*, 47(1), 70–74. https://doi.org/10.1093/bja/47.1.70
8. Mahaley, M. S., Mettlin, C., Natarajan, N., Laws, E. R., & Peace, B. B. (1989). National survey of patterns of care for brain-tumor patients. *J Neurosurg*, 71(6), 826–836. https://doi.org/10.3171/jns.1989.71.6.0826
9. Artru, A. A., Cucchiara, R. F., & Messick, J. M. (1980). Cardiorespiratory and cranial-nerve sequelae of surgical procedures involving the posterior fossa. *Anesthesiology*, 52(1), 83–86. https://doi.org/10.1097/00000542-198001000-00021
10. Hatashita, S., Koike, J., Sonokawa, T., & Ishii, S. (1985). Cerebral edema associated with craniectomy and arterial hypertension. *Stroke*, 16(4), 661–668. https://doi.org/10.1161/01.str.16.4.661
11. Rupp, S. M., Wickersham, J. K., Rampil, I. J., Wilson, C. B., & Donegan, J. H. (1989). The effect of halothane, isoflurane, or sufentanil on the hypertensive response to cerebellar retraction during posterior fossa surgery. *Anesthesiology*, 71(5), 660–663. https://doi.org/10.1097/00000542-198911000-00006
12. Olsen, K. S., Pedersen, C. B., Madsen, J. B., Ravn, L. I., & Schifter, S. (2002). Vasoactive modulators during and after craniotomy: relation to postoperative hypertension. *J Neurosurg Anesthesiol*, 14(3), 171–179. https://doi.org/10.1097/00008506-200207000-00001
13. Lyubashina, O. A., Mamontov, O. V., Volynsky, M. A., Zaytsev, V. V., & Kamshilin, A. A. (2019). Contactless assessment of cerebral autoregulation by photoplethysmographic imaging at green illumination. *Front Neurosci*, 13, 1235. https://doi.org/10.3389/fnins.2019.01235
14. Sharma, D., Bithal, P. K., Dash, H. H., Chouhan, R. S., Sookplung, P., & Vavilala, M. S. (2010). Cerebral autoregulation and CO2 reactivity before and after elective supratentorial tumor resection. *J Neurosurg Anesthesiol*, 22(2), 132–137. https://doi.org/10.1097/ANA.0b013e3181c9fbf1
15. Williams, M., & Lee, J. K. (2014). Intraoperative blood pressure and cerebral perfusion: strategies to clarify hemodynamic goals. *Paediatr Anaesth*, 24(7), 657–667. https://doi.org/10.1111/pan.12401
16. Jian, M., Li, X., Wang, A., Zhang, L., Han, R., & Gelb, A. W. (2014). Flurbiprofen and hypertension but not hydroxyethyl starch are associated with post-craniotomy intracranial haematoma requiring surgery. *Br J Anaesth*, 113(5), 832–839. https://doi.org/10.1093/bja/aeu185
17. Bloomfield, E. L., Schubert, A., Secic, M., Barnett, G., Shutway, F., & Ebrahim, Z. Y. (1998). The influence of scalp infiltration with bupivacaine on hemodynamics and postoperative pain in adult patients undergoing craniotomy. *Anesth Analg*, 87(3), 579–582. https://doi.org/10.1097/00000539-199809000-00015
18. Koerbel, A., Gharabaghi, A., Samii, A., Gerganov, V., von Gösseln, H., Tatagiba, M., & Samii, M. (2005). Trigeminocardiac reflex during skull base surgery: mechanism and management. *Acta Neurochir (Wien)*, 147(7), 727–732; discussion 732-723. https://doi.org/10.1007/s00701-005-0535-1
19. Kross, R. A., Ferri, E., Leung, D., Pratila, M., Broad, C., Veronesi, M., & Melendez, J. A. (2000). A comparative study between a calcium channel blocker (Nicardipine) and a combined alpha-beta-blocker (Labetalol) for the control of emergence hypertension during craniotomy for tumor surgery. *Anesth Analg*, 91(4), 904–909. https://doi.org/10.1097/00000539-200010000-00024
20. Bekker, A., Didehvar, S., Kim, S., Golfinos, J. G., Parker, E., Sapson, A., ... Lee, M. (2010). Efficacy of clevidipine in controlling perioperative hypertension in neurosurgical patients: initial single-center experience. *J Neurosurg Anesthesiol*, 22(4), 330–335. https://doi.org/10.1097/ANA.0b013e3181e3077b
21. Velayutham, P. K., Adhikary, S. D., Babu, S. K., Vedantam, R., Korula, G., & Ramachandran, A. (2013). Oxidative stress-associated hypertension in surgically induced brain injury patients: effects of β-blocker and angiotensin-converting enzyme inhibitor. *J Surg Res*, 179(1), 125–131. https://doi.org/10.1016/j.jss.2012.09.005
22. Fukamachi, A., Koizumi, H., & Nukui, H. (1985). Postoperative intracerebral hemorrhages: a survey of computed tomographic findings after 1074 intracranial operations. *Surg Neurol*, 23(6), 575–580. https://doi.org/10.1016/0090-3019(85)90006-0
23. Palmer, J. D., Sparrow, O. C., & Iannotti, F. (1994). Postoperative hematoma: a 5-year survey and identification of avoidable risk factors. *Neurosurgery*, 35(6), 1061–1064; discussion 1064-1065. https://doi.org/10.1227/00006123-199412000-00007
24. Berger, A., Tzarfati, G., Costa, M., Serafimova, M., Korn, A., Vendrov, I., ... Grossman, R. (2019). Incidence and impact of stroke following surgery for low-grade gliomas. *J Neurosurg*, 134(1), 1–9. https://doi.org/10.3171/2019.10.JNS192301
25. Conner, A. K., Briggs, R. G., Palejwala, A. H., Sali, G., & Sughrue, M. E. (2018). The safety of post-operative elevation of mean arterial blood pressure following brain tumor resection. *J Clin Neurosci*, 58, 156–159. https://doi.org/10.1016/j.jocn.2018.09.001
26. Gempt, J., Förschler, A., Buchmann, N., Pape, H., Ryang, Y. M., Krieg, S. M., ... Ringel, F. (2013). Postoperative ischemic changes following resection of newly diagnosed and recurrent gliomas and their clinical relevance. *J Neurosurg*, 118(4), 801–808. https://doi.org/10.3171/2012.12.JNS12125
27. Linder, A., Rass, V., Ianosi, B.A., Schiefecker, A.J., Kofler, M., Gaasch, M., ... Helbok, R. (2021). Individualized blood pressure targets in the postoperative card of patients with intracerebral hemorrhage. *J Neurosurg*, 135(6), 1656–1665. https://doi.org/10.3171/2020.9.JNS201024

CHAPTER

53

How Do We Best Monitor and Treat for Perioperative Diabetes Insipidus?

Hussain Mahmud, MD, Pouneh K. Fazeli, MD, MPH, Georgios A. Zenonos, MD, & Paul A. Gardner, MD

Case

A 43-year-old woman with a history of acromegaly undergoes an endoscopic transsphenoidal resection of her pituitary tumor. On postoperative day 2, she develops polyuria with associated increase in serum sodium level. What are the management considerations for her condition?

Key Points

- Transient central diabetes insipidus (DI), alternatively known as Arginine Vasopressin Deficiency (AVP-D), is a common complication following transsphenoidal surgery, while persistent DI is relatively rare.
- Protocols for monitoring of incipient DI should be implemented for all patients undergoing transsphenoidal surgeries.
- Distinguishing DI from physiologic polyuria is important.
- In the initial postoperative period, desmopressin should be administered on an as-needed basis when the patient develops polyuria to avoid hyponatremia.
- An open line of communication between the neurosurgical, endocrine, and critical care teams is essential for optimal patient care and outcomes.

BACKGROUND

Diabetes insipidus (DI), or alternatively Arginine Vasopressin Deficiency (AVP-D), is the inappropriate excretion of copious hypotonic urine despite serum hyperosmolality, occurring due to deficiency of antidiuretic hormone (ADH). Permanent DI requiring long-term desmopressin administration is a relatively uncommon complication of transsphenoidal surgical procedures, with the incidence being 2% to 5% after pituitary adenoma surgeries.[1] But dysnatremic processes such as transient DI (18%-31%) and hyponatremia (8%-21%) are far more common and likely underreported due to lack of agreed-upon diagnostic criteria.[2]

Transient DI occurs from mild damage to the pituitary stalk or the posterior pituitary gland. Postoperative DI can often precede an episode of syndrome of inappropriate ADH (SIADH) secretion, which is theorized to occur due to the release of preformed ADH stored inside the affected neurohypophyseal neurons. The typical onset of hyponatremia due to SIADH is approximately 6 to 10 days after surgery.[3] With the biphasic pattern, normal ADH secretion and fluid balance are restored once the SIADH phase is over. With the triphasic pattern, which is uncommon and occurs due to significant posterior pituitary, stalk, or hypothalamic damage, permanent DI will manifest once the excessive ADH, released due to neuronal degeneration, has been metabolized.

Well-established risk factors for the development of DI include large tumor size and Rathke's cleft cysts.[4] Other studies have also identified craniopharyngiomas, Cushing's disease, intraoperative CSF leaks, and pituitary stalk lesions as independent risk factors for postoperative DI.[2,5]

Of note, a move to change the previously established DI nomenclature is currently afoot.[6] It has been proposed that central/neurogenic DI and nephrogenic DI be referred to as arginine vasopressin deficiency (AVP-D) and arginine vasopressin resistance (AVP-R), respectively. The reason behind this name change is the confusion the word "diabetes" causes among patients' and medical providers' minds. There have been cases in which desmopressin was discontinued or insulin was incorrectly administered because medical providers unfamiliar with this uncommon condition assumed that they have a hyperglycemia or carbohydrate metabolism problem rather than a fluid balance problem. This nomenclature change has been endorsed by multiple professional societies, and we expect that it will start appearing in medical literature and clinical documentation over the next few years.

EVIDENCE AND REVIEW

Monitoring

DI surveillance protocols should be instituted among all patients undergoing transsphenoidal surgeries or other skull base procedures with high DI risk. Clinical staff should be instructed to monitor fluid intake and urine output hourly. If the adult patient's urine output exceeds 300 mL/h for 3 consecutive hours, serum sodium and urine osmolality should be measured promptly. At our institution, sodium levels are measured on a daily basis, but more frequent monitoring is considered for patients at high risk of DI, such as those with craniopharyngiomas or pituitary stalk lesions. Among pediatric neurosurgical patients, urine output of >5 mL/kg/h warrants further investigation.[7]

Due to the administration of large volumes of intravenous fluids during surgery, polyuria is quite common during the perioperative period, but the presence of hypotonic polyuria along with hyperosmolality and/or hypernatremia is used to distinguish between physiologic postoperative diuresis and DI. Physiologic polyuria is also seen among patients with acromegaly whose tumors have been adequately resected, as excess growth hormone secretion promotes volume retention. Osmotic diuresis from hyperglycemia (frequently encountered in this patient population due to perioperative administration of high doses of glucocorticoids) should also be excluded as a cause of polyuria. On the other hand, glucocorticoid administration can also "unmask" preexisting DI by impacting ADH release and action.

Diagnosis

Multiple diagnostic criteria, including hourly urine output, daily urine output, urine specific gravity, urine osmolality, serum osmolality, and serum sodium levels, have previously been described in the literature. A recent paper proposed the definition of postoperative DI based on the following mandatory and relative diagnostic criteria, in an effort to improve the reliability of diagnosis and standardize the reporting across literature.[8]

- Urine output > 300 mL/h for 3 consecutive hours
- Urine specific gravity < 1.005

And at least one of the following:

- Excessive thirst (numerical rating scale of ≥6 out of 10)
- Hypernatremia (sodium > 145 mEq/L)
- Serum osmolality > 300 mosmol/kg

Probable transient DI (grade 1) was defined as polyuria meeting the above criteria but only lasting <48 hours after surgery and not requiring the use of desmopressin.[7] Transient DI (grade 2) requires the use of desmopressin and may prolong the hospital stay but will resolve in 2 weeks. Prolonged DI (grade 3) lasts >2 weeks but resolves before 6 months due to recovery of neurohypophyseal function. Chronic or persistent DI (grade 4) will continue to require treatment beyond 6 months indicating permanent neuronal loss from hypothalamic or posterior pituitary damage.[8]

A few studies have demonstrated the use of postoperative copeptin levels to prognosticate development of DI and postoperative hyponatremia.[9,10] Copeptin is secreted in equimolar concentrations along with ADH and neurophysin II upon the depolarization of neurohypophyseal neurons. It is a larger molecule with a longer half-life, which makes its measurement easier and more reliable compared to ADH. Typically, copeptin levels are high as part of the stress response to extubation and postoperative stress, but if copeptin is low in the immediate postoperative period, it is associated with the subsequent development of DI. However, this approach needs further validation before it can be incorporated into routine clinical care.

Management

The management of DI has two components: (1) replacement of ADH to prevent further free water losses and (2) replacement of water losses that have already occurred. Mild postoperative DI typically does not require treatment with desmopressin; therefore, at our institution, we initially attempt to treat with fluids alone. If awake and alert, the patient is encouraged ad-lib fluid intake and a pitcher of water should be placed by the bedside. Transsphenoidal surgical patients are obligate mouth breathers and the presence of dry mouth may confound the thirst and DI symptoms. If the patient is unable to drink and an enteral tube is not present, intravenous hydration with hypotonic fluids such as 0.45% normal saline should be considered. The intravenous fluid rates are based on the calculated free water deficit and as the postoperative hypernatremia is acute, serum sodium can be quickly brought down into the normal range.

Desmopressin is administered if the patient is unable to maintain normal sodium levels despite aggressive hydration, to reduce severe polyuria, and to make patients more comfortable. Our preference is to administer intravenous desmopressin 0.5 mcg on an as-needed basis due to its quick onset of action and predictable bioavailability. Oral desmopressin is also used in some centers as initial treatment, but as desmopressin is "spot dosed" when patient is already polyuric and free-water deplete, the quick onset of action of the intravenous form is more desirable. Among children, continuous intravenous infusion of aqueous vasopressin is often used to treat postoperative DI.[7] Desmopressin is also available for use as an intranasal preparation, but its use should be avoided during the perioperative period due to recent endonasal surgery which may impact its absorption. Larger doses of desmopressin (1 mcg IV or up) do not necessarily lead to a more efficacious antidiuretic response but may prolong its duration of action. Due to the risk of hyponatremia from desmopressin among patients who enter biphasic or triphasic patterns, scheduled desmopressin administration is not recommended until the diagnosis of DI is well established. Patients who likely have prolonged or persistent DI are transitioned to oral desmopressin (typical starting dose being 100 mcg/0.1 mg once or twice daily) before discharge.

Patients with hypothalamic involvement are at risk of developing adipsic DI due to damage to the thirst center in addition to damage to the neurohypophyseal neurons. This is most commonly seen among patients with craniopharyngiomas and surgical clipping of anterior communicating artery aneurysms following subarachnoid hemorrhage.[11] Patients with adipsic DI are likely to develop severe hypernatremia as there is no thirst mechanism to rescue them from the dehydration caused by the inexorable free water loss from DI. These patients are managed by establishing the daily desmopressin dose and then gradually adjusting the daily fluid prescription until optimal fluid balance is achieved. Unfortunately, the risk of water intoxication with hyponatremia or recurrent dehydration with hypernatremia remains high among patients with adipsic DI despite frequent monitoring and fluid prescription adjustments, mainly due to changes in insensible fluid losses.

AVAILABLE GUIDELINES

DI management guidelines have been published by Australian and UK endocrine societies. But in the United States, no national guidelines for DI monitoring and management exist, so there is considerable institutional heterogeneity in DI management.

REFERENCES

1. Paluzzi A, Fernandez-Miranda JC, Tonya Stefko S, Challinor S, Snyderman CH, Gardner PA. Endoscopic endonasal approach for pituitary adenomas: a series of 555 patients. *Pituitary.* 2014 Aug;17(4):307–19. doi: 10.1007/s11102-013-0502-4. PMID: 23907570.
2. Loh JA, Verbalis JG. Diabetes insipidus as a complication after pituitary surgery. *Nat Clin Pract Endocrinol Metab.* 2007 Jun;3(6):489–94. doi: 10.1038/ncpendmet0513. PMID: 17515893.
3. Sane T, Rantakari K, Poranen A, Tähtelä R, Välimäki M, Pelkonen R. Hyponatremia after transsphenoidal surgery for pituitary tumors. *J Clin Endocrinol Metab.* 1994 Nov;79(5):1395–8. doi: 10.1210/jcem.79.5.7962334. PMID: 7962334.
4. Lobatto DJ, de Vries F, Zamanipoor Najafabadi AH, Pereira AM, Peul WC, Vliet Vlieland TPM, Biermasz NR, van Furth WR. Preoperative risk factors for postoperative complications in endoscopic pituitary surgery: a systematic review. *Pituitary.* 2018 Feb;21(1):84–97. doi: 10.1007/s11102-017-0839-1. PMID: 28916976; PMCID: PMC5767215.
5. Devuyst F, Kazakou P, Balériaux D, Alexopoulou O, Burniat A, Salenave S, Chanson P, Corvilain B, Maiter D. Central diabetes insipidus and pituitary stalk thickening in adults: distinction of neoplastic from non-neoplastic lesions. *Eur J Endocrinol.* 2020 Jul 1;181(3):95–105. doi: 10.1530/EJE-20-0058. PMID: 32530258.
6. Working Group for Renaming Diabetes Insipidus; Arima H, Cheetham T, Christ-Crain M, Cooper D, Gurnell M, Drummond JB, Levy M, McCormack AI, Verbalis J, Newell-Price J, Wass JAH. Changing the name of diabetes insipidus: a position statement of The Working Group for Renaming Diabetes Insipidus. *Endocr J.* 2022 Nov 28;69(11):1281–4. Doi: 10.1507/endocrj.EJ20220831.
7. Mak D, Schaller AL, Storgion SA, Lahoti A. Evaluating a standardized protocol for the management of diabetes insipidus in pediatric neurosurgical patients. *J Pediatr Endocrinol Metab.* 2021 Sep 27;35(2):197–203. doi: 10.1515/jpem-2021-0305. PMID: 34563107.
8. de Vries F, Lobatto DJ, Verstegen MJT, van Furth WR, Pereira AM, Biermasz NR. Postoperative diabetes insipidus: how to define and grade this complication? *Pituitary.* 2021 Apr;24(2):284–91. doi: 10.1007/s11102-020-01083-7. Epub 2020 Sep 29. PMID: 32990908; PMCID: PMC7966184.
9. Winzeler B, Zweifel C, Nigro N, Arici B, Bally M, Schuetz P, Blum CA, Kelly C, Berkmann S, Huber A, Gentili F, Zadeh G, Landolt H, Mariani L, Müller B, Christ-Crain M. Postoperative copeptin concentration predicts diabetes insipidus after pituitary surgery. *J Clin Endocrinol Metab.* 2015 Jun;100(6):2275–82. doi: 10.1210/jc.2014-4527. Epub 2015 Apr 29. PMID: 25923040.
10. Berton AM, Gatti F, Penner F, Varaldo E, Prencipe N, Rumbolo F, Settanni F, Gasco V, Ghigo E, Zenga F, Grottoli S. Early copeptin determination allows prompt diagnosis of post-neurosurgical central diabetes insipidus. *Neuroendocrinology.* 2020;110(6):525–34. doi: 10.1159/000503145. Epub 2019 Sep 5. PMID: 31484187.
11. Cuesta M, Hannon MJ, Thompson CJ. Adipsic diabetes insipidus in adult patients. *Pituitary.* 2017 Jun;20(3):372–80. doi: 10.1007/s11102-016-0784-4. PMID: 28074401.

CHAPTER

54

How Should We Dose Corticosteroids to Treat Brain Tumors?

Mary Jane Lim-Fat, MD, MSc, FRCPC & Patrick Y. Wen, MD

Case

A 24-year-old woman presents to the emergency department with a 1-week history of worsening headaches, nausea, and gait difficulties. When examining, she has bilateral papilledema and left-sided leg weakness. A computed tomography (CT) head is done showing a large mass with surrounding vasogenic edema. An MRI brain with and without contrast is also obtained urgently (Figure 54–1). What dose and choice of corticosteroid agent would be the most appropriate to treat vasogenic edema in this patient (1) as a temporizing measure prior to surgery (2) postoperatively following tumor debulking if this is found to be a high-grade glioma?

Key Points

- Corticosteroids can be a useful and potent treatment for symptomatic vasogenic edema in patients with brain tumors.
- Given the potentially deleterious side effects, best practice recommends prescribing the lowest possible effective dose, initiating a taper as soon as possible, prescribing the appropriate prophylactic regimens, and monitoring for possible adverse events.

BACKGROUND

Patients with intracranial lesions in particular brain tumors can suffer from significant morbidity due to vasogenic edema involving surrounding healthy tissue. Vasogenic edema can be associated with primary brain tumors such as gliomas, brain metastases, and central nervous system (CNS) lymphoma among other intracranial processes and is caused by the disruption of the normal blood-brain barrier and accumulation of fluid in the extracellular space. The mechanisms through which the blood-brain barrier is disrupted in brain tumors include (i) increased permeability of vessels due to local production of vascular endothelial growth factor (VEGF), leukotrienes, and glutamate[1,2] and (ii) proliferation of "leaky" tumor blood vessels with absent tight endothelial cell junctions due to the secretion of VEGF and basic fibroblast growth factor.[3]

At a cellular level, vasogenic edema from brain tumors can disrupt synaptic transmission and increase neuronal excitability. Clinically, patients can present with headaches, focal neurological deficits, seizures, and encephalopathy. While these are often subacute in onset, they can also present suddenly as increasing mass effect crosses a symptomatic threshold. In addition, headaches associated with increased intracranial pressure (ICP) can be present (worse in the morning or accompanied by nausea or vomiting). Drowsiness, papilledema, and "plateau waves" (syncope or presyncope related to loss of brain perfusion due to high ICP) also signal a more concerning presentation. If progressing rapidly, cerebral edema can lead to brain herniation and death due to mass effect within the confined space of the cranium.

Dexamethasone, due to its low mineralocorticoid potency and high glucocorticoid activity, has long been the corticosteroid of choice in the management of symptomatic cerebral vasogenic edema. Although the exact mechanisms through which dexamethasone exerts antiedema effects is unclear, it appears to partially restore the blood-brain barrier and promote an anti-inflammatory environment.

EVIDENCE AND REVIEW

Evidence for Dexamethasone Dosing

No randomized control trial has been conducted on the ideal dose and regimen of dexamethasone in brain tumor patients with cerebral edema. While the efficacy of dexamethasone in reducing

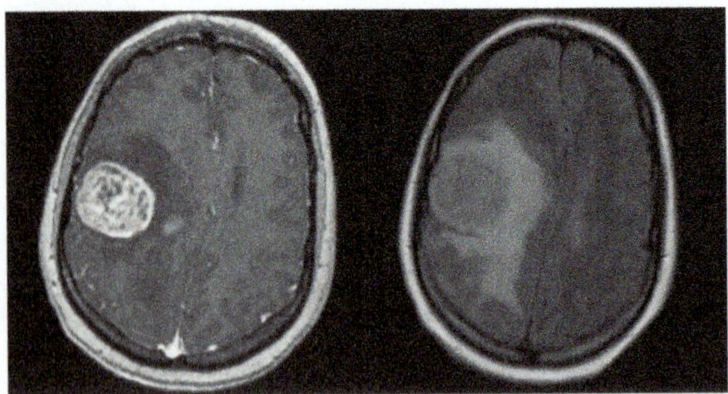

FIGURE 54–1 MRI of brain with and without contrast showing a large contrast enhancing lesion in the left frontoparietal region with surrounding hyperintensity suggestive of vasogenic edema.

vasogenic edema appears to be dose dependent and can often be dramatic, starting at the smallest effective dose and limiting its duration are recommended to reduce the possible adverse effects of corticosteroids. Cushing's syndrome, behavioral changes, myopathy, opportunistic infections, and osteoporosis are all possible steroid-related toxicities. The early use of steroid in primary brain tumors has also been identified as an independent risk factor for increased morbidity and mortality. In glioblastoma, steroid use is related to decreased overall survival, independent of tumor size and performance status.[4] In addition, with newer therapies aimed at augmenting the immune response in the treatment of brain tumors, the use of dexamethasone can be counterproductive.

The ubiquitously adopted "every 6 hour" regimen traces its origin to an often-cited paper by Dr. Joseph Galicich et al from 1961, in which 14 patients with brain-tumor-related edema were treated with an initial bolus of 10 to 40 mg of dexamethasone followed by 4 mg q6h intramuscularly.[5] There is, however, no evidence than a less frequent dosing regimen is inferior, and the biological half-life of dexamethasone is 36 to 54 hours (despite a plasma half-life of 4 hours), with symptomatic benefit for a prolonged duration. More frequent dosing can lead to decreased quality of life related to insomnia, especially if night-time doses are administered on a frequent schedule. A published letter in Neurosurgery, endorsed by several neuro-oncologists and neurosurgeons, advocates for a less liberal use of dexamethasone by opting for once- or twice-daily dosing when possible.[6]

Initiation of Dexamethasone

The most common indications to initiate steroid use in the treatment of vasogenic edema in patients with brain tumors include the symptomatic management of patients perioperatively, during or after radiation therapy, and in the palliative setting following tumor progression. Patients who remain asymptomatic despite the presence of vasogenic edema on imaging do not usually require steroids, unless there is a risk of rapid deterioration (large posterior fossa lesion, tumor-directed therapy with potential for worsening edema, and air travel).

A general approach to dexamethasone use in brain tumor patients is illustrated in Figure 54–2. Dexamethasone is rapidly absorbed and oral or intravenous (IV) dosing can typically be done on a 1:1 conversion ratio.

Frequently, patients with brain lesions are started on steroids as a temporizing measure when they are acutely symptomatic with vasogenic edema. In this setting, a bolus dose of dexamethasone is often initiated in the emergency department or intensive care unit. The use of dexamethasone in this setting is usually as a bridge to surgical debulking or to help with palliative management. While the recommended dose can vary by institution, provider, and patient comorbidities, a typical bolus dose for patients with moderate to severe symptoms include 8 mg IV to 10 mg IV, which is then followed by an oral or IV of up to 16 mg daily in two separate doses. **In patients with mild to moderate symptoms, or who present in a nonemergent setting, 4 to 8 mg divided in one or two daily doses is usually adequate.**

Response Assessment and Steroid Taper

Most patients with steroid-responsive vasogenic edema observe a clinical benefit 1 to 3 days after initiating dexamethasone. An observation period of 3 to 4 days is typically recommended after initiation or dose adjustment to assess for efficacy. After this period, if there is a lack of clinical response, doubling of the dexamethasone dose can be attempted to a maximal total daily dose of 16 mg, and the patient re-evaluated in 72 hours. Lack of a clinical response at this stage would suggest other factors, including tumor progression itself or chronic vasogenic edema, which can be responsible for irreversible neurological deficits in patients with brain tumors.

Altered mental status and headaches have anecdotally been the first symptoms to improve following initiation of dexamethasone, occasionally as quickly as a few hours after the first dose. Focal neurological deficits can often take longer to improve, or may not respond to dexamethasone at all, as they may be the product of direct tumor invasion. As radiological response to steroids can lag by several weeks, clinical response should guide empiric treatment and repeat imaging during this assessment phase is not typically required.

When dexamethasone is found to be ineffective, a rapid taper can usually be used to wean patients off completely within a few days. However, in a previously symptomatic patient with response and stabilization of symptoms on dexamethasone, a gradual taper should be initiated if possible and carefully calibrated to the patient's symptoms. A helpful guide is a reduction by 50% of the total daily dose every 4 days. Many other factors can however affect the speed of tapering, including size of residual tumor, ongoing therapies, duration of steroid use, and adverse effects. Recurrent headaches, lethargy, or worsening focal deficits during steroid reduction may indicate that a dose increase or maintenance is required and warrant a careful and gradual taper. Prednisone, which allows for tapering in smaller increments, can be introduced in patients in whom further reduction of dexamethasone under 1 mg causes rebound symptoms or adrenal insufficiency.

Alternatives to Dexamethasone

Use of dexamethasone should also be avoided when medications specifically directed to symptoms can be used more effectively

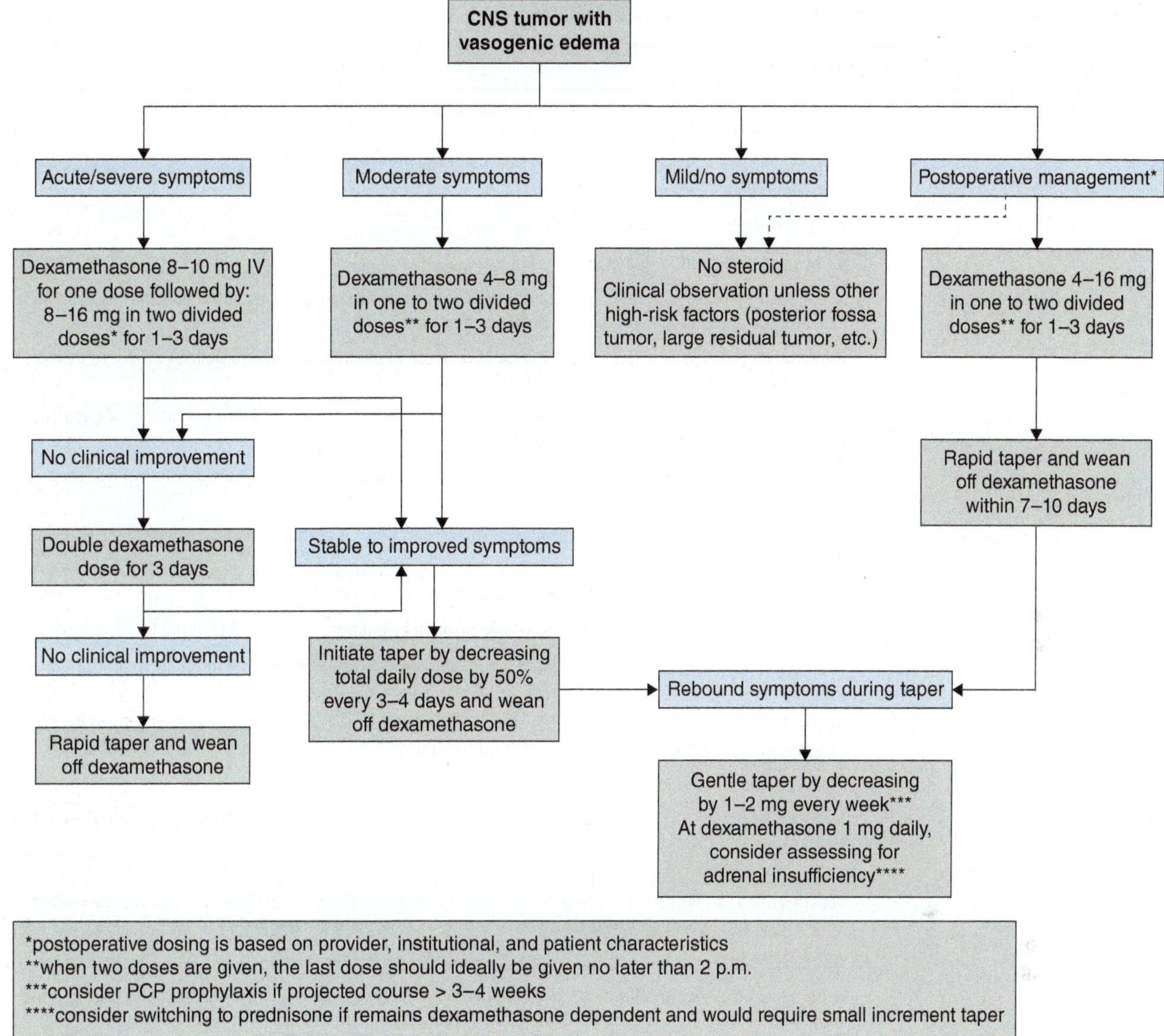

FIGURE 54–2 Proposed algorithm for dexamethasone use in brain tumors.

and in the absence of significant vasogenic edema. For example, optimizing antiseizure medications in a patient with a brain tumor suffering from breakthrough seizures should be prioritized and cannot be substituted with dexamethasone use.

In recent years, bevacizumab (Avastin), a humanized monoclonal antibody inhibiting vascular endothelial growth factor A (VEGF A), has been increasingly introduced as salvage therapy for patients with high-grade gliomas, for the treatment of CNS radiation necrosis, and occasionally in the treatment of patients with brain metastases. While bevacizumab has not been showed to increase overall survival in recurrent high-grade glioma, it can have a dramatic radiological effect on vasogenic edema and confer symptomatic relief of neurological symptoms.[7] Initiation of bevacizumab as salvage tumor-directed therapy needs to be considered very carefully due to possible adverse events (including hypertension, and rarely intracranial hemorrhage, thrombosis, and gastrointestinal [GI] perforation) but can allow steroid-dependent brain tumor patients to be successfully weaned off of dexamethasone.

Word of Caution: The Unidentified CNS Lesion

In patients with a CNS lesion for which a definitive diagnosis has not yet been obtained, caution should be used in the preoperative use of steroids. This is particularly relevant when CNS lymphoma is on the radiological differential. Lymphoma is exquisitely responsive to steroids due to their lymphocytotoxic properties, and any dose of steroid may cause the disappearance of lesions, decrease in the diagnostic yield, and invalidation of the extent of disease evaluation. This in turn delays a definitive diagnosis and treatment plan. Use of steroids in this situation needs to be judicious, accounting for clinical status and timeliness of upcoming interventions or diagnostic procedures.

TABLE 54–1 Management of steroid-related complications.

Complication	Management
Pneumocystis pneumonia (PCP)	• For patients receiving over 2 mg of more of dexamethasone daily for an expected course of >4 weeks, consider the following prophylactic coverage regimens against PCP: 1. trimethoprim-sulfamethoxazole (1 DS [double strength] tablet three times weekly, or 1 SS [single strength] tablet daily) 2. Dapsone (50 mg twice daily or 100 mg daily) 3. Atovaquone (1,500 mg daily). • Respiratory symptoms or fever in a brain tumor patient on dexamethasone should raise the suspicion for PCP and the appropriate workup should be undertaken. • Brain tumor patients who develop PCP should be treated per institutional guidelines similar to other immunocompromised patients with PCP infection.
Gastritis and other GI complications	• Consider prophylactic therapy perioperatively (particularly in patients with known history of gastritis, gastroesophageal reflux, or peptic ulcer disease). • A proton-pump inhibitor such as omeprazole can be prescribed for daily prophylaxis in patients with gastritis or high risk of GI intolerance. • Risk of more severe GI complications is compounded if patients are also on medications such as NSAIDs and concurrent anticoagulation.
Steroid myopathy	• Typically occurs after 9-12 weeks of treatment; onset can be variable. • Typically subacute-onset painless progressive proximal weakness most notable in the lower extremities. • Lowest possible dose of steroid should be used, and every attempt should be made to wean the patient off of steroids. • In steroid-dependent patients, equivalent doses of prednisone (compared to dexamethasone) may cause less severe myopathy and could be used as substitution. • Physical therapy should be encouraged.
Bone health	• Long-term sequelae of steroid use such as osteoporosis and subsequent fractures traditionally do not warrant upfront prophylaxis in brain tumor patients. • Patients early in their disease course, with a longer life expectancy, and additional risk factors (postmenopausal women, known osteoporosis or low bone density, and frequent falls) can be started on calcium supplements (1,500 mg/day) with vitamin D (at least 800 IU daily) should be considered. • Bisphosphonates can be prescribed with the input of an endocrinologist.
Adrenal insufficiency	• Adrenal insufficiency should be screened in patients receiving >20 mg of prednisone daily (about 3 mg of dexamethasone) for over 3 weeks or who have clinical symptoms of Cushing syndrome. • The adrenocorticotropic hormone (ACTH) stimulation test which can be done before dexamethasone is lowered to subphysiological levels (lower than 0.5-1 mg daily of dexamethasone).

Prophylaxis and Management of Complications

Common side effects of corticosteroids such as fluid retention, weight gain, increased appetite, insomnia, and easy bruising can arise after a few days. For patients who are steroid dependent, a protracted course of dexamethasone can, in addition, increase the risk of additional medical complications and adverse effects. In this context, it is essential to consider prophylactic coverage, careful clinical monitoring, and frequent discussions about the risks and benefits of ongoing steroid use (Table 54–1).

REFERENCES

1. Baethmann A, Maier-Hauff K, Schürer L, et al. Release of glutamate and of free fatty acids in vasogenic brain edema. *J Neurosurg*. 1989;70(4):578–591. doi:10.3171/jns.1989.70.4.0578
2. Black KL, Hoff JT, McGillicuddy JE, Gebarski SS. Increased leukotriene C4 and vasogenic edema surrounding brain tumors in humans. *Ann Neurol*. 1986;19(6):592–595. doi:10.1002/ana.410190613
3. Dobrogowska DH, Lossinsky AS, Tarnawski M, Vorbrodt AW. Increased blood-brain barrier permeability and endothelial abnormalities induced by vascular endothelial growth factor. *J Neurocytol*. 1998;27(3):163–173. doi:10.1023/A:1006907608230
4. Pitter KL, Tamagno I, Alikhanyan K, et al. Corticosteroids compromise survival in glioblastoma. *Brain*. 2016;139(Pt 5):1458–1471. doi:10.1093/brain/aww046
5. Galicich JH, French LA, Melby JC. Use of dexamethasone in treatment of cerebral edema associated with brain tumors. *J Lancet*. 1961;81:46–53. http://www.ncbi.nlm.nih.gov/pubmed/13703072. Accessed January 9, 2019.
6. Lim-Fat MJ, Bi WL, Lo J, et al. Letter: When less is more: dexamethasone dosing for brain tumors. *Neurosurgery*. 2019;85(3):E607–E608. doi:10.1093/neuros/nyz186
7. Gerstner ER, Duda DG, di Tomaso E, et al. VEGF inhibitors in the treatment of cerebral edema in patients with brain cancer. *Nat Rev Clin Oncol*. 2009;6(4):229–236. doi:10.1038/nrclinonc.2009.14

CHAPTER

55

How Should We Think About Dysphagia Management in Patients with Cranial Nerve Deficits?

Elliana K. Devore, MD,
Jameson Cooper, MS, CCC-SLP,
Tessa Goldsmith, MA, CCC-SLP, &
Matthew R. Naunheim, MD, MBA

Case

A 44-year-old woman undergoes a posterior fossa approach and resection of a jugular foramen meningioma. Three days out from surgery, she still has persistent dysphagia and clear aspiration of liquids with attempted bedside swallow. How should we think about evaluating and managing her condition?

Key Points

- Cranial nerve deficits, particularly those impacting the hypoglossal and vagus nerves, can result in dysphagia, dysphonia, and aspiration increasing the risk of medical complications and reduced quality of life.
- Optimal diagnosis and management requires thorough evaluation by a multidisciplinary team.
- Management and treatment may include noninvasive therapeutic interventions or surgical interventions selected based off of the pathophysiology of an individual's dysphagia and patient/caregiver goals of care.

BACKGROUND

Oropharyngeal dysphagia is a disorder of deglutition in which there is a disturbance in the sequential and rhythmic transport of liquid and solid materials from the oral cavity, through the pharynx, and into the esophagus. Dysphagia affects over 50 million adults worldwide,[1–4] including those with neuromuscular disorders and neurodegenerative disease, as well as hospitalized, elderly, and chronically ill patients. It is associated with serious mortality and morbidity due to malnutrition and aspiration pneumonia, in addition to a significant social and psychological burden for both patients and caregivers.[5–6] Furthermore, dysphagia contributes to increased length of stay and hospital costs.[7–8] Despite its impact on health and quality of life, oropharyngeal dysphagia remains underdiagnosed and underestimated as a major disorder for several populations, including those recently undergoing neurosurgical procedures and patients admitted to neurocritical care units.

EVIDENCE AND REVIEW

The Normal Swallow

The oropharyngeal swallow is a series of coordinated neuromuscular events that require the integrity of several central and peripheral nervous system structures.[9] Safe swallowing requires intact peripheral sensation, coordination with the respiratory cycle, and the motor reconfiguration of the upper aerodigestive tract into a closed valve system, to allow for adequate and efficient propulsion of food and liquid boluses into the esophagus.[10] Damage to any part of the multiple central or peripheral nervous system structures can result in impaired airway protection increasing the risk for aspiration or pharyngeal residue affecting swallow efficiency.

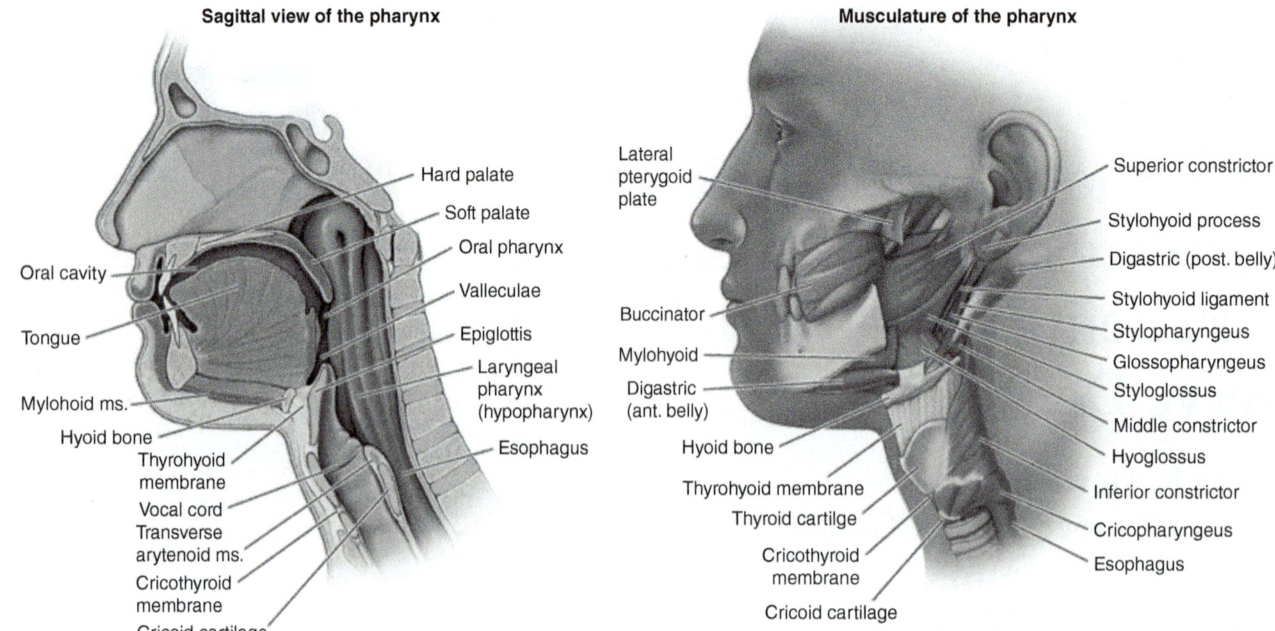

FIGURE 55–1 Anatomy of the oral cavity, pharynx, and larynx. (Reproduced with permission from Dennis L. Kasper, Anthony S. Fauci, Stephen L. Hauser, Dan L. Longo, J. Larry Jameson, Joseph Loscalzo. *Harrison's Principles of internal medicine*. 19th ed. New York: McGraw-Hill Education; 2017).

A primary prerequisite is the patient's cognitive ability to attend to and engage with the bolus within the oral cavity. The swallow begins with the oral phase, during which a bolus (liquid or solid) is manipulated in the oral cavity in preparation for transit through the pharynx (Figure 55–1). During this voluntary phase, bolus formation and control is largely the function of the intrinsic and extrinsic muscles of the tongue, which drives the bolus posteriorly into the pharynx.

Next, taste and mechanoreceptor sensory signals are sent along cranial nerves (CN) IX and X to the rostral portion of the nucleus tractus solitarius in the medulla oblongata,[11] where the central pattern generator triggers a complex motoric sequence from the nucleus ambiguus for the function of protecting the airway and driving the bolus into the esophagus.[12] This rapid cascade of events occurs in <1 second,[13] including contraction of levator veli palatini to close the velopharyngeal port, laryngeal closure to protect the airway, and the gross anterosuperior mobilization of the hyolaryngeal complex and pharynx by way of anterior and posterior muscular slings.[14] This allows the base of tongue and pharyngeal constrictors to drive the bolus through a relaxed upper esophageal sphincter. Intact sensation is not only crucial for triggering timely airway closure to prevent and respond to aspiration but also sends signals to extrapyramidal circuits, modulating motor patterns based on bolus texture, viscosity, size, and environmental conditions.[14]

Manifestations of Cranial Nerve Deficits in Dysphagia

Diseases affecting the base of skull may result in damage to lower CN, causing dysfunction of the larynx and oropharynx manifesting as dysphagia, dysphonia, and aspiration. Although patients may tolerate isolated injury,[15] combined deficits, particularly those involving CN IX, X, and XII, portend devastating disruption to swallow physiology.[16–17] For instance, aspiration is observed in 73% of posttreatment adult patients with posterior fossa lesions.[18–21]

Contribution of CN and their functional supply are listed in Table 55–1. Dysfunction of CN V and VII may contribute to difficulty with jaw depression and rotary mastication, leading to drooling or anterior loss of a bolus from the mouth. Buccinator tone is important to prevent the loss of a bolus to the lateral sulci. Injury to sensory pathways can impact proprioception and awareness of bolus positioning. There are additional contributions to salivation and taste which can lead to dry mouth and poor appetite.

Hypoglossal nerve (CN XII) deficits can result in challenges with bolus preparation, mobilization of the bolus into the pharynx, and overall reduced driving pressures. Base of tongue weakness has been shown to result in incomplete transit of the bolus, leading to residue within the vallecula especially with viscous boluses. Additionally, the base of tongue plays a role in airway protection by assisting with the retroflexion of the epiglottis during the swallow, which serves as one aspect of laryngeal closure.[10]

Glossopharyngeal (CN IX) deficits can affect swallow initiation and impact bolus clearance through reduced pharyngeal elevation and inhibited proprioception. Injury of the vagus nerve (CN X) at the skull base can impact the pharyngeal swallow in several ways, including weakness of the muscles of pharyngeal constriction and elevation, thereby reducing the necessary driving forces within the pharynx, and velopharyngeal insufficiency, resulting in nasal regurgitation. Additionally, CN X injury can impact airway protection through vocal fold paralysis, raising the risk of aspiration due to glottic incompetence, and reducing

TABLE 55–1 Oropharyngeal musculature and innervation for swallowing.

Cranial Nerve	Muscle	Action	Functional Impact
V3 trigeminal motor	Pterygoid lateral	Lateralizes mandible	Mastication
	Pterygoid medial	Elevates mandible	Closes and opens
	Masseter	Elevates and protrudes the mandible	Closes jaw
	Temporalis	Elevation and retraction of the mandible	Closes jaw and moves posteriorly to align with maxilla
	Anterior belly of digastric	Elevates and stabilizes hyoid	Assists in laryngeal closure
	Mylohyoid	Elevates hyoid	Assists in laryngeal movement
	Tensor veli palatini	Stiffens soft palate	Assists in velopharyngeal closure
V3 trigeminal sensory		Senses food in the mouth	Touch, pain, and temperature for anterior tongue, teeth, face
		Proprioception	Jaw and teeth
VII facial	Orbicularis oris	Round and close lips	Contains bolus in the mouth
	Buccinator	Contracts cheek musculature	Prevents boluses in lateral sulci
	Posterior belly of digastric	Depresses mandible, elevates hyoid	
VII facial sensory	Anterior 2/3 tongue	Taste	
IX glossopharyngeal	Stylopharyngeus	Elevates pharynx and larynx during swallowing	
IX glossopharyngeal sensory	Posterior tongue	Taste	
	Upper pharynx	Touch pain, temperature	Assists with swallow initiation
X vagus (pharyngeal branch)	Palatoglossus	Elevates posterior tongue during swallowing	Contains bolus in oral cavity
	Levator veli palatini	Elevates soft palate	Seals off velopharyngeal port
	Palatopharyngeus	Shortens and widens pharynx	
	Salpingopharyngeus		
	Pharyngeal constrictors	Contract medially	Squeeze food and liquid into the esophagus
	True vocal folds	Adduct	Close airway during swallowing
X vagus sensory	Lower pharynx, larynx, esophagus	Temperature, touch, pain	Responds to noxious stimuli
XII hypoglossal	Intrinsic muscles: longitudinal, vertical, transverse	Alters shape of tongue	Positions food or liquid in oral cavity
			Oropharyngeal bolus transport
C1	Geniohyoid	Elevates hyoid forward, depresses mandible	Closes laryngeal vestibule

Adapted from Maynard T, Zohn I, Moody S, LaMantia A-S. Suckling, feeding, and swallowing: behaviors, circuits, and targets for neurodevelopmental pathology. *Annu Rev Neurosci.* 2020;43. 10.1146/annurev-neuro-100419-100636.

the effectiveness of a cough needed to clear aspirate from the lower airway. Injury to vagal sensory pathways can delay timing of airway closure or the pharyngeal swallow itself, leading to laryngeal penetration or aspiration, often with absent sensation (silent aspiration).

Diagnosis

Accurate identification of oropharyngeal dysphagia involves a multidisciplinary team including nurses, intensivists, otolaryngologists, gastroenterologists, pulmonologists, neurologists, neurosurgeons, rehabilitation physicians, dietitians, and radiologists, though it is primarily diagnosed and managed by speech-language pathologists (SLP). In patients at risk of cranial nerve injury, clinical signs of weak cough, dysphonia (particularly breathiness), tongue or facial weakness affecting speech intelligibility, subjective swallowing difficulty, difficulty with secretion management, or oxygen desaturations often prompt evaluation. Screening protocols[22–23] may be used to recognize patients at risk for aspiration and guide diagnostic strategies and are often integrated into various guidelines and auditing systems, especially in stroke units.[24–25] Examples include the Yale Swallow Protocol,[26] or modifications thereof, which can identify concerning features for oropharyngeal dysphagia prompting further workup. Of note, gag reflex testing has demonstrated low sensitivity for detecting dysphagia, limiting its value as a screening tool.[27]

Patients with suspected oropharyngeal dysphagia should be referred to an SLP for evaluation. A Clinical Swallow Evaluation consists of a thorough oral mechanism exam and observation of food/liquid trials. These examinations evaluate manipulation and coordination of bolus formation and identify signs of struggle including coughing, throat clearing, wet vocal quality, or changes in respiratory rate. Tasks to specifically assess cranial nerve dysfunction related to swallowing are summarized in Table 55–2.

Given the high frequency of silent aspiration in patients with neurologically mediated dysphagia, an instrumental assessment may be recommended. Videofluoroscopic Swallow Study (VFSS), also known as Modified Barium Swallow Study, permits direct visualization of oropharyngeal anatomy and physiology during swallowing. The VFSS is performed by the SLP in collaboration with a radiologist to allow real-time continuous fluoroscopic imaging of swallow function using radiopaque barium of different consistencies. The biomechanical causes of the dysphagia are discerned, as well as the patient's response to aspiration into the airway or accumulation of residue in the pharynx. During this exam, there may be a progression from small to larger boluses of progressive liquid and solid consistencies.[28] With the specific pathophysiology identified, the efficacy of targeted compensatory postural strategies or texture modifications can be directly evaluated.

Flexible Endoscopic Evaluation of Swallowing (FEES) is another instrumental assessment that may be performed at the bedside, utilizing a transnasal laryngoscope to visualize the oropharynx and larynx during swallow. The benefits of direct laryngoscopy include visualization of secretion management

TABLE 55–2 Tasks to assess cranial nerve dysfunction related to swallowing.

Cranial Nerve	Sensory	Motor
V	Have the patient close their eyes. Using a swab or similar object, lightly brush across the following: • Forehead (V1) • Zygomatic arch (V2) • Mandible (V3). Have the patient open their mouth and test the following: • Dorsum of the tongue bilaterally (V3) • Interior aspect of the buccal surface Patient should identify the location and relative differences in sensation.	Assess range and strength of mandibular depression and closure during tasks. • Patients should open and close their mouth and move the jaw side to side. Observe maximal incisal opening. • Place fingers under the jaw and instruct patients to open their jaw against clinician resistance. • Patient should open their mouth. Place fingers gently on the chin and instruct the patient to close their jaw against resistance.
VII	Ask targeted questions to identify taste changes, though this is less relevant to swallow function.	Observe facial symmetry at rest and during sustained facial positions for the following: *Zygomatic/buccal branches* Smile, lip seal, lip protrusion (kiss), lip retraction (smile), and cheek puff against pressure (pressing fingers into inflated cheeks). *Temporal branch* Raise and furrow the eyebrows.
IX	Assess gag function by stimulating the anterior faucial pillars, posterior tongue, and lateral/posterior oropharynx with a swab.	
X	Assess voice quality for wetness or gurgling suggestive secretions in the larynx and pharynx. Does the patient require oral/pharyngeal suction? Further testing can include light stimulation of the posterior pharyngeal wall bilaterally with a cotton swab.	Assess voice quality for dysphonia, paying particular attention to breathiness. Observe for velar/palatal asymmetry at rest, during phonation (say *ah ah ah*), and during stimulation of the gag. During stimulation of the gag, observe for medialization of the lateral oropharyngeal walls.
XII		Observe the symmetry and tone of the tongue at rest, noting areas of atrophy, tremulousness, or fasciculations. Observe the symmetry during repeated and sustained tongue protrusion. Test tongue strength with protrusion and lateralization to resistance from a tongue depressor, noting initial strength and vulnerability to fatigue bilaterally.

Adapted from Duffy JR. *Motor speech disorders: substrates, differential diagnosis, and management*. Elsevier, St. Louis, Missouri, USA. 2020.

and assessment of vocal fold function as it relates to swallowing and cough. Liquid and food trials are administered, during which an SLP visualizes the motoric and sensory components of the swallow. Symmetry of pharyngeal and laryngeal function is clearly elucidated with this examination technique. Assessment of laryngeal penetration or aspiration is detected by visualization of the bolus in the laryngeal vestibule or trachea prior to or after the swallow. While FEES has a high sensitivity for aspiration, it does not allow for evaluation of the oral phase of the swallow, nor of airway protection as the swallow occurs. In addition, this test does not provide information about the cervical esophageal stage of swallowing.

Both VFSS and FEES are crucial tools for assessing oropharyngeal swallow function. They are considered complementary evaluations, both with their strengths and limitations. As such, the recommendations to utilize either may consider multiple factors including test availability, patient appropriateness, acuity, and the nature of the clinical suspicion.

Management

Treatment for patients experiencing dysphagia due to cranial nerve injury comprises nonsurgical, surgical adjunctive, and definitive procedures. Once a pathophysiology is identified, treatment and management of dysphagia may use a combined approach of compensatory and therapeutic strategies including diet modifications, positional strategies, and therapeutic exercises.[29–30] Diet modifications can be effective at improving swallow safety and efficiency, although recent review found conflicting evidence regarding impact on airway protection and postswallow residue.[31] Given the documented negative impact diet modifications can have on quality of life and overall nutrition and hydration,[31] dysphagia treatment by a trained SLP is essential to navigate the nuanced decision-making in order find the balance between swallow safety, efficiency, and a patient's specific goals and values.

Surgical adjunctive therapies for cranial nerve deficits are limited. Sensory deficits, hypoglossal injury, and palatal weakness to date have no surgical interventions, whereas vagal deficits can be addressed procedurally, albeit not curatively. Injuries to CNX often begin with injection laryngoplasty to increase the bulk of vocal fold tissue, enabling complete laryngeal closure and airway protection during swallow.[32] Laryngeal framework surgery may be pursued to enhance glottic closure with more permanent intent, usually months after the initial insult if there is no spontaneous improvement.[33] Laryngeal reinnervation represents an emerging surgical option, with preliminary analysis suggesting sustained benefit.[34] For patients with an obstructive pattern at the upper esophageal sphincter, surgical cricopharyngeal myotomy or injection of botulin toxin may be pursued to improve sphincter compliance and reduce strength needed for bolus propulsion.[35] Palatal obturators can enhance velopharyngeal competence in the patient with stable disease.

For patients with significant aspiration or aspiration risk, definitive procedures separate the alimentary tract from the airway. In the immediate hospitalization period, a nasogastric feeding tube offers a short-term solution for nutrition and hydration where improvement in swallow function is expected. Patients with severe alterations in swallowing unresponsive to short-term rehabilitation may require longer term nonoral feeding, such as via gastrostomy tube.[1] The decision to pursue gastrostomy tube placement requires joint discussions between the patient, caretakers, SLP, and primary physicians and may be reassessed at multiple points during a patient's recovery. Gastrostomy tubes do not prevent aspiration of oral secretions or regurgitated gastric contents, and thus risk of aspiration pneumonia persists.[35–36] Tracheostomy placement may be pursued for patients with prolonged intubation or multiple extubation attempts, as well as those with sustained laryngeal dysfunction. Finally, in cases of refractory laryngeal and aerodigestive dysfunction, laryngotracheal separation or total laryngectomy may be considered.

REFERENCES

1. Rofes L, Arreola V, Almirall J, et al. Diagnosis and management of oropharyngeal dysphagia and its nutritional and respiratory complications in the elderly. *Gastroenterol Res Pract.* 2011;2011:818979. doi: 10.1155/2011/818979. Epub 2010 Aug 3. PMID: 20811545; PMCID: PMC2929516.
2. Takizawa C, Gemmell E, Kenworthy J, Speyer R. A Systematic Review of the Prevalence of oropharyngeal dysphagia in stroke, Parkinson's disease, Alzheimer's disease, head injury, and pneumonia. *Dysphagia.* 2016 Jun;31(3):434–41. doi: 10.1007/s00455-016-9695-9. Epub 2016 Mar 12. PMID: 26970760.
3. Ekberg O, Hamdy S, Woisard V, Wuttge-Hannig A, Ortega P. Social and psychological burden of dysphagia: its impact on diagnosis and treatment. *Dysphagia.* 2002 Spring;17(2):139–46. doi: 10.1007/s00455-001-0113-5. PMID: 11956839.
4. Hutcheson KA, Nurgalieva Z, Zhao H, et al. Two-year prevalence of dysphagia and related outcomes in head and neck cancer survivors: an updated SEER-Medicare analysis. Head Neck. 2019 Feb;41(2):479–87. doi: 10.1002/hed.25412. Epub 2018 Dec 7. PMID: 30536748; PMCID: PMC6355350.
5. Falsetti P, Acciai C, Palilla R, et al. Oropharyngeal dysphagia after stroke: incidence, diagnosis, and clinical predictors in patients admitted to a neurorehabilitation unit. *J Stroke Cerebrovasc Dis.* 2009 Sep-Oct;18(5):329–35. doi: 10.1016/j.jstrokecerebrovasdis.2009.01.009. PMID: 19717014.
6. Crary MA, Carnaby GD, Sia I, Khanna A, Waters MF. Spontaneous swallowing frequency has potential to identify dysphagia in acute stroke. *Stroke.* 2013 Dec;44(12):3452–7. doi: 10.1161/STROKEAHA.113.003048. Epub 2013 Oct 22. PMID: 24149008; PMCID: PMC3902546.
7. Qureshi AI, Suri MFK, Huang W, et al. Annual direct cost of dysphagia associated with acute ischemic stroke in the United States. *J Stroke Cerebrovasc Dis.* 2022 May;31(5):106407. doi: 10.1016/j.jstrokecerebrovasdis.2022.106407. Epub 2022 Mar 5. PMID: 35259613.
8. Attrill S, White S, Murray J, Hammond S, Doeltgen S. Impact of oropharyngeal dysphagia on healthcare cost and length of stay in hospital: a systematic review. *BMC Health Serv Res.* 2018 Aug 2;18(1):594. doi: 10.1186/s12913-018-3376-3. PMID: 30068326; PMCID: PMC6090960.
9. Shaw SM, Martino R. The normal swallow: muscular and neurophysiological control. *Otolaryngol Clin North Am.* 2013 Dec;46(6):937–56. doi: 10.1016/j.otc.2013.09.006. Epub 2013 Oct 23. PMID: 24262952.
10. Vose A, Humbert I. "Hidden in Plain Sight": A descriptive review of laryngeal vestibule closure. *Dysphagia.* 2019 Jun;34(3):281–9. doi: 10.1007/s00455-018-9928-1. Epub 2018 Jul 30. PMID: 30062547; PMCID: PMC6408979.
11. AbuAlrob MA, Tadi P. Neuroanatomy, Nucleus Solitarius. 2022 Jul 25. In: StatPearls [Internet]. Treasure Island (FL): StatPearls Publishing; 2022 Jan–. PMID: 31751021

12. Petko B, Tadi P. Neuroanatomy, Nucleus Ambiguus. 2022 Jul 25. In: StatPearls [Internet]. Treasure Island (FL): StatPearls Publishing; 2022 Jan–. PMID: 31613524.
13. Colevas SM, Stalter LN, Jones CA, McCulloch TM. The natural swallow: factors affecting subject choice of bolus volume and pharyngeal swallow parameters in a self-selected swallow. *Dysphagia.* 2022 Oct;37(5):1172–82. doi: 10.1007/s00455-021-10373-6. Epub 2021 Oct 23. PMID: 34687378
14. Pearson WG, Grifeth JV, Ennis JV. Functional anatomy underlying pharyngeal swallowing mechanics and swallowing performance goals. Perspect ASHA SIG. 2019;4(4):1–8.
15. Patel MA, Eytan DF, Bishop J, Califano JA. Favorable swallowing outcomes following vagus nerve sacrifice for vagal schwannoma resection. *Otolaryngol Head Neck Surg.* 2017 Feb;156(2):329–33. doi: 10.1177/0194599816678210. PMID: 27899468.
16. Bennion BR, Herzon F, Clark CR. Rehabilitation of cranial nerve deficits affecting laryngeal and oropharyngeal function. *Oper Tech Otolaryngol Head Neck Surg.* 1996;7(2):200–7.
17. Eibling DE, Boyd EM. Rehabilitation of lower cranial nerve deficits. *Otolaryngol Clin North Am.* 1997 Oct;30(5):865–75. PMID: 9295257.
18. Wadhwa R, Toms J, Chittiboina P, et al. Dysphagia following posterior fossa surgery in adults. *World Neurosurg.* 2014 Nov;82(5):822–7. doi: 10.1016/j.wneu.2013.01.035. Epub 2013 Jan 11. PMID: 23318935.
19. Morgan AT, Sell D, Ryan M, Raynsford E, Hayward R. Pre and post-surgical dysphagia outcome associated with posterior fossa tumour in children. *J Neurooncol.* 2008 May;87(3):347–54. doi: 10.1007/s11060-008-9524-6. Epub 2008 Jan 22. PMID: 18209951.
20. Rajendran S, Antonios J, Solomon B, et al. A prospective evaluation of swallowing and speech in patients with neurofibromatosis type 2. *J Neurol Surg B Skull Base.* 2021 Apr;82(2):244–50. doi: 10.1055/s-0039-1694054. Epub 2019 Sep 18. PMID: 33777639; PMCID: PMC7987378.
21. Best SR, Ahn J, Langmead S, et al. Voice and swallowing dysfunction in neurofibromatosis 2. *Otolaryngol Head Neck Surg.* 2018 Mar;158(3):505–10. doi: 10.1177/0194599817741839. Epub 2017 Nov 21. PMID: 29160153.
22. Fedder WN. Review of Evidenced-based nursing protocols for dysphagia assessment. *Stroke.* 2017 Apr;48(4):e99–101. doi: 10.1161/STROKEAHA.116.011738. Epub 2017 Mar 9. PMID: 28280136.
23. Chen PC, Chuang CH, Leong CP, Guo SE, Hsin YJ. Systematic review and meta-analysis of the diagnostic accuracy of the water swallow test for screening aspiration in stroke patients. *J Adv Nurs.* 2016 Nov;72(11):2575–86. doi: 10.1111/jan.13013. Epub 2016 May 29. PMID: 27237447.
24. Party ISW. *National clinical guideline for stroke*, 5th ed. London, UK: Royal College of Physicians. 2016.
25. Jauch EC, Saver JL, Adams HP, Jr., et al. Guidelines for the early management of patients with acute ischemic stroke. *Stroke.* 2013;44:870–947.
26. Suiter DM, Sloggy J, Leder SB. Validation of the Yale Swallow Protocol: a prospective double-blinded videofluoroscopic study. *Dysphagia.* 2014 Apr;29(2):199–203. doi: 10.1007/s00455-013-9488-3. Epub 2013 Sep 12. PMID: 24026519
27. Ramsey D, Smithard D, Donaldson N, Kalra L. Is the gag reflex useful in the management of swallowing problems in acute stroke? *Dysphagia.* 2005 Spring;20(2):105–7. doi: 10.1007/s00455-004-0024-3. PMID: 16172818.
28. Dhar SI, Nativ-Zeltzer N, Starmer H, et al. The American Broncho-Esophagological Association position statement on swallowing fluoroscopy. *Laryngoscope.* 2022 May 11. doi: 10.1002/lary.30177. Epub ahead of print. PMID: 35543231.
29. Speyer R, Baijens L, Heijnen M, Zwijnenberg I. Effects of therapy in oropharyngeal dysphagia by speech and language therapists: a systematic review. *Dysphagia.* 2010 Mar;25(1):40–65. doi: 10.1007/s00455-009-9239-7. Epub 2009 Sep 17. PMID: 19760458; PMCID: PMC2846331.
30. Chen S, Kent B, Cui Y. Interventions to prevent aspiration in older adults with dysphagia living in nursing homes: a scoping review. *BMC Geriatr.* 2021 Jul 17;21(1):429. doi: 10.1186/s12877-021-02366-9. PMID: 34273953; PMCID: PMC8285814.
31. Steele CM, Alsanei WA, Ayanikalath S, et al. The influence of food texture and liquid consistency modification on swallowing physiology and function: a systematic review. *Dysphagia.* 2015 Feb;30(1):2–26. doi: 10.1007/s00455-014-9578-x. Epub 2014 Oct 25. Erratum in: Dysphagia. 2015 Apr;30(2):272-3. PMID: 25343878; PMCID: PMC4342510.
32. Mallur PS, Rosen CA. Vocal fold injection: review of indications, techniques, and materials for augmentation. *Clin Exp Otorhinolaryngol.* Dec 2010;3(4):177–82. doi:10.3342/ceo.2010.3.4.177
33. Coulter M, Marvin K, Brigger M, Johnson CM. Dysphagia outcomes following surgical management of unilateral vocal fold immobility: a systematic review and meta-analysis. *Otolaryngol Head Neck Surg.* 2022 Jan 12: 1945998211072832. doi: 10.1177/01945998211072832. Epub ahead of print. PMID: 35021908.
34. Baki MM, Clarke P, Birchall MA. Immediate selective laryngeal reinnervation in vagal paraganglioma patients. *J Laryngol Otol.* 2018;132(9):846–51.
35. Panebianco M, Marchese-Ragona R, Masiero S, Restivo DA. Dysphagia in neurological diseases: a literature review. *Neurol Sci.* 2020 Nov;41(11):3067–73. doi: 10.1007/s10072-020-04495-2. Epub 2020 Jun 7. PMID: 32506360; PMCID: PMC7567719.
36. Finucane TE, Bynum JP. Use of tube feeding to prevent aspiration pneumonia. *Lancet.* 1996; 348(9039):1421–4.

SECTION VII SPINE

CHAPTER 56

What Should Be Our Blood Pressure Targets Following Spinal Cord Injury?

Jose A. Torres, BS, Ebubechi Okwumabua, MD, & James Edward Showery, MD

Case

A 55-year-old man falls down the stairs and suffers a fracture dislocation of his cervical spine with a partial spinal cord injury. He is taken for emergent fracture reduction, decompression, and fusion. Afterward, what blood pressure targets should be set to maximize his chance of neurologic recovery?

Key Points

- Achieving a mean arterial pressure (MAP) goal of 80 to 95 mm Hg with volume resuscitation and pharmacologic agents appears to be ideal for optimizing neurologic recovery. MAP events below 70 mm Hg should be minimized as this appears to be the threshold associated with decreased odds of neurologic improvement.
- Negative effects of hypotensive events on neurologic outcomes are most pronounced within the first 72 hours after injury. Hypotensive events after 72 hours after injury through 7 days after injury may negatively impact neurologic outcomes to a lesser extent.
- Norepinephrine appears to be the most effective vasopressor in preserving spinal cord perfusion after cervical and upper thoracic spinal cord injury (SCI).
- Potential risks of the use of vasopressors for MAP support in patients with existing risk factors for adverse effects should be considered on a case-by-case basis prior to initiation of pharmacologic blood pressure support in SCI.

BACKGROUND

Traumatic spinal cord injury (SCI) disrupts normal spinal cord blood flow through several pathophysiological mechanisms. Hypoperfusion and relative hypoxia of the spinal cord in the traumatized and adjacent segments likely impair neurologic recovery after injury. Additionally, SCI frequently results in systemic hypotension through loss of sympathetic tone to the sinoatrial node and peripheral vasculature. Hemorrhage and edema are thought to further contribute to spinal cord hypoxia after injury through mechanical effects on local perfusion. Lastly, hypoperfusion impairs the clearance of inflammatory cytokines that contribute to neuronal apoptosis.

EVIDENCE AND REVIEW

Mean Arterial Pressure (MAP) Targets

Blood pressure targets and avoidance of hypotension have been utilized in the management of SCI since the 1970s. A 1997 study by Vale et al demonstrated better-than-expected neurologic outcomes with the implementation of an institutional SCI management protocol that included MAP maintenance with volume resuscitation and vasopressor support for a minimum of 6 days after injury as well as intravenous (IV) methylprednisolone per NASCIS II protocol.[2] Since the publication of this study, many SCI centers have adopted similar protocols for MAP goals while IV methylprednisolone is no longer recommended.[1] Subsequent studies from many of these centers have attempted to further identify parameters for optimal blood pressure management after SCI. While knowledge gained from more recently published literature may help guide management, there are still many unknowns due to significant limitations in the available studies. The Randomized Trial of Early Hemodynamic Management of Patients Following Acute Spinal Cord Injury (TEMPLE study) comparing MAP goals of 65 to 70 mm Hg to MAP goals of 85 to 90 mm Hg is currently underway and is scheduled to report results in late 2023 (NCT02878850). Until the results of this study complete the peer-review process, the premise that pharmacologic blood pressure augmentation after SCI improves neurologic outcomes remains in question. To date, there is no causal evidence that maintaining MAP through the use of IV vasopressor administration improves neurologic outcomes after SCI.

With this in mind, it is possible to delineate what we know and what we don't in regard to blood pressure goals after SCI. Nearly every study comparing neurologic outcomes and MAP after SCI has occurred in centers with existing protocols for MAP maintenance after injury. Despite best efforts to maintain MAP within goal parameters, episodic hypotension occurred frequently in nearly every study, with Haldrup et al reporting that MAP fell below the goal of 80 mm Hg 18.4% and 35.9% of the time in subjects with cervical and thoracic spine injuries, respectively.[3] In practical application, the intention to maintain MAP above a certain threshold is the intervention, not the actual success in maintaining that goal, and the challenge of consistently maintaining MAP within goal parameters serves as a reflection of the complexity of this patient population. Thus, we suggest that retrospective studies evaluating neurologic outcomes in patients who fell outside MAP parameters should be interpreted with caution (Table 56–1).

TABLE 56–1 Selected studies evaluating effect of MAP goals on neurologic recovery after SCI.

Year	Author	Study Population	*N*	Intervention	Results
1997	Vale et al	Cervical and thoracic SCI	Cervical = 45 Thoracic = 32	MAP >85 mm Hg 6 days minimum in this study • IV fluids • IV dopamine (2.5-5 mg/kg/min), followed by norepinephrine if needed (0.01-0.2mg/kg/min) • All patients received methylprednisolone protocol per NASCIS I	Complete (ASIA A) Cervical • 60% improved 1 ASIA grade • 30% regained the ability to walk Complete (ASIA A) thoracic • 33% improved 1 ASIA grade • 10% regained the ability to walk Incomplete cervical • 92% improved neurologically • 92% regained the ability to walk Incomplete thoracic • 88% improved neurologically • 88% regained the ability to walk
2010	Cohn et al	Complete cervical SCI	17	Outcomes compared to time spent at different MAP thresholds in first 7 days	Time spent in MAP < 65 mm Hg correlated inversely with neurologic improvement No improvement in neurologic outcomes with time in MAP above 75 mm Hg

(Continued)

TABLE 56–1 Selected studies evaluating effect of MAP goals on neurologic recovery after SCI. (Continued)

Year	Author	Study Population	*N*	Intervention	Results
2015	Hawryluk et al	All SCI	Cervical = 46 Thoracic = 17 Lumbar = 3	MAP > 85 mm Hg for 5 days 26.8% first-line phenylephrine 48.5%, first-line dopamine 3.1%, dopamine and phenylephrine were started concurrently 1.0%, Levophed was the first used vasopressor	MAP < 85 events in 0-3 days correlated with less recovery of AIS (ASIA Impairment Score) grade MAP < 70 correlated with worse outcomes Higher MAP correlated with greater recovery Effect was strongest among incomplete SCI
2015	Martin et al	Cervical and thoracic SCI	105	MAP goal of >85 mm Hg for 72 hours. Stratified groups based on episodes of MAP below thresholds of -85 mm Hg -70 mm Hg -65 mm Hg	No difference in neurologic changes with the frequency of hypotensive episodes when controlling for the severity of injury Hypotensive episodes were correlated with the severity of injury
2017	Dakson et al	Cervical and thoracic SCI	Cervical spine = 66 Thoracic spine = 28	MAP goal >85 mm Hg, norepinephrine first line Measured percentage of patients with MAP < 85 mm Hg sustained for 2 h in first 5 days after injury	Patients with MAP < 85 mm Hg for 2 or more hours were 11 times less likely to exhibit at least 1 AIS grade improvement by 4 weeks after injury
2017	Squair et al	Cervical and thoracic SCI	94	Lumbar catheter for SCPP MAP target 80-85 mm Hg Pharmacologic agents • norepinephrine • phenylephrine • dopamine • a combination of two of these vasopressors	Maintaining SCPP (MAP - CSFP) above 50 mm Hg is a strong predictor of improved neurologic recovery • MAP events < 70 was no different in those who recovered and those who didn't • SCPP < 50 events significantly greater in those who did not improve.
2019	Ehsanian et al	All SCI	25	Intraoperative MAP goal > 85 mm Hg	MAP 70-94 mm Hg best neurologic improvement MAP < 70 mm Hg was the threshold for worst odds of neurologic improvement MAP > 94 mm Hg no correlation with improvement
2020	Haldrup et al	All SCI	Cervical = 50 Thoracic = 46 Lumbar = 22	MAP > 80 mm Hg for 7 days Measured percentage of BP events < 80 mm Hg 0%-33% 33%-49.9% 50%-100%	MAP > 80 mm Hg improved neurologic outcomes from 0 to 2 days MAP > 80 mm Hg no difference days 3-7
2020	Weinberg et al	All SCI	Cervical = 102 Thoracic = 29 Lumbar = 5	MAP > 85 mm Hg for 72 hours Vasopressors given to 77.9% of patients NorEpi-Phenylephrine (28.7%) NorEpi (20.6%) Phenylephrine (19.9%) High vasopressor group < 20mg cumulative dose of norEpi equivalents	The proportion of MAP measurements > 85 mm Hg was determined to be an independent predictor of neurological improvement Association between proportion of MAP > 85 and improvement is not sustained at high vasopressor doses 24.9% of MAP measurements below target

IV, intravenous; MAP, mean arterial pressure; SCI, spinal cord injury; SCPP, spinal cord perfusion pressure.

Evidence suggests that avoiding episodic hypotension may improve the odds of neurologic recovery. Cohn et al determined that time spent with MAP < 65 in the first 7 days after injury was inversely associated with neurologic improvement, while time spent with MAP < 75 mm Hg had no association with neurologic improvement.[4] Another study measuring the percentage of patients with MAP < 85 mm Hg for the first 5 days after injury found that patients below this goal for > 2 hours were 11 times less likely to exhibit neurologic improvement.[5] Hawryluk et al further demonstrated that the frequency of MAP events < 85 mm Hg was associated with decreased odds of recovery in the first 3 days after injury. Subgroup analysis of this cohort demonstrated that MAP events < 70 mm Hg were associated with the lowest odds of neurologic recovery and that the effect of MAP goal maintenance was strongest in patients with incomplete SCI.[6] Lastly, one retrospective study found that maintenance of intraoperative MAP of 70 to 94 positively correlated with improvement in motor function. Additionally, the authors found a trend toward decreased neurologic recovery with time spent with MAP > 95 mm Hg that was not statistically significant.[7] In contrast to these studies, Martin et al stratified groups of SCI based on episodes of MAP below thresholds of 85 mm Hg, 75 mm Hg, and 65 mm Hg and found no difference in neurologic outcomes with the frequency of below-goal hypotensive events when controlling for the severity of injury.[8]

Recent efforts have been made to directly target spinal cord perfusion pressure (SCPP) through the use of continuous intrathecal pressure monitoring. The fundamental purpose of targeting MAP is to maintain SCPP to prevent secondary spinal cord ischemia after injury. Squair et al demonstrated that maintaining SCPP (MAP-CSF pressure) above 50 mm Hg was a strong predictor of improved neurologic outcomes after SCI.[9] Interestingly though, MAP events < 70 mm Hg did not predict neurologic recovery in this study. Additionally, this study also found that MAP was not a perfect predictor of SCPP due to variations in CSFP after injury.

Duration of MAP Goals

The duration of MAP goals required to optimize neurologic outcomes has yet to be clearly defined. Current recommendations for the duration of MAP goals in SCI are based on both observational studies and basic science findings indicating that peak spinal cord edema occurs between 3 and 5 days post-SCI.[10] In contrast, Haldrup et al found that neurologic outcome was positively associated with fewer MAP events < 80 mm Hg in the first 48 hours after injury. No association was found with MAP events < 80 mm Hg in the period 3 to 7 days after injury.[3] Similarly, in another study, neurologic outcome correlated with adherence to a MAP goal of > 85 mm Hg during the first 72 hours after injury.[11] Additionally, utilizing high-frequency MAP calculation demonstrated that the average MAP was higher in a group of patients who achieved neurologic improvement compared to a group with no improvement in the first 48 hours after injury.[6] These authors found that patients achieving neurologic improvement had a lower proportion of MAP measures below 85 mm Hg in the first 7 days after admission with diminishing correlation with time after injury.[6] Although only a few studies examining the optimal duration of MAP goals exist, it appears that adherence to MAP goals in the first 72 hours after injury is the most critical, with diminishing effects in days 4 to 7 after injury. Further investigation is required to better understand the optimal duration of MAP goals after SCI.

Vasopressor Agent Selection

It is unclear if the utilization of specific vasopressors in the maintenance of MAP is effective in optimizing neurologic outcomes after SCI. A 2017 study by Dakson et al utilized norepinephrine as a first-line pressor agent over dopamine due to a lower frequency of adverse effects.[5] When examining the efficacy of each agent in maintaining MAP, De Backer et al and Altaf et al both demonstrated that norepinephrine and dopamine are equally effective at maintaining elevated MAP.[12,13] Norepinephrine has also been shown to be superior to dopamine when measuring SCPP. Altaf et al compared MAP and intrathecal pressures to determine SCPP and found that norepinephrine maintained MAP and reduced intrathecal pressure to a greater extent when compared to dopamine.[13]

The adverse effect profile of a pressor agent should be a determining factor when deciding which agent to administer. The inotropic effects of dopamine cannot be understated; De Backer et al and Readdy et al demonstrated the cardiogenic effects that must be considered when utilizing dopamine as more patients experienced arrhythmic events when compared to patients who received either norepinephrine or phenylephrine.[12,14] Phenylephrine, along with dopamine, was also shown to be associated with vasopressor-related complications according to a study by Inoue et al.[15] Complications such as ventricular tachycardia, troponin, elevation, and atrial fibrillation were associated with phenylephrine and dopamine usage. Inoue et al also found an association between high cervical injuries (above C4) and bradycardia after phenylephrine.[15] Importantly, this study found that vasopressor support did not improve neurologic outcomes in their cohort. Readdy et al found that dopamine was associated with a higher risk of complications in patients > 55 years and that 52% and 90% of patients under 55 years and over 55 years, respectively, experienced vasopressor-related complications. Norepinephrine, phenylephrine, and dopamine have all been shown as viable options when trying to elevate MAP. From the currently available evidence, we propose that norepinephrine should be the vasopressor of choice when comparing side effect profiles along with spinal cord physiological advantages demonstrated in animal models[16] (Table 56–2).

Of note, a 2010 systematic review by Ploumis et al found that choice of vasopressor should depend on the level of injury.[10] Cervical and upper thoracic (above T6) injuries benefit the most from chronotropic and inotropic agents like dopamine and norepinephrine. Lower thoracic (below T6) benefit more from the addition of peripheral vasoconstrictors like phenylephrine. The dosage ranges examined by Ploumis et al were dopamine (ug kg^{-1} per min): 2 to 10 (inotropic/chronotropic effects)/10 to

TABLE 56–2 Complications related to vasopressor use after SCI.

Year	Author	Study Population	N	Intervention	Results
2015	Readdy et al	Central cord syndrome	34	MAP goal > 85 mm Hg for 7 days Percentage of patients receiving med • 91% dopamine • 65% phenylephrine Mean time on vasopressors—101 h	Dopamine: 68% cardiogenic complications 29% tachycardia 16% atrial fibrillation 12.9% bradycardia 9.68% ventricular tachycardia 6.45% elevated troponin levels Phenylephrine: 46% cardiogenic complications 13.6% tachycardia 31.82% bradycardia 0 V Tach or a-fib (Ventricular tachycardia or atrial fibrillation) 4% elevated troponin levels 90% of patients over 55 had complications compared to 52% of patients <55 Complications did not affect neurologic recovery
2014	Inoue et al	SCI	131	MAP > 85 mm Hg for 7 days Percentage of patients receiving med • 48.0% dopamine • 45% phenylephrine • 5% norepinephrine • 1.5% epinephrine • 0.5% vasopressin	Odds ratio for complications OR 8.97 with Dopamine OR 5.92 phenylephrine OR 5.16 > 60 y/o OR 3.23 complete SCI High cervical injuries (above C4) were strongly related to bradycardia after phenylephrine

MAP, mean arterial pressure; SCI, spinal cord injury.

20 (vasoconstriction), norepinephrine (ug min^{-1}): 1 to 20 (inotropic effect and peripheral vasoconstriction), and phenylephrine (ug min^{-1}): 10 to 100 (arterial vasoconstriction).[10,17]

AVAILABLE GUIDELINES

Current American Association of Neurological Surgery *Guidelines for the Management of Acute Cervical Spine and Spinal Cord Injuries* from 2002, updated in 2013, recommend the maintenance of MAP between 85 and 90 mm Hg for 7 days after SCI.[1] Due to a lack of well-controlled randomized control trials, this recommendation is based entirely on level III evidence.

REFERENCES

1. Walters BC, Hadley MN, Hurlbert RJ, et al. Guidelines for the management of acute cervical spine and spinal cord injuries: 2013 update. *Neurosurgery.* 2013;60(SUPPL. 1):82–91. doi:10.1227/01.neu.0000430319.32247.7f
2. Vale FL, Burns J, Jackson AB, Hadley MN. Combined medical and surgical treatment after acute spinal cord injury: Results of a prospective pilot study to assess the merits of aggressive medical resuscitation and blood pressure management. *J Neurosurg.* 1997;87(2):239–246. doi:10.3171/jns.1997.87.2.0239
3. Haldrup M, Dyrskog S, Thygesen MM, Kirkegaard H, Kasch H, Rasmussen MM. Initial blood pressure is important for long-term outcome after traumatic spinal cord injury. *J Neurosurg Spine.* 2020;33:256–260. doi:10.3171/2020.1.SPINE191005
4. Cohn J, Wright J, McKenna S, Bushnik T. Impact of mean arterial blood pressure during the first seven days post spinal cord injury. *Top Spinal Cord Inj Rehabil.* 2010;15(3):96–106. doi:10.1310/sci1503-96
5. Dakson A, Brandman D, Thibault-Halman G, Christie SD. Optimization of the mean arterial pressure and timing of surgical decompression in traumatic spinal cord injury: A retrospective study. *Spinal Cord.* 2017;55(11):1033–1038. doi:10.1038/sc.2017.52
6. Hawryluk G, Whetstone W, Saigal R, et al. Mean arterial blood pressure correlates with neurological recovery after human spinal cord injury: Analysis of high frequency physiologic data. *J Neurotrauma.* 2015;32(24):1958–1967. doi:10.1089/neu.2014.3778
7. Ehsanian R, Haefeli J, Quach N, et al. Exploration of surgical blood pressure management and expected motor recovery in individuals with traumatic spinal cord injury. *Spinal Cord.* 2020;58(3):377–386. doi:10.1038/s41393-019-0370-5
8. Martin ND, Kepler C, Zubair M, Sayadipour A, Cohen M, Weinstein M. Increased mean arterial pressure goals after spinal cord injury and functional outcome. *J Emergencies, Trauma Shock.* 2015;8(2):94–98. doi:10.4103/0974-2700.155507
9. Squair JW, Bélanger LM, Tsang A, et al. Spinal cord perfusion pressure predicts neurologic recovery in acute spinal cord injury. *Neurology.* 2017;89(16):1660–1667. doi:10.1212/WNL.0000000000004519

10. Ploumis A, Yadlapalli N, Fehlings MG, Kwon BK, Vaccaro AR. A systematic review of the evidence supporting a role for vasopressor support in acute SCI. *Spinal Cord.* 2010;48(5):356–362. doi:10.1038/sc.2009.150
11. Weinberg JA, Farber SH, Kalamchi LD, et al. Mean arterial pressure maintenance following spinal cord injury: Does meeting the target matter? *J Trauma Acute Care Surg.* 2021;90:97–106. doi:10.1097/TA.0000000000002953
12. De Backer D, Biston P, Devriendt J, et al. Comparison of dopamine and norepinephrine in the treatment of shock. *N Engl J Med.* 2010;362(9): 779–789. doi:10.1056/NEJMoa0907118
13. Altaf F, Griesdale DE, Belanger L, et al. The differential effects of norepinephrine and dopamine on cerebrospinal fluid pressure and spinal cord perfusion pressure after acute human spinal cord injury. *Spinal Cord.* 2017;55(1):33–38. doi:10.1038/sc.2016.79
14. Readdy WJ, Whetstone WD, Ferguson AR, et al. Complications and outcomes of vasopressor usage in acute traumatic central cord syndrome. *J Neurosurg Spine.* 2015;23(5):574–580. doi:10.3171/2015.2.SPINE14746
15. Inoue T, Manley GT, Patel N, Whetstone WD. Medical and surgical management after spinal cord injury: Vasopressor usage, early surgerys, and complications. *J Neurotrauma.* 2014;31(3):284–291. doi:10.1089/neu.2013.3061
16. Streijger F, So K, Manouchehri N, et al. A direct comparison between norepinephrine and phenylephrine for augmenting spinal cord perfusion in a porcine model of spinal cord injury. *J Neurotrauma.* 2018;35(12): 1345–1357. doi:10.1089/neu.2017.5285
17. Gupta R, Bathen ME, Smith JS, Levi AD, Bhatia NN, Steward O. Advances in the management of spinal cord injury. *J Am Acad Orthop Surg.* 2010;18(4):210–222. doi:10.5435/00124635-201004000-00004

CHAPTER

57

Is There Any Role for Corticosteroids in the Management of Spinal Cord Injury?

Troy Q. Tabarestani, BA,
David A.W. Sykes, BA, Kelly R. Wackerle, MD,
Hussein Alshammari, MD, Shreyansh Shah, MD,
& Muhammad M. Abd-El-Barr, MD, PhD

Case

A 25-year-old man is involved in a high-speed motor vehicle collision 2 hours ago. Upon presentation to the emergency room, his initial exam is notable for an American Spinal Injury Association Impairment Scale, grade B injury at the T7 level. Imaging reveals an associated fracture dislocation. Should corticosteroids be started?

Key Points

- The usage of steroids in the setting of acute spinal cord injury (SCI) should be avoided based on the lack of randomized studies with sufficient power to support their benefits in management.
- As discussed, the scientific explanation for why steroids would help patients is sound and has shown promise in animal models; however, the abundance of data suggesting that the usage increases the risk for sepsis, pneumonia, bleeding, and wound infection cannot be overlooked.
- A number of novel neuroprotective and neuroregenerative drugs targeting similar molecular pathways are currently undergoing clinical trials and may offer benefit without the systemic side effects of steroid. These include Riluzole (Phase IIB/III), minocycline (Phase III), Human Hepatocyte Growth Factor (Phase III), and hydrogel scaffolding to name a few. Further studies that assess the differences between various treatment modalities with long-term follow-up are needed before any guidelines should be altered.[1]
- While care for traumatic SCI patients remains complex and multidisciplinary, corticosteroids remains a therapy grounded in pathophysiology and unsupported in practical application due to concern for unwanted side effects.

BACKGROUND

Traumatic spinal cord injury (SCI) can be a potentially devastating event with profound consequences for the lives of both the patient and their families. While there is still no clear superior medical treatment, the role of corticosteroids has been investigated for multiple decades. Although administration of corticosteroids following SCI initially showed potential for neurological recovery, the recent literature has brought to light numerous adverse effects. Due to the lack of knowledge surrounding the pathophysiology and heterogeneity of results, the use of corticosteroids has remained controversial especially with the introduction of novel neuroregenerative treatments.

Here, we review the history of steroid usage in SCI treatment and highlight the perceived risks and benefits surrounding this option of therapy.

EVIDENCE AND REVIEW

From a pathophysiologic standpoint, the use of corticosteroids for SCI is a very promising field. Compression of the spinal cord can induce a rapid change in lipid metabolism of membranes, lipid hydrolysis with release of arachidonate, production of eicosanoids, and loss of cholesterol (Figure 57–1). These disturbances can thereby damage cells and lead to the secondary development of tissue ischemia, edema, and inflammation with neuronophagia.[2] Basic science and animal model studies have proposed two possible pathways by which methylprednisolone may improve neurological recovery. First, methylprednisolone likely suppresses membrane degradation by inhibiting lipid peroxidation and hydrolysis at the site of injury. Additionally, the breakdown of cellular membranes peaks within 8 hours of injury.[3,4] The second pathway is that vasoreactive by-products of arachidonic acid metabolism are reduced with corticosteroids, which improve blood circulation to the injury site.[5–9]

Inspired by these pathophysiologic insights, the use of corticosteroids in the management of SCI dates back to the 1960s with Ducker et al successfully testing the drug in a canine model. Following this, given the drug's inherent potential to reduce swelling, maintain vascular integrity, and minimize the inflammatory response, there were a number of animal studies analyzing the benefits of steroids for the treatment of edema in central nervous system.[11–14] Overall, their initial results were positive: animals had improved functional status with minimal complications. Following these preliminary studies, the National Acute Spinal Cord Injury Study (NASCIS) began a series of three large cohort, multi-institutional analyses of patients treated with corticosteroids for SCI.

In 1984, the first human trial of 330 patients was conducted comparing the efficacy of a high dose of methylprednisolone (1,000-mg bolus and daily thereafter for 10 days) against a standard dose (100-mg bolus and daily thereafter for 10 days). Of note, this study did not have a placebo group since, at the time, glucocorticoid treatment was not allowed to be withheld based on ethical considerations and approved management protocols. Additionally, a standardized neurologic grading scale was not used, which further limited the applicability and generalizability of the study. This study found higher probability of sepsis, pulmonary embolism, and death within 14 days in the high-dose steroid group without neurologic functional difference between the groups. Moreover, it showed an increased rates of wound infection in the high-dose group.[15]

Building off the limitations of their prior study, NASCIS II followed with another multicenter randomized controlled trial of 487 patients treated with either steroids, naloxone, or placebo. Of the 427 patients available for 1-year follow-up, there were no significant differences in motor or sensory scores between any of the groups. However, the 1-year analysis revealed that patients treated with methylprednisolone >8 hours postinjury had worse results than those given placebo. It should be emphasized, however, that this 8-hour cutoff was only established in

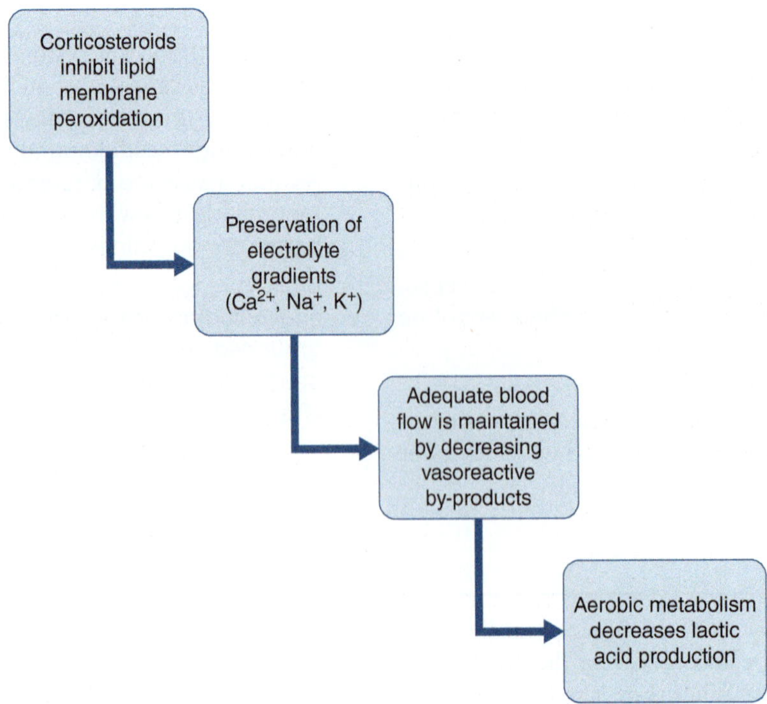

FIGURE 57–1 Proposed mechanism by which corticosteroid therapy can inhibit lipid membrane peroxidation and lead to downstream neuroprotective benefits for patients with acute spinal cord injury.

posthoc analysis and was not part of the original study protocol. Likewise, with early surgical intervention, this study was one of the first to propose that pharmacological timing could be an important factor in determining impact on functional status.[16,17] The NASCIS III study of approximately 500 patients corroborated the prior study's findings, showing that those who received a 48-hour regimen of steroids within 3 to 8 hours of their injury were more likely to improve in neurologic grade, while also showing higher rates of pneumonia and sepsis.[18]

Since these breakthrough studies set the stage for initial management guidelines using corticosteroids, a myriad of other groups have attempted to replicate their work and reassess the drug's efficacy in SCI. Numerous papers have highlighted the benefits of steroids while also providing contradictory data to suggest that there is no link with higher infection rates.[19–23] For instance, both Otani et al and Evaniew et al reviewed randomized controlled trials and found that steroid use was not associated with an increase in adverse events.[20,21] Sauerland et al examined multiple reviews of over 2,000 patients and found no evidence that methylprednisolone increased the risk of gastrointestinal bleeding, wound complication, pulmonary complications, or death. More specifically, Wing et al focused on rates of avascular necrosis and found no difference between the placebo versus the steroid-treated cohorts.[22] Although the NASCIS results showed early infectious complications with treatment, Gerndt et al conversely found a decrease in duration of rehabilitation and no significant impact on other outcomes including mortality.[23]

While there have been results supporting the use of steroids in the management of SCI, the overall literature and international guidelines have shifted away from their acute medical usage.[24–28] For example, Pointillart et al and Sultan et al each analyzed these results, followed similar inclusion criteria, and concluded that steroid therapy within the first 8 hours following SCI failed to show a statistically significant improvement in patients' overall motor or neurological scores when compared to their respective control groups.[29,30] In terms of adverse events, the literature remains controversial on the true risks associated with high-dose steroid therapy. Even within individual studies, there is clear evidence pointing toward a significantly higher risk of infection and bleeding, but simultaneously there is no increase in patient mortality.[31] However, there are obvious limitations to these studies including small sample sizes and confounding variables. Additionally, substantial doubt has been raised regarding the foundational NASCIS trails since there was no actual significant difference in the primary analysis (only after posthoc subgroup) and there was a noticeable trend toward an increase in adverse events for patients receiving high-dose methylprednisolone.

AVAILABLE GUIDELINES

Based on the mixed nature of the above evidence, available guidelines from major spine societies are either mixed or lukewarm on the use of corticosteroids in SCI. AOSpine guidelines state that a 24-hour infusion of corticosteroids can be offered to patients only if they present with 8 hours of their injury.[25] Congress of Neurological Surgeons is more negative, stating that methylprednisolone is not recommended for the treatment of acute SCI and that "Class I, II, and III evidence exists that high-dose steroids are associated with harmful side effects including death."[27]

REFERENCES

1. Fawcett JW, Curt A, Steeves JD, et al. Guidelines for the conduct of clinical trials for spinal cord injury as developed by the ICCP panel: spontaneous recovery after spinal cord injury and statistical power needed for therapeutic clinical trials. *Spinal Cord.* 2007/03/01 2007;45(3):190–205. doi:10.1038/sj.sc.3102007
2. Anderson D, Saunders R, Demediuk P. Lipid hydrolysis and peroxidation in injured spinal cord: partial protection with methylprednisolone or vitamin E and selenium. *Cent Nerv Syst Trauma.* 1985;2:257–267.
3. Braughler JM, Hall ED. Correlation of methylprednisolone levels in cat spinal cord with its effects on (Na+ + K+)-ATPase, lipid peroxidation, and alpha motor neuron function. *J Neurosurg.* Jun 1982;56(6):838–844. doi:10.3171/jns.1982.56.6.0838
4. Braughler JM, Hall ED, Means ED, Waters TR, Anderson DK. Evaluation of an intensive methylprednisolone sodium succinate dosing regimen in experimental spinal cord injury. *J Neurosurg.* Jul 1987;67(1):102–105. doi:10.3171/jns.1987.67.1.0102
5. Young W. Blood flow, metabolic and neurophysiological mechanisms in spinal cord injury. In: Becker DP, J.T., ed. *Central Nervous System Trauma Status Report.* National Institutes of Health; Bethesda, Maryland. 1985:463–473.
6. Young W, Flamm ES. Effect of high-dose corticosteroid therapy on blood flow, evoked potentials, and extracellular calcium in experimental spinal injury. *J Neurosurg.* Nov 1982;57(5):667–673. doi:10.3171/jns.1982.57.5.0667
7. Stys PK. Anoxic and ischemic injury of myelinated axons in CNS white matter: from mechanistic concepts to therapeutics. *J Cereb Blood Flow Metab.* Jan 1998;18(1):2–25. doi:10.1097/00004647-199801000-00002
8. Cui Y, Jin X, Choi JY, Kim BG. Modeling subcortical ischemic white matter injury in rodents: unmet need for a breakthrough in translational research. *Neural Regen Res.* Apr 2021;16(4):638–642. doi:10.4103/1673-5374.295313
9. Chu D, Qiu J, Grafe M, et al. Delayed cell death signaling in traumatized central nervous system: hypoxia. *Neurochem Res.* Feb 2002;27(1-2):97–106. doi:10.1023/a:1014858707218
10. Ducker TB, Hamit HF. Experimental treatments of acute spinal cord injury. *J Neurosurg.* 01 Jan. 1969 1969;30(6):693–697. doi:10.3171/jns.1969.30.6.0693
11. French LA. The use of steroids in the treatment of cerebral edema. *Bull NY Acad Med.* 1966;42:301–311.
12. Long DM, Hartmann J, French LA. The response of experimental cerebral edema to glucosteroid administration. *J Neurosurg.* 1966;24:843–854.
13. Baumann J. Results of treatment of certain diseases of the central nervous system with adrenal cortico-trophic hormone and corticosteroids. *Acta Neurol Scand.* 1965;41:453–461.
14. Burns CM. The history of cortisone discovery and development. *Rheum Dis Clin North Am.* Feb 2016;42(1):1–14, vii. doi:10.1016/j.rdc.2015.08.001
15. Bracken MB, Collins WF, Freeman DF, et al. Efficacy of methylprednisolone in acute spinal cord injury. *JAMA.* Jan 6 1984;251(1):45–52.
16. Bracken MB, Shepard MJ, Collins WF, et al. Methylprednisolone or naloxone treatment after acute spinal cord injury: 1-year follow-up data: results of the second National Acute Spinal Cord Injury Study. *J Neurosurg.* Jan 1 1992 1992;76(1):23–31. doi:10.3171/jns.1992.76.1.0023
17. Fehlings MG, Vaccaro A, Wilson JR, et al. Early versus delayed decompression for traumatic cervical spinal cord injury: results of the Surgical Timing in Acute Spinal Cord Injury Study (STASCIS). *PLoS One.* 2012;7(2):e32037. doi:10.1371/journal.pone.0032037
18. Bracken MB, Shepard MJ, Holford TR, et al. Administration of methylprednisolone for 24 or 48 hours or tirilazad mesylate for 48 hours in the treatment of acute spinal cord injury. Results of the Third National Acute Spinal Cord Injury Randomized Controlled Trial. National Acute Spinal Cord Injury Study. *JAMA.* May 28 1997;277(20):1597–1604.

19. Bracken MB. Steroids for acute spinal cord injury. *Cochrane Database Syst Rev.* Jan 18 2012;1(1):Cd001046. doi:10.1002/14651858.CD001046.pub2
20. Otani K. Beneficial effects of methylprednisolone sodium succinate in the treatment of acute spinal cord injury. *Sekitsui Sekizui.* 1994 1994;7:633–647.
21. Evaniew N, Belley-Côté EP, Fallah N, Noonan VK, Rivers CS, Dvorak MF. Methylprednisolone for the treatment of patients with acute spinal cord jnjuries: a systematic review and meta-analysis. *J Neurotrauma.* Mar 1 2016;33(5):468–481. doi:10.1089/neu.2015.4192
22. Wing PC, Nance P, Connell DG, Gagnon F. Risk of avascular necrosis following short term megadose methylprednisolone treatment. *Spinal Cord.* 1998/09/01 1998;36(9):633–636. doi:10.1038/sj.sc.3100647
23. Gerndt SJ, Rodriguez JL, Pawlik JW, et al. Consequences of high-dose steroid therapy for acute spinal cord injury. *J Trauma.* Feb 1997;42(2): 279–284. doi:10.1097/00005373-199702000-00017
24. O'Toole JE, Kaiser MG, Anderson PA, et al. Congress of Neurological Surgeons systematic review and evidence-based guidelines on the evaluation and treatment of patients with thoracolumbar spine trauma: executive summary. *Neurosurgery.* Jan 1 2019;84(1):2–6. doi:10.1093/neuros/nyy394
25. Fehlings MG, Tetreault LA, Wilson JR, et al. A clinical practice guideline for the management of acute spinal cord injury: introduction, rationale, and scope. *Global Spine J.* Sep 2017;7(3 Suppl):84s–94s. doi:10.1177/2192568217703387
26. Wang TY, Park C, Zhang H, et al. Management of acute traumatic spinal cord injury: a review of the literature. *Front Surg.* 2021;8:698736. doi:10.3389/fsurg.2021.698736
27. Hurlbert RJ, Hadley MN, Walters BC, et al. Pharmacological therapy for acute spinal cord injury. *Neurosurgery.* Mar 2013;72 Suppl 2:93–105. doi:10.1227/NEU.0b013e31827765c6
28. Sayer FT, Kronvall E, Nilsson OG. Methylprednisolone treatment in acute spinal cord injury: the myth challenged through a structured analysis of published literature. *Spine J.* May-Jun 2006;6(3):335–343. doi:10.1016/j.spinee.2005.11.001
29. Pointillart V, Petitjean ME, Wiart L, et al. Pharmacological therapy of spinal cord injury during the acute phase. *Spinal Cord.* Feb 2000;38(2):71–76. doi:10.1038/sj.sc.3100962
30. Sultan I, Lamba N, Liew A, et al. The safety and efficacy of steroid treatment for acute spinal cord injury: a systematic review and meta-analysis. *Heliyon.* Feb 2020;6(2):e03414. doi:10.1016/j.heliyon.2020.e03414
31. Chikuda H, Yasunaga H, Takeshita K, et al. Mortality and morbidity after high-dose methylprednisolone treatment in patients with acute cervical spinal cord injury: a propensity-matched analysis using a nationwide administrative database. *Emergency Medicine Journal.* 2014;31(3):201–206. doi:10.1136/emermed-2012-202058

CHAPTER

58

How Early Should We Do Surgery in Cases of Traumatic Spinal Cord Injury?

Safwan Alomari, MD & Ali Bydon, MD

Case

A 48-year-old man is found at the scene after crashing his motorcycle. Upon presentation to the trauma bay, his polytrauma burden is noted to include several broken ribs, a liver laceration, free intraperitoneal air, and a C6/C7 fracture dislocation. He is noted to have a motor incomplete spinal cord injury at the level of his fracture. How early does this patient need to go for surgical correction of his spine fracture?

Key Points

- There has been growing recognition that early surgical decompression is a reasonable treatment option for patients with acute spinal cord injury (SCI); yet, there remains a lack of class I evidence to support this intervention.[1,2]
- Adaptive stratified designs of clinical trials accounting for the heterogeneity of patients with SCI, differing patterns of injury, and variability in definition of what constitutes an adequate decompression of the spinal cord, among other factors are important to consider in future studies.

BACKGROUND

Traumatic spinal cord injury (SCI), with around 18,000 new cases occurring every year in the United States, leads to a long-term disability, poses risks of medical and surgical complications, and necessitates extensive utilization of health care sectors.[3–5] Despite our expanding knowledge about the pathophysiology of SCI and recent efforts to explore new neuroprotection and regenerative therapies, there remains a lack of high-quality evidence to establish standardized management guidelines.[1] The scope of available treatments has been confined to medical therapy including targeted blood pressure, external immobilization of the spine, or surgical decompression of the cord.[2]

The optimal timing of surgical decompression in acute SCI has been a subject of significant debate over several decades. Early surgical decompression, initially supported by findings from preclinical studies, is based on the potential to reestablish blood flow and improve perfusion to the spinal cord while potentially attenuating the progression of secondary injury cascades.[4,6] However, clinical evidence regarding this matter has been inconclusive, with some studies demonstrating a benefit of early surgical decompression while some others have not. In addition, there exists variability in defining the timing thresholds for early decompressive surgery. The diversity in these definitions, coupled with variations across studies in adjusting for baseline neurological status, has led to a conflict in evidence and, in parallel, to a substantial variability in surgical practice across different institutions.

REVIEW AND DISCUSSION OF THE EVIDENCE

While most studies have used the 24 hours threshold to define what constitutes early surgery, several authors have conducted studies to investigate whether earlier decompression can lead to further benefit.[7,8] Although these few studies have proposed that surgical decompression within 8 hours after injury might lead to improved neurological outcomes when compared to decompression 8-24 hours after injury, these studies were either retrospective in nature, included heterogeneous cohorts of small sample size from single institutions, or accounted for a limited number of predictors and outcome measures.[7,8] Therefore, there remains a lack for high-level evidence for or against such practice.

In 2017, a systematic review analyzed five pertinent studies assessing the impact of decompression within 24 hours.[9] While a trend toward improved neurological outcomes in early surgical decompression was noted, meta-analyses to quantitatively determine treatment effects were deemed unfeasible due to inconsistency in the methodology and outcome reporting in these studies.[9] Hence, the evidence was considered of low quality owing to potential bias and imprecision.[4] Therefore, the derived guidelines offered only a tentative recommendation for decompression within 24 hours as a possible option.[4]

In 2020, Badhiwala et al reported the results of the largest-to-date pooled analysis encompassing data from 1,548 patients with a SCI spanning the years 1991 to 2017.[10] The study was conducted using four independent, prospective, multicenter databases containing important variables including time interval between injury and surgical intervention. These databases were: (1) the National Acute Spinal Cord Injury Study (NASCIS III),[11] (2) the North American Clinical Trials Network (NACTN) SCI Registry,[12] (3) the Surgical Timing in Acute Spinal Cord Injury Study (STASCIS),[13] and (4) the Sygen trial.[14] Based on the timing of surgery, patients were categorized into two cohorts: early (<24 hours post-SCI) and late (≥24 hours post-SCI). Outcome measures included the International Standards for Neurological Classification of Spinal Cord Injury (ISNCSCI) and the American Spinal Injury Association (ASIA). Two major findings were found in this analysis:

1. Firstly, early surgical decompression (<24 hours post-SCI) demonstrated superior 1-year sensorimotor recovery compared to surgical decompression beyond 24 hours.
   - Greater degree of recovery was observed at 1 year in the early decompression group (n = 528) compared to the late decompression group (n = 1020). Specifically, there was a total motor scores improvement of 23.7 points (95% CI 19.2-28.2) within the early decompression cohort compared to 19.7 points (15.3-24.0) in the late decompression cohort (mean difference [MD] 4.0 points [1.7-6.3]; P = .0006). Similarly, improvements were noted in light touch scores 19.0 points (15.1-23.0) versus 14.8 points (11.2-18.4) (MD 4.3 [1.6-7.0]; P = .0021), and pinprick scores 18.3 points (13.7-22.9) versus 14.2 points (9.8-18.6); (MD 4.0 [1.5-6.6]; P = .0020) within respective groups.
   - Individuals who underwent early decompression also exhibited superior ASIA Impairment Scale (AIS) grades at the 1-year mark post-surgery, compared to those who had late decompression.
   - A subgroup analysis on patients with cervical SCI having early decompression found greater magnitude of improvement in total motor scores in the upper extremities as opposed to the lower extremities.
2. Secondly, upon including the time to decompression as a continuous variable in the statistical model, a significant decrease in the change in total motor score was observed with increments in the time elapsed during the initial 24-36 hours following the injury. Beyond the 36-hour mark, the capacity for timely decompressive surgery to yield improved outcome was notably diminished (Figure 58–1).

While this study presents compelling evidence in support of early decompressive surgery, a key limitation, shared with previous studies, is the absence of randomization of patients to early and late decompression groups. Hence, even with controlling for important variables in these analyses, the potential for residual confounding by unmeasured covariates remains a concern.[15] Another limitation of this study is the utilization of data from various sources collected over three decades of patient enrollment, during which significant evolutions in diagnostic methods, surgical approaches, and rehabilitative programs have occurred.[4,16]

Accounting for these limitations, the Optimal Treatment for Spinal Cord Injury Associated with Cervical Canal Stenosis (OSCIS) group from Japan published the results of their multicenter randomized controlled trials in 2021.[17] The trial included a total of 72 individuals with incomplete-motor cervical SCI (with preexisting canal stenosis and without bone injury) and a subgroup of 24 patients with central cord syndrome.[17] To be considered having central cord syndrome, patient needed to have an upper extremity ASIA motor score of ≥10 points lower compared to the respective score in the lower extremity. Patients were randomly allocated to undergo either early surgical decompression (24 hours of admission) or late surgical decompression (after a minimum of 14 days of medical management). The three principal outcome measures were (1) improvement in the mean ASIA motor score, (2) the spinal cord independence measure score, and (3) the percentage of individuals achieving independent ambulation at 1 year post-SCI. The analysis showed that, among individuals without central cord syndrome, early decompression produced accelerated recovery within the first 6 months post-injury when compared to late decompression, but both early and late surgery demonstrated similar motor recovery at 12 months (Figure 58–2). Confounding factors in the study included the inability to collect comprehensive data regarding severity or extent of cord compression, variability of surgical approaches in both groups, and the lack of standardized rehabilitation programs in the included institutions.[17] Therefore, future work remains essential to validate these results.

AVAILABLE GUIDELINES

Currently available guidelines from the Congress of Neurological Surgeons corroborate the mixed nature of these results.[18] They note that there is insufficient evidence on the timing of surgical intervention. Moreover while "early" surgery can be considered an option, they caution that the definition of "early" is inconsistent in the literature, ranging from within 8 hours to within 72 hours.

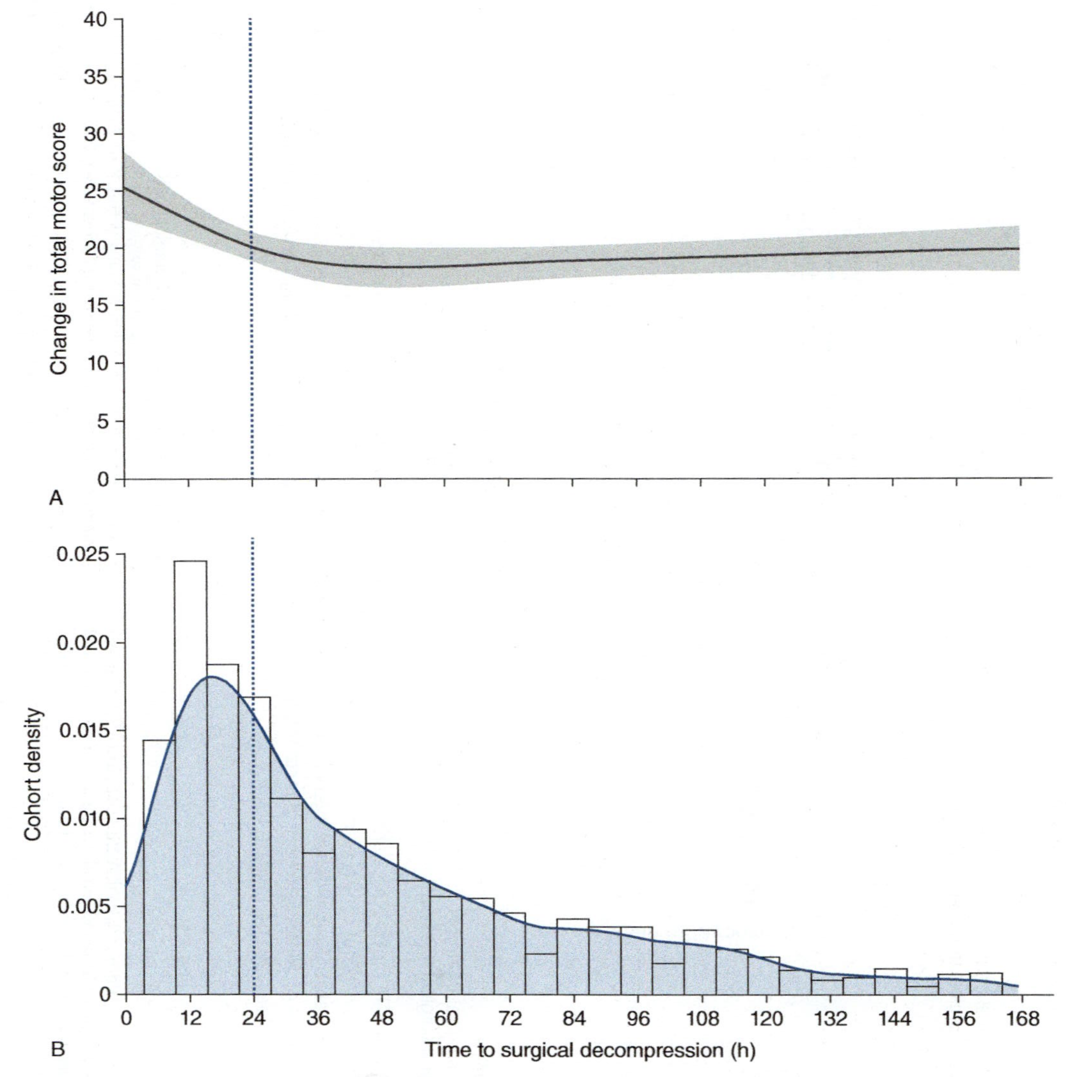

FIGURE 58–1 Risk-adjusted relationship of time to surgical decompression with change in total motor score from baseline to 1-year of follow-up in patients with acute spinal cord injury.[10] **(A)** Change in total motor score by time to surgical decompression adjusted for baseline total motor score, age, mechanism of injury, AIS grade, spinal level of injury, and administration of methylprednisolone; the shaded area indicates 95% CI. **(B)** Density plot of the frequency distribution of time to surgical decompression within the study cohort. CI, confidence interval. (Reproduced with permission from Badhiwala JH, Wilson JR, Witiw CD, et al. The influence of timing of surgical decompression for acute spinal cord injury: a pooled analysis of individual patient data. The Lancet Neurology. 2021;20(2):117-126).

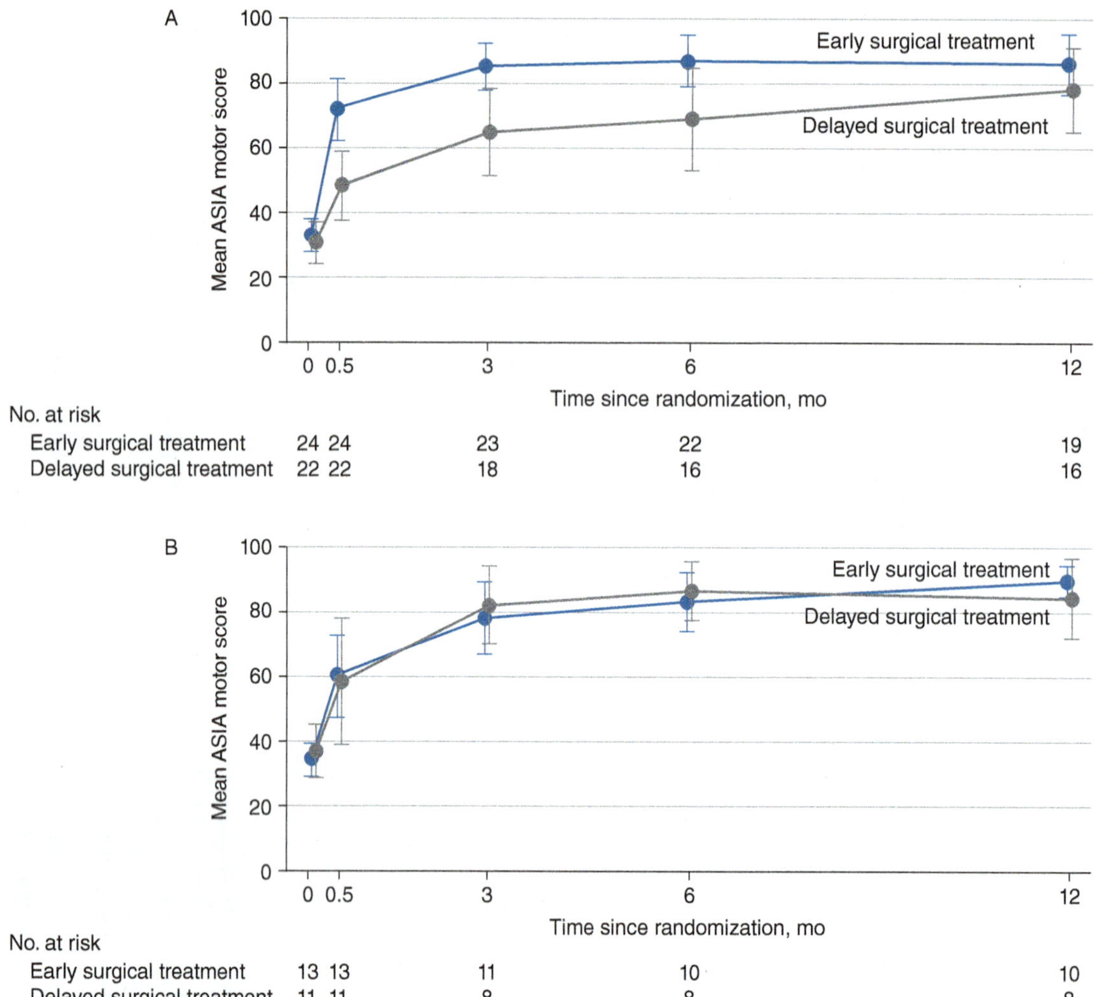

FIGURE 58–2 Mean ASIA motor score during the study period, according to treatment group, among patients with and without central cord syndrome. (**A**) Patients without central cord syndrome. (**B**) Patients with central cord syndrome. ASIA indicates American Spinal Injury Association; error bars indicate 95% confidence intervals (CIs).[17] (Reproduced from Chikuda H, Koyama Y, Matsubayashi Y, et al. Effect of Early vs Delayed Surgical Treatment on Motor Recovery in Incomplete Cervical Spinal Cord Injury With Preexisting Cervical Stenosis: A Randomized Clinical Trial. JAMA Netw Open. 2021;4(11):e2133604).

REFERENCES

1. Fehlings MG, Tetreault LA, Wilson JR, et al. A clinical practice guideline for the management of patients with acute spinal cord injury and central cord syndrome: recommendations on the timing (≤24 hours versus >24 hours) of decompressive surgery. *Global Spine Journal.* 2017;7(3_suppl):195S–202S.
2. Fehlings MG, Pedro K, Hejrati N. The management of acute spinal cord injury: where have we been? Where are we now? Where are we going? *Journal of Neurotrauma.* 2022;39(23-24):1591–1602.
3. Ropper AE, Ropper AH. Acute spinal cord compression. *New England Journal of Medicine.* 2017;376(14):1358–1369.
4. Ahuja CS, Wilson JR, Nori S, et al. Traumatic spinal cord injury. *Nature Reviews Disease Primers.* 2017;3(1):17018.
5. El Masri WS, Kumar N. Traumatic spinal cord injuries. *Lancet.* 2011;377(9770):972–974.
6. Yao C, Cao X, Yu B. Revascularization after traumatic spinal cord injury. *Frontiers in Physiology.* 2021;12:631500.
7. Grassner L, Wutte C, Klein B, et al. Early decompression (< 8 h) after traumatic cervical spinal cord injury improves functional outcome as assessed by spinal cord independence measure after one year. *Journal of Neurotrauma.* 2016;33(18):1658–1666.
8. Jug M, Kejžar N, Vesel M, et al. Neurological Recovery after traumatic cervical spinal cord injury is superior if surgical decompression and instrumented fusion are performed within 8 hours versus 8 to 24 hours after injury: a single center experience. *Journal of Neurotrauma.* 2015;32(18):1385–1392.
9. Wilson JR, Tetreault LA, Kwon BK, et al. Timing of decompression in patients with acute spinal cord injury: a systematic review. *Global Spine Journal.* 2017;7(3_suppl):95S–115S.
10. Badhiwala JH, Wilson JR, Witiw CD, et al. The influence of timing of surgical decompression for acute spinal cord injury: a pooled analysis of individual patient data. *The Lancet Neurology.* 2021;20(2):117–126.
11. Bracken MB, Shepard MJ, Holford TR, et al. Administration of methylprednisolone for 24 or 48 hours or tirilazad mesylate for 48 hours in the treatment of acute spinal cord injury: results of the third national acute spinal cord injury randomized controlled trial. *JAMA.* 1997;277(20):1597–1604.
12. Grossman RG, Toups EG, Frankowski RF, Burau KD, Howley S. North American clinical trials network for the treatment of spinal cord injury: goals and progress. *Journal of Neurosurgery: Spine.* 2012;17(Suppl1):6–10.
13. Fehlings MG, Vaccaro A, Wilson JR, et al. Early versus delayed decompression for traumatic cervical spinal cord injury: results of the Surgical Timing in Acute Spinal Cord Injury Study (STASCIS). *PLoS One.* 2012;7(2):e32037.

14. Geisler FH, Coleman WP, Grieco G, Poonian D, Group SS. The Sygen® multicenter acute spinal cord injury study. *Spine.* 2001;26(24S): S87–S98.
15. Bhatt DL, Mehta C. Adaptive Designs for Clinical Trials. *New England Journal of Medicine.* 2016;375(1):65–74.
16. Ducker TB. Treatment of spinal-cord injury. *New England Journal of Medicine.* 1990;322(20):1459–1461.
17. Chikuda H, Koyama Y, Matsubayashi Y, et al. Effect of early vs delayed surgical treatment on motor recovery in incomplete cervical spinal cord injury with preexisting cervical stenosis: a randomized clinical trial. *JAMA Network Open.* 2021;4(11):e2133604.
18. Eichholz, KM, Rabb, CH, Anderson PA, et al. Congress of neurological surgeons systematic review and evidence-based guidelines on the evaluation and treatment of patients with thoracolumbar spine trauma: timing of surgical intervention. *Neurosurgery.* 2019;84(1):E53–E55.

CHAPTER

59

What Are the Surgical Indications for Spinal Metastases?

Andreas Seas, BS, Emily Luo, BS, Antoinette Charles, BS, Meghan Price, MD, & C. Rory Goodwin, MD, PhD

Case

A 58-year-old woman with a history of locally invasive renal cell carcinoma now presents with worsening axial mid-back pain. Imaging demonstrates a solitary expansile lesion in the T8 vertebral body, with abutment of the cord and no clear cerebrospinal fluid (CSF) plane between the tumor. Her exam is notable for 4+/5 strength distal to the lesion. Is spine surgery appropriate for such a patient?

Key Points

- Neurologic, oncologic, mechanical, and systemic (NOMS) has provided a reliable framework for identifying patients for whom surgery is indicated—primarily those with spinal cord compression and/or instability.
- Outside of NOMS, several risk factors have been associated with poor survival, but these should always be considered on a case-by-case basis, with the ultimate treatment course based on reaching patient goals of care.
- Frailty is an emerging metric that has found use in clinical decision-making for patients with spinal metastasis and should become a part of the standard of care for all patients.
- It is important to assess surgical indications in the context of individual patient priorities, considering the role of surgery and radiation in palliative care.

BACKGROUND

Spinal metastases are the most common tumors of the spine. They occur when cancer of another origin spreads to the vertebral body or invades the spinal cord. Spinal metastases are diagnosed through thorough history, physical exam, and radiographic imaging. The initial presentation of spine metastases can vary considerably. Some patients are asymptomatic while approximately 10% to 20% of patients present with symptoms that significantly impact their quality of life (QoL).[1]

Primary symptoms include back pain, spinal cord compression, gait instability, loss of bladder/bowel function, paresthesia, and weakness or paralysis of the extremities.[2] Physical exam findings typically correspond with tumor location and the extent of spinal cord compression. It is important to assess for weakness, sensory changes, impaired reflexes, ataxia, and point tenderness on exam.[3] Magnetic resonance imaging (MRI) is the preferred method to visualize and characterize spinal metastases; however, computed tomography (CT) allows assessment of spine biomechanical integrity.[4] Immunohistological and clinicopathological sampling of the tumor through CT-guided biopsy can also help determine the primary source of the metastasis.[5]

Treatment for metastatic spine tumors requires a multidisciplinary approach incorporating medical/interventional pain management, chemotherapy, radiation, and surgical intervention.[6,7] The primary goals of therapy are pain control, improved QoL, mitigation of mass effect on the neural elements, local tumor control, and stabilization of the underlying spinal column. Spinal metastases are most effectively managed by multidisciplinary teams consisting of medical oncologists, neurosurgeons, orthopedic surgeons, radiation oncologists, interventional radiologists, palliative care (PC) providers, and physical therapists. This team-based approach can both potentially prolong survival while improving patient QoL through increased mobility, reduction of back pain, recovery of bowel/bladder function, and support for cognitive and psychosocial impairments.[8,9]

The purpose of this chapter is to outline the management pathway for spinal metastasis with a focus on patient-centered care and prioritization of QoL. We discuss the indications for surgical intervention using the neurologic, oncologic, mechanical, and systemic (NOMS) framework, outline the role of prognostication in spinal metastasis, describe situations in which surgery may not be beneficial, and finally explore the roll of PC in the treatment of this patient population.

EVIDENCE AND REVIEW

The Neurologic, Oncologic, Mechanical, and Systemic (NOMS) Decision Framework

Developing a framework for the treatment of metastatic spinal tumors is complex and requires a multidisciplinary approach. For the past 15 years, the NOMS framework developed by Memorial Sloan Kettering Cancer Center has been a leading decision-making schema for treating spinal tumors.[10] Combining this framework with other prognostic algorithms and scoring tools offers a powerful system to optimize treatment for patients (Figure 59-1).

Neurologic: Epidural Spinal Cord Compression

The neurologic criteria of NOMS serve to evaluate the degree of epidural spinal cord compression (ESCC), myelopathy, and/or functional radiculopathy primarily by radiographic assessment of ESCC and physical exam. Based on the seminal work of Patchell et al, which demonstrated a higher likelihood of ambulation after surgery, as well as higher rates of regaining and retaining the ability to walk after surgery as opposed to radiotherapy alone, one of the main indications for surgery in metastatic spine is the degree of ESCC as they demonstrated that surgical decompression has superior outcomes compared to radiation therapy alone in patients with ESCC.[11] To guide assessment of neural involvement, a six-point grading system is used to grade axial T2-weight images at the site of the most severe compression. Radiation is the recommended first-line treatment for lower grades that have an absence of mechanical instability. Surgical decompression prior to radiation therapy is optimal for higher grades unless the tumor is highly radiosensitive. The combination of the clinical assessment of myelopathy/functional radiculopathy and radiographic parameters dictates the influence of neurologic status on the decision-making paradigm.[10]

Oncologic: Tumor Radiosensitivity

Radiation therapy is a mainstay treatment for spinal metastases and is often combined with surgery.[12] Radiosensitivity is determined via tumor histology, and most radiosensitive tumors (ie, multiple myeloma, lymphoma, breast, and prostate) are treated with conventional external beam radiation therapy (cEBRT) regardless of ESCC grade or neurologic deficit.[10,13,14] For radioresistant tumors (ie, renal cell carcinoma, melanoma, and sarcoma), cEBRT is not as effective due to limitations in delivering efficacious tumoricidal doses without toxicity to the spinal cord or nearby organs.[10,15,16] Instead, low-ESCC-grade radioresistant tumors should be treated with stereotactic body radiation therapy (SBRT) without surgical decompression, whereas high-ESCC-grade radioresistant tumors should undergo surgical decompression and stabilization before SBRT treatment.[10] In the case of high-ESCC-grade radioresistant tumors, surgery allows for separation of between the tumor and spinal cord for optimal radiation dosing and has led to improved local control.[17]

Mechanical: Spinal Instability Neoplastic Score (SINS)

Mechanical instability is evaluated separately and is viewed as an indication for surgery regardless of the neurologic and oncologic assessment.[10] One method of assessing neoplastic instability is through the 18-point SINS, which assigns a score based on location of instability, pain, alignment, osteolysis, vertebral body collapse, and posterior element involvement.[18,19] Low scores (0-6) denote stability whereas high scores (13-18) denote instability, and intermediate scores (7-12) denote intermediate instability and require further assessment.[10]

Systemic: Assessment of Patient Ability to Tolerate Intervention

The systemic axis of the NOMS assessment considers factors that may indicate a patient's ability to tolerate intervention. These include but are not limited to the extent of tumor spread, histology, and patient comorbidities. Additionally, certain factors such as tumor histology have been correlated with shortened survival and thus surgery may not be as beneficial from a recovery and palliative standpoint.[12,20] Patient prognosis can be assessed via various tools, scoring systems, nomograms, and machine learning algorithms.[21–23] However, physicians should exercise caution against relying on prognostic tools as no perfect tool exists for this patient population.[20] Ultimately, if tumor progression is predicted to not impede postoperative recovery, patients should be considered as candidates for surgery if they are expected to survive greater than 3 months, although studies exist demonstrating patients surviving less than 3 months demonstrate significant improvement as well.[24]

The Role of Prognostication in Metastatic Spine Surgery

There has been an increasing role of prognostication tools across many medical and surgical practices. Specifically, the field of metastatic spine surgery has seen a large volume of new scoring and prognostication tools, some even introducing novel machine learning approaches into the field. A 2018 comparison of

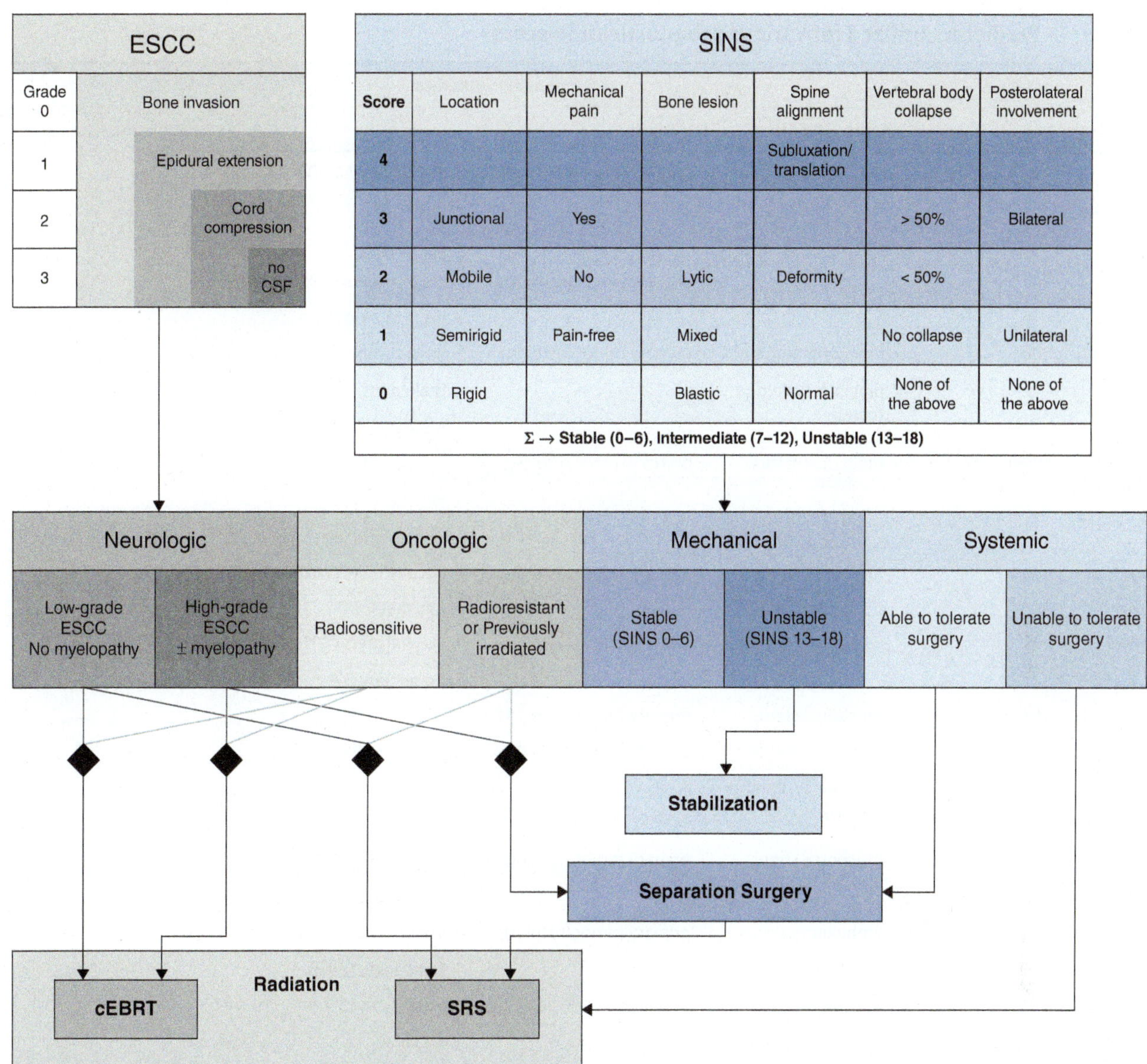

FIGURE 59–1 NOMS criteria.

several of these prognostication tools illustrated variable performance depending on the source of metastasis, with the Skeletal Oncology Research Group (SORG) nomogram most accurately predicting 30- and 90-day survival. The Tokuhashi scoring system most accurately predicted 1-year survival (Table 59–1).[23] More recently, the SORG group updated their algorithm to utilize a machine learning approach.[25] This is still a developing field, and new models must undergo rigorous external validation prior to incorporation into treatment algorithms.

Clinical Decision-Making Beyond NOMS

Historically, the NOMS criteria have provided a framework for the evaluation and care of patients with spinal metastases; however, there are many additional factors to consider in the evaluation of individual patients. Cohort studies have demonstrated that certain factors can be associated with worse outcomes and poor survival for patients with spinal metastases. Specifically, high tumor burden, rapid tumor growth, poor ambulation, and Karnofsky Performance Score (KPS) < 70 have all been associated with reduced postoperative survival in multiple studies.[26] While these risk factors are important to consider when deciding whether to perform surgery, it is important to contextualize them in the overall understanding of each patient's goals of care. Thus, these factors are important aspects of shared decision-making but should not preclude any one specific patient from therapy.

Considering Patient Frailty

Increasingly, patient frailty is considered a critical factor in medical and surgical decision-making and has become important in the evaluation of metastatic spine lesions. This is reflected in the development of frailty assessment scores

TABLE 59-1 Predictors utilized for various prognostication scores.

		Model Predictors					
Score	**Year**	**Demo**	**History and Exam**	**Pathology**	**Imaging**	**Laboratory Data**	
Tokuhashi	1990		• functional status	• primary tumor histology	• visceral mets (Y/N) • #VB mets • bone mets (Y/N)		
Tomita	2001			• primary tumor histology	• visceral mets (Y/N) • bone mets (Y/N)		
Katagiri	2005		• functional status • previous systemic therapy	• primary tumor histology	• visceral mets (Y/N) • brain mets (Y/N) • bone mets (Y/N)		
Revised Tokuhashi	2005		• functional status	• primary tumor histology	• visceral mets (Y/N) • #VB mets • bone mets (Y/N)		
Linden	2005		• functional status	• primary tumor histology	• visceral mets (Y/N)		
Sioutos	2005		• functional status	• primary tumor histology	• #VB mets		
Modified Bauer				• primary tumor histology	• visceral mets (Y/N) • bone mets (Y/N)		
ORI	2013		• functional status	• primary tumor histology			
Revised Katagiri	2014		• functional status • previous systemic therapy	• primary tumor histology	• visceral mets (Y/N) • brain mets (Y/N) • bone mets (Y/N)		
Bollen	2014		• functional status	• primary tumor histology	• visceral mets (Y/N) • brain mets (Y/N)		
NESMS	2015		• ambulatory status	• primary tumor histology	• visceral mets (Y/N) • bone mets (Y/N)		
SORG Nomogram	2016	• Age	• functional status • previous systemic therapy	• primary tumor histology	• visceral mets (Y/N) • #VB mets • brain mets (Y/N)	• WBC • Hgb	
SORG Scoring	2016	• Age	• functional status • previous systemic therapy	• primary tumor histology	• visceral mets (Y/N) • #VB mets • brain mets (Y/N)	• WBC • Hgb	
SORG ML	2019	• BMI	• functional status • neurologic deficit • previous systemic therapy • comorbidity severity	• primary tumor histology	• visceral mets (Y/N) • #VB mets • brain mets (Y/N)	• Hgb/Hct • platelet count • abs lymphocyte • abs neutrophil • NLR	• PLR • albumin • alk phos • creatinine • INR

abs, absolute; alk phos, alkaline phosphatase; BMI, body mass index; CRP, C-reactive protein; Demo, demographics; Hgb, hemoglobin; HCT, hematocrit; INR, international normalized ratio; LDH, lactate dehydrogenase; ML, Machine Learning; mets, metastasis; NESMS, New England Spine Metastasis Score; NLR, neutrophil to lymphocyte ratio; ORI, Oswestry Risk Index; PLR, platelet to lymphocyte ratio; SORG, Skeletal Oncology Research Group; VB, vertebral body; WBC, white blood cell count.

including the Hospital Frailty Risk Score (HFRS)[27] and the Modified Frailty Index (MFI)[28] for general use in hospital and the Metastatic Spinal Tumor Frailty Index (MSTFI)[29] for use in the metastatic spine population (Figure 59–2). The MFI and HFRS were both developed using general hospital datasets, identifying patients with high resource utilization and various diagnoses associated with frailty. The HFRS has recently been used to prognosticate for patients with metastatic spine

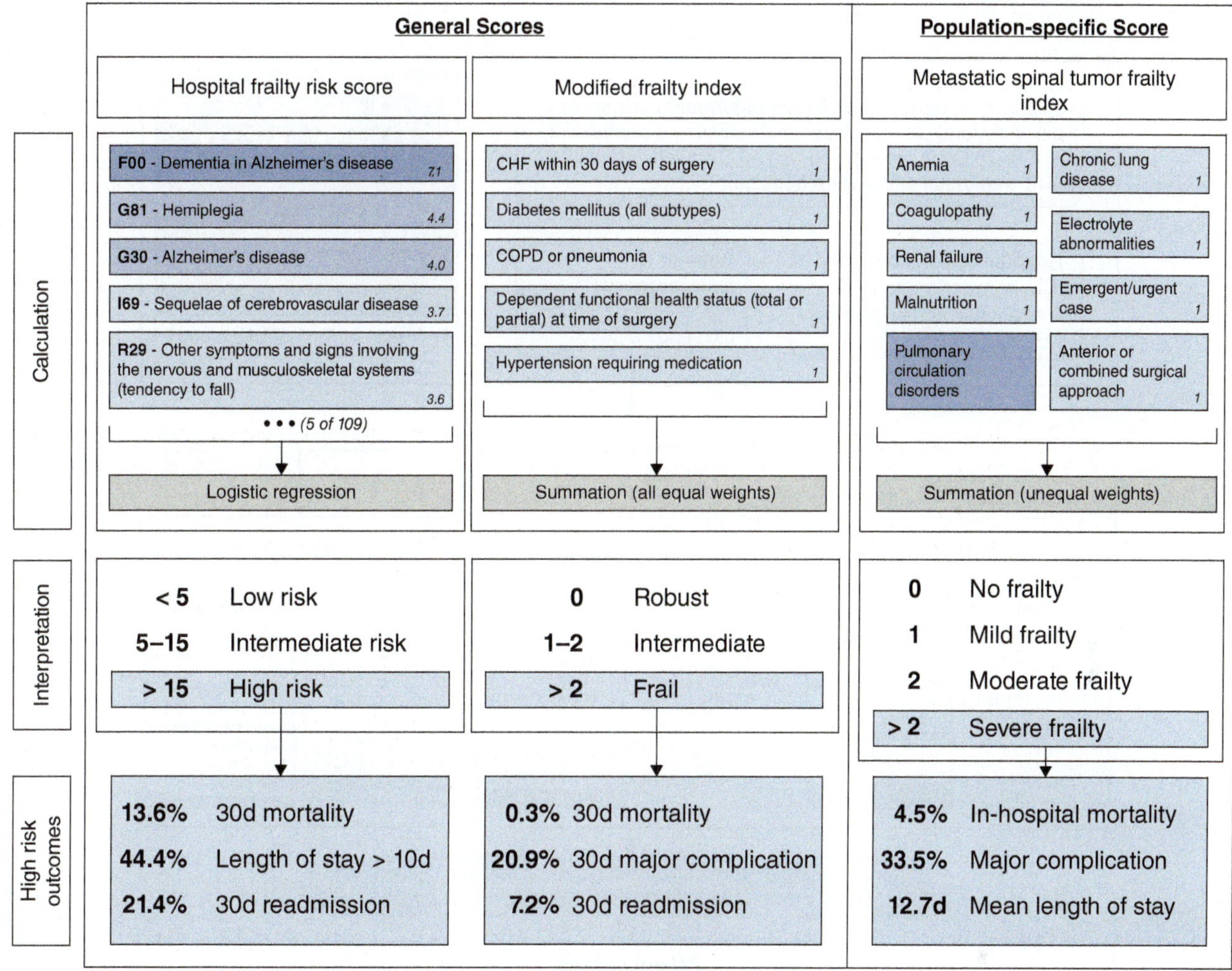

FIGURE 59–2 Frailty scores delineated by patient factors, severity of scores, and outcomes.

tumors; specifically, intermediate or high-risk scores were associated with increased length of stay, more nonroutine discharges, and increased hospital costs.[30] Similarly, the MSTFI was developed from a metastatic spinal tumor patient database using independent parameters associated with frailty. It has been shown to predict inpatient mortality and complications as well as increased length of stay.[29] Additionally, machine learning approaches have recently been implemented to quantify patient frailty using patient radiologic data to approximate body composition.[31]

Palliation and Shared Decision-Making

The Emerging Role of Palliative Care

While recent studies increasingly demonstrate that surgery is not only a feasible but also beneficial treatment option for patients with spine metastases, it is important to ensure that the decision to proceed with surgery and its potential outcomes and/or complications align with patients' priorities and goals of care.[32] Establishing this understanding is particularly important for patients who have poor prognoses and high symptom burdens. For some patients who may not be appropriate surgical candidates, less invasive spinal procedures including vertebroplasty, kyphoplasty, and percutaneous stabilization can be good palliative procedure options.[19,32–35] While not as well studied as palliative procedures, specialty PC can also be a critical aspect of the multidisciplinary care team by helping improve QoL, ensure goal-concordant care, and provide psychosocial, emotional, and/or spiritual support for patients and families along with assisting in pain/symptom management.[36–42]

Across many oncologic patient populations, the importance of PC utilization has been well established. Randomized controlled trials (RCTs) and meta-analyses have demonstrated that early integration of PC can both improve patient QoL and increase survival.[36–42] Despite these demonstrated benefits, uptake of PC, specifically early, outpatient PC, is generally low.[43–46] Surgical patient populations in particular are less likely to have PC incorporated into their care.[44,47–49] However, PC integrates seamlessly into the recommended shared decision model for spine metastasis surgery and should be considered an essential aspect of the care team of patients with spine metastases. Regarding implementation, studies demonstrate the

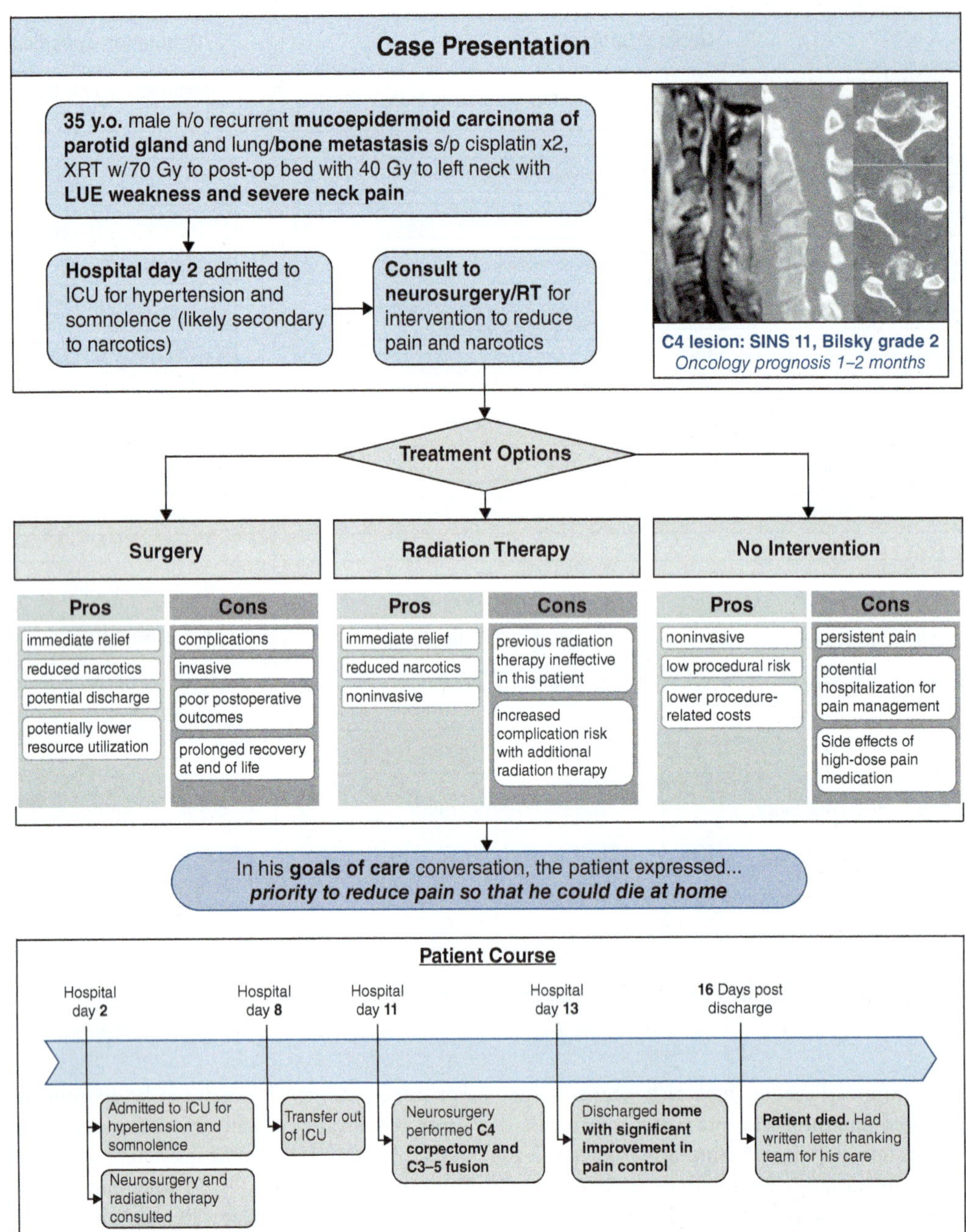

FIGURE 59–3 Case presentation and decision making for a patient who underwent surgery at the end of life for spine metastases.

importance of using multidisciplinary efforts to incorporate PC into the care of oncologic patient populations.[46,50–53] Preliminarily, at our institution, where spine metastasis patients are presented at a multidisciplinary tumor board, we have shown that rates of outpatient PC are significantly higher than those reported in the literature. This trend is even more dramatic for patients receiving surgery for their metastases. The decision to proceed with surgery is often multifactorial and differs among patients; having a care team that intentionally incorporates PC early to support patients as they navigate through both the decision-making processes and the postoperative course can be critical (Figure 59–3).

REFERENCES

1. Nater, A., Martin, A. R., Sahgal, A., Choi, D. & Fehlings, M. G. Symptomatic spinal metastasis: A systematic literature review of the preoperative prognostic factors for survival, neurological, functional and quality of life in surgically treated patients and methodological recommendations for prognostic studies. *PLoS One* 12, e0171507, doi:10.1371/journal.pone.0171507 (2017).
2. Chiu, R. G. & Mehta, A. I. Spinal Metastases. *JAMA* 323, 2438, doi:10.1001/jama.2020.0716 (2020).
3. Dugas, A. F., Lucas, J. M. & Edlow, J. A. Diagnosis of spinal cord compression in nontrauma patients in the emergency department. *Acad Emerg Med* 18, 719–725, doi:10.1111/j.1553-2712.2011.01105.x (2011).
4. MacVicar, D. Imaging of the spine in patients with malignancy. *Cancer Imaging* 6, S22–S26, doi:10.1102/1470-7330.2006.9002 (2006).

5. Feroz, I., Makhdoomi, R. H., Khursheed, N., Shaheen, F. & Shah, P. Utility of computed tomography-guided biopsy in evaluation of metastatic spinal lesions. *Asian J Neurosurg* 13, 577–584, doi:10.4103/ajns.AJNS_192_16 (2018).
6. Wagner, A. *et al.* Comprehensive surgical treatment strategy for spinal metastases. *Sci Rep* 11, 7988, doi:10.1038/s41598-021-87121-1 (2021).
7. Porras, J. L. *et al.* Radiotherapy and surgical advances in the treatment of metastatic spine tumors: a narrative review. *World Neurosurg* 151, 147–154, doi:10.1016/j.wneu.2021.05.032 (2021).
8. Barzilai, O., Fisher, C. G. & Bilsky, M. H. State of the art treatment of spinal metastatic disease. *Neurosurgery* 82, 757–769, doi:10.1093/neuros/nyx567 (2018).
9. Li, J. *et al.* Clinical therapy of metastatic spinal tumors. *Front Surg* 8, 626873, doi:10.3389/fsurg.2021.626873 (2021).
10. Laufer, I., Hanover, A., Lis, E., Yamada, Y. & Bilsky, M. Repeat decompression surgery for recurrent spinal metastases. *J Neurosurg Spine* 13, 109–115, doi:10.3171/2010.3.Spine08670 (2010).
11. Patchell, R. A. *et al.* Direct decompressive surgical resection in the treatment of spinal cord compression caused by metastatic cancer: a randomised trial. *Lancet* 366, 643–648, doi:10.1016/s0140-6736(05)66954-1 (2005).
12. Wang, J. C. *et al.* Single-stage posterolateral transpedicular approach for resection of epidural metastatic spine tumors involving the vertebral body with circumferential reconstruction: results in 140 patients. Invited submission from the Joint Section Meeting on Disorders of the Spine and Peripheral Nerves, March 2004. *J Neurosurg Spine* 1, 287–298, doi:10.3171/spi.2004.1.3.0287 (2004).
13. Gilbert, R. W., Kim, J. H. & Posner, J. B. Epidural spinal cord compression from metastatic tumor: diagnosis and treatment. *Ann Neurol* 3, 40–51, doi:10.1002/ana.410030107 (1978).
14. Gerszten, P. C., Mendel, E. & Yamada, Y. Radiotherapy and radiosurgery for metastatic spine disease: what are the options, indications, and outcomes? *Spine (Phila Pa 1976)* 34, S78–92, doi:10.1097/BRS.0b013e3181b8b6f5 (2009).
15. Katagiri, H. *et al.* Clinical results of nonsurgical treatment for spinal metastases. *Int J Radiat Oncol Biol Phys* 42, 1127–1132, doi:10.1016/s0360-3016(98)00288-0 (1998).
16. Maranzano, E. & Latini, P. Effectiveness of radiation therapy without surgery in metastatic spinal cord compression: final results from a prospective trial. *Int J Radiat Oncol Biol Phys* 32, 959–967, doi:10.1016/0360-3016(95)00572-g (1995).
17. Rock, J. P. *et al.* Postoperative radiosurgery for malignant spinal tumors. *Neurosurgery* 58, 891–898; discussion 891-898, doi:10.1227/01.Neu.0000209913.72761.4f (2006).
18. Fisher, C. G. *et al.* A novel classification system for spinal instability in neoplastic disease: an evidence-based approach and expert consensus from the Spine Oncology Study Group. *Spine (Phila Pa 1976)* 35, E1221–1229, doi:10.1097/BRS.0b013e3181e16ae2 (2010).
19. Fourney, D. R. *et al.* Percutaneous vertebroplasty and kyphoplasty for painful vertebral body fractures in cancer patients. *J Neurosurg* 98, 21–30, doi:10.3171/spi.2003.98.1.0021 (2003).
20. Laufer, I. *et al.* The NOMS framework: approach to the treatment of spinal metastatic tumors. *Oncologist* 18, 744–751, doi:10.1634/theoncologist.2012-0293 (2013).
21. Cui, Y., Lei, M., Pan, Y., Lin, Y. & Shi, X. Scoring algorithms for predicting survival prognosis in patients with metastatic spinal disease: the current status and future directions. *Clin Spine Surg* 33, 296–306, doi:10.1097/bsd.0000000000001031 (2020).
22. Shah, A. A. *et al.* Updated external validation of the SORG machine learning algorithms for prediction of ninety-day and one-year mortality after surgery for spinal metastasis. *Spine J* 21, 1679–1686, doi:10.1016/j.spinee.2021.03.026 (2021).
23. Ahmed, A. K. *et al.* Predicting survival for metastatic spine disease: a comparison of nine scoring systems. *Spine J* 18, 1804–1814, doi:10.1016/j.spinee.2018.03.011 (2018).
24. Dea, N. *et al.* Metastatic spine disease: should patients with short life expectancy be denied surgical care? An international retrospective cohort study. *Neurosurgery* 87, 303–311, doi:10.1093/neuros/nyz472 (2020).
25. Karhade, A. V. *et al.* Discharge disposition after anterior cervical discectomy and fusion. *World Neurosurg* 132, e14–e20, doi:10.1016/j.wneu.2019.09.026 (2019).
26. Luksanapruksa, P. *et al.* Prognostic factors in patients with spinal metastasis: a systematic review and meta-analysis. *Spine J* 17, 689–708, doi:10.1016/j.spinee.2016.12.003 (2017).
27. Gilbert, T. *et al.* Development and validation of a Hospital Frailty Risk Score focusing on older people in acute care settings using electronic hospital records: an observational study. *Lancet* 391, 1775–1782, doi:10.1016/s0140-6736(18)30668-8 (2018).
28. Abellan van Kan, G. *et al.* The assessment of frailty in older adults. *Clin Geriatr Med* 26, 275–286, doi:10.1016/j.cger.2010.02.002 (2010).
29. De la Garza Ramos, R. *et al.* Development of a metastatic spinal tumor frailty index (MSTFI) using a nationwide database and its association with inpatient morbidity, mortality, and length of stay after spine surgery. *World Neurosurg* 95, 548–555.e544, doi:10.1016/j.wneu.2016.08.029 (2016).
30. Elsamadicy, A. A. *et al.* Hospital Frailty Risk Score and healthcare resource utilization after surgery for primary spinal intradural/cord tumors. *Global Spine J*, 21925682211069937, doi:10.1177/21925682211069937 (2022).
31. Massaad, E. *et al.* Evaluating frailty, mortality, and complications associated with metastatic spine tumor surgery using machine learning–derived body composition analysis. *Journal of Neurosurgery: Spine*, 37(2), 263–273. doi:10.3171/2022.1.spine211284 (2022).
32. Williamson, T., Painter, B., Howell, E. P. & Goodwin, C. R. Top ten tips palliative care clinicians should know about spinal tumors. *J Palliat Med* 22, 84–89, doi:10.1089/jpm.2018.0608 (2019).
33. Samala, R. V., Lagman, R. L. & Steinmetz, M. P. Palliative spine surgery in a patient with advanced cancer: a case report and decision-making guide. *J Palliat Med* 24, 793–796, doi:10.1089/jpm.2020.0219 (2021).
34. Ishida, Y. *et al.* Impairment-driven cancer rehabilitation in patients with neoplastic spinal cord compression using minimally invasive spine stabilization. *World J Surg Oncol* 18, 187, doi:10.1186/s12957-020-01964-y (2020).
35. Itagaki, M. W. *et al.* Percutaneous vertebroplasty and kyphoplasty for pathologic vertebral fractures in the Medicare population: safer and less expensive than open surgery. *J Vasc Interv Radiol* 23, 1423–1429, doi:10.1016/j.jvir.2012.08.010 (2012).
36. Bakitas, M. A. *et al.* Early versus delayed initiation of concurrent palliative oncology care: patient outcomes in the ENABLE III randomized controlled trial. *J Clin Oncol* 33, 1438–1445, doi:10.1200/jco.2014.58.6362 (2015).
37. Borelli, E. *et al.* Changes in cancer patients' and caregivers' disease perceptions while receiving early palliative care: a qualitative and quantitative analysis. *Oncologist* 26, e2274–e2287, doi:10.1002/onco.13974 (2021).
38. Vogt, J. *et al.* Symptom burden and palliative care needs of patients with incurable cancer at diagnosis and during the disease course. *Oncologist* 26, e1058–e1065, doi:10.1002/onco.13751 (2021).
39. Fulton, J. J. *et al.* Integrated outpatient palliative care for patients with advanced cancer: a systematic review and meta-analysis. *Palliat Med* 33, 123–134, doi:10.1177/0269216318812633 (2019).
40. Zimmermann, C. *et al.* Early palliative care for patients with advanced cancer: a cluster-randomised controlled trial. *Lancet* 383, 1721–1730, doi:10.1016/s0140-6736(13)62416-2 (2014).
41. Ferrell, B. *et al.* Interdisciplinary Palliative Care for Patients With Lung Cancer. *J Pain Symptom Manage* 50, 758–767, doi:10.1016/j.jpainsymman.2015.07.005 (2015).
42. Temel, J. S. *et al.* Longitudinal perceptions of prognosis and goals of therapy in patients with metastatic non-small-cell lung cancer: results of a randomized study of early palliative care. *J Clin Oncol* 29, 2319–2326, doi:10.1200/jco.2010.32.4459 (2011).
43. Yeh, J. C. *et al.* Different associations between inpatient or outpatient palliative care and end-of-life outcomes for hospitalized patients with cancer. *JCO Oncol Pract*, Op2100546, doi:10.1200/op.21.00546 (2021).
44. Price, M. *et al.* Inpatient palliative care utilization for patients with brain metastases. *Neurooncol Pract* 8, 441–450, doi:10.1093/nop/npab016 (2021).
45. Kubendran, S. *et al.* Trends in inpatient palliative care use for primary brain malignancies. *Support Care Cancer* 29, 6625–6632, doi:10.1007/s00520-021-06255-0 (2021).
46. Sedhom, R. *et al.* Oncology fellow-led quality improvement project to improve rates of palliative care utilization in patients with advanced cancer. *JCO Oncol Pract* 16, e814–e822, doi:10.1200/jop.19.00714 (2020).

47. Gani, F., Enumah, Z. O., Conca-Cheng, A. M., Canner, J. K. & Johnston, F. M. Palliative care utilization among patients admitted for gastrointestinal and thoracic cancers. *J Palliat Med* 21, 428–437, doi:10.1089/jpm.2017.0295 (2018).
48. Nguyen, M. T. *et al.* Differential utilization of palliative care consultation between medical and surgical services. *Am J Hosp Palliat Care* 37, 250–257, doi:10.1177/1049909119867904 (2020).
49. Moroney, M. R. & Lefkowits, C. Evidence for integration of palliative care into surgical oncology practice and education. *J Surg Oncol* 120, 17–22, doi:10.1002/jso.25454 (2019).
50. Mathews, J., Hannon, B. & Zimmermann, C. Models of integration of specialized palliative care with oncology. *Curr Treat Options Oncol* 22, 44, doi:10.1007/s11864-021-00836-1 (2021).
51. Einstein, D. J. *et al.* Improving end-of-life care: palliative care embedded in an oncology clinic specializing in targeted and immune-based therapies. *J Oncol Pract* 13, e729–e737, doi:10.1200/jop.2016.020396 (2017).
52. Blum, D., Seiler, A., Schmidt, E., Pavic, M. & Strasser, F. Patterns of integrating palliative care into standard oncology in an early ESMO designated center: a 10-year experience. *ESMO Open* 6, 100147, doi:10.1016/j.esmoop.2021.100147 (2021).
53. Boddaert, M. S. *et al.* Specialist palliative care teams and characteristics related to referral rate: a national cross-sectional survey among hospitals in the Netherlands. *BMC Palliat Care* 20, 175, doi:10.1186/s12904-021-00875-3 (2021).

Index

Page numbers followed by "f" denote figures and "t" denote tables.

T

U

V